Schizophrenia

Schizophrenia
An overview and practical handbook

Edited by

David J. Kavanagh
Senior Lecturer in Psychology
University of Sydney, Australia

CHAPMAN & HALL
London · Glasgow · New York · Tokyo · Melbourne · Madras

Published by Chapman & Hall, 2–6 Boundary Row, London SE1 8HN

Chapman & Hall, 2–6 Boundary Row, London SE1 8HN, UK

Blackie Academic & Professional, Wester Cleddens Road, Bishopsbriggs, Glasgow, G64 2NZ, UK

Chapman & Hall, 29 West 35th Street, New York NY10001, USA

Chapman & Hall Japan, Thomson Publishing Japan, Hirakawacho Nemoto Building, 7F, 1-7-11 Hirakawa-cho, Chiyoda-ku, Tokyo 102, Japan

Chapman & Hall Australia, Thomas Nelson Australia, 102 Dodds Street, South Melbourne, Victoria 3205, Australia

Chapman & Hall India, R. Seshadri, 32 Second Main Road, CIT East, Madras 600 035, India

Distributed in the USA and Canada by Singular Publishing Group Inc., 4284 41st Street, San Diego, California 92105

First edition 1992

© 1992 Chapman & Hall

Typeset in 10/12 Times by Mews Photosetting, Beckenham, Kent
Printed in Great Britain by Clays Ltd, Bungay, Suffolk

ISBN 0 412 38900 2   1 56593 054 1 (USA)

To the sufferers of schizophrenia and their families,
whose courage and hope are an inspiration to us all.

Contents

Contents

Contributors

Paul Bebbington PhD, MRCpsych
MRC Social and Community Psychiatry
    Unit, Institute of Psychiatry
London, UK

Richard P. Bentall, **MClin. Psychol,
PhD**
Department of Clinical Psychology,
    University of Liverpool
Liverpool, UK

Max Birchwood, PhD
All Saints Hospital and University of
    Birmingham
Birmingham, UK

Keith Clements, PhD
Department of Psychology, Polytechnic
    South West
Plymouth, UK

**David L. Copolov, MB, BS, DPM,
MPM, MRANZCP, FRACP**
NH and MRC
Schizophrenia Research Unit, and Mental
    Health Institute of Victoria, Royal Park
    Hospital
Melbourne, Australia

Tom K.J. Craig, MB, BS, PhD, MRCPsych,
Professor, Department of Community
    Psychiatry, United Medical and Dental
    Schools, St Thomas' Hospital
London, UK

Alan J. Cross PhD
Astra Neuroscience Research Unit
London, UK

Jane Edwards, MA (Clin. Psychol.)
NH and MRC
Schizophrenia Research Unit, Royal Park
    Hospital, and Albert Park Clinic
Melbourne, Australia

**Ian R.H. Falloon, MB, ChB, DPM,
MRCPsych**
Buckingham Hospital, Buckingham and
    University of California at Los Angeles
Los Angeles, USA

Doug Farnill, PhD
Department of Behavioural Science in
    Medicine
University of Sydney, Australia

Shirley M. Glynn, PhD
West Los Angeles VA Medical Center,
    Brentwood Division
California, USA

Michael F. Green, PhD
Department of Psychiatry and Biobehavioral
    Sciences, University of California at Los
    Angeles
California, USA

**Hugh M.D. Gurling, MD, MPhil,
MRCPsych**
Molecular Psychiatry Laboratory, Academic
    Department of Psychiatry, University
    College and Middlesex School of
    Medicine, University of London
London, UK

Dušan Hadži-Pavlović, BSc, MPsychol
The Prince Henry and Prince of Wales
    Hospitals and School of Psychiatry
University of NSW, Australia

W. Kim Halford, PhD
Department of Psychiatry
University of Queensland, Australia

Robyn L. Hayes, MOccTher
Department of Psychiatry
University of Queensland, Australia

**Henry J. Jackson, PhD, MA (Clin.
Psychol.)**
Department of Psychology, University of
    Melbourne
Melbourne, Australia

Terry L. Jernigan, PhD
Department of Veterans Affairs Medical
    Center, Department of Psychiatry,
    University of California
San Diego, USA

David J. Kavanagh, Dip.Psychol. PhD
Department of Psychology
University of Sydney, Australia

Liz Kuipers, PhD, FBPS
Department of Psychology, Institute of
    Psychiatry
London, UK

Marc Laporta, MD
Royal Victoria Hospital, Allan Memorial
    Institute
Montreal, Canada

**Patrick D. McGorry, MB, BS, MRCP,
FRANZCP**
NH and MRC
Schizophrenia Research Unit, Royal Park
    Hospital and Associate Professor of
    Psychological Medicine, Monash
    University
Melbourne, Australia

Sally MacKain, PhD
Neuropsychiatric Institute, University of
    California at Los Angeles
California, USA

Fiona Macmillan, MD, MRCPsych
All Saints Hospital
Birmingham, UK

Stephen R. Marder, MD
West Los Angeles VA Medical Center,
    Brentwood Division, and Department of
    Psychiatry and Biobehavioral Sciences,
    University of California at Los
    Angeles, USA

**Matthijs Muijen, MSc, PhD, MO,
MRCPsych**
RDP
134–138 Borough High Street
London SE1 1LB, UK

Kim T. Mueser, PhD
Medical College of Pennsylvania at Eastern
    Pennsylvania Psychiatric Institute
Pennsylvania, USA

Paul E. Mullen, FRCPsych, FRANZCP
Professor, Department of Psychological
    Medicine, University of Otago Medical
    School
New Zealand

Frank Owen, PhD
Professor, Department of Physiological
    Sciences, University of Manchester
Manchester, UK

Gordon Parker MD, PhD, FRANZCP
Professor, The Prince Henry and Prince of
    Wales Hospitals and School of
    Psychiatry, University of NSW
Australia

Olga Piatkowska, BA, Dip. Psychol.
Manly-Warringah Area Health Service
Sydney, Australia

**M. Potter, BMedSci, MB, BS,
    MRCPsych**
Middlesex Hospital
London, UK

T. Read, BSc, MB, BS, MRCPsych
Middlesex Hospital
London, UK

**Alan Rosen, MB, BS, MRCPsych,
    FRANZCP, DPM**
School of Psychiatry
University of NSW
Prince of Wales Hospital
Randwick, Australia

Margaret S.D. Sayers, MA
Medical College of Pennsylvania at Eastern
    Pennsylvania Psychiatric Institute
Pennsylvania, US

**Bruce S. Singh, MB, BS, PhD, FRACP,
    FRANZCP**
NH and MRC
Professor in Community Medicine, Monash
    University and Schizophrenia Research
    Unit, Royal Park Hospital
Melbourne, Australia

Jo Smith, PhD
All Saints Hospital
Birmingham, UK

Nicholas Tarrier, PhD
Professor, School of Psychiatry and
    Behavioural Sciences
University of Manchester, UK

Graham Turpin, PhD
Department of Psychology, University of
    Sheffield
Sheffield, UK

John K. Wing, MD, PhD, FRCPsych
Royal College of Psychiatrists Research
    Unit and Emeritus Professor of Social
    Psychiatry, University of London,
London UK

Til Wykes, DPhil
Department of Psychology, Institute of
    Psychiatry
London, UK

Joseph Zubin, PhD
US Veterans Administration and
    Distinguished Research Professor,
    University of Pittsburgh School of
    Medicine
Pennsylvania, USA

Preface

This book has ambitious objectives. The intention was to develop a work that not only reviewed the current status of research on the nature of schizophrenia, but would provide information on the range of assessment and treatment issues that practitioners would encounter. I wanted it to have a readable style and offer detailed practical suggestions, but at the same time I wanted it to offer a sound treatment of the theoretical issues and a review of the literature that was current and reasonably comprehensive. The chapters would provide descriptions of current research by the contributors, but their reviews would also be wide-ranging and the whole book would incorporate a coherent development of concepts rather than comprising a set of disparate and unconnected papers.

The characteristics of the target audience were just as broad: postgraduate students to experienced practitioners who were interested in a current review of the area. I had a specific interest in providing a text for trainee clinical psychologists, but wanted the book to be relevant to social workers, medical practitioners and other health professionals. I hoped that the book would offer an introduction to the area as well as examining some current issues that would interest the seasoned researcher.

All of this was a rather tall order, and I leave it to you to decide whether it has been successful. In the tradition of Kurt Lewin, I hope that the book will demonstrate the practicality of a good theory. I also hope that you will catch some of the enthusiasm that contributors have had for the concept.

The book is composed of three sections: Part One presents an overview of current knowledge on the nature of schizophrenia and the aetiology of its onset and recurrence. Because of the interest that is attracted by the idea that schizophrenia may increase the likelihood of criminal behaviour, a chapter is also provided on that subject. Part Two examines assessment strategies for a range of problem behaviours and risk factors. Part Three reviews the current status of interventions for treating and preventing episodes, controlling recurrent symptoms and increasing functional behaviours. The whole book is heavily influenced by a stress–vulnerability view of the disorder, and I am delighted that Dr Joseph Zubin, one of the pioneers of this perspective, has written an introduction to Part One. This is one of the final contributions that Dr Zubin was able to make in his long and illustrious career. Dr Zubin, who died quietly on December 18, 1990, will be remembered as a pioneer in our understanding of schizophrenia and as a gentle and warm person. He will be sorely missed by the scientific community.

I offer the authors my congratulations for their excellent contributions, and thank them for their cooperation and patience throughout this venture. I gratefully acknowledge the support of John Wing, Julian Leff, Paul Bebbington and other staff of the MRC Social Psychiatry Unit at the Institute of Psychiatry, London where the book began during my study leave in 1989. I also thank David Rosenhan and Nick Tarrier for their suggestions and encouragement as well as Christine Birdsall and Terri Cooper of Chapman & Hall whose assistance has been inestimable.

David J. Kavanagh

Editors' Note

This is one of the final contributions that Dr Zubin was able to make in his long and illustrious career. Dr Zubin, who died quietly on December 18, 1990, will be remembered as a pioneer in our understanding of schizophrenia and as a delightfully gentle and warm person. He will be sorely missed by the scientific community.

Dr. Zubin had apparently intended to write in more detail about other chapters, but was prevented from doing so by his death.

Part One
Overview of Schizophrenia

Introduction

JOSEPH ZUBIN

Historically, the various past attempts at presenting an overview of schizophrenia suffered from the fact that there was no compelling synthesis of the multidisciplinary approaches that dominate the field. The only major classification separated the approaches into descriptive vs. aetiological domains. This volume presents a more integrated approach, in that while the domains remain, the individual authors have extended descriptive findings to aetiological bases through the use of models of schizophrenic function.

The descriptive approach is introduced by John Wing in Chapter One on The Differential Diagnosis of Schizophrenia, and is followed by Richard P. Bentall on the Typology of Schizophrenia. These chapters are essentially phenomenological in their approach based on investigations utilizing interviewing and observation methods to arrive at a systematic descriptive classification.

The aetiological approach is represented there by a wider scope, which does not lend itself readily to categorization. The chapters on aetiology comprise a survey of Psychophysiological Contributions to Clinical Assessment and Treatment (Turpin and Clements), which could easily fall into the previous descriptive domain, and it also introduces some explanatory principles for the causes of the observed deviations by appealing to the vulnerability

MODEL. A more direct theoretical approach to aetiology is provided in the chapter on Information Processing in Schizophrenia (Green). Building on the well-developed knowledge base of normal information processing, an attempt is made to determine just where the deviations in information processing occur in schizophrenia. Perhaps the most basic approach to aetiology is provided by the chapters on biochemistry (Owen and Cross), Neuroanatomy (Jernigan) and Genetics (Read *et al.*).

Midway between the two extremes of the spectrum of description vs. aetiology lies the chapter by Bebbington and Kuipers addressing psychosocial factors. While making no aetiological claims, they point out the role of life events in triggering episodes, and the impact of the environment on the course of the illness, with special attention to the role of expressed emotion in relapse. In a sense these psychosocial factors may be viewed as mediating factors. They serve as catalysts to permit the interaction between endogenous aetiology and the exogenous environment.

An introduction to a set of chapters should set the stage for a systematic perspective on what these contain so that the readers could be guided in their journey in a systematic way. In an attempt to carry out this intention, it becomes necessary to conceive of three aspects that are represented in this section of the book –

description, aetiology, and mediating variables in the form of scientific models with parsimonious structures, well-defined parameters and hypotheses which can be submitted to tests of tenability. The author of this introduction has provided such a framework in previous publications (Zubin and Spring, 1977; Zubin and Steinhauer, 1981). The framework begins with a presentation of some seven models of aetiology which range from environmental field forces impinging on the ecological niche the person occupies (physical and cultural factors) through primarily psychological and social experiences (developmental and learning models) to internal biological models (genetic, internal environment, neurophysiological, neuroanatomical and neurohumoral and immunological). In order to provide a theatre for the interaction of these models an integrating model is required, and the vulnerability model has been offered for this purpose. The model proposes that the various separate aetiological sources contribute to a threshold vulnerability. When stresses exceed the threshold, symptoms are present, but decreasing the impact of life stresses, symptoms subside. In addition, the model proposes that there are markers of vulnerability to schizophrenia, occurring in the patient even when free of symptoms. Moreover, these markers may be present even in unaffected family members. The search for markers assists us in predicting those individuals who may be most vulnerable to the disorder. The vulnerability model has a strong heuristic utility, and several of the authors (Turpin and Clements; Green) utilized it as a framework for interpreting current research findings.

In order to test the empirical tenability of any model, we need to define the universe of patients we are concerned with. For this purpose the descriptive approach is introduced and systematic interviewing methods and observations are developed for examining the phenomenology of the patient and criteria for accepting or rejecting the diagnosis of schizophrenia are established.

Once the diagnosis is established, the search for vulnerability markers can proceed and the role of the mediating factors in eliciting vulnerability determined. Wing reminds us that the attempt to diagnose patients consists of two goals – to find who they resemble as well as those from whom they differ – these are the essential elements in a differential diagnosis. In searching for the disorder category to which a patient belongs we follow the ancient dictum of Aristotle that every category has an essence and the problem is to see whether this essence is found in the patient. This approach, which the ancient Greeks referred to as the ontological approach, specified that disorders, like any other objects of entities, can be defined rigorously and exist as specific independent entities. This is similar to the species in animals and plants, in that membership in a given category of disorder is determined by criteria which the patient must meet. In contrast to this was the approach of Hippocrates, who did not believe in these entities and did not see his function as treating disorders. Instead he focused on the individual and his specific response to whatever was interfering with health, and aimed at removing these obstacles to health by engaging the natural tendency to self-healing. Thus, instead of the procrustean approach of searching for similarities in the patients expected on the basis of a rigidly specified diagnosis, he was more protean in his approach, dealing with the individual differences exhibited by the patients, and tailored his treatment accordingly regardless of the alleged disorder entity. Thus, the ontological approach was more categorical while the Hippocratic approach could be regarded as more dimensional.

A current example is provided in this volume. It is the dimensional approach that Wing prefers and provides two dimensions as the basic domains in schizophrenia – positive and negative symptoms. It is likely that the need for these dimensions arose because the overall diagnosis of schizophrenia was too global to permit its utilization in the selection of treatment regimes. In order to tailor the treatment to the patient, a more subtle differentiation into dimensional classification was needed and the negative vs. positive domains seemed promising, since, for example, positive symptoms were more responsive to neuroleptics. That the positive symptoms seem to go along with the presence of an episode, and hence, are state variables, seems to be generally accepted. The negative symptoms seem to be more like traits not as readily amenable to change as the positive. While the positive symptoms seem to be firmly attached to the episode, waxing and waning with it, the negative symptoms seem less mutable and may not be as closely inter-digitated with schizophrenia. They may, in many cases, be a premorbid characteristic which persists after the episode is ended.

Negative symptoms may be the earmarks of the chronicpostepisode state, and may turn out to be independent of schizophrenia.

The conceptual approaches provided by the authors of Part One provide a contemporary view of research findings and clinical overviews. They provide the reader with a firm basis for our current understanding of schizophrenia, and point the directions towards which we must now progress.

REFERENCES

Zubin, J. and Spring, B. (1977) Vulnerability: A new view of schizophrenia. *J. Abnorm. Psychol.*, **86**, 103–26.

Zubin, J. and Steinhauer, S.R. (1981) How to break the logjam in schizophrenia: A look beyond genetics. *J. Nerv. Ment. Dis.* **169**, 477–92.

Chapter 1

Differential diagnosis of schizophrenia

J.K. WING

1.1 SUMMARY

The way that the phenomena of the major psychoses have been classified and conceptualized has fluctuated markedly during the past 150 years. Kraepelin's formulation, and Eugen Bleuler's extension of it, have been clinically influential and scientifically fruitful although alternative models have always been available. The negative symptoms, for example, are well-known to neurologists in the form of akinetic mutism, catatonia and abulia. They occur in a wide range of psychiatric conditions, including dementia, the autistic spectrum, schizophrenia and bipolar disorders, in an approximate dimension of severity. The positive symptoms appear clinically to lie near the top of an approximate hierarchy. Symptoms of conditions lower down, such as the affective psychoses and neuroses, are commonly associated.

Differential diagnosis is most conveniently considered, first in terms of the positive and negative symptoms separately and then in terms of the relationship between them at different cross-sectional levels. The various ways in which schizophrenia can be formulated as a category, and the overlap with other symptoms, can then be identified and used to test alterna-tive hypotheses concerning causes, pathology, treatment and course.

The classifying rules in the tenth edition of the *International Classification of Diseases* should be used as a general standard of comparison but it is important to apply all sets of rules to a clinical database that allows a flexible approach to the investigation of co-morbidity.

1.2 TWO APPROACHES TO DIAGNOSIS

The title of this chapter contains a semantic trap. In everyday conversation the natural way to define a concept is from 'left to right'. An example might be: 'Schizophrenia is . . .', followed by a formula defining a disease entity. Students are often taught in this way because it is a convenient method of memorizing facts. Aristotle stated that the term to be defined 'is the name of the essence of a thing', and this kind of definition is called 'essentialist'.

Scientific definitions, by contrast, are much less natural. To define one's terms scientifically means no more than to say that a term will be used in a particular way, using words and measurements as precisely as possible in order that other scientists who wish to do so can check the observations or try to replicate the results of experiments. The right hand part of the definition is a technical specification designed to be useful in testing theories. It carries no significance in itself and the term so defined is only a shorthand label for the specification. This is 'empirical' definition. Karl Popper (1945) calls it 'right to left'.

These two approaches can be discerned throughout the history of medicine. Sir Henry Cohen suggested that the essentialist type of definition might have sprung from the notion of demoniacal possession. In various forms, notably the Galenic humoral theory, it was the main approach to diagnosis for 2000 years. It maintains that there are innumerable disease entities, each with its individual and recognizable characteristics and natural history. This concept of disease 'still dominates our textbook descriptions, as illustrated by the so-called classical pictures of typhoid fever, influenza, disseminated sclerosis and the rest. Many of these are little more helpful in diagnosis than would be a composite portrait of a Cabinet or a Test Team in revealing whether a given individual is a member of either' (Cohen, 1961).

The empirical approach to diagnosis often begins with observations of a previously undescribed abnormality by an intuitive clinician. If they can be repeated accurately and independently, they appear to take on a 'validity' of their own. The fact that the elements occur in an observable pattern, together and/or over time, suggests that there is a non-random structure, the nature of which can be investigated. Such disorders (often eponymously named) are used as a starting point for hypotheses that they are manifestations (symptoms or syndromes) or deviations from one or more cycles of normal biological functioning. This kind of medicine could only develop when some of the factors that keep bodily systems within defined functional limits had been demonstrated. Knowledge does not reside where Aristotle thought it did, in essentialist definitions, but in hypotheses that survive the most severely designed tests to disprove them. This is what 'validation' should strictly mean, and even that knowledge must remain provisional.

Medical terminology is also conventionally used when a biological basis has been postulated but not fully demonstrated. This carries dangers since the problems presented to psychiatrists and clinical psychologists by disorders such as schizophrenia are far from exclusively biological. Biological abnormalities can have social causes. Many biological systems depend for their proper functioning on interaction with the psychosocial environment. The extent to which an individual is socially disabled depends partly on psychosocial factors such as disadvantage, and on public, family and self-attitudes. Psychosocial methods of treatment and care are founded on such observations (Chapter 24). It will be suggested later that some features of psychosis are elaborations and explanations (affected by personal and cultural factors) of simpler 'primary' experiences.

Social definitions of abnormality must nevertheless be distinguished from concepts of biological deviation; if they are not, and particularly if the two are equated, both types of concept can be (and have been) misapplied. These issues have been discussed in detail elsewhere (Wing, 1991a,b).

Once knowledge of normal anatomical, biochemical, physiological and psychological functioning began to be accumulated, tests of clinical theories in terms of deviations from the normal became possible. Scientific medicine in this sense is barely a century old and many symptoms and syndromes are still in process of evolution from intuitive observation to theories with a firm basis in replicated fact. This is particularly evident in psychological medicine. Although deviations from normal psychological functioning (Lewis, 1953) are accepted as scientifically interesting, progress has been slow.

The shorthand labels used in this chapter should, except where stated, be understood in the empirical and not in the essentialist sense.

Terms like 'psychosis', 'neurosis', 'functional', 'organic', 'schizophrenia', 'bipolar disorder', and so on, either have a technical descriptive content intended to facilitate the testing of biological, psychological or social theories, or are used more generally to indicate common clinical usage. The theories themselves, whether of causation, pathology or treatment, and whether biological, psychological or social in nature, are considered in other chapters.

1.3 SCHIZOPHRENIA AS A DISEASE ENTITY

In the late nineteenth century, the discovery of the anatomical and physiological concomitants of clinically identified syndromes, sometimes together with what appeared to be a single causal agent such as the tubercle bacillus or the cholera vibrio, proved irresistible to neurologists and psychiatrists who were also carving more specific syndromes out of the global concepts of dementia, delirium and insanity that preceded them. The proliferation of syndromes among the conditions that later became known as 'functional' psychoses, side by side with the old ideas, threatened to become chaotic (Berrios, 1987; Berrios and Hauser, 1988).

In the fifth and sixth editions of his textbook Emil Kraepelin introduced a simple distinction between conditions characterized by mental deterioration, such as catatonia, hebephrenia and dementia phantastica (which became subdivisions of the disorder), and more periodic forms of mania and melancholia. The two new 'disease entities' were thought to be justified because of a unity of cause, course and outcome. The formulation was thankfully adopted because of its simplicity but it was evident from the beginning that the two forms could coexist, and Kraepelin himself eventually (1920) agreed.

The form in which dementia praecox has remained a dominant feature of psychiatric nosology is, of course, Eugen Bleuler's creation. It retains the separation from bipolar disorder but Bleuler did point out that affective symptoms could coexist. The convenience of the new name must have played a large part in its acceptance, as did the fact that the connotations of the term 'dementia' for the course of the disease seemed to have been dropped. But Bleuler gives his interpretation of dementia praecox at the very beginning of his monograph. After noting that 'some are baffled by the manifold external clinical manifestations presented by this disease', he states that all the cases have much in common. Although the course is not always towards complete deterioration, 'each case nevertheless reveals some significant residual symptoms . . . not quantitatively, but qualitatively . . .' (Bleuler, 1913).

Bleuler's primary symptom was cognitive – loosening of the associations. This was his link to the biological origins of schizophrenia and also, through psychic complexes, to the disorders of affectivity, ambivalence, autism, attention and will, which he tentatively designed as secondary. All these disorders were 'fundamental' in the sense that they could be observed in every case. Catatonia, delusions, hallucinations and behavioural disturbance he regarded as accessory, because they could occur in other disorders. These theoretical assumptions held true also for Bleuler's largest sub-group, latent schizophrenia, in which none of the accessory symptoms need be present. In this way Bleuler greatly extended Kraepelin's concept. The first descriptions of dementia praecox and schizophrenia are now available in English translation and are worth reading for comparison and contrast (Bleuler, 1908; Kraepelin, 1896).

Bleuler's concept was, in effect, dimensional. It was subsequently used in markedly different ways. Under the influence of psychoanalysis in the US, the least differentiated forms – latent and simple schizophrenia – dominated diagnosis to such an extent that descriptive psychopathology was derided and neglected. In the USSR, the biological implications of the primary and fundamental symptoms were exploited. The concept of 'sluggish schizophrenia', often applied to people with politically deviant behaviour, was developed directly from Bleuler's 'hidden or latent' form. Smulevich (1989) points out that pseudoneurotic and borderline schizophrenia are analogous constructs. The possibility of misusing such vague concepts has been discussed elsewhere (Wing, 1978a). Kendler (Kendler *et al.*, 1989) has recently described an improved technique of operationalizing 'schizotypy' that should provide a means of investigating the concept of a 'schizophrenia spectrum' (Kety *et al.*, 1978), separate from bipolar disorder.

Jaspers (1962, Chapter 13) provided a critique of the concept of disease entity, as applied to psychiatric disorders, that articulated the views of many clinicians, both before and after these two pioneers. Werner Janzarik (1987), the present occupant of the chair formerly held by Kraepelin and Schneider, has recently made the point explicitly. The position taken in this chapter is that, both from a clinical and scientific point of view, it is wise to approach the classification of psychiatric disorders rather as a meteorologist approaches the classification of clouds. Cumulus and stratus do have different shapes but there is also cumulostratus. The barometric factors underlying these and other cloud formations are dimensional rather than categorical, and a scientist must be able to pass easily from one mode of analysis to the other.

Although many modifications to Kraepelin's and Bleuler's concepts, great and small, have been put forward, they are nearly all variations on one or both of two great underlying themes — the positive and the negative syndromes. The simplest way to make sense of differential diagnosis, therefore, is to consider each of these syndromes within the context of a descriptive dimension of clinical severity. Both dimensions can be described in terms of unusual subjective experiences and/or behavioural abnormalities in movement, language and affect. But the positive symptoms are most clearly recognized when an articulate patient is describing the inner experiences, while the negative symptoms (or signs) are mainly behavioural. The relationship between the two groups will be considered later.

1.4 POSITIVE SYMPTOMS

1.4.1 KURT SCHNEIDER'S SYNDROME

Schneider (1959, 1976) described a group of abnormal experiences that he and, he suggested, most psychiatrists, would usually call schizophrenic if they occurred in clear consciousness and the absence of overt brain disease. The symptoms include thoughts experienced as spoken aloud or echoed or removed or broadcast or alien; voices heard commenting on the patient's thoughts or coming from some part of the body or making references in the third person; feeling that the patient's bodily functions, movements, emotions or will are under the influence or control of some external force or agency. Delusional perceptions and delusional mood are also described but difficult to operationalize sufficiently to obtain good reliability between observers. Persistent auditory hallucinations not congruent with affect can probably be added to this list. Differential definitions can be found in the PSE9 glossary (Wing *et al.*, 1974) and are updated and expanded in the PSE10 glossary available from the World Health Organization.

Schneider did not think the symptoms had any particular theoretical or even prognostic significance. The interest of the syndrome is that it consists mainly of experiences that appear to be what Jaspers (1962, p. 584) called 'primary', in the sense that they cannot be reduced to other psychological components or explanations. The experience of loud or echoed thoughts is probably a primordium for auditory hallucinations and all the first rank symptoms can be elaborated or explained in delusional terms, often of a bizarre kind.

Delusions and hallucinations can therefore be divided according to whether or not they appear to be based on primary phenomena such as these, although the clinical information necessary to make the distinction is often not available. The first rank symptoms tend to fade with time and to be replaced by secondary phenomena. If they are thought to be, or to have been, present, schizophrenia becomes part of the differential diagnosis. (Other types of delusion or hallucination are discussed below.)

1.4.2 ORGANIC EXCLUSION FACTORS

For a long time it has been a convention of clinical diagnosis that symptoms and signs of an 'organic' psychosis take precedence in classification over those of 'functional' conditions. Application of this rule means that clouding of consciousness, delirium, memory disorders and gross cognitive deficits, especially in the presence of overt brain disease or intoxication, are used as superordinate classifying criteria even in the presence of first rank symptoms or marked mood swings.

Severe dementia and profound mental retardation are obvious examples of this hierarchical principle, but are not interesting because these patients are by definition incapable of describing inner experiences. In delirium, speech is so incoherent or fragmented, and the patient's attention so distractable, that it is usually unwise to be dogmatic about the presence or absence of first rank symptoms. However, they are clearly described from time to time in association with a wide variety of cerebral disorders, for example, as early prodromata of Huntington's and Alzheimer's diseases.

Temporal lobe epilepsy, particularly if left-sided, is a specific example. First rank symptoms can also be precipitated by amphetamine intoxication. Evelyn Waugh's autobiographical novel, *The Ordeal of Gilbert Pinfold*, describes the symptom of third-person hallucinosis in detail. In his case it was probably precipitated by a regime of alcohol and potassium bromide, the tranquillizers of the time, and was not diagnosed as schizophrenia. Hallucinosis in the absence of clouding, when associated wiith alcohol consumption, is often classified separately from schizophrenia. Such clues to aetiology are lost in a top-down rule-based nosology. A multi-axial system would be preferable.

A different kind of exclusion criterion should, however, always be considered. It is essential to remember, when examining for positive symptoms, that any serious deficit or disorder of language, from whatever cause, imposes serious limitations on the respondent's understanding of questions and the examiner's interpretation of the answers. Disorders of intelligence or language make communication difficult or impossible and it is most unwise to make a diagnosis of schizophrenia in such circumstances (Strömgren, 1982). Asperger's syndrome and other disorders within the autistic spectrum (see below) are particularly likely to give rise to false positives.

Another problem of recognition is that patients are often asked about experiences of 'control', which may lead to affirmative replies from people who for occupational or religious reasons or because they belong to certain sects, cultivate analogous experiences. An example was that of a Taoist priestess who was examined during the International Pilot Study of Schizophrenia (WHO, 1973, pp. 275–6).

1.4.3 DIFFERENTIATION FROM AFFECTIVE PSYCHOSES

Schneider contended that first rank symptoms, in the absence of gross 'organic' disorders, are likely to determine diagnosis whatever 'functional' disorders appear to be present. This clinical convention was confirmed in the IPSS, using the eighth edition of the PSE to establish the presence or absence of a comprehensive range of symptoms irrespective of clinical diagnosis. The other major international study to use the PSE, the US–UK Diagnostic Project, gave a similar result. For example, delusions of control were rated in 224 out of 1177 IPSS patients. Of these, 97% were given a clinical diagnosis of schizophrenia, 2% of mania and 1% of depression. However, it is difficult to find any symptom highly predictive of mania until the schizophrenic disorders are removed from the analysis, since obvious candidates such as elation, flight of ideas and grandiose ideas are quite common in schizophrenia as well (Wing *et al.*, 1974; Chapter 7). This is even more true of depression. A recent report on a series of first admissions in Finland, using PSE9, provides tables showing frequencies of syndromes by clinical diagnosis (Pakaslahti, 1986).

In the IPSS, most of the few discrepancies between first rank symptoms and clinical diagnosis could have been due to the use of broader definitions than Schneider would have approved of (WHO, 1973, Chapter 11; Wing and Nixon, 1975). An example of a symptom that, if included, could lead to a discrepancy with clinical diagnosis was provided by a patient whose condition in every other respect fitted the pattern of recurrent mania. He said that at the height of his latest episode he had experienced his thoughts bursting like tiny stars around his head. He was fully aware that they were his own thoughts, though he could not explain the experience. This description does not fit the conventional definition of a first rank symptom: 'The essence of the symptom is that the subject experiences thoughts *which are not his own* intruding into his mind . . . the thoughts *themselves* are not his' (Wing *et al.*, 1974). In general, first rank symptoms are experienced passively, as deficits, whereas analogous experiences in mania are expressed as expansions of the patient's powers: 'My thoughts are so powerful it's just like they are God's'.

'Secondary' delusions of reference and persecution, often with religious or subcultural or bizarre content, are quite common in mania and severe depression as well as in schizophrenia but usually the content is congruent with the mood. If, for example, a severely depressed woman described a voice accusing her of unnamable crimes, for which she accepted the guilt, the symptoms would be regarded as mood-congruent.

George Winokur *et al.* (1985a) investigated the extent to which delusions and hallucinations were congruent with mood in patients diagnosed as schizophrenic, schizoaffective, bipolar, or unipolar depressive, and concluded that there was a good distinction between schizophrenia and affective disorders but that congruent and incongruent symptoms tended to occur together in schizoaffective conditions. The authors' assumption is that non-congruent psychotic symptoms can 'trump' the congruent symptoms in forming a diagnosis, but not *vice versa*. However they provide no external evidence to this effect.

1.4.4 DELUSIONAL PSYCHOSES

Continuing along a hypothetical hierarchy of positive symptoms, there still remains a small group of psychotic disorders characterized by mood-incongruent delusions (rarely, hallucinations) but not by first rank experiences (Winokur, 1977). These may be 'monosymptomatic', as in the case of a man whose only psychotic symptom is that he thinks other people say that he gives off an unpleasant smell, although he himself denies it and, so far as one can tell, is right to do so. Other examples are litigious delusional ideas or morbid jealousy, not associated with first rank or psychotic affective psychoses. Other examples seem unlikely to be 'primary' in Jaspers' sense; e.g. the fixed belief of a long institutionalized woman that she is married to some royal personage, or the false accusations sometimes made by people who are becoming deaf or blind or losing their memory. A mentally retarded man thought that when he flushed the toilet, everyone else in the street did the same. Such beliefs tend to be called 'delusional ideas'. In the large international studies they tended to be diagnosed as part of schizophrenia but that removes the possibility of testing alternative hypotheses.

1.4.5 NEUROTIC SYMPTOMS

A further problem of diagnosis can occur when it is difficult to distinguish between a delusion and an obsession, although this is unusual. The occurrence of obsessional symptoms in post-encephalitic disorders and Tourette's syndrome muddies the already dubious distinctions between 'organic', 'psychotic' and 'neurotic' disorders. However, there is rarely any problem of differential diagnosis if there is no suspicion of the presence of delusions or hallucinations. Perhaps the sudden unavailability of thoughts in an attack of panic (well known to students in oral examinations) is a form of 'blocking' that, like a freezing of movement, has analogies with a first rank and with a catatonic symptom. 'Non-specific' symptoms such as worrying or muscular tension pose no diagnostic difficulty. They are very common in all the foregoing conditions.

1.4.6 A POSITIVE HIERARCHY

It is possible, therefore, to adopt conventions of diagnosis that allow three groups of 'functional psychotic' symptoms to be distinguished with reasonable clinical clarity, each of which can be designated part of a schizophrenic, affective or delusional complex. Much statistical expertise has been put into trying to separate the two larger complexes, without much success in finding a 'point of rarity' between them (Kendell, 1989). Such attempts deliberately leave out of account the loading that clinicians place on some symptoms at the expense of others, because it is assumed that it is a bias derived from diagnostic preconceptions. The possibility that there is a natural hierarchy is thereby discounted.

There is no doubt that the positive phenomena **can** be placed approximately into a non-reflexive hierarchy of scarcity-ubiquity, in which items higher in the order tend to be associated with items lower down but not *vice versa*. Sturt (1981) demonstrated an empirical hierarchy in data collected by lay interviewers using PSE9 to assess a community sample. Diagnostic bias was thereby eliminated. The rarest symptoms were associated with high total PSE scores and, to a lesser extent, with more social disablement. Heading the hierarchy were symptoms such as pathological guilt, loss of libido and suicidal ideas, loss of interest, morning depression and self-depreciation. Sturt also showed that total PSE9 score could be regarded as a measure of severity throughout a range of samples of patients contacting specialist services, including many with psychotic disorders.

A difficulty in interpreting data from almost all samples is that they contain individuals at different points in the course of disorder, many of whom will not display a full complement of positive symptoms. There is some evidence, for example, that these can appear and disappear 'up and down' a hierarchy, as the disorder waxes and wanes (Herz *et al.*, 1982; Hirsch *et al.*, 1987; Knights *et al.*, 1980; Winokur, 1985b). A second problem is that disorders higher in any postulated hierarchy, because they are likely to be more severe than those lower down, may have a precipitating action. Certainly, it is not clinically surprising if first rank symptoms are experienced as exciting, depressing, terrifying or worrying by turns. But a biological chain reaction down the hierarchy is a further possibility. Thirdly, it may well be that there are varieties of disorder that do not fit into any hierarchy but cannot at the moment be clinically identified and can thus contribute only noise to the system.

1.5 THE AUTISTIC SPECTRUM

A brief reference to the autistic spectrum is of

relevance to the theme of this chapter for three reasons. First, because of the word 'autism'. Second, because people with such disorders who have understandable, if odd, speech are often called 'schizophrenic' because clinicians interested in adult disorders tend not to be able to take a good developmental history. Third, because it throws new light on the concept of negative symptoms and catatonia.

The best description of the syndrome is still that written in two reports soon after the French revolution, by J.M.G. Itard (Lane, 1977), concerning the characteristics and treatment of Victor, a boy discovered in 1799 living wild in the woods of Aveyron. Pinel had come to the conclusion that Victor was a congenital idiot and was abandoned because of this. Itard (a man of the Enlightenment) thought the child was the prototype of the natural savage, a human being untouched by education, but in spite of his best efforts (Itard was the first experimental psychologist) Victor never learned to speak and his comprehension remained severely limited. Itard probably came to the conclusion in the end that Pinel had been right, and it may be for that reason that he did not name the syndrome he described (Wing, 1976).

It was left to Leo Kanner (1943) to describe 11 cases in detail, fill in the developmental history, and apply the label 'early infantile autism' to them. Leaving the actual name aside, this step was of immense value. Nearly 150 years had passed before Itard's syndrome was recognized as such and his insights applied to other children with the condition. Tests could then be made of the validity of increasingly crucial hypotheses. This is not essentialist 'labelling' in the sense that sociologists such as Scheff (1966) use the term (Wing, 1978a; Chapter 5).

In the year following Kanner's first publication, Hans Asperger (1944) independently published a monograph on a syndrome with remarkable resemblances but also differences, which he called 'autistic psychopathy'. This group was characterized by a lack of intuitive understanding of the rules of social interaction, naïve and tactless behaviour, pedantic and literal understanding and use of language, difficulty in co-ordinating complex movements, and one or a few circumscribed and often odd interests (Frith, 1989; Tantam, 1988; Wing, 1981, 1982).

Lorna Wing has suggested that 'social impairment' is at the centre of the observable clinical manifestations of Kanner's, Asperger's, and a number of other eponymous syndromes that lie within an autistic spectrum. Social impairment is not just social withdrawal. It is technically specifiable in terms of a triad of difficulties affecting reciprocal social interaction, verbal and non-verbal language, and imaginative activities, and can be reliably measured by trained workers. The spectrum is usefully described in terms of three clinical subgroups: those who are aloof and indifferent to others, who avoid contact except for simple physical needs or pleasures (such as tickling); those who make no spontaneous social contacts but passively accept the approaches of others; and those who initiate contacts but in an odd, one-sided way, unaffected by the reaction of the person approached (Wing and Gould, 1979). This last 'active but odd' pattern is particularly likely to be confused with 'schizophrenia'.

Nowadays, in psychiatric practice, catatonic symptoms are more often observed in people with disorders in the autistic spectrum than in people with schizophrenia. For example, only one person with signs of catatonia was found in a recent survey of 172 long-term attenders at psychiatric day care units serving a district in southeast London. These were people with an average of 15 years in contact with services. Many had been long-stay inpatients (Brugha *et al.*, 1988).

The patient was a single man of 26 with a long history of social inadequacy. He moved awkwardly, with his left arm held to his chest and the fingers of the right hand held in odd positions that must have been quite difficult to maintain voluntarily. He rocked to and fro throughout the interview and swayed his legs from side to side. He imitated the examiner's gestures in mirror image fashion. His affect was flat, there was virtually no eye contact or other body language, and speech was limited to absolutely concrete one-or-two-word answers. Occasionally there was no answer but an effect of trying without success to reply. (In another case, the patient could only begin to reply when the examiner made as if to get up and leave). All positive symptoms were denied. His only interest was a pile of Presley records. His IQ (WAIS Full Scale) was 86. He walked late, had always been very slow, and had spent a year in hospital as a child, the diagnosis being 'schizoid personality'. The case notes carried no record of a developmental history. His father was said to have been 'schizophrenic' but no symptoms were specified. All physical investigations were normal.

This man would certainly have been diagnosed schizophrenic 20 years ago and would still be so diagnosed in many psychiatric clinics. His symptoms fit Bleuler's description of catatonia. The phenomenon of apparent suspension of the will is quite often observed in autistic people. A slight prompt, such as a brief pressure with a finger, may be sufficient to unlock a temporarily frozen posture, for example when a spoonful of food is held motionless between plate and mouth.

The name Kanner gave to his syndrome was therefore not without its problems, since the 'autistic aloneness' he described was different from that of the autism of Bleuler. The lack of fantasy and creative inner life so clearly observed and described by Kanner himself, is the opposite of a flight into fantasy. In fact, the general concept of 'autism' is altogether too complex to be of much value in understanding either Kanner's or Kraepelin's disorder unless it is unpacked (Wing, 1976). The differences in developmental and family history between Kanner's and Asperger's syndromes, on the one hand, and 'schizophrenia' on the other, are the main reason for differentiating the two groups

clinically. Part of schizophrenia may well be a developmental disorder but it clearly is not of the same severity or type. That does not mean that there are no underlying biological similarities. The matter will only be resolved by experimental evidence. Meanwhile, it is important not to prevent the possibility of distinguishing between the two by submerging them under rubrics such as 'schizoid personality' (Wolff and Chick, 1980) or 'simple schizophrenia' (Cutting and Shepherd, 1987).

1.6 NEGATIVE SYMPTOMS

1.6.1 'ORGANIC' DISORDERS

The neurologist, C.M. Fisher, noted that, 'prior to 1900, when neurological and psychiatric syndromes were being delineated, the symptoms of psychomotor retardation, slowness, apathy and lack of spontaneity were universally regarded as manifestations of abulia' (Fisher, 1983). Auerbach (1902), for example, referred to the syndrome associated with a frontal lobe tumour as abulia. Much of the literature was concerned with the most severe state, akinetic mutism, which occurred most frequently with infarction of the cingulate gyrus or mesodiencephalon. The phenomena associated with postencephalitic parkinsonism, particularly the elements of catatonia, are similar (Sachs, 1976). The autistic spectrum has been mentioned above. Fisher was more interested in lesser, though still severe degrees, which he called 'abulia minor'. The descriptions of poverty of speech and movement are virtually identical to those of equivalent items in PSE9.

1.6.2 NEGATIVE SYMPTOMS IN SCHIZOPHRENIA

The distinction between positive and negative symptoms became abundantly clear when conducting research into the social milieu of long-stay 'schizophrenic' patients in the late 1950s (Wing, 1959; Wing and Brown, 1970), and applying the results to systems of rehabilitation. It became even more obvious when the ideas derived from this research were applied to the manifestations observed in acute episodes. Testing the hypothesis that characteristics of the environment could cause amplification of either kind of symptom meant that a series of measuring instruments with publicly specified technical standards were required.

The negative symptoms were visible deficits in behaviour, such as emotional blunting, slowness of speech and movement, poverty of speech, poor use of non-verbal 'body' language and lack of motivation — all summed up in a score called SW, for social withdrawal, which was the central behavioural item (Wing, 1989). From the third edition onward the PSE contained equivalent items, including a motor examination based on the descriptions of classical German authors. Although there was a strong motor component to the negative syndrome, and overactivity was clearly related (Venables, 1957), cognition, affect and will were all deeply involved. Incoherence of speech (and presumably, therefore, of thought) was kept separate, although behaviourally it was highly correlated with social withdrawal.

Catatonia was already uncommon and, in retrospect, it is questionable how far those patients who did show such behaviour had ever experienced positive psychotic symptoms of the kind described by Schneider. There was, however, a wide range of severity of the negative symptoms, which was correlated with measures of social disablement (Catterson *et al.*, 1963; Wing and Freudenberg, 1961) and social environment (Wing and Brown, 1970).

1.7 RELATION OF POSITIVE TO NEGATIVE SYMPTOMS AND THE SIGNIFICANCE FOR 'SCHIZOPHRENIA'

Thus both positive and negative symptoms can tentatively be placed along a dimension of severity, according to degree of clinical and social disablement (Wing, 1990). The first can clinically be ranked in terms mainly of abnormal subjective experiences. The second is more of a continuum, measurable mainly in terms of behaviour, affect and speech. The items in each series can be technically defined. There is some evidence for an empirical non-reflexive ordering of types of positive symptoms, in line with clinical judgements of severity but independent of diagnostic loading; this, however, remains speculative.

An interesting hypothesis can therefore be put forward to the effect that the negative and positive symptoms are connected, cross-sectionally, in descending order of severity. At the top of both dimensions are severe global dementia and profound mental retardation. After that on the negative side come other abnormalities of the brain that seriously disrupt experience and behaviour, including disorders in the autistic spectrum. Then there are the well-attested negative behavioural characteristics (often also experienced by afflicted individuals) associated with first rank phenomena and their elaborations. The social course and outcome are better predicted by the negative symptoms. If the positive symptoms erupt suddenly and are precipitated (as in the case of Gilbert Pinfold) the outcome is more favourable (Zubin *et al.*, 1961).

Motor slowness, underactivity, and deficits in various bodily, affective and cognitive functions are also characteristically observed in severe depression. One of the most severe, which is given great diagnostic weight in German phenomenology, is subjective 'feeling of loss of feeling'. The definition in PSE10 is taken from Manfred Bleuler's edition of his father's textbook: 'The loss of feeling is felt, the numbness perceived, the lifelessness experienced' (Bleuler, 1983). Finally, even anxiety can 'paralyse' occasionally.

There are, of course, many specific neurological features (e.g. within the autistic spectrum, the dementias, parkinsonism, etc), that do not form part of a general negative dimension. If there is a biological as well as a clinical continuity underlying these manifestations, there are also many specific syndromes that do not form part of it.

Differential diagnosis can therefore be considered from a dimensional or from a cross-sectional point of view. From the former perspective, the old idea of a unitary psychosis seems still plausible. Seen in transverse section, the conventional clinical typology is more evident. Considering the dimensional with the categorical sequences brings out some of the anomalies of their relationships in 'schizophrenia' in a constructive way. It was obvious from a five-year retrospective follow-up study of patients admitted to three district psychiatric hospitals in 1956 (Brown *et al.*, 1966), from subsequent medication trials (Leff and Wing, 1971; Hirsch *et al.*, 1973; Stevens, 1973), and from the WHO follow-up studies (1979), that negative and positive symptoms frequently occur together but that either can occur independently of the other within the same clinical course.

Environmental conditions, for example the degree of understimulation of the milieu, appear to amplify the manifestation of negative symptoms. People with communication disorders are probably particularly vulnerable (Wing and Freudenberg, 1961; Wing and Brown, 1970). Socially overstimulating conditions seem more likely to precipitate disorders characterized by positive symptoms. The best known example — high 'expressed emotion' (Leff, 1987) — is manifested by persons close to the patient; by no means only, or always, relatives. It is associated with relapse of positive symptoms and possibly with the timing of the first onset (Chapter 8). These are part of a more general susceptibility to stressful environmental pressures, such as life events (Brown and Birley, 1968) and over-enthusiastic attempts at rehabilitation (Wing *et al.*, 1964). Neither effect, therefore, is specific to schizophrenia

but depends on underlying vulnerabilities.

The necessity for people with disorders such as schizophrenia to walk a tightrope between the different dangers of under- and over-stimulation led us to suggest methods of coping with long-term vulnerability (Wing, 1978b). Together with the usefulness of the phenothiazine medications, it was also suggested that part of the vulnerability must be associated with the arousal mechanisms of the brain (Wing *et al.*, 1973). Recent theories that involve the processing of information via the arousal system, mid-brain, hippocampus and frontal lobes, and the various pathologies associated with these areas (Beckmann, 1991; Roberts and Crow, 1987), point a plausible way forward for research. These spatial analogies are complicated by the fact that severe negative symptoms are likely to be associated with pathology lower in the anatomical chain, while severe positive symptoms (the first rank syndrome for example) are likely to be associated with abnormality in the temporal and frontal cortex.

'One of the reasons for lack of progress in unravelling the secrets of schizophrenia may be that it is difficult to understand how the experience of hearing one's thoughts aloud in one's head, or of knowing that one's own will has been replaced by the will of some other agency, can have an anatomical or biochemical representation' (Medical Research Council, 1987). One of the tasks of disciplines such as neuropsychology is to try to provide some of the intermediate links in this chain, particularly in terms of theories of normal cognitive, affective and conative processes and how they may be disturbed to produce the features of schizophrenia and its neighbouring disorders.

A serious attempt to tackle the problems at this intermediate level has been made by Chris and Uta Frith (C. Frith, 1987, 1991; U. Frith, 1989). Their ideas on possible neuropsychological mechanisms that could form links between the clinical manifestations of both the autistic and the schizophrenic disorders, and possible abnormalities in neurological

16

pathways, suggest that order and coherence might be brought into part at least of an area where few theories have previously been sufficiently clinically specific.

1.8 DIFFERENTIAL DIAGNOSIS OF SCHIZOPHRENIA

Janzarik (1987) stated that the history of schizophrenia 'is a history, not of medical discoveries but of the intellectual models on which the orientation of psychiatry is based'. Models need a few 'hard, obstinate facts' to turn them into knowledge. We are not there yet.

The somewhat unconventional approach to differential diagnosis, via two clinical dimensions, presented here does, however, keep the options open. The more familiar categorical approach is now enshrined in the rule-based systems of DSM–III-R (American Psychiatric Association, 1987) and the new ICD-10 (WHO, 1990), which represent compromises between scientists with the most influential theories and the practice of senior clinicians at national and international level. The rules are specified in fair detail (Tables 1.1 and 1.2). The two lists of symptoms and signs are quite similar, though not identical in detail.

Both allow, among other options, a preliminary diagnosis on the basis of catatonic behaviour plus flatness of affect only. However, DSM–III-R requires a symptomatic period of at least 6 months, compared with 1 month for ICD-10. This is enough to exclude more acute disorders, even if the symptoms are identical. Another important difference is the clause in DSM–III-R that excludes autistic disorder unless there are prominent and persistent hallucinations. What neither system provides is definitions of the symptoms on which the rules operate. Also, many of the anomalies of differential diagnosis that are obvious when longitudinal and transverse sections are compared are not addressed. DSM–IV is promised shortly.

In retrospect, Kraepelin's syndrome probably included, among others, conditions that could now be specified more precisely; for example, postencephalitic disorders or conditions within the autistic spectrum. The assumption that symptoms of bipolar disorder could not be associated was incorrect. With these two caveats, it is still possible to delineate a syndrome that would fit his descriptions quite well. With its emphasis on negative characteristics, associated with course, it would look not unlike DSM–III-R. Bleuler's concept placed

Table 1.1 Summary of ICD-10, diagnostic criteria for research, draft of February 1990

Schizophrenia (F20)

A. *One of the symptoms under A1*
    OR two of the symptoms under A2
    must be present for most of an episode lasting at least a month

  A1a. Thought echo, insertion, withdrawal, broadcasting
  A1b. Delusions of control, influence, passivity, delusional perception
• A1c. Verbal hallucinations, with running commentary or discussing patient, or coming from a part of the body
  A1d. Delusions that are persistent and culturally implausible
  A2e. Persistent hallucinations with half-formed delusions without clear affective content
  A2f. Breaks in train of thought, giving rise to incoherent or irrelevant speech, neologisms
  A2g. Catatonic behaviour
  A2h. Negative – apathy, paucity of speech, blunted or incongruent affect, not due to depression or medication

B. *If manic or depressive episode*, Criterion A must be met *before* mood disturbance developed

C. Not attributable to organic brain disease (F0) or substance misuse (F1)

All three conditions, A, B, and C, must be satisfied

Table 1.2 Summary of DSM–III-R, criteria of schizophrenia (295)

A.   *Active phase: 1 of A1, A2 or A3 must be present for at least a week*
   A1.   Two of the following five:
      (a) delusions
      (b) prominent hallucinations
      (c) incoherence of speech
      (d) catatonic behaviour
      (e) flat or grossly inappropriate affect
   A2.   Bizarre delusions
   A3.   Prominent verbal hallucinations not related to depression or elation OR running commentary on behaviour or thoughts OR voices conversing with each other

B.   *During disturbance: work, social, self-care functioning lowered*

C.   *Absence of schizoaffective disorder and mood disturbance with psychotic features* (Total duration of all mood episodes brief relative to that of active and residual)

D.   *Continuous disturbance for 6 months, including:*

An active phase (A above) at least a week, unless successfully treated

A prodromal phase. Deterioration in functioning before active phase, not due to mood disorder or alcohol/drug use, including two of the following nine symptoms:
(1) marked social isolation or withdrawal
(2) marked impairment in occupational role
(3) markedly peculiar behaviour
(4) markedly impaired self-care
(5) blunted or inappropriate affect
(6) odd speech, poverty of speech, poverty of content of speech
(7) odd or magical beliefs incompatible with cultural norms
(8) unusual perceptual experiences
(9) marked lack of initiative, interests, energy

A residual phase. Following the active phase, persistence of at least two symptoms from the nine listed above

E.   *No organic factor initiated or maintained the disorder*

F.   *If autistic disorder:*
   Diagnose only if criteria of schizophrenia are met and, in addition, there are prominent delusions or hallucinations.

All six criteria, A, B, C, D, E, and F, must be met.

less emphasis on dementia but, by designating minor, vaguely defined, extensions of his fundamental symptoms as the commonest subgroup, he allowed the concept to expand beyond the boundaries of what was (and probably still is) technically specifiable. This is legitimate in theory but not when acted upon in clinical practice.

Some of the mysteries of 'schizophrenia' are due to the sheer difficulty of the problems posed. The ways in which information is processed in the brain, and the links between deviations from normal processing and clinical manifestations, are immensely complex. A rigid 'left to right' approach to definition leads to an inefficient scientific strategy. Other problems have been due to the failure of researchers to use standards of reference, both for a comprehensive phenomenology and for the classifying rules. The consequence has been a mass of unreplicated data. The longitudinal and cross-sectional approach adopted here shows how easy it is to designate (quite legitimately) different areas of phenomenology as 'schizophrenias'. But trying to avoid classification altogether would be even more crippling clinically and scientifically.

Some recent (but rather soft) epidemiological data suggest that the frequency and course of 'schizophrenia' may have fluctuated markedly during the past two centuries and that its severity may now be different in different parts of the world. Part of this fluctuation might be due to changing conceptions of what symptoms should be included. 'Organic' disorders and the autistic spectrum are better recognized today. Part may be due to a genuine fluctuation in perinatal morbidity, or infections such as encephalitis lethargica, or to other possible environmental causes. Part might well be due to the fact that some 'schizophrenias', not at the moment clinically specifiable, are more reactive to changing environmental conditions than others. Certainly there is a wide range of prognosis, particularly varying with severity of premorbid abnormalities.

The sensible way to proceed, for anyone who seriously wishes the results of observations or experiments to be compared with those produced elsewhere, is to use the two international nosologies, together perhaps with a local variant, for which an algorithm should be provided. This fulfils the public health function of diagnosis and the necessity for clinical responsibility. The approach adopted here is not based on an assumption that schizophrenia does not exist or that the whole concept should be abandoned. On the contrary, it assumes that 'schizophrenias' do represent important clinical problems and a fertile source for research. However, none of the rules represent disease entities, nor could they. Anyone who disagrees with them should specify precisely how, so that comparability is still possible. These rules should act upon a comprehensive phenomenological database, the items of which are differentially defined. SCAN (Schedules for Clinical Assessment in Neuropsychiatry) which includes PSE10, associated with modules for the developmental, social and clinical history and personality disorder, attempts to meet this requirement (Wing *et al.*, 1990; WHO, 1992).

Studies of possible causes or underlying psychological or biological deviations can then be used to try to refine syndromes 'bottom up', as well as investigating the properties of those defined 'top down'. In this way, various 'schizophrenias' (Bleuler's word) will eventually be specified from the general area of overlapping disorders that have at various times been called 'schizophrenia', and their interrelationships will finally be understood.

REFERENCES

American Psychiatric Association (1987) *Diagnostic and Statistical Manual of Mental Disorders*, third edition-revised. Washington, DC.

Asperger, H. (1944) Die autistischen Psychopathen im Kindesalter. *Arch. Psychiatr. Nerv.*, **117**, 76–136.

Auerbach, S. (1902) Beitrag zur Diagnostik der Geschwulste des Stirnhirn. *Deutsche Zeitung Nervenheilkunde*, **22**, 312–22.

Beckmann, H. (1991) Schizophrenia and the limbic system. In *Schizophrenia and Youth. Etiology and Therapeutic Consequences*. C. Eggers (ed), Springer-Verlag, Heidelberg.

Berrios, G.E. (1987) Historical aspects of psychoses. Nineteenth century issues. *Br. Med. Bull.*, **43**, 484–98.

Berrios, G.E. and Hauser, R. (1988) The early development of Kraepelin's ideas on classification. A conceptual history. *Psychol. Med.*, **18**, 813–21.

Bleuler, E. (1908) The prognosis of dementia praecox. The group of schizophrenias. Translated into English, 1987. In *The Clinical Roots of the Schizophrenia Concept*. J. Cutting and M. Shepherd, (eds), Cambridge, Cambridge University Press.

Bleuler, E. (1913) *Dementia Praecox or the Group of Schizophrenias*. Translated into English, 1950. International Universities Press, New York.

Bleuler, E. (1983) *Lehrbuch der Psychiatrie. Funfzehnte Auflage neubearbeitet von Bleuler M*, **233**. Springer-Verlag, Heidelberg.

Brown, G.W. and Birley, J.L.T. (1968) Crises and life changes and the onset of schizophrenia. *J. Health Soc. Behav.*, **9**, 203.

Brown, G.W., Bone, M., Dalison, B. and Wing, J.K. (1966) *Schizophrenia and Social Care*. Oxford University Press, London.

Brugha, T.S., Wing, J.K., Brewin, C.R. *et al.* (1988) The problems of people in long-term psychiatric day care. *Psychol. Med.*, **18**, 443–56.

Catterson, A., Bennett, D.H. and Freudenberg, R.K. (1963) A survey of long-stay schizophrenic patients. *Br. J. Psychiatry*, **111**, 750–7.

Cohen, H. (1961) The evolution of the concept of disease. In *Concepts of Medicine*. Lush, B. (ed), Pergamon Press, Oxford, UK, pp. 159–69.

Cutting J. and Shepherd, M. (eds) (1987) *The Clinical Roots of the Schizophrenia Syndrome*. Cambridge University Press, Cambridge.

Fisher, C.M. (1983) Abulia minor versus agitated behaviour. *Clin. Neurosurg.*, **31**, 9–31.

Frith, C.D. (1987) The positive and negative symptoms of schizophrenia reflect impairments in the perception and initiation of action. *Psychol., Med.* **17**, 631–48.

Frith, C.D. (1991) Schizophrenia. Second order representation in the brain. In *Schizophrenia and Youth. Aetiology and Therapeutic Consequences*. C. Eggers (ed), Springer-Verlag, Heidelberg.

Frith, U. (1989) *Autism. Explaining the Enigma*. Blackwell, London.

Herz, M.I., Szymanski, H.V. and Simon, J. (1982) Intermittent medication for stable schizophrenic out-patients. *Am. J. Psychiatry*, **139**, 918–22.

Hirsch, S., Gaind, R., Rohde, P. *et al.* (1973) Outpatient maintenance of chronic schizophrenic patients with long-acting fluphenazine. Double blind placebo trial. *Br. Med. J.*, **1**, 633–7.

Hirsch, S.R., Jolley, H.G., Manchanda, R. and McRink, A. (1987) Early intervention medication as an alternative to continuous depot treatment in schizophrenia. In *Psychological Treatment of Schizophrenia*. J.S. Strauss, W. Böker and H.D. Brenner (eds), Huber, Stuttgart.

Janzarik, W. (1987) The concept of schizophrenia. History and problems. In *Search for the Causes of Schizophrenia*, H. Hafner, W.F. Gättz and W. Janzarik (eds), Springer-Verlag, Heidelberg, pp. 11–18.

Jaspers, K. (1962) *General Psychopathology*. Translated into English from the 7th edition. Manchester University Press, Manchester, UK.

Kanner, L. (1943) Autistic disturbances of affective contact. *Nerv. Child*, **2**, 217–50.

Kendell, R.E. (1989) Clinical validity. *Psychol. Med.*, **19**, 45–55.

Kendler, K.S., Lieberman, J.A. and Walsh, D. (1989) The structured interview for schizotypy. *Schizophr. Bull.* **15**, 559–71.

Kety, S.S., Rosenthal, D., Wender, P.H., *et al.* (1978) The biologic and adoptive families of adopted individuals who became schizophrenic. In *The Nature of Schizophrenia*. L. Wynne, R.L. Cromwell and S. Matthysse (eds), Wiley, New York, pp. 25–37.

Knights, A., Hirsch, S.R. and Platt, S.D. (1980) Clinical change as a function of brief admission to hospital in a controlled study using the PSE. *Br. J. Psychiatry*, **137**, 170–80.

Kraepelin, E. (1896) Dementia praecox. Translated into English, 1987. In *The Clinical Roots of the Schizophrenia Concept*. J. Cutting and M. Shepherd (eds) Cambridge University Press, Cambridge.

Kraepelin, E.(1920) Die Erscheinungsformen des Irreseins. *Zeitschrift Neurol. Psychiatr.*, **62**, 1–29.

Lane, H. (1977) *The Wild Boy of Aveyron*. Allen and Unwin, London.

Leff, J.L. (1987) A model of schizophrenic vulnerability to environmental factors. In *Search for the Causes of Schizophrenia*, H. Häfner, W.F. Gattaz and W. Janzarik (eds), Springer-Verlag, Heidelberg, pp. 317–330.

Leff, J.L. and Wing, J.K. (1971) Trial of maintenance therapy in schizophrenia. *Br. Med. J.*, **3**, 599–604.

Lewis, A. (1953) Health as a social concept. *Br. J. Sociol.*, **4**, 109–24.

Medical Research Council (1987) *Research into Schizophrenia*. MRC, London.

Pakaslahti, A. (1986) *Principles and Practices in Diagnosing Schizophrenia*. Research Institute for Social Security, Helsinki.

Popper, K. (1945) *The Open Society and its Enemies. Volume II. The High Tide of Prophesy.* Routledge, London, pp. 9–20.

Roberts, G.W. and Crow, T. (1987) The neuropathology of schizophrenia. *Br. Med. Bull.*, **43**, 599–615.

Sachs, O. (1976) *Awakenings*. Pelican, London.

Scheff, T. (1966) *Being Mentally Ill*. Aldine, Chicago, IL.

Schneider, K. (1959) *Clinical Psychopathology*. Translated by M.W. Hamilton, Grune and Stratton, New York.

Schneider, K. (1976) *Klinische Psychopathologie*. 9te Auflage. Thieme, Stuttgart.

Smulevich, A.B. (1989) Sluggish schizophrenia in the modern classification of mental illness. *Schizophr. Bull.*, **15**, 553–40.

Stevens, B.C. (1973) Role of fluphenazine decanoate in lessening the burden of chronic schizophrenics in the community. *Psychol. Med.*, **3**, 141–58.

Strömgren, E. (1982) Differential diagnosis of schizophrenia. In *Psychoses of Uncertain Aetiology*. J.K. Wing and L. Wing (eds), Cambridge University Press, Cambridge.

Sturt, E. (1981) Hierarchical patterns in the distribution of psychiatric symptoms. *Psychol. Med.*, **11**, 783–94.

Tantam, D. (1988) Asperger's syndrome. *J. Child Psychol. Psychiatry*, **29**, 245–55.

Venables, P.H. (1957) A short scale for 'activity-withdrawal' in schizophrenics. *J. Ment. Sci.*, **103**, 197–9.

Wing, J.K. (1959) The measurement of behaviour in chronic schizophrenia. *Acta Psychiatr. Neurol.*, **35**, 245–54.

Wing, J.K. (1976) Kanner's syndrome. A historical introduction. In *Early Childhood Autism*, L. Wing (ed), Pergamon Press, Oxford. Chapter 1.

Wing, J.K. (1978a) *Reasoning about Madness*. Oxford University Press, London.

Wing, J.K. (1978b) Social influences on the course of schizophrenia. In *The Nature of Schizophrenia*. L. Wynne, R.L. Cromwell and S. Matthysse (eds), Wiley, New York, pp. 599–617.

Wing, J.K. (1989) The measurement of social disablement. The MRC Social Behaviour and Social Performance Schedules. *Soc. Psychiatry Psychiatr. Epidemiol.*, **24**, 173–8.

Wing. J.K. (1990) Meeting the needs of people with psychiatric disorders. *Soc. Psychiatry Psychiatr. Epidemiol.*, **25**, 2–8.

Wing, J.K (1991a) Social psychiatry. In *Social Psychiatry. Theory, Methodology and Practice*. P. Bebbington (ed), Transaction Publishers, New Brunswick NJ.

Wing, J.K (1991b) Measuring and Classifying Psychiatric Disorders. Learning from the PSE. In *Social Psychiatry. Theory, Methodology and Practice* P. Bebbington (ed), Transaction Publishers, New Brunswick NJ.

Wing, J.K., Babor, T., Brugha, T. *et al.* (1990) SCAN; Schedules for clinical assessment in neuropsychiatry. *Arch. Gen. Psychiatry*, **47**, 589–93.

Wing, J.K., Bennett, D.H. and Denham, J. (1964) *The Industrial Rehabilitation of Long-stay Schizophrenic Patients*. MRC Memorandum No. 42. Medical Research Council, London.

Wing, J.K. and Brown, G.W. (1970) *Institutionalism and Schizophrenia*. Cambridge University Press, London.

Wing, J.K. Cooper, J.E. and Sartorius, N. (1974) *The Description and Classification of Psychiatric Symptoms. An Instruction Manual for the PSE and CATEGO System*. Cambridge University Press, London.

Wing, J.K. and Freudenberg, R.K. (1961) The response of severely ill chronic schizophrenic patients to social stimulation. *Am. J. Psychiatry*, **118**, 311–22.

Wing, J.K., Leff, J.L. and Hirsch, S. (1973) Preventive treatment of schizophrenia. Some theoretical and methodological issues. In *Psychopathology and Pharmacology*. J.O. Cole, A.M. Freedman and A.J. Friedhoff (eds), Johns Hopkins University Press, Baltimore, MD.

Wing, J.K. and Nixon, J. (1975) Discriminating symptoms in schizophrenia. *Arch. Gen. Psychiatry*, **32**, 853–9.

Wing, L. (1981) Asperger's syndrome. *Psychol. Med.*, **11**, 115–29.

Wing, L. (1982) Development of concepts, classification and relationship to mental retardation. In *Psychoses of Uncertain Aetiology*. J.K. Wing and L. Wing (eds), Cambridge University Press, Cambridge.

Wing, L. and Gould, J. (1979) Severe impairments of social interaction and associated abnormalities in children. Epidemiology and classification. *J. Autism Dev. Disord.*, **9**, 11–29.

Winokur, G. (1977) Delusional disorder (paranoia). *Compr. Psychiatry*, **18**, 511–21.

Winokur, G. (1985) Stability of psychotic symptomatology over episodes in remitting psychoses. *Eur. Arch. Psychiatr. Neurol. Sci.*, **234**, 303–7.

Winokur, G., Scharfetter, C. and Angst, J. (1985) The diagnostic value in assessing mood congruence in delusions and hallucinations and their relationship to the affective state. *Eur. Arch. Psychiatr. Neurol. Sci.*, **234**, 299–302.

Wolff, S. and Chick, J. (1980) Schizoid personality in childhood. A controlled follow-up study. *Psychol. Med.*, **10**, 85–100.

World Health Organization (1973) *The International Pilot Study of Schizophrenia*. WHO, Geneva.

World Health Organization (1979) *Schizophrenia. An International Follow-up Study*. Wiley, New York.

World Health Organization (1990) *International Classification of Diseases*, tenth edition, WHO, Geneva.

World Health Organization (1992) SCAN; *Schedules for Clinical Assessment in Neuropsychiatry* WHO, Geneva.

Zubin, J., Sutton, S., Salzinger, K. *et al.* (1961) A biometric approach to prognosis in schizophrenia. In *Comparative Epidemiology of the Mental Disorders*. P.H. Hoch and J. Zubin (eds), Grune and Stratton, New York, pp. 143–203.

Chapter 2

The classification of schizophrenia

RICHARD P. BENTALL

2.1 INTRODUCTION

In his essay, 'John Wilkin's analytical language', the Argentinian writer Borges (1960) remarks on the classification which Franz Kuhn attributes to a certain Chinese encyclopaedia, *Celestial Emporium of Benevolent Knowledge*:

In those remote pages it is stated that animals can be divided into the following classes:

(a) Belonging to the Emperor
(b) Embalmed
(c) Trained
(d) Sucking pigs
(e) Mermaids
(f) Fabulous
(g) Stray dogs
(h) Included in this classification
(i) With the vigorous movements of madmen
(j) Innumerable
(k) Drawn with a very fine camel hair brush
(l) Etcetera
(m) Having just broken a large vase
(n) Looking from a distance like flies.
 (Borges, 1960; trans. M.E. Dewey)

In this way Borges reminds us of some of the errors that we may fall victim to when attempting to divide and classify natural phenomena.

The purpose of this chapter is to outline some of the arguments and empirical findings that have been invoked in the attempt to classify psychotic phenomena. I will attempt to address two issues: the question of whether or not the diagnostic concept of schizophrenia is scientifically meaningful; and the related question of whether or not schizophrenic disorders can be divided into valid subtypes. In the course of discussing these problems I hope to show that there is a much greater need for new organizing principles in the science of psychopathology than there is a need for new facts. Before proceeding to discuss these issues, however, it will be useful to place them within their proper historical and scientific context.

Kraepelin first outlined his concept of dementia praecox in 1896 (it was Bleuler in 1911 (1950), who later substituted the term 'schizophrenia' to denote Kraepelin's concept). When developing his classification of psychotic illnesses, Kraepelin relied on a combination of phenomenological and outcome data (Berrios and Hauser, 1988), arguing that dementia praecox could be distinguished from the manic-depressive psychoses by its poor outcome. Close examination of Kraepelin's work, however, reveals many inconsistencies in his use of clinical evidence relevant to his hypotheses (Boyle, 1990). Central to his method was his assumption that phenomenological, course and outcome data would converge to reveal aetiologically distinct diseases, an assumption that set the agenda for future research into psychosis:

> Judging from our experience in internal medicine it is a fair assumption that similar disease processes will produce identical symptom pictures, identical pathological anatomy and an identical aetiology. If, therefore, we possessed a comprehensive knowledge of any one of these three fields — pathological anatomy, symptomatology, or aetiology — we would at once have a uniform and standard classification of mental diseases. A similar comprehensive knowledge of either of the other two fields would give us not just as uniform and standard classifications, but all of these classifications would exactly coincide (Kraepelin, 1907, p. 117).

Nearly 100 years after Kraepelin first outlined his theory, approximately 0.5% to 1% of individuals in the industrial societies can expect to be diagnosed as schizophrenic at some point in their lives (Torrey, 1987). Considerable efforts have therefore been directed towards discovering the cause or causes of schizophrenic breakdowns. Aetiological hypotheses have pointed to genetic endowment (Gottesman and Shields, 1982), abnormalities of brain structure (Pincus and Tucker, 1978) and neurochemistry (Green and Costain, 1981), diet (Singh and Kay, 1976), viral agents (Crow, 1984), birth complications (Lewis *et al.*, 1989), the socioeconomic environment (Faris and Dunham, 1939); unpleasant life events (Brown and Birley, 1968) and family structure (Bateson, *et al.*, 1956). Indeed, virtually every variable known to influence human conduct has at one time been implicated as a potential cause of schizophrenia.

Partly because of the continuing absence of a known aetiology for the disorder some authors have questioned the value of the diagnosis. In the 1960s and 1970s in particular, a number of writers turned their attention to the concept of schizophrenia as a means of expressing a more general dissatisfaction with the medical approach towards explaining and treating severe psychiatric disorder. Some argued that the diagnosis of schizophrenia is used to justify the social control of deviant individuals (Scheff, 1966: Szasz, 1976) that schizophrenics are the victims of conspiracies between their families and the medical establishment (Laing and Esterson, 1970) or that they are particularly creative individuals capable of undergoing psychedelic experiences (Laing, 1967). Behaviourist psychologists (e.g. Ullmann and Krasner, 1975), perhaps naïvely, held that schizophrenic behaviour is governed by exactly the same lawful processes that govern normal conduct, and therefore advocated behaviour modification programmes as the treatment of choice for all psychotic patients.

It is doubtful whether these critiques have had any lasting effects on the way in which psychopathologists think about schizophrenic behaviour. By far the majority of research studies into psychosis continue to use the presence or absence of the diagnosis of schizophrenia as an independent variable (Sarbin and Mancuso, 1980). Precisely because the criticisms of the schizophrenia concept were perceived to be philosophical and ethical rather than empirical in nature, responses tended to focus on the meanings of the words 'illness' and 'disease' (Hamilton, 1973; Roth, 1973; Kendell, 1975). In the course of this debate the question of whether or not the concept of schizophrenia is scientifically useful was almost forgotten. Yet, if researchers are to continue to investigate psychotic phenomena with the hope of finding out something about the causes of insanity this question remains of paramount importance. The traditional psychopathology research paradigm, which involves comparing people with one diagnosis (for example, 'schizophrenia') with control subjects with another diagnosis (or no diagnosis at all) rests on the assumption that those with the target diagnosis have something in common which is absent in the case of the controls. If this assumption is invalid, the traditional research paradigm cannot hope to yield meaningful findings.

I have reviewed evidence relevant to this issue elsewhere (Bentall *et al.*, 1988; Bentall, 1990a) but it will be useful to repeat the main findings here. It should be noted that the term 'schizophrenic' is employed in the following discussions to denote anyone with a diagnosis of schizophrenia; similarly the term 'schizophrenia' will often be used to denote the broadest range of phenomena normally covered by the term and does not imply the existence of a unitary schizophrenia disease entity in the absence of justifying data.

2.2 THE SCIENTIFIC VALIDITY OF THE SCHIZOPHRENIA CONCEPT

To determine whether or not the concept of schizophrenia is scientifically meaningful it is necessary to decide if it meets acceptable criteria for **reliability** and **validity**. Reliability refers to the extent to which different observers can agree about the application of a concept; in schizophrenia this amounts to the question of whether or not different clinicians and researchers can agree about who is schizophrenic and who is not. Validity is a more complex requirement and cannot be satisfied by any one test (Robins and Guze, 1970; Kendell, 1989). In order to be valid a concept must be useful. For example, it is important to know whether the diagnosis of schizophrenia identifies a specific set of related phenomena and whether it predicts important observations about aetiology, response to treatment and outcome. From the account given above it should be apparent that Kraepelin believed that the diagnosis of schizophrenia met all of these criteria.

Various different sources of disagreement about the assignment of the diagnosis of schizophrenia have become apparent from research. For example, early studies not only showed that there was poor agreement between clinicians about who merited the diagnosis (Blashfield, 1984) but that there were also important differences between the diagnostic practices

of psychiatrists in different countries (Kendell *et al.*, 1971), with American psychiatrists diagnosing schizophrenia much more often than their British counterparts. In response to these observations, attempts were made to construct structured psychiatric interviews (such as the Present State Examination) whereby clinical data can be systematically collected, and operational criteria (such as those found in DSM–III) for reaching diagnoses. There is no doubt that operationalized definitions of schizophrenia enjoy higher inter-rater reliabilities than non-operationalized criteria, but problems still remain. For example, many different sets of operational criteria for schizophrenia have been proposed by different authors and the concordance between the different definitions is not impressive; in other words the different criteria tend to diagnose different people as schizophrenic (Brockington *et al.*, 1978). Moreover, when the stability of the operationalized diagnoses has been studied the results have also proved to be unimpressive. On re-examination with the same criteria after several years many patients are assigned to a different diagnosis than the one they originally received (Kendell *et al.*, 1979).

As reliability is a necessary but insufficient requirement for validity it is to be expected that the concept of schizophrenia will perform poorly on validity assessments. Attempts to use multivariate statistical techniques such as factor analysis (Slade and Cooper, 1979; Blashfield, 1984) and cluster analysis (Everitt *et al.*, 1971) have not yielded convincing evidence either of a naturally occurring group of correlated psychotic traits or of discrete groups of individuals who share a common set of schizophrenic symptoms. In a recent factor analysis of Present State Examination data, for example, evidence was found that suggested the existence of three independent dimensions of psychosis (Liddle, 1987; see Section 2.5). Moreover, when discriminant function analysis has been used to try to discriminate, on the basis of symptoms, between groups diagnosed as schizophrenic and those with other diagnoses (such as affective disorder) the results have not been encouraging (Kendell and Gourlay, 1970; Brockington and Wainwright, 1980; Kendell and Brockington, 1980). Taken together, these findings cast doubt on the existence of a unique schizophrenia syndrome.

Available research findings also call into question the predictive validity of the schizophrenia diagnosis. The short-term outcome for patients diagnosed as schizophrenic is highly variable and better predicted by sociopyschological factors than symptom variables (Hawke *et al.*, 1975; Sartorius *et al.*, 1987). This observation is mirrored by the results of long-term studies of 30 years or more which also show an extremely variable outcome for schizophrenic patients, with approximately one third completely recovering from their illnesses, one third showing an intermediate outcome, and only one third showing the deteriorating course held by Kraepelin to be one of the hallmarks of the disorder (Bleuler, 1978; Ciompi, 1980, 1984). Although there is a tendency for patients with predominantly schizophrenic symptoms to have a worse outcome than patients with predominantly affective symptoms, the overlap in outcome is sufficient to suggest that psychotic disorders exist along a continuum running from the affective disorders to schizophrenia (Kendell and Brockington, 1980).

It is also unclear whether the diagnosis of schizophrenia is a good predictor of response to treatment. Although neuroleptic drugs are usually considered to be the treatment of choice for the disorder perhaps half of all patients so diagnosed show little or no response to them (Warner, 1985), whereas some respond to lithium (Delva and Letemendia, 1982), normally used to treat the affective disorders, or even to benzodiazapines (Lingjaerde, 1982), usually employed to treat anxiety. There have in fact been few studies in which the effects of different medications have been studied with patients having a range of diagnoses. However,

in an early study by Overall *et al.* (1964) no evidence was found that phenothiazines or tricyclic antidepressants were diagnostically specific in their action. More recently, Johnstone *et al.* (cited in Kendell, 1989) gave pimozide, lithium or both to psychotic patients regardless of diagnosis. Although the pimozide was found to have a specific therapeutic effect on hallucinations, delusions, incoherence of speech and incongruity of affect, and although lithium proved to be effective against elevated mood, neither of these effects was specific to diagnosis and the results in general failed to support the hypothesis that schizophrenia and the affective psychoses are distinct entities.

Finally, although the search for a common aetiology of schizophrenia continues, the wide range of theories which have been proposed to account for the disorder are testament to the fact that this goal has yet to be achieved.

2.3 STUDYING THE HETEROGENEITY OF SCHIZOPHRENIA

In the face of evidence of this sort, and because of the continued lack of progress in aetiological research, many clinicians and researchers have embraced the idea (at least implicitly) that schizophrenia is a heterogeneous phenomenon.

In a thoughtful discussion of the problem of heterogeneity, Tsuang *et al.* (1990) argued that researchers should distinguish between different types of indicators of schizophrenia. In Tsuang *et al.*'s view, these indicators may be at three levels: aetiology (e.g. environmental effects, birth complications, genetic factors), pathophysiology (e.g. drug response; neuroanatomical findings), and symptoms. It is notable that Reider (1974) criticized Kraepelin precisely because he assumed that these levels must be directly related, so that classifications based on one level of indicators were assumed to map directly onto classifications based on indicators at other levels. Tsuang *et al.*, in contrast to Kraepelin, have argued that heterogeneity may occur relatively independently

Symptom

		Hallucinations	Delusions	Thought disorder	Depression
Perception	Perceptual acuity	Slow loss of acuity related to vulnerability	Deafness related to vulnerability	Not implicated	Not implicated
	Perceptual judgement	Rapid search for meaning	Rapid search for meaning	Not implicated	Not implicated
Cognition	Detection of covariation	Not implicated	Overdetection of covariation	Not implicated	Realistic under-detection of covariation
	Attributions	Not implicated	External, global and stable for negative events	Not implicated	Internal, global and stable for negative events
Metacognition	Confidence in judgements	Over-confident	Over-confident	Not known to be implicated	Under-confident
	Reality discrimination	Impaired	Not implicated	Impaired	Not implicated

Figure 2.1 Tsuang *et al.*'s conceptual models for the heterogeneity of schizophrenia. From Tsuang *et al.* (1990), reproduced with permission of the authors.

at any one level, and have therefore gone a long way towards completely abandoning a Kraepelinian disease model of schizophrenic breakdowns. Indeed, they note that the relationships between the indicators at the different levels may be highly complex (Figure 2.1).

At the first level most attention has been devoted to the implications of genetic findings for the identification of subtypes. The recent report of a genetic linkage between schizophrenia and a locus on chromosome–5 (Sherrington *et al.*, 1988) and subsequent failures to replicate this finding (e.g. Kennedy *et al.*, 1988; St Clair *et al.*, 1989) have been interpreted by some authors as evidence of the genetic heterogeneity of schizophrenic phenomena (Lander, 1988). Data from family studies have been consulted by some authors in an attempt to identify sub-types of schizophrenia. Kendler and Davis (1981), in a review of studies addressing this question found some evidence that Kraepelinian sub-types (see Section 2.4.2) breed true, although the data obtained from later and methodologically tighter studies were found to be rather less compelling than the data collected by earlier and scientifically less sophisticated investigators. Kendler *et al.* (1988) failed to find evidence in favour of Kraepelin's sub-types in a subsequent family study. Using family data in a different way, Kendler and Hays (1982) divided a group of schizophrenics into those with a first-degree relative suffering from schizophrenia ('familial schizophrenics') and those without ('non-familial schizophrenics') and found that the familial group were more often thought disordered.

Clearly, genetic studies could provide useful clues about different aetiological pathways to psychotic breakdown but caution is necessary when interpreting the results of particular studies. McGuffin *et al.* (1987) have pointed out that apparent heterogeneity at the level of symptoms might result if sub-types represent different thresholds of expression of a single underlying polygenically determined

continuum of psychosis. On the basis of their own review of the relevant genetic evidence, McGuffin *et al.* (1987) rather pessimistically concluded:

> Rather than providing a means of 'carving nature at the joints', the systems of classifying sub-types which are so far available appear to offer different ways of slicing up the salami. Undoubtedly the salami has more genetic content at one end than the other, but as yet there is no convincing evidence that we are dealing with two or more completely different varieties of sausage (p. 589).

Other variables could be studied in attempts to identify sub-types at the level of aetiology. For example, it is clear from the discordance rates observed in twin studies that there must be a substantial environmental contribution to schizophrenic breakdowns, yet environmental contributions to psychosis have received comparatively little attention from schizophrenia researchers, although recent findings do suggest that overly hostile or controlling family environments may have a role in determining psychotic breakdown in vulnerable individuals (Goldstein, 1988). Whether there can be said to be a subtype of reactive psychosis remains a matter of conjecture.

At the level of pathophysiology the possibilities for research into sub-types are also considerable, although researchers need to be sophisticated when thinking about the relationship between pathophysiology and symptoms (for example, there are no *a priori* reasons for assuming that causal abnormalities of neurophysiology must lie at the root of **all** forms of abnormal behaviour). If neuroleptic medication acts to correct abnormal brain states the observed variable response to medication, rather than being a source of despair, might yield important information. Brown and Herz (1989) have reviewed some of the methodological requirements for identifying sub-types in this way and have argued that there must first be a reliable and valid way of identifying neuroleptic nonresponders, there must be evidence that individuals are consistent in their response to treatment, and it must be possible to relate drug response to other meaningful variables. Brown and Herz tentatively concluded that these requirements could in principle be met in studies of neuroleptic response but that data on responders and nonresponders is currently too limited to allow firm conclusions to be drawn. Thus, although it has been claimed that only certain ('positive') symptoms respond to neuroleptics, relevant empirical findings are by no means unambiguous (Section 2.4.2). However, there is at least fragmentary evidence that nonresponders are more likely to show evidence of neurological impairment than responders (Marder *et al.*, 1984; Schulz *et al.*, 1989).

Again, other indicators of pathophysiology could be studied in the attempt to identify meaningful sub-types. Biochemical variables other than drug response are obvious candidates: for some time it was thought that there might be an association between blood platelet monoamine oxidase levels and delusional symptoms (Potkin *et al.*, 1978) although subsequent research did not substantiate this apparent indicator of a paranoid sub-type (Kendler and Davis, 1981). The wide ranging and often inconsistent neurological findings reported for schizophrenics (Seidman, 1984) could also be studied for evidence of sub-types. In this vein, Reveley and Murray (1984) and Reveley and Chitkara (1985) reported that, in twins discordant for schizophrenia, the affected twin typically showed enlargement of the cerebral ventricles, as revealed by CT scan, suggesting that ventricular enlargement might be indicative of an environmentally determined sub-type. Unfortunately, these findings have not been replicated in subsequent studies (e.g. Owen *et al.*, 1989). Weiss (1989) has recently raised the possibility of studying psychological processes such as attention and arousal in the attempt to develop more meaningful

classifications of psychotic phenomena, and there is at least some evidence that particular results on certain psychological tests reflect the type of symptomatology experienced by psychotic patients (Section 2.4).

At the level of symptomatology, multivariate statistical tools (identical to those which have been applied in the attempt to identify a schizophrenia syndrome) are clearly applicable. Attempts to identify sub-types by using cluster analysis have been made by a number of authors (e.g. Carpenter *et al.*, 1976; Farmer *et al.*, 1983), although the results of these endeavours have been compromised by the inconsistency of the findings, by the tendency for the majority of subjects to fall in one large cluster and by the limitations of existing cluster analytic techniques.

2.4 SPECIFIC SUB-TYPE PROPOSALS

At this point it might be useful to consider some specific proposals for sub-typologies of schizophrenia. Two main proposals will be considered: Kraepelin and Bleuler's division of schizophrenic disorders into simple, catatonic, hebephrenic and paranoid sub-types; and more recent attempts to distinguish between two types of schizophrenic disorder characterized by positive and negative symptoms.

2.4.1 KRAEPELINIAN SUB-TYPES

Kraepelin (1907) recognized three main sub-types of schizophrenia: catatonic, hebephrenic and paranoid. **Catatonic** schizophrenia was characterized by pronounced motor symptoms and swings from stupor to extreme excitement; **hebephrenic** schizophrenia by over-scrupulousness about trivial matters, emotional indifference, laughing and immature speech; and **paranoid** schizophrenia by suspiciousness and well-organized delusions, usually of persecutory or grandiose content. Bleuler, who regarded abnormalities of psychological processes as fundamental to schizophrenia, added a fourth sub-type of **simple** schizophrenia, characterized by mixed psychotic symptoms which did not fit into any of the sub-types outlined by Kraepelin. Despite persisting doubts about the value of these sub-types, they continue to be used widely, and modern equivalents have found a place in DSM–III.

As already indicated, the data from a range of genetic studies have been examined to see whether the Kraepelinian sub-types breed true in families, but the evidence from the better studies is not impressive (Kendler and Davis, 1981; Kendler et al., 1988). Nonetheless, some twin studies have yielded evidence of a modest concordance between the sub-type diagnoses of affected twins (Fisher, 1973).

The reliability of neo-Kraepelinian sub-types was studied by Gruenberg et al. (1985), who examined data collected from 500 admissions, 187 of whom were classified as schizophrenic. Four different criteria for assigning these subjects were applied: DSM–III (paranoid, hebephrenic, catatonic and undifferentiated); RDC (paranoid, hebephrenic, catatonic, and undifferentiated); ICD–9 (paranoid, hebephrenic, catatonic and other); and criteria proposed by Tsuang and Winokur (paranoid, hebephrenic and undifferentiated). Inter-rater reliabilities, assessed on a sub-sample, were acceptable for all four systems, but the systems differed widely in the frequency with which they assigned subjects to sub-types. For example, 69 subjects were diagnosed as paranoid by ICD–9 but only 22 by the Tsuang and Winokur criteria. The Tsuang and Winokur criteria, on the other hand, diagnosed nearly two thirds of the patients as undifferentiated. The concordances between the four systems were generally quite low, echoing the observations reported by Brockington et al. (1978) for different sets of criteria for schizophrenia. It is notable that a high level of concordance was found only between the DSM–III and RDC systems, which is unsurprising given that DSM–III was developed on the basis of the RDC criteria.

Because the admission data on their subjects had been collected many years previously, Kendler et al. (1985) were also able to examine the stability of the different sub-types. Case note data were used to reclassify the patients at follow-up using the same four systems. Concordances were not good when all the subjects were taken into account but became modestly acceptable when only those patients who had not improved and could be assigned a sub-type at both admission and follow-up were included. The best results were obtained for the diagnosis of paranoid sub-type. Kendler et al. (1985) concluded that the stability of the sub-types was only modest overall, and that the shift over time of individuals between sub-types might account for inconsistencies in the data obtained from family and twin studies.

Evidence which might shed further light on the value of Kraepelinian sub-types is available from the International Pilot Study of Schizophrenia (WHO, 1973). Using the Present State Examination to yield ICD–9 diagnoses on 1202 patients from nine countries, it was found that the symptom profiles of the different sub-types did not vary across countries. However, this was because there was very little difference between the symptom profiles of the different sub-types. Carpenter et al. (1976) subsequently reanalysed the IPSS data, reducing the 350 PSE items to 27 dimensions of psychopathology in the hope that this would allow a more meaningful estimate of any differences between sub-types; profile analyses of variance still failed to reveal significant differences, confirming that the individuals assigned to the different sub-types suffered from a comparable range of symptoms. Their subsequent cluster analysis of the data (briefly mentioned in Section 2.3) generated sub-types quite different from those proposed by Kraepelin.

Taking the available findings together, there seems to be no solid evidence that the Kraepelinian sub-types represent distinct entities at either of the three levels of indicators described by Tsuang et al. (1990).

2.4.2 POSITIVE AND NEGATIVE SYMPTOMS

In recent years, a number of investigators have distinguished positive and negative schizophrenia symptoms in the hope that this might help to define scientifically meaningful sub-types of psychotic disorder. Positive symptoms are those notable by their presence (e.g. delusions, hallucinations and disordered speech) whereas negative symptoms are those which are evident by a lack of appropriate behaviour (e.g. social withdrawal, anhedonia, poverty of speech). Crow (1980) proposed that schizophrenic psychoses could be subdivided into two syndromes: Type I schizophrenia consisting mainly of positive symptoms and Type II schizophrenia consisting mainly of negative symptoms. Crow argued that these two syndromes often overlap but maintained that they are nonetheless aetiologically distinct: Type I schizophrenia being caused by dopamine abnormalities in the brain and Type II schizophrenia reflecting ventricular enlargement (perhaps due to birth complications, early brain injury or viral infection).

In contrast to the Kraepelinian sub-types, it is clear that the presence or absence of both positive and negative symptoms can be assessed with a reasonable degree of reliability (Andreasen and Olsen, 1982). However, the results of more complex multivariate analyses do not provide clear support for Crow's typology. Thus, when Liddle (1987) factor analysed symptom data collected using the Present State Examination, he obtained not two factors but three, the first and last reflecting positive and negative symptoms respectively but the second reflecting cognitive and verbal disorganization.

There have been comparatively few attempts to investigate the role of genetic factors in Crow's hypothesized sub-types. Dworkin and Lenzenweger (1984) attempted to classify twins from previous twin studies as either high or low in negative symptoms and found that, in the majority of studies, concordance rates were higher for the high negative symptom twins. In a more recent study, McGuffin *et al.* (1987) used operational criteria derived from Crow's work to reclassify patients and family members previously examined by Gottesman. They found a modest tendency for the two types to breed true but this was not sufficient to allow McGuffin and his colleagues to interpret their findings as supporting Crow's model.

A number of investigators have attempted to study demographic and psychological correlates of positive and negative symptoms but the results have not always been consistent. Some studies revealed evidence that cognitive deficits, a history of low educational attainment and a later age of hospitalization are associated with negative symptoms (Andreasen and Olsen, 1982; Opler *et al.*, 1984) but these findings have not been replicated by others (Pogue-Geile and Harrow, 1984). Although attentional impairment is classified among the negative symptoms on some rating scales, psychological studies have found experimental measures of attentional impairment to correlate both with positive thought disorder and total positive symptom score (Bilder *et al.*, 1985; Cornblatt *et al.*, 1985). Early visual information processing deficits, on the other hand, have been observed to correlate with the severity of negative symptoms (Green and Walker, 1986).

As Crow hypothesized that only Type I schizophrenia is caused by abnormalities of the dopamine pathways in the brain his model carries the implication that neuroleptic drugs should be effective only on positive symptoms. Some investigators have therefore studied drug response in attempts to validate Crow's typology. Contrary to Crow's model, Goldberg (1985) found that data from a number of studies indicated that negative symptoms are responsive to neuroleptic drugs. On the basis of Crow's typology it might also be expected that Type I patients would have their symptoms exacerbated by amphetamine (which stimulates dopamine turnover); contrary to the theory

Kornetsky (1976) found predominantly positive symptom patients to be hyporesponsive to the effects of amphetamine.

Overall, it would seem that the distinction between positive and negative symptoms has been a useful one in that it has allowed investigators to explore relationships between dependent variables and symptomatology. However, as yet there is no clear evidence that positive and negative symptoms are indicative of scientifically meaningful sub-types of schizophrenic disorder. Moreover, some of the predictions made by Crow on the basis of his model — for example, that the negative symptoms would be neuroleptic resistant and that the positive symptoms would be vulnerable to exacerbation by amphetamine — have not survived testing.

Just because there is little or no evidence favouring the sub-typologies of Kraepelin and Crow it should not be assumed that no meaningful sub-types of schizophrenia will ever be found. Some research strategies — for example, the division of patients into neuroleptic responders and nonresponders — have been far from exhausted. On the other hand, investigators should accept that there are no *a priori* reasons for assuming that meaningful sub-types await identification, other than the inconsistent findings of aetiological research into schizophrenia in general. Although it is impossible not to recognize the need for new organizing principles in schizophrenia research, it is possible that the most useful frameworks for future research will not be categorical in nature.

2.5 DIMENSIONAL CLASSIFICATIONS

Given the failure to identify meaningful sub-types of schizophrenic disorder so far, some authors have argued that dimensional models might better describe psychotic phenomena. Taking this view, people might be expected to be more or less schizophrenic along a continuum or a series of continua. Various arguments in favour of dimensional models have been proposed and can only be summarized here. First, many authors have suggested that the observed results of genetic studies can best be accounted for by assuming that what it is inherited is a polygenically determined vulnerability to schizophrenia which a person may have to greater or lesser degree (Meehl, 1962; Claridge, 1987, 1990). Second, a major series of genetic investigations (the Danish-American adoption studies, Rosenthal *et al.*, 1971; Kety *et al.*, 1975) failed to find evidence that schizophrenia is inherited when only breakdowns leading to hospitalization were considered, leading the investigators to broaden their diagnostic criteria to include various quasi-schizophrenic states which they labelled 'schizophrenia spectrum disorders.' Largely as a result of their efforts 'schizotypal personality disorder' was included as a new classification in DSM–III (APA, 1980). Third, a number of investigators found that a considerable minority of apparently well-adjusted people would report schizophrenia-like experiences and behaviour if required to complete relevant questionnaires (e.g. Chapman *et al.*, 1976; Launay and Slade, 1981; Claridge and Broks, 1984). There is now substantial evidence that these people perform similarly to some schizophrenics on a wide range of experimental measures (Claridge, 1987, 1990). Finally, a number of authors have argued on theoretical and psychometric grounds that psychotic traits are best regarded as one of a small number of fundamental dimensions which account for individual differences in temperament and personality (Eysenck and Eysenck, 1968). In an attempt to integrate these kinds of observations, Claridge (1987) drew a parallel between systemic diseases (such as hypertension) and schizophrenic traits, arguing that such traits might be distributed normally in the population, only becoming manifest as illness in those individuals who are endowed with them in greater measure and who are subjected the right kinds of environmental stresses.

Taken together, the evidence that subclinical variants of schizophrenic behaviour can be observed in otherwise 'normal' people cannot be ignored. However, some attempts to describe these variants are probably seriously misleading. For example, DSM–III includes descriptions of not only schizotypal personality but also other personality disorders, placing them on a separate axis to the major mental illnesses. This amounts to something of a compromise between the categorical and the dimensional approach which does little to clarify the true nature of the subclinical states. Not surprisingly, there is evidence of a considerable degree of overlap between the different personality disorders described in DSM–III, particularly between schizotypal personality disorder, borderline personality disorder and antisocial (psychopathic) personality disorder (Spitzer *et al.*, 1979; Hare and Forth, 1985) with many individuals scoring as 'cases' on more than one disorder. These observations strongly suggest that the criteria given for the personality disorders in DSM–III do not accurately reflect the structure of the psychopathology which they were designed to describe.

Dimensional models of schizophrenia therefore lead to similar questions to those which are raised by the categorical models: how many dimensions are required and how might they best be described? Although many authors, following the works of Eysenck and Eysenck (1968), seem to assume that one psychosis dimension is sufficient to account for the available data, there is at least some evidence that one dimension will not suffice. For example, Liddle's (1987) factor analysis of PSE data can be interpreted as consistent with a model requiring three dimensions: positive symptomatology; cognitive disorganization; and negative symptomatology. Questionnaire studies carried out on normal individuals similarly suggest that a multidimensional model of schizotypal traits (and by implication schizophrenia) is required to account for the distribution of schizophrenic phenomena (Chapman

et al., 1982; Muntaner *et al.*,1988; Bentall *et al.*, 1989; Venables *et al.*, 1990). Interestingly, a consistent finding of these studies has been that positive and negative schizotypal features load on different dimensions, lending weight to the hypothesis that positive and negative symptoms of psychosis reflect different dimensions of psychopathology. Unfortunately, much of the research on dimensional aspects of psychosis has been carried out either on patients defined as personality disordered, or on non-patients (often university students). In order for dimensional models of psychosis to be properly evaluated it will be necessary to use research strategies which allow the comparison of data collected from patients suffering from fully developed psychotic illnesses with data collected from both personality disordered and normal subjects.

2.6 SHOULD WE ABANDON THE ATTEMPT TO CLASSIFY PSYCHOSES?

The attempt to identify sub-types or dimensions of schizophrenic behaviour, like Kraepelin's attempt to identify specific disease entities, has been driven by the perceived need to identify homogeneous groups of psychotic people about whom clinicians can make succinct communications, who share a common aetiology, and for whom common predictions about outcome and response to treatment can be made. The evidence I have outlined suggests that this goal has yet to be achieved. Although dimensional models may hold more promise for the future than categorical models, a considerable amount of research will be required before it is possible to specify a dimensional structure for psychotic phenomena. Of course, it is possible that a typology of schizophrenic disorders will be achieved at some future point in time, following the collection of yet further data — it should be apparent from the above discussion that the evaluation of typological proposals is a complex matter and many avenues for research remain relatively unexplored. Nonetheless, it is equally possible that nature provides no easy joints along which psychotic phenomena can be unambiguously dismembered, that there are no naturally occurring sub-types of psychosis and that further attempts to classify and sub-classify psychotic behaviour will therefore fail. This prospect is one which clinicians and researchers are usually reluctant to accept (perhaps because the alternative to using diagnoses is usually believed to be some form of theoretical anarchy) but after nearly 100 years of schizophrenia research it is a prospect which should at least be considered carefully. In the remaining pages of this chapter I will attempt to outline a strategy for carrying out research into psychosis which is scientific, which does not rely on psychiatric diagnoses or the determination of sub-types, but which nonetheless allows the psychopathologist to proceed in an an orderly fashion without falling into the Laingian abyss.

There is a perfectly logical alternative to using diagnostic classifications as independent variables in research into psychopathology: researchers could abandon the attempt to classify psychotic illness (at least for the time being) and make the actual phenomena they encounter in the clinic, that is to say particular types of complaints or behaviours (usually described as 'symptoms') the focus of their efforts. For example, investigators might study hallucinations, delusions, disordered discourse, flat affect, or any other symptom. This kind of research has at least two advantages. First, psychotic behaviours and experiences are interesting in their own right and, whatever the merits of any particular system of classification, no model of psychosis can be complete without an account of them (Persons, 1986). Second, research into symptoms is not inconsistent with the hope that an adequate system of classification will one day be devised (indeed it may yield data that will be helpful in that regard) but it is not dependent on classification (Bannister, 1968; Bentall *et al.*, 1988).

For symptom-orientated research to proceed certain methodological difficulties must be overcome. For example, it must be possible to determine which patients have which symptoms. Although this is sometimes difficult the problem is not insurmountable and structured psychiatric interviews such as the PSE can be used to obtain the necessary information. Elsewhere I have outlined the symptom-orientated reseach strategy in detail and have tried to show that research into particular symptoms can rapidly lead to meaningful results (Bentall, 1990a). For reasons of space, only the barest account of the relevant findings can be given here. I will therefore focus the following discussion on three symptoms: hallucinations, delusions and disordered discourse.

2.6.1 HALLUCINATIONS

A considerable amount is known about the determinants of hallucinatory experiences (Asaad and Shapiro, 1986; Slade and Bentall, 1988). Hallucinations are especially likely to be experienced under conditions of stress (Slade, 1972; Cooklin *et al.*, 1983) or unpatterned environmental stimulation (Margo *et al.*, 1981). There is also evidence that psychotic hallucinations can be influenced by suggestions (Mintz and Alpert, 1972; Alpert, 1985; Young *et al.*, 1987). EEG data indicate that auditory hallucinations are of left-hemisphere origin (Stevens and Livermore, 1982), a finding which is consistent with the observation that they are accompanied by subvocalization, i.e. micromovements of the speech muscles (McGuigan, 1966; Inouye and Shimizu, 1970).

Although a number of theories have been proposed to account for hallucinations several authors have recently suggested that hallucinations are thoughts misattributed to an external source (Heilbrun, 1980; Hoffman, 1986; Bentall, 1990b). This hypothesis is consistent with the subvocalization data as micromovements of the speech muscles accompany ordinary verbal thinking (McGuigan, 1978).

Direct evidence in favour of this hypothesis was reported by Heilbrun (1980), who observed that hallucinators in comparison with controls were poor at recognizing their own thoughts. However, this result was only partially replicated by Bentall *et al.* (1991) who, using a methodologically tighter reality monitoring paradigm, found that hallucinators were more likely than non-hallucinating paranoid controls to confuse effortfully generated thoughts with external stimuli. Clearer evidence in favour of the hypothesis was found by Bentall and Slade (1985) using a signal detection task, who found that hallucinators have normal perceptual sensitivity (an observation also made by Collicut and Hemsley, 1981) but, under conditions of uncertainty, have a greater bias towards believing that an external stimulus is present. This latter finding is consistent with the observation that hallucinations are more likely to occur under noisy conditions when there is a poor signal to noise ratio. The hypothesis that hallucinations result from a difficulty in distinguishing between thoughts and events in the world also helps to explain why hallucinations can be influenced by suggestions, as it seems likely that judgements of reality are made partly on the basis of contextual information and the individual's expectations about what kinds of events are likely to be experienced. A consistent picture of the cognitive processes involved in hallucinations is therefore emerging. However, further research is necessary to determine the biological and environmental causes of the hallucinator's inability to discriminate internal and external events.

2.6.2 DELUSIONS

There has been very little research into delusional beliefs (Winters and Neale, 1983). This is surprising given that cognitive and social psychologists have extensively studied the acquisition of normal beliefs and attitudes. For simplicity, the process of belief acquisition can be thought of as occurring in stages: first, data has to be perceived; second, on the basis of the perceived data the individual may make an inference or a series of inferences using heuristic (non-logical rule-of-thumb) strategies much studied by social psychologists — this will lead to the generation of a belief; finally, the individual may or may not seek out further information (research suggests that normal individuals rarely proceed scientifically in this regard).

In an influential paper, Maher (1973) proposed that all delusions are products of anomalous experiences (such as hallucinations) and that there is nothing abnormal about the reasoning of deluded people. The only evidence presented by Maher in favour of this hypothesis is the observation that schizophrenic patients (defined by broad diagnostic criteria and therefore not necessarily deluded) perform normally on syllogistic reasoning tasks (Williams, 1964). The significance of this observation is reduced when it is noted that cognitive psychologists have generally rejected syllogistic reasoning as a good model or measure of reasoning processes (Johnson-Laird, 1989). Some case study evidence (Johnson *et al.*, 1977; Maher and Ross, 1984) does seem to be consistent with the idea that delusions are sometimes rational attempts to account for unpleasant or disturbing perceptions. However, given that many hallucinators do not develop complex delusional systems it seems most unlikely that perceptual abnormalities alone are sufficient for the acquisition of abnormal beliefs (Chapman and Chapman, 1988).

Clearly, research on the reasoning of deluded subjects should focus on domains of reasoning likely to be implicated in the genesis or maintenance of abnormal beliefs. Hemsley and Garety (1986) have argued that the probabilistic reasoning of deluded patients is particularly worthy of investigation because an inability to adequately weigh evidence is likely to make an individual vulnerable to developing irrational beliefs in the face of contrary evidence. Consistent with this hypothesis, Brennan and Hemsley (1986) found that paranoid as opposed to non-paranoid schizophrenics were more likely to judge randomly covarying events to be causally related. Subsequently, Huq *et al.* (1988) studied the performance of deluded patients on a probabilistic reasoning task and observed that the deluded subjects searched for less evidence than controls before making a decision; they were also abnormally confident about their performance on the task.

Focusing more on social reasoning, Kaney and Bentall (1988) demonstrated that patients with persecutory delusions have an abnormal attributional style (the subjects studied had the opposite bias to depressives, systematically attributing unpleasant outcomes to causes external to themselves and pleasant outcomes to their own abilities). This result was substantially replicated by Candido and Romney (1990) and is consistent with the hypothesis that persecutory delusions are a defence against depression and poor self-esteem (Zigler and Glick, 1988).

In a further test of this hypothesis, Kaney and Bentall (in press) exposed persecuted patients and depressed and normal controls to computer games which were rigged to give either a 'win' or a 'lose' outcome; as predicted the deluded subjects claimed very little control over the outcome of the game in the lose condition but a great deal of control in the win condition. Bentall *et al.* (1991) were able to show that deluded patients make abnormal inferences when explaining the behaviour of other people, particularly when the behaviour is threatening. One possible explanation for these biases is that deluded subjects preferentially process threat-related information. Consistent with this hypothesis, the results of two further studies showed that deluded individuals selectively attend to threat-related stimuli (Bentall and Kaney, 1989) and preferentially recall threat-related propositions (Kaney *et al.*, 1992).

It is not difficult to see how an inability to weigh evidence adequately, a reluctance to attribute failure to the self, or an abnormal understanding of the intentions of others might make a person vulnerable to persecutory delusions. However, the relationship between these abnormalities remains unclear. Further research is required to establish whether these abnormalities are manifestations of a common abnormal process or alternatively (as seems more likely) reflect cognitive biases which additively contribute to the formation and maintenance of delusions. Once the cognitive contribution to delusions is understood more adequately further research will be also be required to determine the biological and environmental determinants of the deluded person's abnormal cognitive organization.

2.6.3 THOUGHT DISORDER OR DISORDERED DISCOURSE

In thought disorder (or, to use a more accurate term, disordered discourse) there has been an abundance of research, most of which has been compromised by the use of broad diagnostic criteria in the selection of subjects with the consequent failure to determine whether the subjects tested were actually exhibiting the relevant symptomatology (Harvey and Neale, 1983).

Considerable efforts have been directed towards determining the key features of the disordered discourse of psychotic patients. Rochester and Martin (1979), in an influential attempt to analyse the speech of thought-disordered patients diagnosed as schizophrenic, showed that their subjects exhibited many referential failures, so that there were few links between clauses and few clear references to previously presented ideas. In a well controlled study, Harvey (1983) was able to replicate this finding with patients diagnosed as schizophrenic and also with thought-disordered patients diagnosed as manic.

Although the causes of the thought disordered person's reference failures remain unclear, Harrow and Prosen (1978) were able to show that many thought-disordered segments of speech included intermingled associations from the past, indicating that thought-disordered patients suffer from an impairment of perspective which prevents them from taking into account the needs of the listener and deciding whether or not their speech is appropriate to the circumstances.

Hoffman *et al.* (1982) suggested that the thought-disordered patient suffers from a disorder of discourse planning, where discourse planning is a hypothetical pre-verbal stage in which speech is planned before being uttered. However, Hoffman *et al.*'s method of determining the structure of a speaker's discourse plans has been criticized for being unreliable and subjective (Beveridge and Brown, 1985). Harvey (1985) hypothesized that reference failures in disordered speech might result from a patient's failure to discriminate between thoughts and statements that he or she has already made. The results of a study designed to test the ability of thought-disordered patients to discriminate between their thoughts and their own speech was consistent with this hypothesis. Interestingly, in an attempt to study the possible contribution of heredity to thought-disorder evidence was found suggesting that some aspects of disordered speech are familial but non-genetic (Berenbaum *et al.*, 1985).

2.7 THE SYMPTOM-ORIENTATED APPROACH VS. CLASSIFICATION

These all too brief accounts must suffice to demonstrate the possibility of achieving progress in psychopathology by studying particular types of psychotic behaviour independently of diagnosis. Whether research into specific symptoms will ever converge with attempts to classify psychotic phenomena is moot; I have argued elsewhere that symptoms might be taken at face value and mapped directly onto a taxonomy of cognitive processes without recourse to conventional classificatory schemes. The result of such an exercise would be an organizing principle analogous to the Periodic Table in chemistry. Just as the Periodic Table explains the properties of elements according to their underlying structure, so a 'cognitive table' of psychotic phenomena would explain those phenomena in terms of combinations of abnormal cognitive processes (Bentall, 1990a; Figure 2.2). These abnormalities of cognition might, in turn, be the products of a range of biological and environmental factors which would be the targets of further scientific inquiry.

This position is not very different from that taken by Tsuang *et al.* (1990) as discussed earlier in this chapter. Indeed, once that it is recognized that the relationships between different indicators of psychopathology (at the levels of aetiology, pathophysiology, cognition and symptomatology) may be very complex, the model of psychosis that inevitably results shows very little resemblance to the simple classificatory models outlined in standard textbooks of psychiatry. Abandoning Kraepelin's expectation that classifications based on aetiology, pathological anatomy and symptomatology must exactly coincide therefore amounts to abandoning his concept of schizophrenia, at least implicitly. It is perhaps not surprising that both psychological and biological considerations should independently lead to this conclusion. The concept of schizophrenia, though useful in its time, is now so old and tired that it is surely wrong to expect it to bear upon its back the burden of modern scientific research findings.

2.8 CONCLUSION

Arguably, there is no shortage of facts in schizophrenia research. Biological, psychological and sociological investigations have generated a virtual deluge of information, much of which is contradictory or inconsistent, but all of which says something about the people we continue to lump together under the label 'schizophrenia'. What has been lacking since

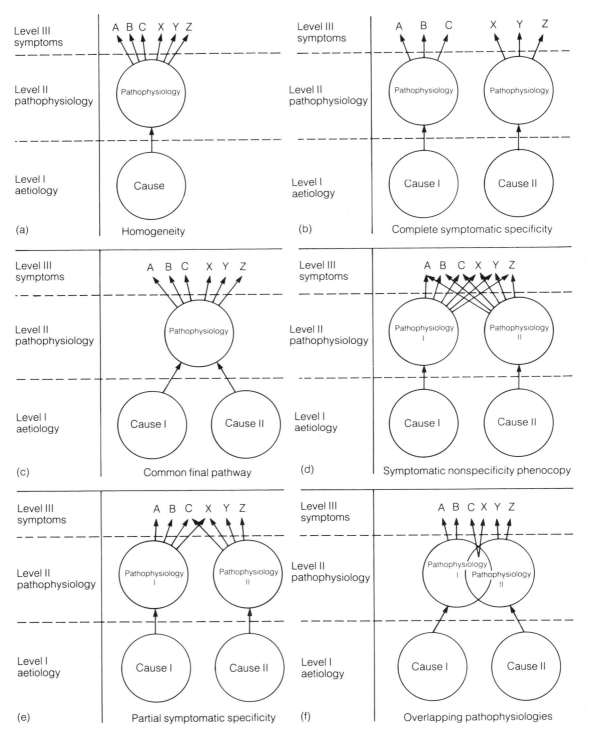

Figure 2.2 A schematic 'cognitive table' relating some symptoms of mental disorder to specific abnormalities of different cognitive processes, after Bentall (1990a). A particular cognitive abnormality may not be either necessary or sufficient to make a person vulnerable to a particular symptom. Also, some cognitive abnormalities may cause vulnerability to more than one symptom. The table is not meant to be definitive or complete, and evidence for each of the suggested relationships between abnormal cognition and symptomatology is outlined in the source paper, which should be consulted for details. A clearer understanding of the structure of human cognitive processes would be needed to allow a more exact construction of the table.

Kraepelin's time is a way of organizing this information. It therefore seems unlikely that progress in schizophrenia research will result from a sudden discovery or scientific breakthrough, from the application of new techniques (bigger and better scanners) or from the mindless repetition of well-tried strategies in the hope that further methodological refinements will add clarity to data already obtained. Rather, what is required is new ways of thinking about schizophrenic phenomena. The problem of classifying these phenomena lies at the heart of this difficulty. Until this problem is adequately resolved we may expect slow progress in the understanding of psychosis.

REFERENCES

Alpert, M. (1985) The signs and symptoms of schizophrenia. *Compr. Psychiatry*, **26**, 103–12.

American Psychiatric Association (1980) *Diagnostic and Statistical Manual for Mental Disorders*. APA Washington, DC.

Andreasen, N.C. and Olsen, S. (1982) Negative vs positive symptoms of schizophrenia: Definition and validation. *Arch. Gen. Psychiatry*, **39**, 780–94.

Asaad, G. and Shapiro, M.D. (1986) Hallucinations: Theoretical and clinical overview. *Am. J. Psychiatry*, **143**, 1088–97.

Bannister, D. (1968) The logical requirements of research into schizophrenia. *Br. J. Psychiatry*, **114**, 181–8.

Bateson, G., Jackson, D.D., Haley, J. and Weakland, J. (1956) Towards a theory of schizophrenia. *Behav. Sci.*, **1**, 251–64.

Bentall, R.P. (1990a) The syndromes and symptoms of psychosis: Or why you can't play twenty questions with the concept of schizophrenia and hope to win. In *Reconstructing Schizophrenia*, R.P. Bentall (ed), Routledge, London, pp. 23–60.

Bentall, R.P. (1990b) The illusion of reality: A review and integration of psychological research on hallucinations. *Psychol. Bull.*, **107**, 82–95.

Bentall, R.P., Baker, G.A. and Havers, S. (1991) Reality monitoring and psychotic hallucinations. *Br. J. Clin. Psychol.*, **30**, 213–22.

Bentall, R.P. Claridge, G.S. and Slade, P.D. (1989) The multidimensional nature of schizotypal traits: A factor analytic study with normal subjects. *Br. J. Clin. Psychol.*, **28**, 363–75.

Bentall, R.P., Jackson, H.F. and Pilgrim, D. (1988) Abandoning the concept of 'schizophrenia': Some implications of validity arguments for psychological research into psychotic phenomena. *Br. J. Clin. Psychol.*, **27**, 303–24.

Bentall, R.P. and Kaney, S. (1989) Content specific information processing and persecutory delusions: An investigation using the emotional Stroop test. *Br. J. Med. Psychol.*, **62**, 355–64.

Bentall, R.P., Kaney, S. and Dewey, M. (1991) Paranoia and social reasoning: An attribution theory analysis. *Br. J. Clin. Psychol.*, **30**, 13–23.

Bentall, R.P. and Slade, P.D. (1985) Reality testing and auditory hallucinations: A signal detection analysis. *Br. J. Clin. Psychol.*, **24**, 159–69.

Berenbaum, H., Oltmanns, T.F., and Gottesman, I. (1985) Formal thought disorder in schizophrenics and their twins. *J. Abnorm. Psychol.*, **94**, 3–16.

Berrios, G.E. and Hauser, R. (1988) The early development of Kraepelin's ideas on classification: A conceptual history. *Psychol. Med.*, **18**, 813–21.

Beveridge, A.W. and Brown, K. (1985) A critique of Hoffman's analysis of schizophrenic speech. *Brain Lang.*, **24**, 174–81.

Bilder, R., Mukherjee, S., Reider, R. and Pandurangi, A. (1985), Symptomatic and neuropsychological components of defect states. *Schizophr. Bull.*, **11**, 409–19.

Blashfield, K. (1984) *The Classification of Psychopathology: NeoKraepelinian and Quantitative Approaches*. Plenum, New York.

Bleuler, E. (1950) *Dementia Praecox or the Group of Schizophrenias*. International Universities Press, New York.

Bleuler, M. (1978) The long-term course of schizophrenic psychoses. In *The Nature of Schizophrenia*, L.C. Wynne, R.L. Cromwell and S. Matthysse (eds), Wiley, New York, pp. 631–40.

Borges, J. (1960) El idioma analítico de John Wilkins in *Otras inquisiciones*, Emecé, Buenos Aires, 631–40.

Boyle, M. (1990) The non-discovery of schizophrenia: Kraepelin and Bleuler reconsidered. In *Reconstructing Schizophrenia*, R.P. Bentall (ed), Routledge, London, pp. 3–22.

Brennan, J.H. and Hemsley, D.R. (1984) Illusory

correlations in paranoid and non-paranoid schizophrenia. *Br. J. Clin. Psychol.*, **23**, 225–6.

Brockington, I.F., Kendell, R.E. and Leff, J.P. (1978) Definitions of schizophrenia: Concordance and prediction of outcome. *Psychol. Med.*, **8**, 399–412.

Brockington, I.F. and Wainwright, R.S. (1980) Depressed patients with schizophrenic or paranoid symptoms. *Psychol. Med.*, **10**, 665–75.

Brown, G.W. and Birley, J.L.T. (1968) Crises and life changes and the onset of schizophrenia. *J. Health Soc. Behav.*, **9**, 203–14.

Brown, W.A. and Herz, L.R. (1989) Response to neuroleptic drugs as a device for classifying schizophrenia. *Schizophr. Bull.*, **15**, 123–9.

Candido, C.L. and Romney, D.M. (1990) Attributional style in paranoid vs depressed patients. *Br. J. Med. Psychol.*, **63**, 355–63.

Carpenter, W.T., Bartko, J., Carpenter, C.L. and Strauss, J.S. (1976) Another view of schizophrenia subtypes: A report from the International Pilot Study of Schizophrenia. *Arch. Gen. Psychiatry*, **33**, 508–16.

Chapman, L.J. and Chapman, J.P. (1988) The genesis of delusions. In *Delusional Beliefs*, T.F. Oltmanns and B. Maher (eds), Wiley, New York, pp. 167–83.

Chapman, L.J., Chapman, J.P. and Miller, E.N. (1982) The reliabilities and intercorrelations of eight measures of proneness to psychosis. *J. Consult. Clin. Psychol.*, **50**, 187–95.

Chapman, L.J., Chapman, J.P. and Raulin, M.L. (1976) Scales for measuring physical and social anhedonia. *J. Abnorm. Psychol.*, **85**, 374–82.

Ciompi, L. (1980) The natural history of schizophrenia in the long term. *Br. J. Psychiatry*, **136**, 413–20.

Ciompi, L. (1984) Is there really a schizophrenia?: the long-term course of psychotic phenomena. *Br. J. Psychiatry*, **145**, 636–40.

Claridge, G.S. (1987) The schizophrenias as nervous types revisited. *Br. J. Psychiatry*, **151**, 735–43.

Claridge, G.S. (1990) Can a disease model of schizophrenia survive? In *Reconstructing Schizophrenia*. R.P. Bentall (ed), Routledge, London, pp. 157–83.

Claridge, G.S. and Broks, P. (1984) Schizotypy and hemisphere function I: Theoretical considerations and the measurement of schizotypy. *Pers.*

Indiv. Diff., **5** 633–48.

Collicut, J.R. and Hemsley, D.R. (1981) A psychophysical investigation of auditory functioning in schizophrenia. *Br. J. Clin. Psychol.*, **20**, 199–204.

Cooklin, R., Sturgeon, D. and Leff, J.P. (1983) The relationship between auditory hallucinations and spontaneous fluctuations in skin conductance in schizophrenia. *Br. J. Psychiatry*, **142**, 47–52.

Cornblatt, B., Lezenweger, M., Dworkin, R. and Erlenmeyer-Kimling, L. (1985) Positive and negative symptoms in schizophrenia: Attention and information processing. *Schizophr. Bull.*, **11**, 397–408.

Crow, T.J. (1980) Molecular pathology of schizophrenia: more than one disease process. *Br. Med. J.*, **280**, 66–8.

Crow, T.J. (1984) A re-evaluation of the viral hypothesis: Is psychosis the result of retroviral integration at a site close to the cerebral dominance gene? *Br. J. Psychiatry*, **148**, 120–7.

Delva, N.J. and Letemendia, F.J.J. (1982) Lithium treatment in schizophrenia and schizo-affective disorders. *Br. J. Psychiatry*, **141**, 387–400.

Dworkin, R.H. and Lenzenweger, M.F. (1984) Symptoms and the genetics of schizophrenia: Implications for diagnosis. *Am. J. Psychiatry*, **141**, 1541–6.

Eysenck, S.B. and Eysenck, H.J. (1968) The measurement of psychoticism: A study of factor stability and reliability. *Br. J. Soc. Clin. Psychol.*, **7**, 286–94.

Everitt, B.S., Gourlay, A.J. and Kendell, R.E. (1971) An attempt at validation of traditional psychiatric syndromes by cluster analysis. *Br. J. Psychiatry*, **119**, 399–42.

Faris, R.E.I. and Dunham, H.W. (1939) *Mental Disorders in Urban Areas: An Ecological Study of Schizophrenia and Other Psychoses*. Chicago University Press, Chicago, IL.

Farmer, A.E., McGuffin, P. and Spitznagel, E.L. (1983) Heterogeneity in schizophrenia: A cluster-analysis approach. *Psychiatry Res.*, **8**, 1–12.

Fisher, M. (1973) Genetic and environmental factors in schizophrenia: A study of schizophrenic twins and their families. *Acta Psychiatr. Scand.*, Supp. 238.

Goldberg, S.C. (1985) Negative and deficit symptoms do respond to neuroleptics. *Schizophr. Bull.*, **11**, 453–6.

Goldstein, M.J. (1988) The family and psycho-pathology. *Ann. Rev. Psychol.*, **39**, 283–300.

Gottesman, I. and Shields, J. (1982) *Schizophrenia: The Epigenetic Puzzle*. Cambridge University Press, Cambridge.

Green, A.R. and Costain, D.W. (1981) *Pharmocology and Biochemistry of Psychiatric Disorders*. Wiley, London.

Green, M. and Walker, E. (1986) Symptom correlates of backward masking in schizophrenia. *Am. J. Psychiatry*, **143**, 181–6.

Gruenberg, A.M., Kendler, K.S. and Tsuang, M.T. (1985) Reliability and concordance in the subtyping of schizophrenia. *Am. J. Psychiatry*, **142**, 1355–8.

Hamilton, M. (1973) Psychology in society: Ends or ends? *Bull. Br. Psychol. Soc.*, **26**, 185–9.

Hare, R.D. and Forth, A.E. (1985) Psychopathy and lateral preference. *J. Abnorm. Psychol.*, **94**, 541–6.

Harrow, M. and Prosen, M. (1978) Intermingling and disordered logic as influences on schizophrenic thought. *Arch. Gen. Psychiatry*, **35**, 1213–18.

Harvey, P.D. (1983) Speech competence in manic and schizophrenic psychoses: The association between clinically rated thought disorder and cohesion and reference. *J. Abnorm. Psychol.*, **92**, 368–77.

Harvey, P.D. (1985) Reality monitoring in mania and schizophrenia: the association of thought disorder and performance. *J. Nerv. Ment. Dis.*, **173**, 67–73.

Harvey, P.D. and Neale, J.M. (1983) The specificity of thought disorder to schizophrenia: Research methods in their historical perspective. In *Progress in Experimental Personality Research*. B. Maher (ed), **Vol. 12**, Academic Press, New York, pp. 153–77.

Hawke, A.B., Strauss, J.S. and Carpenter, W.T. (1975) Diagnostic criteria and five-year outcome in schizophrenia. *Arch. Gen. Psychiatry*, **32**, 343–7.

Heilbrun, A.R. (1980) Impaired recognition of self-expressed thought in patients with auditory hallucinations. *J. Abnorm. Psychol.*, **89**, 728–36.

Hemsley, D.R. and Garety, P.A. (1986) The formation and maintenance of delusions: A Baysian analysis. *Br. J. Psychiatry*, **149**, 51–6.

Hoffman, R.E. (1986) Verbal hallucinations and language production in schizophrenia. *Behav. Brain Sci.*, **9**, 503–48.

Hoffman, R.E., Kirstein, L., Stopek, S. and Cicchetti, V. (1982) Apprehending schizophrenic discourse: A structural analysis of the listener's task. *Brain Lang.*, **15**, 207–33.

Huq, S.F., Garety, P. and Hemsley, D.R. (1988) Probabilistic judgements in deluded and non-deluded subjects. *Q. J. Exp. Psychol.*, **40A**, 801–12.

Inouye, T. and Shimizu, A. (1970) The electromyographic study of auditory hallucination. *Folia Psychiatr. Japon.*, **29**, 123–43.

Johnson, W.G., Ross, J.M. and Mastria, M.A. (1977) Delusional behaviour: An attributional analysis of development and modification. *J. Abnorm. Psychol.*, **86**, 421–6.

Johnson-Laird, P. (1989) *The Computer and the Mind*, Fontana, London.

Kaney, S. and Bentall, R.P. (1989) Persecutory delusions and attributional style. *Br. J. Med. Psychol.*, **62**, 191–8.

Kaney, S. and Bentall, R.P. (in press) Persecutory delusions and the self-serving bias: evidence from a contingency judgement task. *J. Nerv. Ment. Dis.*

Kaney, S., Wolfenden, M., Dewey, M.E. and Bentall, R.P. (1992) Persecutory delusions and the recall of threatening and non-threatening propositions. *Br. J. Clin. Psychol.*, **31** 8–27.

Kendell, R.E. (1975) *The Role of Diagnosis in Psychiatry*. Blackwell, Oxford.

Kendell, R.E. (1989) Clinical validity. In *The Validity of Psychiatric Diagnosis*, L.N. Robins and J.E. Barrett (eds) Raven Press, New York, pp. 305–21.

Kendell, R.E. and Brockington, I.F. (1980) The identification of disease entities and the relationship between schizophrenic and affective psychoses. *Br. J. Psychiatry*, **137**, 324–31.

Kendell, R.E., Brockington, I.F. and Leff, J.P. (1979) Prognostic implications of six different definitions of schizophrenia. *Arch. Gen. Psychiatry*, **36**, 25–31.

Kendell, R.E., Cooper, J.E. and Gourlay, J.A. (1971) Diagnostic criteria of British and American psychiatrists. *Arch. Gen. Psychiatry*, **25**, 123–30.

Kendell, R.E. and Gourlay, J.A. (1970) The clinical distinction between the affective psychoses and schizophrenia. *Br. J. Psychiatry*, **117**, 261–6.

Kendler, K.S. and Davis, K.L. (1981) The genetics and biochemistry of paranoid schizophrenia and other paranoid psychoses. *Schizophr. Bull.*, **7**, 689–709.

Kendler, K.S., Gruenberg, A.M. and Tsuang, M.T. (1985) Sub-type stability in schizophrenia. *Am. J. Psychiatry*, **142**, 827–32.

Kendler, K.S., Gruenberg, A.M. and Tsuang, M.T. (1988) A family study of the sub-types of schizophrenia. *Am. J. Psychiatry*, **145**, 57–62.

Kendler, K.S. and Hays, P. (1982) Familial and sporadic schizophrenia: A symptomatic, prognostic and EEG comparison. *Am.J. Psychiatry*, **139**, 1557–162.

Kennedy, J.L., Giuffra, L.A., Moises, H.W. *et al.* (1988) Evidence against linkage of schizophrenia to markers on chromosome 5 in a northern Swedish pedigree. *Nature*, **336**, 167–70.

Kety, S.S., Rosenthal, D., Wender, P.H. *et al.* (1975) Mental illness in the biological and adoptive families of adopted individuals who have become schizophrenic. In *Genetic Research in Psychiatry*. R. Fiove, D. Rosenthal and H. Brill (eds), Johns Hopkins University Press, Baltimore, MD, pp. 147–65.

Kornetsky, C. (1976) Hyporesponsivity of chronic schizophrenic patients to dextroamphetamine. *Arch. Gen. Psychiatry*, **33**, 1425–8.

Kraepelin, E. (1907) *Textbook of Psychiatry*, (seventh ed.), Macmillan, London.

Laing, R.D. (1967) *The Politics of Experience*. Penguin, Harmondsworth.

Laing, R.D. and Esterson, A. (1970) *Sanity, Madness and the Family: Families of Schizophrenics*. Basic Books, New York.

Lander, E.S. (1988) Splitting schizophrenia. *Nature*, **336**, 105–6.

Launay, G. and Slade, P.D. (1981) The measurement of hallucinatory predisposition in male and female prisoners. *Pers. Indiv. Diff.*, **2**, 221–34.

Lewis, S.W., Owen, M.J. and Murray, R.M. (1989) Obstetric complications and schizophrenia: Methodology and measurement. In *Schizophrenia: Scientific Progress*, S.C. Schulz and C.A. Tamminga. (eds), Oxford University Press, Oxford, pp. 56–8.

Liddle, P. (1987) The symptoms of chronic schizophrenia: A re-examination of the positive-negative dichotomy. *Br. J. Psychiatry*, **151**, 145–51.

Lingjaerde, O. (1982) Effects of the benzodiazapine estazdam in patients with auditory hallucinations: A multi-centre double-blind cross-over study. *Acta Psychiatr. Scand.*, **63**, 339–54.

Maher, B.A. (1973) Delusional thinking and perceptual disorder. *J. Indiv. Psychol.*, **30**, 98–113.

Maher, B.A. and Ross, J.S. (1984) Delusions. In *Comprehensive Handbook of Psychopathology*. H.E. Adams and P. Suther (eds), Plenum, New York, pp. 383–408.

Marder, S.R., Asarnow, R.F. and van Putten, T. (1984) Information processing and neuroleptic response in acute and stabilized schizophrenic patients. *Psychiatry Res.*, **13**, 41–9.

Margo, A., Hemsley, D.R. and Slade, P.D. (1981) The effects of varying auditory input on schizophrenic hallucinations. *Br. J. Psychiatry*, **139**, 122–7.

McGuigan, F.J. (1966) Covert oral behaviour and auditory hallucinations. *Psychophysiology*, **3**, 73–80.

McGuigan, F.J. (1978) *Cognitive Psychophysiology: Principles of Covert Behavior*. Prentice-Hall, Englewood Cliffs, NJ.

McGuffin, P., Farmer, A.M. and Gottesman, I. (1987) Is there really a split in schizophrenia? The genetic evidence. *Br. J. Psychiatry*, **150**, 581–92.

Meehl, P. (1962) Schizotaxia, schizotypy and schizophrenia. *Am. Psychol.*, **17**, 827–38.

Mintz, S. and Alpert, M. (1972) Imagery vividness, reality testing and schizophrenic hallucinations. *J. Abnorm. Psychol.*, **79**, 310–6.

Muntaner, C., Garcia-Sevilla, L., Fernandez, A. and Torrubia, R. (1988) Personality dimensions, schizotypal and borderline personality traits and psychosis proneness. *Pers. Indiv. Diff.*, **9**, 257–68.

Opler, L., Kay, S. and Rosado, V. (1984) Positive and negative syndromes in schizophrenic patients. *J. Nerv. Ment. Dis.*, **171**, 317–87.

Overall, J.E. Hollister, L.E., Meyer, F., *et al.* (1964) Imipramine and thioridazine in depressed and schizophrenic patients. *J. Am. Med. As.*, **189**, 605–8.

Owen, M.J., Lewis, S.W. and Murray, R.M. (1989) Family history and cerebral ventricular enlargement in schizophrenia: A case control study. *Br. J. Psychiatry*, **154**, 629–34.

Persons, J.B. (1986) The advantages of studying

psychological phenomena rather than psychiatric diagnoses. *Am. Psychol.*, **41**, 1252–60.

Pincus, J.H. and Tucker, G.J. (1978) *Behavioural Neurology*. Oxford University Press, New York.

Pogue-Geile, M. and Harrow, M. (1984) Negative and positive symptoms in schizophrenia and depression: A follow-up study. *Schizophr. Bull.*, **10**, 371–87.

Potkin, S.G., Cannon, H.E., Murray, D.L. and Wyatt, R.J. (1978) Are paranoid schizophrenics biologically different from other schizophrenics? *New Engl. J. Med.*, **298**, 61–6.

Reider, R.O. (1974) The origins of our confusion about schizophrenia. *Psychiatry*, **37**, 197–208.

Reveley, A.M. and Chitkara, B. (1985) Subtypes in schizophrenia. *Lancet*, i, 1503.

Reveley, A.M. and Murray, R.M. (1984) Cerebral ventricular enlargement in non-genetic schizophrenia: A controlled twin study. *Br. J. Psychiatry*, **144**, 89–93.

Robins, E. and Guze, S.B. (1970) Establishment of diagnostic validity in psychiatric illness: Its application to schizophrenia. *Am J. Psychiatry*, **126**, 107–11.

Rochester, S. and Martin, J.R. (1979) *Crazy Talk: A Study of the Discourse of Schizophrenic Speakers*. Plenum, New York.

Rosenthal, D., Wender, P.H., Kety, S.S., Welner, J. and Schulsinger, F. (1971) The adopted away offspring of schizophrenics. *Am. J. Psychiatry*, **128**, 307–11.

Roth, M. (1973) Psychiatry and its critics. *Br. J. Psychiatry*, **122**, 374.

StClair, D., Blackwood, D., Muir, W. *et al.* (1989) No linkage of chromosome 5q11–q13 markers to schizophrenia in Scottish families. *Nature*, **339**, 305–9.

Sarbin, T.R. and Mancuso, J.C. (1980) *Schizophrenia: Medical Diagnosis or Moral Verdict?* Pergamon, Oxford.

Sartorius, N., Jablensky, A. Ernberg, G. *et al.* (1987) Course of schizophrenia in different countries: Some results of a WHO international collaborative 5-year follow-up study. In *Search for the Causes of Schizophrenia*. H. Hafner, W.G. Gattaz and W. Janzarik (eds), Berlin, Springer-Verlag, pp. 107–13.

Scheff, T. (1966) *Being Mentally Ill: A Sociological Theory*. Weidenfeld and Nicholson, London.

Schulz, S.C., Conley, R.R., Kahn, E.M. and Alexander, J. (1989) Nonresponders to neuroleptics: A distinct subtype. In *Schizophrenia: Scientific Progress*. S.C. Schulz and C.A. Tamminga (eds), Oxford University Press, New York, pp. 341–50.

Seidman, L. (1984) Schizophrenia and brain dysfunction: An integration of recent neurodiagnostic findings. *Psychol. Bull.*, **94**, 195–238.

Sherrington, R., Brynjolfsson, J., Pertursson, H. *et al.* (1988) Localization of a susceptibility locus for schizophrenia on chromosome 5. *Nature*, **336**, 164–7.

Singh, M.M. and Kay, S.R. (1976) Wheat gluten as a pathogenic factor in schizophrenia. *Science*, **191**, 401–2.

Slade, P.D. (1972) The effects of systematic desensitisation on auditory hallucinations. *Behav. Res. Ther.*, **10**, 85–91.

Slade, P.D. and Bentall, R.P. (1988) *Sensory Deception: A Scientific Analysis of Hallucinations*. Croom Helm, London.

Slade, P.D. and Cooper, R. (1979) Some conceptual difficulties with the term 'schizophrenia': an alternative model. *Br. J. Soc. Clin. Psychol.*, **18**, 309–17.

Spitzer, R.L., Endicott, J. and Gibbon, M. (1979) Crossing the border into borderline personality and borderline schizophrenia: The developmnent of criteria. *Arch. Gen. Psychiatry*, **36**, 17–24.

Stevens, J.R. and Livermore, A. (1982) Telemetered EEG in schizophrenia: Spectral analysis during abnormal behaviour episodes. *J. Neurol. Neurosurg. Psychiatry*, **45**, 385–95.

Szasz, T. (1976) *Schizophrenia: The Sacred Symbol of Psychiatry*, Basic Books, New York.

Torrey, E.F. (1987) Prevalence studies in schizophrenia. *Br. J. Psychiatry*, **150**, 598–608.

Tsuang, M.T., Lyons, M.J. and Faraone, S. (1990) Heterogeneity in schizophrenia: Conceptual models and analytic strategies. *Br. J. Psychiatry*, **156**, 17–26.

Ullmann, L. and Krasner, L. (1975) *A Psychological Approach to Abnormal Behaviour*. Appleton-Century-Crofts, New York.

Venables, P.H., Wilkins, S., Mitchell, D.A. *et al.* (1990) A scale for the measurement of schizotypy. *Pers. Indiv. Diff.*, **11**, 481–95.

Warner, R. (1985) *Recovery from Schizophrenia: Psychiatry and Political Economy*. Routledge, London.

Weiss, K.M. (1989) Advantages of abandoning symptom-based diagnostic systems of research in schizophrenia. *Am. J. Orthopsychiatry*, **59**, 324–30.

Williams, E.B. (1964) Deductive reasoning in schizophrenia. *J. Abnorm. Soc. Psychol.*, **69**, 47–61.

Winters, K. and Neale, J.M. (1983) Delusions and delusional thinking: A review of the literature. *Clin. Psychol. Rev.*, **3**, 227–53.

World Health Organization (1973) *International Pilot Study of Schizophrenia*, **vol. 1**. WHO, Geneva.

Young, H.F., Bentall, R.P., Slade, P.D. and Dewey, M. (1987) The role of brief instructions and suggestibility in the elicitation of hallucinations in normal and psychiatric subjects. *J. Nerv. Ment. Dis.*, **175**, 41–8.

Zigler, E. and Glick, M. (1988) Is paranoid schizophrenia really camouflaged depression? *Am. Psychol.*, **43**, 284–90.

Chapter 3

Information processing in schizophrenia

MICHAEL FOSTER GREEN

In therapy I worked on the developmental issues I missed in prep school and college. My negative self-image was a large issue. I developed a close relationship with a very skillful therapist who became an important father figure. But my depression continued to be a major concern, and I discovered other problems too — most significantly, sensory overload and paranoia. I had at least two psychotic episodes in the city but was not hospitalized there. During these episodes I formed delusions that completely absorbed my thinking and took over my life. For example, I believed that there was an undeclared city-wide civil war going on and that I played an important but undefined part in it. I also believed that I had telepathic powers and spent hours lying on my bed 'communicating' with my therapist and his wife, whom I had never met. (Anonymous, 1989, p. 636).

This passage is a first-person account of the initial psychotic experiences of a young man. The writer is trying to understand the origins of these experiences and he suggests that early developmental factors might have contributed to his episode which was characterized by delu-sions of reference and paranormal delusions. In addition to the early developmental and familial factors, we now know that genetic, bio-chemical, and neuroanatomical factors are also associated with the initiation of psychotic episodes. How did these various factors con-verge and lead to schizophrenic symptoms? Most likely, these factors interacted to produce alterations in **cognitive processes** which underly the development of psychotic symptoms. The writer alludes to a breakdown of cognitive functioning when he refers to a 'sensory overload'. Cognitive processes are often seen as mediators between underlying factors (such as biochemistry) and phenomenology. As Holzman (in press) pointed out, studies that have ignored cognitive processes by jumping directly from behavioural to biological variables have not typically been successful in finding relationships:

An approach that systematically works its way by degrees from behavior towards physiological, biochemical, and genetic levels will be most fertile. Great leaps from behavioural events to biochemical events have not worked well in the past and are not likely to work in the future (p. 50).

Such a systematic approach would need to consider the role of cognitive functioning. Interest in cognitive deficits in schizophrenia dates back to the early part of this century. Kraepelin not only established a highly influential classification of psychiatric disorders, he also distinguished between different types of attentional dysfunctions in schizophrenia (Kraepelin, 1913/1919). Kraepelin's interest in psychological factors probably resulted from his training with Wilhelm Wundt, who is credited with establishing the world's first psychology laboratory. Kraepelin differentiated between *auffassung* (the passive registration of information), and *aufmerksamkeit* (active, voluntary attention). He proposed that schizophrenia was characterized by a consistent deficit in active attention, but passive attention was disrupted only in the acute and terminal stages of the disorder (Nuechterlein and Asarnow, 1989). This distinction between active and passive attention turns out to be remarkably similar to modern distinctions between automatic and effortful cognitive processes.

Traditionally, two general approaches have been employed to study cognitive processes in schizophrenia. One approach used *clinical neuropsychological* techniques in an effort to discriminate between patients with schizophrenia and those with brain damage. Many of these studies were primarily concerned with 'hit rates' (i.e. placing subjects into the correct diagnostic categories) and perfecting measures that could aid in diagnosis. A second approach borrowed from experimental psychology in an effort to characterize and understand the nature of cognitive deficits that are central to psychotic disorders. More recently this second approach has relied heavily on *information processing* models and has been viewed in the context of *vulnerability issues*. Let us begin our discussion with the first approach, clinical neuropsychology.

3.1 CLINICAL NEUROPSYCHOLOGY AND DIFFERENTIAL DIAGNOSIS

Traditionally, neuropsychologists were asked whether abnormalities in patients were 'organic' or 'functional' in origin. Such a question is fraught with conceptual and practical problems. Unfortunately, this type of referral question is still seen all too frequently in many psychiatric centres. The term 'functional' refers to signs and symptoms that stem from psychiatric, but not neurological factors. 'Organic' refers to signs and symptoms mediated by brain damage and not attributable to psychosis alone. Neuropsychologists tended to receive this type of referral question so it is not surprising that many of them set out to find tests that could distinguish between schizophrenic and brain-damaged patients. Although this task appears formidable, it was frequently simplified (actually oversimplified) by considering brain damage as a single category regardless of the type or location of the injury. Let us consider a series of questions that illustrate the problems of using neuropsychological tests for psychiatric diagnoses.

Question 1: Is it possible to discriminate between schizophrenic and brain-damaged patients on the basis of neuropsychological tests?

Heaton *et al.* (1978) reviewed 94 studies published between 1960 and 1975 that compared patients with brain injury to patients with various psychiatric disorders on the basis of neuropsychological assessment. The studies differed substantially in their psychiatric and neurological diagnostic procedures. In addition, most studies did not conduct neurological examinations with the psychiatric patients and hence could not have sufficiently ruled out neurological factors. Hit rates were determined by selecting a cut-off score for a given test and classifying anyone with a better score as 'schizophrenic' and anyone with a worse score

Table 3.1 Mean hit rates (schizophrenia vs. brain-damaged)

Disorder	%	Attempts
Mixed psychiatric	77	29
Affective	77	10
Mixed psychotic	70	8
Acute schizophrenic	77	14
Chronic schizophrenic	54	34

Adapted from Heaton *et al.* (1978).

as 'brain-injured'. After subjects were classified according to test results, the cut-off score diagnoses were compared to the actual diagnoses and the percentage of correct detections became the hit rate. Many of the studies that were reviewed used a single neuropsychological test to determine a hit rate.

Table 3.1 is adapted from the Heaton *et al.* (1978) study. The median hit rates are respectable for the mixed psychiatric, affective and acute schizophrenic patients. The hit rate is also sufficient for the mixed psychotic patients. But the hit rate for the chronic schizophrenic patients is little better than flipping a coin (for two groups, a hit rate of 50% is chance).

The conclusion from this review is that neuropsychological tests cannot adequately discriminate between chronic schizophrenic patients and brain-damaged patients. Although the hit rate is better for patients called 'acute schizophrenic', it is unlikely that most of these patients would be diagnosed with schizophrenia according to DSM–III (American Psychiatric Association, 1980) or DSM–III-R (American Psychiatric Association, 1987) because these systems require a minimum six-month duration. Hence, it appears that based on level of test performance, neuropsychological tests do not distinguish between brain-injured subjects and schizophrenic patients diagnosed by current criteria.

Question 2: Why are the tests unable to distinguish brain-damaged from schizophrenic patients?

These two groups of patients differ dramatically in aetiology and clinical presentation, so initially it may seem surprising that neuropsychological tests cannot distinguish between them. One possible explanation is that the neuropsychological measures were not sensitive enough to detect relatively subtle differences between the two patient groups. However, the neuropsychological measures have previously been shown to be highly sensitive to the presence of brain damage.

Alternatively, the two groups may perform at comparable levels, but for entirely different reasons. The brain-damaged patients may be *unable* and the schizophrenic patients may be *unwilling* to perform better. The question of sufficient motivation is a constant problem in the assessment of schizophrenic patients who sometimes appear apathetic in testing situations. Deficit symptoms (negative symptoms) are generally considered part of the schizophrenic disorder and could contribute to reduced performance. In addition, most schizophrenic in-patients are medicated at the time of testing, which has raised concerns about the effects of neuroleptic medications on neuropsychological performance. However, neuroleptics seem to improve performance on many information processing tests (Spohn *et al.*, 1977; Braff and Saccuzzo, 1982; Spohn and Strauss, 1989). Nonetheless, some other aspect of the hospitalization or treatment could conceivably account for performance deficits.

A third reason why neuropsychological tests do not discriminate between schizophrenic and brain-damaged patients may be because the distinction is illusory: schizophrenic patients may in fact be brain damaged. Numerous imaging studies have reported that schizophrenic patients (as a group) show abnormalities in brain structure and brain function, such as enlarged lateral ventricles and reduced metabolism in the frontal regions (Buchsbaum and Haier, 1987; Suddath *et al.*, 1990). Neuropathology studies have revealed abnormalities in neuronal orientation (Kovelman and Scheibel, 1984) and brain volume (Bogerts *et al.*, 1985). Schizophrenic patients with enlarged lateral ventricles on CT scans tend to have more neuropsychological deficits which suggests that the structural brain changes may be related to some of the observed cognitive deficits (e.g. Golden *et al.*, 1980). Although several types of neuropathology and several regions have been implicated in schizophrenia, it should be emphasized that no single region or abnormality can be found in all (or even most) cases of schizophrenia. It appears that schizophrenia is associated with a heterogeneous type of brain disorder, or the damage is very diffuse. These topics are covered in Chapters 5 and 6 on biochemistry and neuroanatomy.

Question 3: Is a specific pattern of cognitive deficits associated with schizophrenia?

Perhaps schizophrenic patients differ from brain-damaged patients in the *pattern* of their neuropsychological deficits, but these differences are obscured when only cut-off scores are considered. Some investigators have reported characteristic profiles of schizophrenic patients, but these reports tend not to be replicated. Even expert clinical neuropsychologists could not discriminate between brain-damaged and schizophrenic patients by using a full neuropsychological battery (Halsted-Reitan) and intelligence scales (Watson *et al.*, 1968). After reviewing this literature, Goldstein (1986) concluded: 'Thus, in my view, no one has been able to successfully derive a characteristic performance pattern on standard neuropsychological tests that is specific to schizophrenia' (p. 154).

The inability to find a specific cognitive pattern in schizophrenia should be predictable after we consider some relevant issues. Cognitive deficits in schizophrenia show tremendous variability between and within individuals. Some of the within-subject variability appears to correspond to fluctuations in the patient's clinical state. However, certain cognitive deficits seem to remain fixed and stable across

different clinical states for a given patient. Considering the potpourri of stable and unstable cognitive deficits in schizophrenia, it requires a large amount of optimism to search for a cognitive profile that consistently characterizes schizophrenia across time and individuals.

In summary, the contributions of clinical neuropsychology to the study of schizophrenia appear to be modest at best. This approach has focused on differential diagnosis in separating schizophrenic from brain-damaged patients. Such an endeavour has been unsuccessful for various reasons including poor methodologies, inadequate neurological and psychiatric diagnostic procedures, and unsophisticated conceptualizations of the role of brain functioning in schizophrenia. Let us now consider the information processing approach which has been concerned with identifying and conceptualizing the cognitive impairments that are central to schizophrenia.

3.2 INFORMATION PROCESSING APPROACH

Since the 1930s several centres (such as the New York State Psychiatric Institute) in the US have incorporated advances in the field of experimental psychology with the study of schizophrenia. One goal of these investigations has been to describe and measure cognitive impairment in schizophrenia within theoretical frameworks of experimental psychology. Recently, the predominant framework in experimental psychology has come from information processing theory. The studies that have used information processing techniques attempt to identify deficits that are central to schizophrenia and not merely the result of hospitalization or the presence of psychotic processes. A second and related goal of this approach has been to search for indices of genetic vulnerability to schizophrenia (Nuechterlein and Asarnow, 1989). Some understanding of vulnerability/stress theory is necessary to appreciate these goals.

3.3 VULNERABILITY/STRESS THEORY

In its most simple form, the vulnerability/stress theory of schizophrenia states that certain individuals are predisposed to developing schizophrenia and that various environmental factors influence the expression of the predisposition (Zubin and Spring, 1977). The predisposition is usually considered to be genetic in origin, but additional factors such as pre- and perinatal complications may also contribute to one's predisposition. The interaction between predisposition and environmental stress is represented in Figure 3.1 (adapted from Mirsky and Duncan, 1986). In this diagram, an individual with substantial predisposition (toward the right of the x-axis) requires relatively little environmental stress to be pushed over the threshold into schizophrenia. Hence, a person with such a predisposition would be 'at risk' for developing schizophrenia. Conversely, someone with relatively little predisposition would require substantially more environmental stress to cross the threshold for schizophrenia. It is also reasonable to expect that individuals with unusually low predisposition might never become schizophrenic regardless of the amount of stress they encounter.

Although the vulnerability/stress formulation of schizophrenia is widely accepted, it needs to be understood in a more specific fashion to be practically applied. The goal of many current investigations is to identify the particular vulnerability factors and the specific environmental stressors that are relevant to schizophrenia. How would we know if a cognitive deficit reflects vulnerability to schizophrenia? If a deficit is a vulnerability indicator, it should be found more frequently in schizophrenic patients than in the general population. The deficit should be present before and after a schizophrenic episode, not only during psychotic periods. Lastly, the deficit should be found in a disproportionate number of first-degree relatives of schizophrenic patients, even if the relatives do not develop schizophrenia

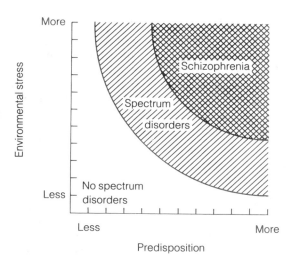

Figure 3.1 'Vulnerability/stress model'. Adapted from Mirsky and Duncan (1986).

themselves. The last prediction is based on the notion that only some of the first degree relatives will carry the predisposition for schizophrenia. Whether or not these predisposed relatives develop the illness depends upon their coping skills and the environmental stresses they encounter. The vulnerability indicator will reflect the underlying predisposition, not the presence of an illness.

Vulnerability indicators can be contrasted with episode indicators. An episode indicator would be a cognitive deficit that appears during the psychotic episode and normalizes during remission. Such a pattern could occur if the deficit was initially due to psychotic processes, confusion, overmedication, or a variety of factors that are specific to the episode period. A vulnerability indicator is theoretically quite interesting because the deficit is likely to be central to schizophrenia and not an 'epiphenomenon' resulting from the psychosis or the treatment of the psychosis. In addition to episode and vulnerability indicators, Nuechterlein and Dawson (1984a) have suggested that some deficits fit a 'mediating vulnerability' pattern. A mediating vulnerability indicator is a deficit that is slightly deviant during remission and becomes more deviant during psychotic episodes. Figure 3.2 shows the hypothetical results from a group of patients who have received

some cognitive measure during an episode and again during remission. The figure shows the characteristic patterns of performance that we would expect from each of the three types of indicators.

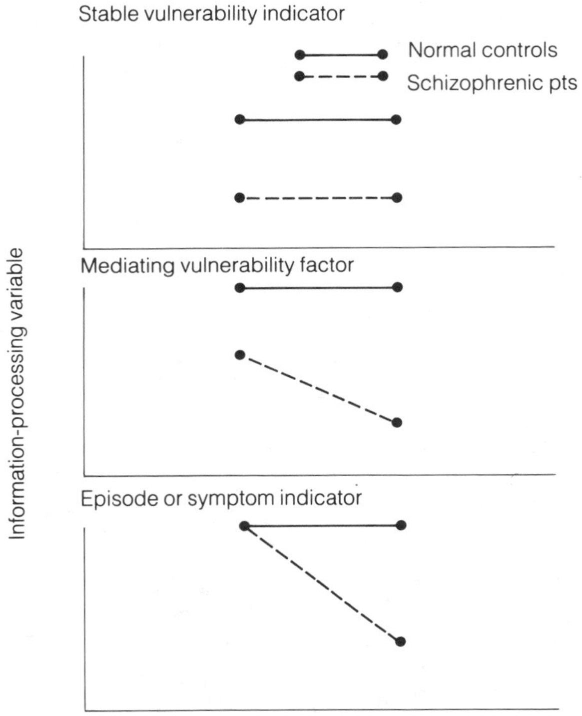

The search for vulnerability indicators in schizophrenia has direct clinical applications. First, if particular vulnerability factors can be determined, they could be used to identify individuals who are at risk for developing schizophrenia. According to the vulnerability/ stress model, these individuals can avoid the illness if certain 'protective factors' are present. These protective factors can be within the person (e.g. effective coping abilities) or social/environmental (e.g. supportive family). Hence, identification of vulnerable individuals allows for early intervention techniques that could prevent the development of schizophrenia. A second clinical application would be in the area of cognitive rehabilitation. If certain cognitive deficits are considered primary (e.g. they precede and lead to psychotic symptoms), remediation of these deficits should serve a prophylactic function by reducing the chances of developing an episode. Moreover, a residual attention deficit would be likely to interfere with social and occupational functioning; so remediation of underlying cognitive deficits should also improve functioning during periods of relative remission.

3.4 INFORMATION PROCESSING MEASURES: POTENTIAL VULNERABILITY INDICATORS

Deficits on several information processing measures have been implicated as vulnerability indicators of schizophrenia including: The Continuous Performance Test, The Span of Apprehension, the Digit-Span Distractibility Test, Dichotic Listening Test, and the Backward Masking Procedure. This list of measures is representative, but not exhaustive. In addition, some abnormalities on psychophysiological procedures (e.g. eye movements) are

Characteristic patterns across clinical states for stable vulnerability indicators, mediating vulnerability factors, and episode or symptom indicators

Figure 3.2 'Vulnerability and episode indicators' from Nuechterlein *et al.*, (1990). Reproduced by permission of Springer-Verlag, Heidelberg.

likely to be vulnerability indicators. To illustrate how information processing tests are studied within a vulnerability/stress framework, two measures, the Continuous Performance Test and the Backward Masking Procedure will be described in more detail.

Studies with information processing measures have been viewed within two separate (but overlapping) frameworks: *capacity models* and *stage models*. Processing capacity models emphasize the overall processing capacity of an individual (Kahneman, 1973). Within this type of model, deficits in cognition are attributed to decreases in amount of processing capacity (possibly due to deviant levels of arousal), or to inefficient allocation of the available processing resources. Processing capacity models are particularly relevant for understanding the Continuous Performance Test. In contrast, stage models of information processing emphasize a series of processing stages so that the output from one stage is fed to the subsequent stage where the information becomes transformed or elaborated. When considering cognitive deficits (as in schizophrenia), this model leads to a search for the earliest dysfunctional stage of processing that presumably disrupts processing in subsequent stages in a type of cascade effect. Stage models of processing are appropriate for discussions of the backward masking procedure.

3.4.1 CONTINUOUS PERFORMANCE TEST

First developed by Rosvold *et al.* (1956) the Continuous Performance Test (CPT) has become the standard index of vigilance or 'sustained attention'. Interest in vigilance stemmed from a practical problem. During World War II, the Royal Air Force requested laboratory experiments to determine the optimal length of time that a radar operator could be on anti-submarine patrol. There was concern that the radar operators were overstrained and that potential U-boat contracts were being

missed. Mackworth initiated a series of vigilance studies with airborne radar operators and found that a marked deterioration in accuracy occurred after about 30 minutes (Davies and Parasuraman, 1982).

Although there are now several different versions of the CPT, they are still designed to approximate the experience of a radar operator searching for enemy U-boats. Typically, the CPT uses a computer screen where a series of stimuli are presented one at a time to a subject. Some of the stimuli are targets that require a response by the subject (typically a button press); the rest of the stimuli are 'noise' and are to be ignored. The target can be a single letter or digit, or it can be a target sequence (e.g. a 7 only when it follows a 3). The duration of the target is brief (usually less than two tenths of a second) and each target occurs relatively rarely, ranging from 10% to 25% of the total stimuli (Nuechterlein and Zaucha, 1990). Measures from the CPT include errors of omission (missed targets), errors of commission (responses to non-targets), hit rate, false alarm rate (responding to a non-target) and sensitivity (ability to distinguish targets from noise).

Interpretation of performance on the CPT often rests on processing capacity models (Kahneman, 1973). Figure 3.3 represents Kahneman's capacity model. In this model, attention is viewed as a limited pool of processing resources that can be allocated to one task or divided among several different tasks. The model assumes that the amount of resources is not entirely fixed, but is partially determined by the individual's arousal level. Of all possible activities, the individual can devote processing resources to only a few, and therefore must decide how to allocate the available resources. If a person is performing two tasks at the same time and the demands of the tasks exceed the total amount of available processing capacity, then task performance will decrease. Both momentary intentions (e.g. demands of the test) and enduring dispositions (e.g. tendency for people to process their

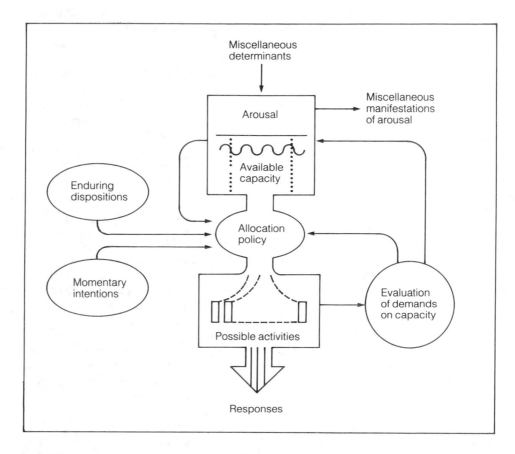

Figure 3.3 'Kahneman's Capacity Model of Attention' from D. Kahneman *Attention and Effort.* © 1973. Reproduced by permission of Prentice-Hall Inc., Englewood Cliffs, NJ.

own names when they hear them) influence the allocation policy.

The versions of the CPT differ to the extent that they place demands on information processing. For example, if the target is a single, clear digit, the processing load is relatively small. However, blurring the digit so that it is more difficult to identify places a higher processing load on the subject. Likewise, adding a short-term memory demand by having the subject respond to a target sequence imposes a greater processing load than a single target.

During a schizophrenic episode, patients perform poorly on both high- and low-load versions of the CPT compared with normal controls and other clinical populations (Orzack and Kornetsky, 1966). However, this finding by itself is not surprising because actively psychotic schizophrenic patients tend to perform poorly on almost all cognitive measures. To determine if CPT deficits are vulnerability indicators we need to consider the performance of remitted patients and of first degree relatives of schizophrenic patients.

Several studies have found that schizophrenic patients in remission continue to show deficits on the CPT, but only on versions of the CPT with relatively high processing loads (Asarnow and MacCrimmon, 1978; Wohlberg and Kornetsky, 1973; Nuechterlein *et al.*, 1989). The studies of first-degree relatives of schizophrenic patients have used offspring of schizophrenic mothers ('high risk' offspring) and compared them with age-matched controls. The offspring of schizophrenic mothers showed deficits on the high-processing load versions of the CPT compared with controls (Rutschmann *et al.*, 1977; Nuechterlein, 1983). Studies of other first-degree relatives (e.g. siblings and parents) are currently under way, but have not yet been published. Taken together, it appears that both high- and low-processing load versions of the CPT (e.g. single clear stimuli) reveal deficits in symptomatic schizophrenic patients, but only the high-processing load versions show deficits in remitted and high-risk groups. This pattern of results suggests that deficits on the CPT versions with high processing loads might indicate vulnerability to schizophrenia (Nuechterlein and Dawson, 1984b; Nuechterlein and Zaucha, 1990).

In the past decade, there has been increasing interest in the relationship between cognitive functioning and certain symptom dimensions in schizophrenia. Most often, this type of study takes the form of contrasting positive (florid) to negative (deficit) symptoms. At first glance, such studies may seem reminiscent of the unsuccessful searches for a characteristic pattern of cognitive deficits in schizophrenia. However, the newer studies have looked for associations of cognitive patterns with symptoms *in particular*, not with schizophrenia *in general* and the results have been more promising. Nuechterlein *et al.* (1986) found that deficits on the high load versions of CPT were associated with negative, but not positive

symptoms at the inpatient phase. Although CPT performance and negative symptoms were not related during the outpatient testing, outpatient CPT performance was related to inpatient level of negative symptoms. These results were interpreted to suggest that deficits on the high load versions of the CPT may serve as a vulnerability factor for negative symptoms of schizophrenia. Note that this interpretation suggests that certain indicators might reflect vulnerability to a specific symptom cluster instead of vulnerability to schizophrenia in general.

Low levels of arousal typically result in suboptimal attentional functioning, hence there has been some speculation that abnormalities in arousal in schizophrenia might lead to both negative symptoms and attentional deficits. Indirect support for this explanation comes from findings that negative symptoms are associated with low levels of skin conductance, which is an index of activity of the sympathetic nervous system (Green *et al.*, 1989).

3.4.2 BACKWARD MASKING

Imagine that you are seated in front of a screen and an experimenter is presenting letters to you one at a time with a type of projector. Although the duration of each letter is very brief (perhaps 10 msec), you can easily identify each letter with perfect accuracy. The experimenter pauses and tells you that he/she will continue to show you letters at the same duration, but there will be one difference: after you are shown each letter, the screen will go blank for a short time and some crossed lines will appear where the letters had been. Your job is only to report the letter and to ignore the crossed lines. The task probably sounds quite easy because you had no difficulty identifying the letters before, and the duration of the letters will not change. However, when the stimuli are presented, you might find that you can see the crossed lines, but no letter at all. This is the backward masking effect. A brief discussion of the information processing model of memory will be helpful for understanding this effect.

Figure 3.4 represents the major components of one information processing model of memory. The first structure is the sensory register which is extremely brief (up to 250 msec), has a large capacity, and occurs automatically. The term for the sensory register in vision is the 'icon' (Neisser, 1967). The implications of such a store are somewhat surprising because the model predicts that when you see a complex display (e.g. a list a words), all of the information in the display is available to you for a brief period after the stimulus presentation. However the store decays quickly, so that it is not possible to report the entire display. Some of the information in the sensory register can be selected for additional analysis and transferred to a more durable store called the short-term memory.

Short-term memory has limited capacity so that we can only be working on a relatively small amount of information at any point in time. The short-term store typically lasts for about 15 seconds, but it can last indefinitely if the material is maintained by rehearsal. For example, suppose someone tells you their phone number and you have no place to write it down. If the number is fairly short (e.g. seven digits) you can keep the number in mind by constantly repeating it. If someone interrupts you before you have a chance to write the number down, you might find that the number has disappeared. Hence, the information decays in a relatively brief time unless it is maintained by rehearsal. If the phone number is in a foreign country and

has many digits, you might not be able to successfully rehearse it. This observation suggests that the capacity of short-term store is limited.

Information in short-term memory can be transferred to long-term memory which, like the sensory register has a very large capacity. Once in long-term memory, the information is very durable, and could last for years even without rehearsal. The information is believed to be organized semantically so that material of similar meaning is organized together. In more recent years, it has been argued that the three structures in this model of memory (sensory register, short-term and long-term memory) are probably not truly distinct. However, the model still provides a useful heuristic for understanding backward masking.

In the backward masking paradigm, a target stimulus (the letter) can be easily identified when presented alone. Hence, the information (the features of the letter) was transferred from the sensory register to short-term memory so that the subject could extract enough information to correctly name the letter. When the mask (the crossed lines) was presented, it presumably disrupted the information from the target as it was being transferred. Due to the mask, the information from the target did not arrive at the short-term store, so the subject did not have any recollection of the letter. When a mask prevents identification of a target that was presented earlier in time, it is called backward masking. If the mask comes before the target, it is called forward masking.

Using this view of the backward masking procedure, we can hypothetically measure a subject's speed in visual information processing. The interval between the offset of the target and the onset of the mask (the inter-stimulus interval, ISI) can be varied so that the identification becomes easier or harder. At short ISIs, (e.g. the mask occurs 20 msec after the target) subjects are rarely able to identify the target above chance performance, but as we increase the ISI, subjects gradually become

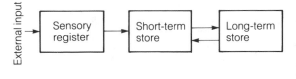

Figure 3.4 'Hypothetical memory structures'.

aware of the target. At some ISI, the subject is able to correctly identify the letter, and we say that the target has been 'unmasked'. Suppose that we test two subjects: one subject experiences unmasking at an ISI of 50 msec and another unmasks at an ISI of 70 msec. The subject who unmasked at 50 msec would be considered a faster visual processor because the information was transferred from the sensory register to a durable store within 50 msec, but the information for the other subject was still 'in transit' and susceptible to disruption at 50 msec.

Not surprisingly, schizophrenic patients show deficits on the backward masking procedure. Patients consistently require a longer ISI to correctly identify a target compared with normal controls (Saccuzzo and Braff, 1981, 1986). These deficits have been interpreted to indicate that schizophrenic patients are slower processors and require a longer time to transfer their information to a more durable store (Braff, 1981). Although many researchers believe that masking deficits reflect a 'slow-down' in processing, alternative hypotheses (such as deficits in perceptual organization; Knight *et al.*, 1985) are also plausible. The backward masking deficit appears not to be due to antipsychotic medication, which may actually reduce the deficit (Braff and Sacuzzo, 1982).

Studies with remitted patients and first-degree relatives are necessary to determine if the backward masking deficit observed in schizophrenia is a vulnerability or episode indicator. However, very few studies have considered vulnerability issues with this procedure. So far no published study has considered masking performance in first degree relatives of schizophrenic patients. Only one study (Miller *et al.*, 1979) has examined masking deficits in remitted schizophrenic patients. They found that a small group (*n* = 10) of remitted patients showed masking deficits compared with normal controls. This result should be interpreted cautiously because the patients were presumed to be asymptomatic

according to staff reports, but they were living in board and care homes and still exhibited poor social functioning. Hence, we have suggestive evidence that backward masking is a vulnerability indicator, although the question is far from settled.

What about the relationship between masking deficits and positive and negative symptoms? The deficits on backward masking have been related to the presence of negative, but not positive symptoms (Braff, 1989; Green and Walker, 1984, 1986). In addition, Braff (1989) found that the negative symptom patients needed a substantially longer stimulus duration to identify the target **without** the mask. The results of these studies suggest that negative symptoms are associated with deficits in the very early stages of visual input. The deficits in such early stages are impressive given the largely automatic nature of the task. For example, naming a single letter does not seem to require complex strategies or much effort. These early processing deficits could cascade and lead to processing deficits at later stages of cognition.

3.4.3 INFORMATION PROCESSING IN SCHIZOPHRENIA: WHAT HAVE WE LEARNED?

We have discussed two substantially different approaches to the study of cognitive processes in schizophrenia. The first was the use of clinical neuropsychological techniques to differentially diagnose schizophrenia from brain damage. This effort was largely misguided for conceptual and methodological reasons and the resulting database has not led to meaningful theoretical developments. Even the practical gains from this approach have been unimpressive. After all, if you really wanted to know if someone was brain damaged or schizophrenic, the easiest and most reliable way is for a diagnostician to simply ask them what sorts of problems they are having.

The second aproach has incorporated developments from experimental psychology to study the nature of cognitive deficits in schizophrenia. These approaches have relied on information processing models which currently direct research in cognitive psychology. Two laboratory based methods were discussed in some detail (CPT and backward masking) because they emphasize different information processing models (capacity models for the CPT, and stage models for backward masking). To adequately interpret the information processing studies, the results need to be viewed within a vulnerability/stress framework. Studies of remitted patients and unaffected first-degree relatives help separate fact from artefact by determining which deficits reflect vulnerability to the disorder and which deficits result from the psychosis.

By combining information processing models with vulnerability theory, we are in a stronger position to suggest which deficits **underlie** the development of psychotic episodes. The writer of the passage at the beginning of this chapter might have been able to avoid his initial psychotic experiences if we only knew which factors placed him at risk for the episode. The information processing research from the CPT suggests that he might have had a reduced capacity or a poor allocation policy that led to his sensory overload. Alternatively, results from backward masking suggests that his overload resulted from a very early slowdown in visual processing that disrupted subsequent processing stages. The two theories are not incompatible, and perhaps in the near future we will see an integration of models and techniques that will allow for early detection and intervention. Such investigations (in combination with advances in genetics, social factors, and epidemiology) offer hope for something that has never been possible before: a truly preventative mental health programme for schizophrenia.

ACKNOWLEDGEMENTS

The author thanks Genie Cynn, Ph.D., for her thoughtful comments, and Donna Gaier and Cathy Phipps for their help in the preparation of this manuscript.

REFERENCES

American Psychiatric Association (1980) *Diagnostic and Statistical Manual of Mental Disorders*, third ed. (DSM–III). American Psychiatric Association, Washington, DC.

American Psychiatric Association (1987) *Diagnostic and Statistical Manual of Mental Disorders*, third ed. revised (DSM–III–R). American Psychiatric Association, Washington, DC.

Anonymous (1989) First person account: How I've managed chronic mental illness: *Schizophr. Bull.*, **15**, 635–40.

Asarnow, R.F. and MacCrimmon, D.J. (1978) Residual performance deficit in clinically remitted schizophrenics: A marker of schizophrenia? *J. Abnorm. Psychol.*, **87**, 597–608.

Bogerts, B., Meertz, E. and Schonfeldt-Bausch, R. (1985) Basal ganglia and limbic system pathology in schizophrenia: A morphometric study of brain volume and shrinkage. *Arch. Gen. Psychiatry*, **42**, 784–90.

Braff, D.L. (1981) Impaired speed of information processing in non-medicated schizotypal patients. *Schizophr. Bull.*, **7**, 499–508.

Braff, D.L. (1989) Sensory input deficits and negative symptoms in schizophrenic patients. *Am. J. Psychiatry*, **146**, 1006–11.

Braff, D.L. and Saccuzzo, D.P. (1982) Effect of antipsychotic medication on speed of information processing in schizophrenic patients. *Am. J. Psychiatry*, **139**, 1127–30.

Buchsbaum, M.S. and Haier, R.J. (1987) Functional and anatomical brain imaging: Impact on schizophrenia research. *Schizophr. Bull.*, **13**, 115–32.

Davies, D.R. and Parasuraman, R. (1982) *The Psychology of Vigilance*. Academic Press, London

Golden, C.G., Moses, J.A., Zelazowski, R., *et al.* (1980) Cerebral ventricular size and neuropsychological impairment in young chronic schizophrenics. *Arch. Gen. Psychiatry*, **37**, 619–23.

Goldstein, G. (1986) The neuropsychology of schizophrenia. In *Neuropsychological Assessment of Neuropsychiatric Disorders*, I. Grant and K.M. Adams (eds), Oxford University Press, New York, pp. 147–71.

Green, M.F., Nuechterlein, K.H. and Satz, P. (1989) The relationship of symptomatology and medication to electrodermal activity in schizophrenia. *Psychophysiology*, **26**, 148–57.

Green, M. and Walker, E. (1984) Susceptibility to backward masking in schizophrenic patients with positive and negative symptoms. *Am. J. Psychiatry*, **141**, 1273–5.

Green, M. and Walker, E. (1986) Symptom correlates of vulnerability to backward masking in schizophrenia. *Am. J. Psychiatry*, **143**, 181–6.

Halstead-Reitan, R.M. and Davison, L.A. (1974) *Clinical Neuropsychology: Current Status and Applications*. Hemisphere, New York.

Heaton, R.K., Baade, L.E. and Johnson, K.L. (1978) Neuropsychological test results associated with psychiatric disorders in adults. *Psychol. Bull.*, **85**, 141–62.

Holzman, P.S. (1987) Recent studies of psychophysiology in schizophrenia. *Schizophr. Bull.*, **13**, 49–76.

Kahneman, D. (1973) *Attention and Effort*. Prentice-Hall, Englewood Cliffs, N.J.

Knight, R.A., Elliot, D.S. and Freedman, E.G. (1985) Short-term visual memory in schizophrenics. *J. Abnorm. Psychol.*, **94**, 427–42.

Kovelman, J.A. and Scheibel, A.B. (1984) A neurohistological correlate of schizophrenia. *Biol. Psychiatry*, **19**, 1601–21.

Kraepelin, E. (1913/1919) *Dementia Praecox and Paraphrenia*. (R.M. Barclay, trans). E. and S. Livingston, Edinburgh.

Miller, S., Saccuzzo, D. and Braff, D. (1979) Information processing deficits in remitted schizophrenics. *J. Abnorm. Psychol.*, **88**, 446–9.

Mirsky, A.F. and Duncan, C.C. (1986) Etiology and expression of schizophrenia: Neurobiological and psychosocial factors. *Ann. Rev. Psychol.*, **37**, 291–319.

Neisser, U. (1967) *Cognitive Psychology*. Appleton-Century-Crofts, New York.

Nuechterlein, K.H. (1983) Signal detection in vigilance tasks and behavioral attributes among offspring of schizophrenic mothers and among hyperactive children. *J. Abnorm. Psychol.*, **92**, 4–28.

Nuechterlein, K.H. and Asarnow, R.F. (1989) Cognition and perception. In *Comprehensive Textbook of Psychiatry/V*. H.I. Kaplan and B.J. Sadock (eds), Williams and Wilkins, Baltimore, pp. 241–56.

Nuechterlein, K.H. and Dawson, M.E. (1984a) A heuristic vulnerability/stress model of schizophrenic episodes. *Schizophr. Bull.*, **10**, 300–12.

Nuechterlein, K.H. and Dawson, M.E. (1984b) Information processing and attentional functioning in the developmental course of schizophrenic disorders. *Schizophr. Bull.*, **10**, 160–203.

Nuechterlein, K.H. and Zaucha, K.M. (1990) Similarities between information-processing abnormalities of acutely symptomatic schizophrenic patients and high-risk children. In *Schizophrenia: Concepts, Vulnerability and Intervention*. E. Straube and K. Halweg (eds), Springer-Verlag, Heidelberg, pp. 77–96.

Nuechterlein, K.H., Dawson, M.E., Ventura, J. *et al.* (1989) *Are schizophrenic deficits in signal detection during vigilance and span of apprehension vulnerability or episode indicators?* Presented at The International Congress on Schizophrenia Research, San Diego, CA.

Nuechterlein, K.H., Dawson, M.E, Ventura, J. *et al.* (1990) Testing vulnerability models: Stability of potential vulnerability indicators across clinical state. In *Search for the Causes of Schizophrenia, Vol 2*. H. Hafner and W.F. Gattaz (eds), Springer-Verlag, Heidelberg, 177–91.

Nuechterlein, K.H., Edell, W.S., Norris, M. and Dawson, M.E. (1986) Attentional vulnerability indicators, thought disorder, and negative symptoms. *Schizophr. Bull.*, **12**, 408–26.

Orzack, H.M. and Kornetsky, C. (1966) Attention dysfunction in chronic schizophrenia. *Arch. Gen. Psychiatry.*, **14**, 323–6.

Rosvold, H.E., Mirsky, A.F., Sarason, I., Bransome, E.D. and Beck, L.H. (1956) A continuous performance test of brain damage. *J. Consult. Psychol.*, **20**, 343–50.

Rutschmann, J., Cornblatt, B. and Erlenmeyer-Kimling, L. (1977) Sustained attention in children at risk for schizophrenia: Report on a continuous performance test. *Arch. Gen. Psychiatry*, **34**, 571–5.

Saccuzzo, D.P. and Braff, D.L. (1981) Early information processing deficit in schizophrenia. *Arch. Gen. Psychiatry*, **38**, 175–9.

Saccuzzo, D.P. and Braff, D.L. (1986) Information-processing abnormalities. *Schizophr. Bull.*, **12**, 447–59.

Spohn, H.E., Lacoursiere, R.B., Thompson, K. and Coyne, L. (1977) Phenothiazine effects on psychological and psychophysiological dysfunction in chronic schizophrenics. *Arch. Gen. Psychiatry*, **34**, 633–44.

Spohn, H.E. and Strauss, M.E. (1989) Relation of neuroleptic and anticholinergic medication to cognitive functions in schizophrenia. *J. Abnorm. Psychol.*, **98**, 367–80.

Suddath, R.L., Christian, G.W., Torrey, E.F., Casanova, M.F. and Weinberger, D.R. (1990) Anatomical abnormalities in the brains of monozygotic twins discordant for schizophrenia. *New Engl. J. Med.*, **322**, 789–94.

Watson, C.G., Thomas, R.W., Andersen, D. and Felling, J. (1968) Differentiation of organics from schizophrenics at two chronicity levels by use of the Reitan-Halstead organic test battery. *J. Consult. Clin. Psychol.*, **32**, 679–84.

Wohlberg, G.W. and Kornetsky, C. (1973) Sustained attention in remitted schizophrenics. *Arch. Gen. Psychiatry*, **28**, 533–7.

Zubin, J. and Spring, B. (1977) Vulnerability: A new view of schizophrenia. *J. Abnorm. Psychol.*, **86**, 103–26.

Chapter 4

Psychophysiological contributions to clinical assessment and treatment

GRAHAM TURPIN and KEITH CLEMENTS

4.1 INTRODUCTION

Psychophysiological measures have been extensively used by clinical researchers to investigate phenomena associated with the psychiatric construct of 'schizophrenia'. In contrast, practising clinicians have rarely resorted to such measures either during assessment or the course of treating these disorders. The major purpose of this chapter, therefore, is to attempt to construct a bridge between clinical research and clinical practice. This will necessitate examining, first of all, the historical application of psychophysiological research to schizophrenia. The various rationales for the use of psychophysiological measures adopted by clinical researchers will be identified and critically appraised. It will be argued that in order to provide an explanatory framework with which to view the plethora of research findings in this area, theoretical models will need to be developed which explain both the production of schizophrenic symptoms and also the role of psychophysiology in their study. Particular emphasis will be given to vulnerability models such as those proposed by Zubin and Spring (1977) and Nuechterlein and Dawson (1984). The use of psychophysiological measures to explore such models will be reviewed. Finally, the disparity between the use of psychophysiological measures in clinical research and practice will be addressed. On one hand, the limitations and obstacles relating to the application of psychophysiological measures to clinical practice will be discussed, on the other hand the potential advantages of adopting such measures for assessment and treatment evaluation will be outlined from the perspective of vulnerability models.

Since this chapter will attempt to evaluate the potential contribution of psychophysiological measures to clinical practice, an exhaustive review of clinical research in this area will not be undertaken. However, it is our intention to provide examples of both previous and current psychophysiological research into schizophrenia, which if supplemented by the numerous excellent reviews of this topic published elsewhere (e.g. Bernstein, 1987; Dawson et al., 1989; Steinhauer et al., in press) should provide the reader with a reasonably comprehensive account of psychophysiological endeavours in this area.

4.2 OVERVIEW OF PSYCHO-PHYSIOLOGICAL APPROACHES TO SCHIZOPHRENIA RESEARCH

From about the time of Kraepelin (1919) it has been speculated that schizophrenic disorders may be related to some underlying biological dysfunction. It is not surprising, therefore, that with the growth of psychophysiology as a scientific discipline (Turpin, 1989), clinical researchers would have adopted non-invasive physiological measures in order to investigate the origins of such a presumed biological substrate. However, psychophysiology also emphasizes the importance of psychological constructs and theories for the explanation of essentially behavioural phenomena (Turpin, 1989). Accordingly, it can be distinguished from *pathophysiology* which seeks purely to identify physiological dysfunction *per se* (Shagass, 1976). True psychophysiological studies have utilized generally non-invasive measures of the peripheral and central nervous system to investigate psychological constructs such as attention, arousal and vigilance. It is this adoption of presumably objective measures (Levenson, 1983), together with an emphasis upon psychological processes, which has presumably motivated clinical researchers to employ psychophysiological techniques in order to study the complex biological and physiological dysfunctions said to subsume schizophrenic disorders.

Early studies of people identified as schizophrenic were directed at resolving essentially diagnostic questions relating to differences in, for example, arousal (Lang and Buss, 1965), attention (Bernstein, 1967), autonomic balance (Wenger, 1966) or autonomic hyperactivity (Malmo and Shagass, 1952). Since these early forays into schizophrenia research, psychophysiological studies have become increasingly more diverse and sophisticated. Whereas early research was restricted largely to peripheral autonomic variables (skin conductance and heart rate activity) and measures of somatic tension (electromyographic activity, EMG), more recent research has employed a wide range of psychophysiological indices. These have included peripheral autonomic measures, central measures (the quantitative electro-

encephalogram, EEG; evoked potentials, EPs; electromagnetography; brain mapping), motoric measures (EMG, smooth pursuit eye movements, SPEMs; startle and blink responses), biochemical assays (e.g. monoamine oxidase metabolites or adrenaline and noradrenaline), radiographic and computerized tomographic techniques (e.g. CT, PET scans), together with a wide range of cognitive performance (e.g. the Continuous Performance Task, reaction time, orienting/habituation paradigms) and neuropsychological tasks. A detailed review of these techniques and their principal findings is beyond the scope of this chapter but they are covered in many reviews. Specifically, the general application of psychophysical measures have been previously reviewed exhaustively by other authors (e.g. Spohn and Patterson, 1979; Venables and Bernstein, 1983; Dawson and Nuechterlein, 1984; Zahn, 1986; Dawson *et al.*, 1989). Specific response systems have also been reviewed such as electrodermal activity (Ohman, 1981), the EEG (Saletu, 1980), evoked potentials (Duncan, in press; Roth *et al.*, 1986), smooth pursuit eye movements (Holzman and Levy, 1977; Cegalis *et al.*, 1982; Levy *et al.*, 1988) and orienting paradigms (Venables and Bernstein, 1983; Bernstein, 1987). Data on cognitive testing and information processing are reviewed in Chapter 3.

Before attempting any synthesis of these diverse findings, it is necessary to clarify the different rationales underlying various psychophysiological research questions. In addition, it is necessary to identify some general limitations which have raised problems for both the implementation and interpretation of psychophysiological measures.

4.2.1 RATIONALES FOR EMPLOYING PSYCHOPHYSIOLOGICAL MEASURES

Essentially, three inter-related but distinct rationales have driven psychophysiological research relating to schizophrenia. These concern diagnosis and discrimination, the study of psychological dysfunction *per se*, and the investigation of vulnerability models.

4.2.1.1 Diagnosis and discrimination

Perhaps the most influential rationale has concerned the questions of diagnosis and discrimination. The identification and subsequent classification of psychiatric syndromes have been largely based upon careful observational and phenomenological accounts of behaviours associated with abnormal mental states which accompany presumed psychiatric disorders (Wing *et al.*, 1974). However, psychiatric diagnosis has been fraught with numerous methodological difficulties such as limited construct and predictive validity, poor inter-observer reliability, and poorly operationalized criteria and assessment techniques (Morey *et al.*, 1986). Moreover, the construct of schizophrenia tends to illustrate the extremes of the controversies which surround the utility of psychiatric diagnoses (see Chapters 1 and 2). Accordingly, many researchers have proposed the use of more objective measures such as biological or cognitive variables which might help to operationalize what is said to be a poorly specified and heterogenous group of psychiatric disorders (e.g. Neale and Oltmanns, 1980). The adoption of 'biological markers' has, therefore, been advocated to strengthen both the construct and predictive validity of psychiatric disorders (Usdin and Hanin, 1982). Psychophysiological measures, given their non-invasive nature and relative ease of application, have been frequently adopted in attempts to discriminate the boundaries of schizophrenia. Early attempts generally focused on the possible identification of differences between physiological functioning (e.g. autonomic balance; Wenger, 1966) in schizophrenia and other psychiatric disorders. Later attempts have concerned putative psychophysiological dysfunctions such as arousal or attention which might account for the production of specific schizophrenic symptoms and help demarcate a particular schizophrenic entity.

Unfortunately, several substantial barriers exist which limit the easy application of psychophysiological measures to the diagnostic process (Turpin, 1989). Two major problems exist: methodological imprecision and the lack of diagnostic specificity.

As has already been alluded to, the diagnostic process is beset with methodological inconsistencies. Controversy still surrounds the exact operationalization and reliability of schizophrenic diagnoses (Chapters 1 and 2). Given the past existence of different diagnostic criteria, particularly between North American and European diagnostic practices, and the development of diverse diagnostic procedures and interview schedules, both the uniformity and reliability of individual schizophrenic diagnoses might be questioned. This is particularly true of studies conducted prior to the introduction of more standardized diagnostic procedures in the 1970s. Hence, equivocal findings from different studies may reflect methodological inconsistencies arising from the use of incompatible diagnostic criteria or dissimilar but undifferentiated subject populations.

Another source of methodological error concerns the assumption that psychophysiological measures provide objective and reliable diagnostic measures. In reality, psychophysiological measures are prone to numerous confounding variables such as diet, medication, activity levels, gender and ethnic differences, and situational and environmental variables (Iacono and Ficken, 1989; Turpin, 1989). In practice, careful consideration is required if these potential confounding influences are to be successfully controlled.

The second major problem relating to the adoption of psychophysiological diagnostic markers concerns their sensitivity and specificity. Sensitivity refers to the likelihood that a marker will consistently identify a specific disorder (i.e. the hit rate), whereas specificity concerns the ratio of specific cases identified versus non-related cases (i.e. the false alarm rate). For example, electrodermal hypo-responsibility and hyporeactivity are commonly obtained in schizophrenic samples (Ohman, 1979, 1981; Bernstein *et al.*, 1982). While this indicates a reasonable degree of sensitivity to schizophrenic characteristics, these electrodermal characteristics may also be observed in other diagnostic groups such as depression (e.g. Dawson *et al.*, 1977) and eating disorders (Callaway *et al.*, 1983). Consequently, the specificity of electrodermal activity for schizophrenia has to be considered to be low. Low specificity [1] may indicate a common psychopathological process. Alternatively, it may suggest the presence of some common and non-specific antecedent or consequent of psychopathological dysfunction such as inattention, poor motivation, non-specific affective change, psychological distress or discomfort.

In summary, a useful psychophysiological marker should be easily standardized and demonstrate high sensitivity and specificity. In practice, few measures yield this degree of diagnostic precision. However some measures may yield putative 'vulnerability' markers (see Iacono and Ficken, 1989) and this will be discussed in section 4.2.1.3. Moreover, it may be possible that multivariate combinations of psychophysiolological measures may provide greater predictive power than the use of single criterion measures (e.g. Shagass *et al.*, 1985).

4.2.1.2 Study of psychological dysfunction

It would be misleading to presume that most psychophysiological studies in schizophrenia have been prompted by the aim of developing biological diagnostic markers. Much published research in the last two decades has been directed at gaining a fuller understanding of the psychopathological processes underlying schizophrenia. Although this has invariably taken the form of identifying various differences between schizophrenic, non-schizophrenic psychiatric, and 'normal' control groups, the principle purpose has been to identify some underlying dysfunction subsuming the production of symptoms and hence, characterizing the essential nature of the disorder. Much of this research has been directed to the notion that schizophrenia may involve a fundamental filtering deficit within the information processing chain (Dawson and Neuchterlein, 1984; Zahn, 1986). Consequently much psycho-physiological research has been conducted employing paradigms designed to investigate information processing within experimental studies of non-pathological populations.

The most widely used approach has been the orienting response (OR) paradigm whereby simple stimuli, usually auditory tones of around 1000 Hz and 50–75 dB, are presented at inter-trial intervals of around 25–45 sec for up to 12 to 30 repetitions. In experimental psycho-pathology this is considered to represent a simple learning task whereby the subjects attend to the first few 'novel' stimulus presentations and demonstrate response habituation to the continued presentation of the stimulus series (Siddle, 1983). Although a range of autonomic and central measures may be employed as indices of orienting activity (Turpin, 1983), research into schizophrenia has predominantly utilized electrodermal responses. Studies of the OR in schizophrenic subjects have yielded a variety of findings (see Ohman, 1979, 1981; Venables and Bernstein, 1983; Dawson and Neuchterlein, 1984; Zahn, 1986; Bernstein, 1987). However, it appears that two distinct groups of schizophrenic response types emerge. First, a predominance of people fail to respond to the simple tone stimuli (around 40%) when compared with non-pathological, usually undergraduate populations (around 10%). Second, a smaller proportion of schizophrenic subjects demonstrates continued responding and a failure to habituate. This distinction between responder and non-responder subgroups has been said to suggest the possible existence of two distinct schizophrenic sub-types which may differ with respect to symptomatology (Gruzelier, 1976), task performance (Straube, 1979) and possible biological substrates (Alm *et al.*, 1984). Although we shall return to the detailed implications of this distinction for assessment later in the chapter, the interested reader should consult Bernstein (1987) for a greater in-depth discussion of the significance of the responder/non-responder dichotomy.

Psychological interpretations of electro-dermal habituation data have included 'overly permeable' versus 'closed' filters (Zahn, 1986); a dysfunction in the initiation of information processing in a limited capacity central processor (Ohman, 1979; Bernstein *et al.*, 1988; Dawson *et al.*, 1989) and the possibility of an 'arousal' regulation dysfunction (e.g. Rubens and Lapidus, 1978).

Central measures, such as evoked potentials (EP), have also been widely applied to the study of attentional deficits in schizophrenia. Evoked potentials are derived from the electroencephalogram (EEG) and consist of averages of stimulus evoked responses within the EEG (Callaway *et al.*, 1978; Donchin *et al.*, 1986; Hillyard and Hansen, 1986). The early or endogenous components reflect the physical attributes of the stimulus, whereas the later or exogenous components (e.g. P300, which is a positive wave occurring at 300 msec after the stimulus) are sensitive to psychological variables specifically associated with the experimental paradigm and include stimulus attributes such as novelty, expectancy, target *vs* non-target, distractability etc. A variety of paradigms have been employed ranging from 'odd ball' procedures, through to choice reaction time and dichotic listening tasks. The 'odd ball' paradigm is essentially a signal detection task where the target is a rare stimulus occurring in the context of more frequent stimuli. The range of paradigms employed relative to studies which have adopted autonomic measures such as skin conductance or heart rate, provides for a more sophisticated means to examine different attentional hypo

theses in schizophrenia research. Evoked potentials also yield more information concerning the timing and topography of brain-related events which in some circumstances can be related to cognitive processes, especially in the presence of accompanying behavioural data relating to task performance (e.g. reaction times, detection rates). The existence of behavioural data is also important since it helps rule out non-specific explanations of EP deficits such as general effects of motivation, task difficulty or distraction (e.g. Grillon *et al.*, 1990).

Much research which has adopted evoked potentials has been directed towards characterizing the specific nature of the 'filtering deficit' which has so frequently been postulated to exist in schizophrenia (Venables and Bernstein, 1983; Zahn, 1986). Some proponents of the filter deficit have emphasized an early 'stimulus set' dysfunction in pre-attentive processing resulting in a failure to inhibit responses to irrelevant stimuli. There is some evidence which is consistent with this interpretation concerning early to middle EP components (Shagass, 1979; Zahn, 1986). Studies which examined later EP components such as the P300 place greater emphasis on response set or pigeon-holing dysfunctions associated with subsequent categorical processing of stimuli (Baribeau, 1986). A consistent finding in schizophrenia is the reduced P300 (Zahn, 1986; Dawson *et al.*, 1989; Grillon *et al.*, 1990) which has been interpreted in terms of an overall reduced processing capacity, an inability to allocate processing capacity appropriately to relevant stimuli, or competition in processing demands between external and internal stimuli. Other explanations focus on the effects of an early pre-attentive deficit upon subsequent processing (e.g. Callaway and Naghdi, 1982). Recent studies have also related P300 changes in schizophrenia to symptom characteristics or medication and to state-trait vulnerability markers (Duncan, 1988; Pfefferbaum *et al.*, 1989). Although the potential of central measures for clinical assessment will be discussed later in this chapter, their major contribution to research in this area has undoubtedly been to provide what Duncan (1988) describes as 'a window on information processing'.

Although a major impetus for psychophysiological research has been directed mainly at investigating information processing deficits in schizophrenia, other important areas of study also exist. For example, many studies have obtained phasic and tonic autonomic measures, such as heart rate and electrodermal activity, in an attempt to quantify different arousal levels in schizophrenic sub-types (e.g. Fowles *et al.*, 1970). Similarly, quantitative EEG research using spectral analysis of the various different frequency wavebands present in the EEG has also focused upon arousal interpretations of differences between schizophrenic and control groups (Itil, 1977; Saletu, 1980). These have frequently been considered from the perspective of laterality differences (Gruzelier and Flor-Henry, 1979).

Despite the persistent conceptual problems which surround 'arousal' or 'activation' constructs (Turpin, 1989; Venables, 1984), the concept has frequently been used in schizophrenia research. Recently it has been proposed that arousal might represent a common pathway whereby psychosocial stressors such as expressed emotion (EE) or other life events (LE) might trigger schizophrenic episodes or the exacerbation of persistent schizophrenic symptoms (Turpin and Lader, 1986; Turpin *et al.*, 1988; Dawson *et al.*, 1989; Tarrier and Turpin, in press). This avenue of research was prompted by a study by Tarrier *et al.* (1978) of electrodermal and cardiovascular activity in a group of remitted schizophrenics living with their relatives. The patients were studied when socially interacting with their relatives who had previously been rated in terms of their expressed emotion. Ratings of expressed emotion are based upon a semi-structured interview with the patient's key relative, and are said to predict the likelihood that patients

will relapse in the future (Turpin *et al.*, 1988; Chapter 8). This study yielded an important finding that patients living with high expressed emotion relatives demonstrated greater levels of skin conductance responding than those living with low expressed emotion relatives. This was interpreted in terms of excessive arousal in the patients of high EE relatives which contributed to their subsequent relapse. This study has now been partially replicated several times (Sturgeon *et al.*, 1984; Tarrier 1989a, 1989b) and has important clinical implications which are discussed in Section 4.3.

In summary, psychophysiological measures have contributed to an understanding of the psychopathological process underlying production of psychotic phenemona and the manifestation of episodes of schizophrenia.

4.2.1.3 High-risk research

The majority of studies of psychological dysfunction described above adopted cross-sectional designs whereby groups of schizophrenic patients were compared either across different conditions or with different patient or control groups. The basis for this is the underlying assumption that specific differences in psychophysiological activity between the groups might be related to differences in symptoms that are used to define the groups in terms of psychiatric nosologies. In contrast, psychophysiological measures have sometimes been employed in longitudinal designs in order to examine for example, relationships between changes in symptomatology, risk of morbidity or familial aggregation. Essentially, such designs are directed towards questions concerning aetiology and the identification of casual explanations of the origins of schizophrenic disorders.

Recent examples to account for the origins of schizophrenia have emphasized the importance of multifactorial models (e.g. Zubin and Spring, 1977) which stress the interaction of many diverse domains including biological, developmental, social and interpersonal factors. Accordingly, these models have frequently been termed psychosociobiological or vulnerability models. Not only do these models seek to explain differences in functioning between pathological and normal groups, but also the development of the disorder within the population. Consequently, the models have distinguished between the expression of the disorder within the population, as indicated by the onset of symptoms, and the transmission of risk or predisposition in those individuals vulnerable to developing the disorder (cf. Turpin and Lader, 1986; Turpin *et al.*, 1988). Early examples of theoretical accounts which emphasize the interaction of predispositional and triggering factors have included Meehl's (Meehl, 1989) classical paper entitled 'Schizotaxia, schizotypy and schizophrenia' and the stress-diathesis models of genetic expression in schizophrenia (Garmezy and Streitman, 1974; Rosenthal, 1970).

In order to identify risk factors which might predispose individuals to develop schizophrenia sometime in their lives, it is necessary to study people at risk for schizophrenia longitudinally. This approach is termed 'high risk research' and has frequently employed psychophysiological markers. At risk groups for developing schizophrenia are frequently identified in terms of their family relationship to individuals already diagnosed schizophrenic (Watt *et al.*, 1984; Goldstein and Tuma, 1987). An early example was a study by Mednick and Schulsinger (1973) who employed autonomic orienting and conditioning measures to predict later risk for the development of psychopathology. Risk itself has also been defined with respect to psychophysiological variables (e.g. Venables, 1978). Autonomic indices of risk which have been suggested from high-risk research include electrodermal hyperactivity (Ohman, 1981), skin conductance conditioning and recovery rates (Mednick and Schulsinger, 1973), and in more recent studies, even electrodermal hyporesponsivity (Erlenmeyer-Kimling

et al., 1985). Central measures have also been employed in high risk research, but to a lesser degree (Zahn, 1986; Dawson *et al.*, 1989). Another psychophysiological measure which has been specifically identified as a possible genetic marker is known as smooth pursuit eye movements (SPEM). Subjects are required to track a small visual target whilst eye movements are recorded using either electro-oculographic (EOG) or infra-red eye movement techniques. The accuracy of tracking is either assessed qualitatively or quantitatively (Dawson *et al.*, 1989). According to some authors (e.g. Holzman *et al.*, 1974) SPEM abnormalities are prevalent in the relatives of people diagnosed schizophrenic, and may therefore represent a form of genetic marker. The problems associated with categorizing and identifying biological markers have been discussed at length elsewhere (Iacono, 1983; Iacono and Fricken, 1989).

Psychophysiological measures have been adopted in other types of prospective research design. These include the identification of putative risk in non-patient populations using schizotypy personality measures (e.g. Simons, 1981, 1982; Miller, 1986).

4.3 THE NEED FOR THEORETICAL MODELS TO GUIDE DEVELOPMENTS IN PSYCHOPHYSIOLOGICAL RESEARCH

We have attempted to review some of the principal findings and rationales associated with psychophysiological research in schizophrenia. Even within the limitations of such a cursory review, the range of studies and their sometimes equivocal outcomes present a formidable task for those intent on integrating these data into the general body of schizophrenic research. Psychophysiological measures have frequently been employed within a context of 'mini-theories' seeking to explain schizophrenic deficits associated with psychological concepts such as orienting, attention or arousal. However, this poses a problem both to the theoretically minded researcher and the practising clinician who wish to extrapolate from these observations to an overall understanding of schizophrenia. For example, with regard to psychosomatic disorders, Weiner (1977) identified three important questions which need to be addressed if an understanding of a proposed 'disease' process is to be found. These are the ability to identify factors associated with the risk of the disorder within the population, the factors that mediate the expression of risk, and the processes and mechanisms which account for the specific production of symptoms. In order to provide a more comprehensive account of psychophysiological research within schizophrenia, the contribution of this approach to these three questions needs to be clearly specified. Unfortunately, until recently the 'mini-theories' which have guided psychophysiological investigations have lacked the scope to address these issues. However, recent theoretical developments are beginning to yield more heuristic models within which the role of psychophysiology can be addressed.

Perhaps the most influential turning point within schizophrenia research during the last three decades has been the development of vulnerability models. These models stress the multifactorial contribution of a variety of aetiological factors including genetic, developmental and social factors that may contribute to population risk for schizophrenia. They also adopt a longitudinal perspective and distinguish between factors associated with the development of risk (causal or formative influences) and those factors that account for the expression of risk as individual schizophrenic episodes (precipitant or triggering factors). Finally, they also attempt to identify the psychological processes that mediate these events and seek to identify markers which can be adopted to study the differential impact of formative and precipitant influences on the expression of schizophrenia. A classic example of such an approach is the 'stress vulnerability model'

proposed by Zubin and his colleagues (Zubin and Spring, 1977; Zubin and Steinhauer, 1981; Spring and Coons, 1982). The model relies on the notion of a trait-like vulnerability factor which determines the population risk for schizophrenia. The actual manifestation of the illness is the result of challenging and/or stressful environmental events interacting with this vulnerability factor. The model is essentially a threshold model whereby the individual crosses the boundary from 'well' to 'ill' (displaying schizophrenic symptoms) if the level of environmental stress exceeds a threshold value for any particular level of vulnerability. The model also broadly defines the factors which determine vulnerability and the events associated with the initiation of illness onset. The utility of this and other psychobiological models for psychopathology research has been discussed elsewhere (Turpin and Lader, 1986; Turpin *et al.*, 1988).

Vulnerability models have imposed a structure within which psychophysiological research may be examined. Indeed, many authors have identified psychophysiological measures as being potentially useful markers for dissociating the processes underlying vulnerability and the expression of schizophrenic symptoms (Ohman, 1981; Zubin and Steinhauer, 1981; Nuechterlein and Dawson, 1984; Iacono and Ficken, 1989; Meehl, 1989). Until recently they have lacked any specific psychophysiological focus. Nuechterlein and Dawson (1984) have proposed a revised 'stress vulnerability' model for schizophrenia which is essentially based upon psychophysiological research and theory. This model is illustrated in Figure 4.1. It is a significant advance upon Zubin and Spring's original vulnerability model since it attempts to specify in detail the processes that mediate the expression of risk into the manifestation of schizophrenic symptoms. As can be seen from Figure 4.1, vulnerability is characterized by factors such as reduced processing capacity, hyperarousal and poor social competence, which result in an increased risk of an individual

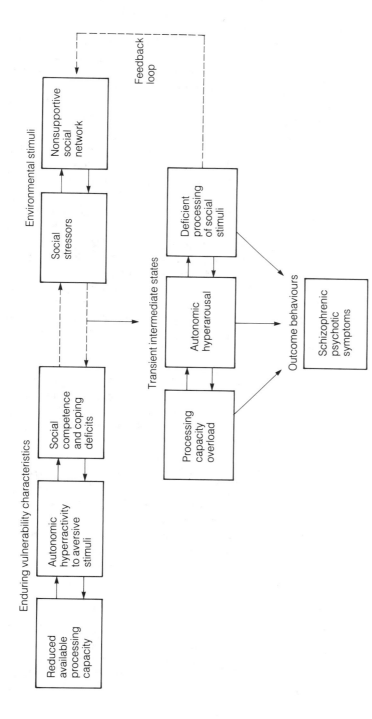

Figure 4.1 Nuechterlein and Dawson's 'tentative, interactive vulnerability/stress model for the development of schizophrenic episodes'. (Reproduced by permission of the *Schizophrenia Bulletin* from Nuechterlein and Dawson, 1984.)

exhibiting symptoms of schizophrenia if exposed to social stressors such as expressed emotion, life events or inadequate social supports etc. In order to describe the process underlying this interaction, Nuechterlein and Dawson (1984) define several 'transient states' which may, in the absence of reduced social stressors or enhanced coping, develop into the full manifestation of schizophrenic symptoms and their associated disabilities and social handicaps.

It has been previously argued (Turpin *et al.*, 1988) that the above model provides a sound basis for psychophysiological research in schizophrenia. It would appear that a 'final common pathway' in the expression of symptoms can be identified in psychophysiological terms. For example 'autonomic hyperarousal' is associated with both vulnerability (e.g. reduced processing capacity) and psychosocial stressors (e.g. life events and expressed emotion), and with intermediate transient states (e.g. processing capacity overload, deficient processing of social stimuli). It would appear, therefore, that psychophysiology is well placed to evaluate the presence of this 'final common pathway' (Tarrier and Turpin, in press; Turpin *et al.*, 1988).

We propose, therefore, that the above model provides a framework for general understanding which has utility both for the researcher and clinician alike. From a theoretical perspective, it provides a broad scenario within which the contribution of psychophysiology and its associated 'mini-theories' can be incorporated and tested. It also helps to impose a structure upon the interpretation of schizophrenic psychophysiological deficits. For example, should cross-sectional psychophysiological differences be considered as indicators of vulnerability or mediational-vulnerability, as episode markers or as responses to psychosocial stressors? The complex pattern of markers differentially associated with the model requires a more sophisticated interpretation of psychophysiological differences across different patient groups than existing diagnostic formulations. At the very least, state-trait distinctions

need to be made (Duncan, 1988) which will require longitudinal research strategies which result in data from at-risk groups, patients who are floridly ill, and patients in remission. This problem will be discussed in Section 4.4. Unfortunately, it can also be argued that the breadth and scope of the model gives rise to difficulties in empirically testing the model and ensuring that it is falsifiable. Such an argument has been made by Dimsdale (1982) in relation to other broadly conceived psychobiological models. In addition, schizophrenia is treated in a general, if not an even unitary fashion. Issues relating to sub-type differences (e.g. positive vs. negative symptoms) and the general controversy surrounding the 'psychosis continuum vs. discrete syndrome categories' argument, perhaps, need to be incorporated into future versions of the model.

From a clinical perspective, vulnerability models pose several advantages. Firstly, given their multifactorial view of aetiology, they provide the potential for an acceptable 'melting pot' of ideas which may be accessible to different professionals working within multidisciplinary teams, each tending to have separate and distinct philosophical models and outlooks. At an anecdotal level, such models often provide an accessible and non-controversial middle-ground which facilitates communication and clinical decision making both between different professions and with clients themselves. Secondly, vulnerability models provide both a structure and means with which psychophysiological measures might be incorporated within clinical assessments and interactions. This approach will form the basis of the remainder of this chapter.

4.4 PSYCHOPHYSIOLOGY AND CLINICAL PRACTICE

The purpose of this section is to construct a bridge between clinical research and practice. In Section 4.3 we have identified some of the major research findings and have outlined a general vulnerability model which might provide a basis for establishing the relevance of the psychophysiological approach to the general study of schizophrenia. We now wish to examine the clinical implications of both this approach and the existing psychophysiological database associated with schizophrenia. For example, the enthusiastic and optimistic, if not to say naïve, reader of Section 4.3 might assume that psychobiological measures ought to be able to define population risk, yield reliable diagnoses, discriminate between different sub-groups and effectively monitor treatments and interventions. Unfortunately, few examples of such a progressive psychophysiological approach to clinical practice exist. It should be stressed, therefore, from the outset, that this section is primarily concerned with the *potential* for clinical applications. Clinical psychophysiology, although well-represented in applied research, is rarely adopted in clinical practice (Turpin, 1989, 1991). We aim, first of all, to identify some of the obstacles which have prevented the widespread use of psychophysiological measures in clinical settings. We will then go on to suggest some possible applications for both assessment and intervention. Examples of the potential use of psychophysiological measures will be drawn from the clinical research literature, and these will be critically assessed with respect to their possible clinical utility and feasibility.

4.4.1 OBSTACLES TO THE IMPLEMENTATION OF CLINICAL PSYCHOPHYSIOLOGY

Assuming that sound rationales, together with reliable and valid psychophysiological measures exist [2] what other factors might account for the lack of the widespread implementation of psychophysiological measures? Perhaps the major issue concerns access. Most psychophysiological research is laboratory-based requiring sophisticated facilities and equipment whereas clinicians tend to be in centres that

have little or no laboratory facilities. Similarly, psychophysiology requires sophisticated technical and academic expertise which is rarely available to clinicians. Finally, there is the question of the relationship between laboratory research and research based within the 'real world' (in the clinic or the patients' social environment). In order to optimize the potential of clinical psychophysiology, it will be essential that methods can be adopted and used within clinical settings. However, this presents two problems. First, from a practical perspective, how feasible is it to transfer laboratory-based paradigms and measures into the clinical setting? Second, if this is achieved what is the relationship between laboratory results and psychophysiological observations obtained in the real world? This issue concerns the 'generalizability' of psychophysiological data across diverse situations. Findings from other areas of study such as hypertension might suggest that laboratory assessments may have a limited or restricted generalizability to the 'real world'. For example, laboratory-based measures of cardiovascular reactivity to cognitive stressors may not always relate to naturalistic assessments of reactivity throughout a 24-hour period (Johnston *et al.*, 1990).

How can these potential obstacles be overcome? First, there should be a greater awareness of psychophysiology in the training of clinicians. Previous surveys of graduate and clinical psychology training within the USA reveal that this is frequently quite variable (Feuerstein and Schwartz, 1977; Jones and Collins, 1989). Second, in order to facilitate the use of psychophysiological measures in clinical settings laboratory procedures need to be either modified or simplified. An example of the former approach includes the development of ambulatory recording whereby psychophysiological measures are obtained using miniaturized equipment from the free-moving and unrestricted patient (Turpin, 1985; 1990). An example of the latter approach is the development of simple measures, such as the Palmar Sweat Index, which can be easily and economically used in field settings (Clements *et al.*, in press; Koehler and Voegele, 1989). Tarrier's use of social-interaction settings also provides an alternative approach (Tarrier *et al.*, 1978). Once measures can be obtained in both laboratories and the 'real world', questions concerning generalizability and the possible reactivity of laboratory assessment (Turpin, 1989; 1990) can then be examined. Finally, it is important that psychophysiologists address issues of clinical relevance, in addition to examining issues of theoretical importance. For instance, if psychophysiological measures could be developed to identify 'at risk' groups for the early onset of schizophrenia, or to predict differential treatment outcomes, or to identify individual episodes of schizophrenic relapse prior to behavioural indicators, clinicians might show greater interest in the adoption of these measures.

4.4.2 APPLICATIONS TO ASSESSMENT

Psychophysiological measures are frequently identified as having potential to play a major role in clinical assessment (Haynes *et al.*, 1989; Turpin, 1989). For a detailed discussion of the issues surrounding their use in clinical assessment, albeit from a behavioural analysis perspective, the interested reader should consult a recent review (Turpin, 1990). With respect to schizophrenia, the issue of assessment will be approached from both a traditional diagnostic approach and also from the perspective of vulnerability models.

4.4.2.1 Diagnostic applications

As has already been discussed, psychophysiological measures have frequently been adopted in the hope that they might provide sensitive and specific markers with which to separate different diagnostic categories. When examining their diagnostic utility, a distinction

should be made (cf. Turpin, 1989) between attempts to discriminate between different diagnostic entities such as schizophrenic and affective disorders, and applications directed at prognostic information concerning different schizophrenic sub-types (e.g. positive vs. negative, process vs. reactive etc). Given the common proposal that schizophrenia is an imprecisely defined, and possibly heterogeneous collection of disorders of diverse aetiologies, this distinction is probably more apparent than real. However, from a clinical perspective it is highly relevant since it might help demarcate the limits of the boundary conditions for using psychophysiological measures as practical assessment instruments.

Most research which attempted to demonstrate major diagnostic differences in psychophysiological variables was conducted several decades ago. For example, many authors (e.g. Bernstein, 1967) had attempted to observe differences in 'arousal' which might be specifically related to schizophrenia. As already discussed, 'arousal' differences that have been observed are frequently inconsistent, highly dependent upon sub-types and not specific to schizophrenic disorders. Other attempts that have used more sophisticated measures, such as evoked potentials, have proved more successful. Shagass (1985) examined the *potential* clinical utility of somatosensory, visual and auditory EPs recorded from 253 unmedicated patients representing a broad range of psychiatric diagnoses and 99 non-patients. Multivariate statistical methods were employed to reduce the EP amplitude measurements into a set of factor scores which were subsequently used to discriminate between the various diagnostic groups. The data from this study suggested possible clinical applications of EP measurement to the discrimination of schizophrenic from other mainly non-psychiatric groups. The increase in the widespread availability of multichannel, computerized EEG systems or brain mappers (e.g. Karson *et al.*, 1988; Maurer, 1989; Sampson-Dollfus, 1989) may see a renewed interest in the use of central psychophysiological measures as possible tools to unravel differential psychiatric diagnoses.

More recent applications of psychophysiology to questions of discrimination and diagnosis have focused upon identifying sub-types within the spectrum of schizophrenic disorders. Sub-types can either be defined with respect to symptoms or to biological markers (Turpin, 1989). Perhaps the most widely known example concerns electrodermal responsivity and non-responsivity (e.g. Gruzelier and Venables, 1975; Bernstein *et al.*, 1982). As discussed in Section 4.2 it has been claimed that at least two distinct types of electrodermal deficit may be present in schizophrenia: electrodermal non-responsivity and electrodermal hyper-reactivity (Ohman, 1981; Venables and Bernstein, 1983; Dawson and Nuechterlein, 1984; Bernstein, 1987). It is possible that these electrodermal deficits may be related to positive vs. negative syndromes of schizophrenia (Bernstein, 1987; Tarrier and Turpin, in press). Moreover, it has also been suggested that symptom ratings on scales such as the Brief Psychiatric Rating Scale (Overall and Gorham, 1962) may also be generally related to electrodermal activity (Gruzelier and Manchanda, 1982; Olbrich and Mussgay, 1987; Dawson *et al.*, 1989). Similar claims have also been made for sub-type differences in relation to P300. For example, Baribeau (1986) has observed that the P300 was more abnormal in a formally thought-disordered schizophrenic group than inpatients not displaying formal thought disorder. Similarly, several authors have associated P300 attenuation with the severity of negative symptoms in schizophrenia (e.g. Pfefferbaum *et al.*, 1989). Moreover, Shenton *et al.* (1989) have suggested that the topographical distribution of P300 deficits may be associated with two distinct schizophrenic syndromes. If different symptomatic sub-types in schizophrenia can be assumed to be associated with diverse aetiologies, outcomes and response to treatment, then the ability to distinguish between such sub-types on the basis of psychophysiological responding would certainly possess clinical advantages.

4.4.2.2 Vulnerability markers

The majority of the distinctions made above have been based on cross-sectional studies of various psychiatric groups. If a prospective approach is adopted in conjunction with a 'stress-vulnerability' approach, it is necessary to identify additional categories of marker than those based exclusively upon the presence of different psychiatric symptoms. In particular, the detection of psychophysiological deficits in high-risk groups that are defined either on the basis of familial association (Watt *et al.*, 1984) or putative premorbid personality types (e.g. Simons, 1981, 1982; Buchsbaum and Haier, 1983) may indicate the presence of vulnerability markers. Similarly, the presence of psycho-physiological deficits in people already diagnosed schizophrenic but in the absence of symptoms when the disorder is in remission may also be indicative of a psychophysiological vulnerability marker (Iacono, 1982). As discussed above, several psychophysiological indices have been identified as possible vulnerability markers for schizophrenia in general or for particular schizophrenic sub-types. These include electrodermal non-responsivity (Bernstein, 1987), electrodermal hyper-reactivity (Ohman, 1981), the auditory P300 (Duncan, 1988) and SPEMs (Holzman *et al.*, 1974). The presence of such markers might help to identify vulnerable individuals present in the population. Vulnerability models also identify the importance of episode markers which are associated with the presence of schizophrenic symptoms. Once again, episode or state markers might include the visual P300 (Duncan, 1988) or certain electrodermal variables (Dawson *et al.*, 1989).

Psychophysiological measures may also be sensitive to other factors described by the 'stress-vulnerability' model. The presence of psychosocial stressors such as life events (e.g. Nuechterlein *et al.*, 1989) or expressed emotion (Sturgeon *et al.*, 1984) may also be reflected by psychophysiological indices such as electrodermal activity. If such differences are only evident in vulnerable individuals, this might be evidence of 'vulnerability-mediational' markers as described by Nuechterlein and Dawson (1984).

4.4.2.3 Clinical implications

It could be argued that the inclusion of psychophysiological measures within clinical assessment might have several distinct advantages. First, they might help identify individuals at risk for schizophrenia and hence lead on to primary and secondary forms of prevention. They may also yield potential for helping to decide between various differential dignoses. For people already identified as schizophrenic in terms of behavioural symptoms, psychophysiological measures might help define distinct sub-types which could be associated with differential outcomes and treatment methods. Finally, the increased risks associated with exposure to psychosocial stressors such as EE or LE might also be identified by psychophysiological variables (e.g. Tarrier and Barrowclough, 1984).

Unfortunately, the full potential of clinical psychophysiology for the clinical assessment of schizophrenia has yet to be realized. The reasons for this have alredy been identified at the beginning of this section. Nevertheless, it is hoped that some of these obstacles might be overcome, and the clinical utility of psychophysiological measures be explored in a thorough but cost-effective manner.

4.4.3 APPLICATIONS TO TREATMENT

To a large extent the distinction between assessment and treatment is artificial. The choice of different treatments may depend exclusively upon information derived from a clinical assessment, and hence, psychophysiological methods may have some bearing upon both. For example, if psychophysiological measures could identify individuals at risk for developing schizophrenia, some early intervention or primary prevention strategy might be indicated. Unfortunately, our lack of knowledge concerning the early developmental processes associated with the development of schizophrenia is not sufficient to identify effective interventions (Asarnow and Goldstein, 1986). Moreover, the sociopolitical consequences of such an approach might also need to be carefully considered.

The major area where psychophysiological assessment might influence treatment is in the determination of the clinical course and outcome for individuals already diagnosed as experiencing schizophrenia. Methods for the prediction of outcome in schizophrenia have not received much support in the past (e.g. Bland, 1982). However, psychophysiologically diferentiated sub-types such as electrodermal responders/non-responders might identify important sub-groups of patients with quite distinct outcomes. As discussed by Tarrier and Turpin (in press), elevated electrodermal activity (slow habituation and high levels of SCL and NS-SCRs) seems to be predictive of short-term outcome as regards the reappearance of symptoms, or response to neuroleptic medication. For example, Straube (1989) has replicated a previous finding that habituation rate and NS-SCR frequency are associated with the number of days of hospitalization for patients receiving short-term treatment. Similarly, Sturgeon *et al.* (1984) presented data consistent with the view that elevated SCR frequency was associated with both high EE and future risk for symptomatic relapse. However, it has also been argued by Alm *et al.* (1984) that non-responding might be associated with vulnerability for a particular schizophrenic sub-type characterized by poor premorbid functioning, family-linkage, poor neuroleptic treatment response, and a negative symptom profile. Indeed, recent data by Ohman *et al.* (1989) suggest that electrodermal non-responding is indicative of poor social outcomes as measured by unemployment and restricted social contacts. The apparent inconsistency between electrodermal findings and outcome may be dependent upon the nature of the outcome measure that is employed (Tarrier and Turpin, in press). Other psychophysiological measures have also been used as outcome indicators, particularly in relation to predicting the response to neuroleptic treatment (Zahn, 1986).

Psychophysiological assessment may in the future be able to focus interventions by identifying particular sub-groups at risk for poor neuroleptic treatment response, high expressed emotion or poor social adjustment. Such information may inform the clinician as regards the particular choice of medication and psychosocial interventions. Further research is required to establish the unique contribution of those measures to the overall prediction of outcome.

Finally, the use of prospective psychophysiological measures may also have potential for helping to determine not only the choice of intervention but also its timing. The prediction of individual episodes of relapse has recently been said to be facilitated by the longitudinal measurement of 'early signs' which are commonly based upon the patients self-report or those of either clinicians or relatives (Subotnik and Nuechterlein, 1986; Birchwood *et al.*, 1989; see also Chapter 6). This approach has two aims: to enhance the involvement of patients and significant others in being able to cope with schizophrenic episodes and to provide a potentially more effective delivery of neuroleptic treatment via the use of low-dose or intermittent medication regimes (Chiles *et al.*, 1989; see also Chapter 19). It is possible that psychophysiological measures might also aid in the detection of early signs of relapse. For example, it has already been suggested that electrodermal activity in some patients might predict short-term outcome and incipient

relapse. Moreover, some preliminary data by Dawson would appear to demonstrate elevations in skin conductance level that precede the onset of relapse or exacerbation of symptoms in a small sample of individual patients (Dawson *et al.*, 1989; Dawson, 1990). If electrodermal data could be together with observations and self-reports of symptoms collected on a regular (weekly or bi-weekly?) basis, the utility of a psychophysiological 'early signs' approach might be tested. However, as with all psychophysiological procedures, the expertise and equipment required might seriously threaten the cost-effectiveness of such an approach. The development of simpler and more economic analogues of electrodermal assessment, such as the PSI, might present an alternative, although rather speculative, approach (Clements *et al.* 1990).

4.5 CONCLUSION

We have attempted to provide a broad overview of the application of psychophysiology to enhancing the understanding of schizophrenia. It is important when evaluating psychophysiological methods that the rationales for their use are clearly identified. It has been argued that from the perspective of the clinical researcher, psychophysiological studies have yielded unique and useful data concerning basic processes subserving schizophrenia (e.g. attention) and have also contributed to the development of heuristic psychosociobiological models of aetiology. From the clinical viewpoint, it has to be recognized that few if any of the applications from this research have been implemented or even recognized. It is hoped that clinical researchers might address this discrepancy by also focusing upon research questions with direct and demonstrable clinical benefits.

NOTES

1. In the case of electrodermal non-responding, it has also been argued that the cause for

this autonomic dysfunction may differ in schizophrenia and depression. In schizophrenia, non-responding is observed in other autonomic measures such as finger pulse amplitude and appears to be differentially affected by instructions compared with findings from depressive disorders (Bernstein *et al.*, 1988). A possible explanation, therefore, is that non-responding in schizophrenia results from an information processing deficit at a central level, whereas in depression it may reflect a more peripheral cholinergic deficit.

2. For a fuller and general discussion of these assumptions see Turpin (1989, 1990).

REFERENCES

Alm, T., Lindstrom, L., Ost, L.G., and Ohman, A. (1984) Electrodermal non-responding in schizophrenia: relationships to attentional, clinical, biochemical and computed tomographical and genetic factors. *Int. J. Psychophysiol.*, **1**, 195–208.

Asarnow, J.R. and Goldstein, M.J. (1986) Schizophrenia during adolescence and early adulthood: a developmental perspective on risk research. *Clin. Psychol. Rev.*, **6**, 211–35.

Baribeau, J. (1986) Current evoked potential research and information processing in schizophrenics. *Integ. Psychiatry*, **4**, 109–13.

Bernstein, A.S. (1967) Electrodermal base level, tonic arousal and adaptation in chronic schizophrenics. *J. Abnorm. Psychol.*, **72**, 221–32.

Bernstein, A.S. (1987) Orienting response research in schizophrenia: where we have come from and where we might go. *Schizophr. Bull.*, **13**, 623–41.

Bernstein, A.S., Frith, C.D., Gruzelier, J.H. *et al.* (1982) An analysis of skin conductance orienting responses in samples of British, American and German schizophrenics. *Biol. Psychol.*, **14**, 155–211.

Bernstein, A.S., Riedel, J.A., Graae, F. *et al.* (1988) Schizophrenia is associated with altered orienting response; depression with electrodermal (cholinergic?) deficit and normal orienting response. *J. Abnorm Psychol.*, **97**, 3–12.

Birchwood, M., Smith, J., MacMillan, F. *et al.* (1989) Predicting relapse in schizophrenia: the development and implementation of an early signs monitoring system using patients and families as observers, a preliminary investigation. *Psychol. Med.*, **19**, 649–56.

Bland, R.C. (1982) Predicting the outcome in schizophrenia. *Can. J. Psychiatry*, **27**, 52–62.

Buchsbaum, M.S. and Haier, R.J. (1983) Psychopathology: biological perspectives. *Ann. Rev. Psychol.*, **34**, 401–30.

Callaway, E. and Naghdi, S. (1982) An information processing model for schizophrenia. *Arch. Gen. Psychiatry*, **39**, 339–47.

Callaway, E., Tueting, P. and Koslow, S. (1978) (eds) *Event Related Brain Potentials in Man*, Academic Press, New York.

Callaway, P., Fonagy, P. and Wakeling, A. (1983) Autonomic arousal in eating disorders: further evidence for the clinical subdivision of anorexia nervosa. *Br. J. Psychiatry*, **142**, 38–42.

Cegalis, J.A., Sweeney, J.A. and Dellis, E.M. (1982) Reflex saccades and attention in schizophrenia. *Psychiatry Res.*, **7**, 189–98.

Chiles, J.A., Sterchi, D., Hyde, T. and Herz, M.I. (1989) Intermittent medication for schizophrenic outpatients: who is eligible. *Schizophr. Bull.*, **15**, 117–21.

Clements, K., Romer, M., Turpin, G. and Hahlweg, K. (in press) Symptomatic correlates of palmar sweat gland activity in schizophrenic individuals. *Psychophysiology*, **27**.

Dawson, M.E. (1990) Psychophysiology at the interface of clinical science, cognitive science and neuroscience. *Psychophysiology*, **27**, 243–55.

Dawson, M.E., Liberman, R.P. and Mintz, L.I. (1989) Sociophysiology of expressed emotion in the course of schizophrenia. In *Sociophysiology of Social Relationships*. P. Barchos (ed), Oxford Press, New York.

Dawson, M.E. and Nuechterlein, K.H. (1984) Psychophysiological dysfunctions in the developmental course of schizophrenic disorders. *Schizophr. Bull.*, **10**, 204–32.

Dawson, M.E., Nuechterlein, K.H. and Adams, R.E. (1989) Schizophrenic disorders. In *Handbook of Clinical Psychophysiology*. G. Turpin (ed), Wiley, Chichester, pp. 393–418.

Dawson, M.E., Schell, A.M. and Catania, J.J. (1977) Autonomic correlates of depression and clinical improvement following electroconvulsive shock therapy. *Psychophysiology*, **14**, 569–78.

Dimsdale, J.E. (1982) Appraising psychobiological approaches to the influences of stress on depression, *Behav. Brain. Sci.*, **5**, 104–5.

Donchin, E., Karis, D., Bashore, T.R., Coles, M.G.H. and Gratton, G. (1986) Cognitive psychophysiology and human information processing. In *Psychophysiology: Systems, Processes and Applications*. M.G.H. Coles, E. Donchin and S.W. Portes (eds), Guilford, New York, pp. 244–67.

Duncan, C.C. (1988) Event-related brain potentials: a window on information processing in schizophrenia. *Schizophr. Bull.*, **14**, 200–3.

Duncan, C.C. (in press) Current issues in the application of P300 to research on schizophrenia. In *Schizophrenia: Models, Vulnerability and Intervention*. E. Straube and K. Hahlweg (eds), Springer-Verlag, New York.

Erlenmeyer-Kimling, L., Friedman, D., Cornblatt, B. and Jacobsen, R. (1985) Electrodermal recovery data on children of schizophrenic parents. *Psychiatry Res.*, **14**, 148–61.

Feuerstein, M. and Schwartz, G.E. (1977) Training in clinical psychophysiology? Present trends and future goals. *Am. Psychol.*, **32**, 560–8.

Fowles, D.C., Watt, N.F., Maher, B.A. and Grinspoon, L. (1970) Autonomic arousal in good and poor premorbid schizophrenics. *Br. J. Soc. Clin. Psychol.*, **9**, 135–47.

Garmezy, N. and Streitman, S. (1974) Children at risk: the search for the antecedents of schizophrenia. Part 1. Conceptual models and research methods. *Schizophr. Bull.*, **1**, 14–90.

Goldstein, M.J. and Tuma, A.H. (1987) High-risk research: editors' introduction. *Schizophr. Bull.*, **13**, 369–72.

Grillon, C., Courchesne, E., Ameli, R., Geyer, M.A. and Braff, D.L. (1990) Increased distractibility in schizophrenic patients: electrophysiologic and behavioural evidence. *Arch. Gen. Psychiatry*, **47**, 171–9.

Gruzelier, J.H. (1976) Clinical attributes of schizophrenic skin conductance responders and non-responders. *Psychol. Med.*, **6**, 245–9.

Gruzelier, J.H. and Flor-Henry, P. (eds) (1979) *Hemisphere Asymmetries of Function in Psychopathology*. Elsevier, Amsterdam.

Gruzelier, J.H. and Manchanda, R. (1982) The syndrome of schizophrenia: relations between electrodermal response lateral asymmetries and clinical ratings. *Br. J. Psychiatry*, **141**, 488–95.

Gruzelier, J.H. and Venables, P.H. (1975) Evidence of high and low levels of physiological arousal in schizophrenia. *Psychophysiology*, **12**, 66–73.

Haynes, S.N., Falkin, S. and Sexton-Radek, K. (1989) Psychophysiological assessment in behaviour therapy. In *Handbook of Clinical Psychophysiology*. G. Turpin (ed), Wiley, Chichester, pp. 69–102.

Hillyard, S.A. and Hansen J.C. (1986) Attention: electrophysiological approaches. In *Psychophysiology: Systems, Processes and Applications*. M.G.H. Coles, E. Donchin and S.W. Porges (eds), New York, Guilford, pp. 227–43.

Holzman, P.S. and Levy, D.L. (1977), Smooth pursuit eye movements and functional psychoses: A review. *Schizophr. Bull.*, **3**, 15–27.

Holzman, P.S., Proctor, L.R., Levy, D.L., Yasillo, N.J., Meltzer, H.Y. and Hurt, S.W. (1974) Eye-tracking dysfunctions in schizophrenic patients and their relatives. *Arch. Gen. Psychiatry*, **31**, 143–51.

Iacono, W.G. (1982) Bilateral electrodermal habituation-dishabituation and resting EEG in remitted schizophrenics. *J. Nerv. Ment. Dis.*, **170**, 91–101.

Iacono, W.G. (1983) Psychophysiology and genetics: a key to psychopathology research, *Psychophysiology*, **20**, 371–83.

Iacono, W.G. and Ficken, J.W. (1989) Research strategies employing psychophysiological measures: identifying and using psychophysiological markers. In *Handbook of Clinical Psychophysiology*. G. Turpin (ed), Wiley, Chichester, pp. 45–70.

Itil, T.M. (1977) Qualitative and quantitative EEG findings in schizophrenia. *Schizophr. Bull.*, **3**, 61–79.

Johnston, D.W., Anastasiades, P. and Wood, C. (1990) The relationship between cardiovascular responses in the laboratory and in the field. *Psychophysiology*, **27**, 34–44.

Jones, G. and Collins, S.W. (1989) Survey of training opportunities in psychophysiology. *Psychophysiology*, **26**, (Suppl.), S36.

Karson, C.N., Coppola, R., Daniel, D.G. and Weinberger, D.R. (1988) Computerized EEG in schizophrenia. *Schizophr. Bull.*, **14**, 193–7.

Koehler, T. and Voegele, C. (1989) Laboratory studies on a potential stress indicator in field research: the palmar sweat index. In *Psychobiology: Issues and Applications*. N. Bond and D.A.T. Siddle (eds), North Holland, Amsterdam, pp. 337–45.

Kraepelin, E. (1919) *Dementia Praecox and Paraphrenia*, 1971 ed., R.B. Barclay (trans.), Krieger, Huntington, NY.

Lang, P.J. and Buss, A.H. (1965) Psychological deficit in schizophrenia: II. Interference and activation. *J. Abnorm. Psychol.*, **70**, 77–126.

Levenson, R.W. (1983) Personality research and psychophysiology: general considerations. *J. Res Pers.*, **17**, 1–21.

Levin, S., Luebke, A., Zee, D.S. *et al.* (1988) Smooth pursuit eye movements in schizophrenics: quantitative measurements with the search-coil technique. *J. Psychiatry Res.*, **22**, 195–206.

Malmo, R.B. and Shagass, C. (1952) Studies of blood pressure in psychiatric patients under stress. *Psychosom. Med.*, **14**, 82–93.

Maurer, K. (ed) (1989) *Topographic Brain Mapping of EEG and Evoked Potentials*. Springer-Verlag, London.

Mednick, S.A. and Schulsinger, F. (1973) Studies of children at high risk for schizophrenia. In *Schizophrenia: The First Ten Dean Award Lectures*. S.R. Dean (ed), MSS Information Corp., New York.

Meehl, P.E. (1962) Schizotaxia, schizotypy, schizophrenia. *Am. Psychol.*, **17**, 827–38.

Meehl, P.E. (1989) Schizotaxia revisited. *Arch. Gen. Psychiatry*, **46**, 935–44.

Miller, G.A. (1986) Information processing deficits in anhedonia and perceptual aberration: A psychophysiological analysis. *Biol. Psychiatr.*, **21**, 100–15.

Morey, L.C., Skinner, H.A. and Blashfield, R.K. (1986) Trends in the classification of abnormal behaviour. In *Handbook of Behaviour Assessment. 2nd ed.* A.R. Ciminero, K.S. Calhoun and H.E. Adams (eds), Wiley, New York, pp. 47–75.

Neale, J.M. and Oltmanns, T.F. (1980) *Schizophrenia*. Wiley, Chichester.

Nuechterlein, K.H. and Dawson, M. (1984) A heuristic vulnerability/stress model of schizophrenic episodes. *Schizophr. Bull.*, **10**, 300–12.

Ohman, A. (1979) The orienting response, attention and learning: an information processing perspective. In *The Orienting Reflex in Humans*. H.D. Kimmel, E.H. van Olst and J.F. Orlebeke (eds), Erlbaum, Hillsdale, NJ, pp. 443–71.

Ohman, A. (1981) Electrodermal activity and vulnerability to schizophrenia: A review. *Biol. Psychol.*, **123**, 87–145.

Ohman, A., Ohlund, L.S., Alm, T., Wieselgren, I.M., Ost, L.G. and Lindstrom, L.H. (1989) Electrodermal non-responding, premorbid adjustment and symptomatology as predictors of long-term social functioning in schizophrenics. *J. Abnorm. Psychol.*, **98**, 426–35.

Olbrich, R. and Mussgay, L. (1987) Spontaneous fluctuations of electrical skin conductance and the actual clinical state in schizophrenia, *Psychopathology*, **20**, 18–22.

Overall, J.E. and Gorham, D.R. (1962) The brief psychiatric rating scale. *Psychol. Reports*, **10**, 799–812.

Pfefferbaum, A., Ford, J.M., White, P. and Roth, W.T. (1989) P3 in schizophrenia is affected by stimulus modality, response requirements, medication status, and negative symptoms. *Arch. Gen. Psychiatry*, **46**, 1035–44.

Rosenthal, D. (1970) *Genetic Theory and Abnormal Behaviour*. McGraw-Hill, New York.

Roth, W.T., Duncan, C.C., Pfefferbaum, A. and Timsit-Berthier, M. (1986) Applications of cognitive ERPs in psychiatric patients. In *Cerebral Psychophysiology: Studies in Event-Related Potentials. (EEG Supplement 38)* W.C. McCallum, R. Zappoli and F. Denoth (eds), Elsevier, Amsterdam, pp. 419–38.

Rubens, R.L. and Lapidus, L.B. (1978) Schizophrenic patterns of arousal and stimulus barrier functioning. *J. Abnorm. Psychol.*, **87**, 199–211.

Saletu, B. (1980) Central measures in schizophrenia. In *Handbook of Biological Psychiatry: Part II. Brain Mechanisms and Abnormal Behaviour – Psychophysiology*. H.M. Van Praag, M.H. Lader, O.J. Rafaelsen and E.J. Sachar (eds), Marcel Dekker, New York, pp. 97–144

Sampson-Dollfus, D. (ed) (1989) *Statistics and Topography in Quantitative EEG.* Elsevier, Amsterdam.

Shagass, C. (1976) An electrophysiological view of schizophrenia. *Biol. Psychol.*, **11**, 3–30.

Shagass, C. (1979) Sensory evoked potentials in psychosis. In *Evoked Brain Potentials and Behavior*, (Vol. 2). H. Begleiter (ed), Plenum, New York.

Shagass, C., Roemer, R.A., Straumaris, J.J. and Josianssen, R.C. (1985) Combinations of evoked potential amplitude measurements in relation to psychiatric diagnosis. *Biol. Psychiatry*, **20**, 701–22.

Shenton, M.E., Ballinger, R., Marcy, B. *et al.* (1989) Two syndromes of schizophrenic psychopathology associated with left *vs* right deficits in P30 amplitude. *J. Nerv. Ment. Dis.*, **177**, 219–25.

Siddle, D. (1983) *Orienting and Habituation: Perspectives in Human Research.* Wiley, Chichester.

Simons, R.F. (1981) Electrodermal and cardiac orienting in psychometrically defined high-risk subjects. *Psychiatry Res.*, **4**, 347–56.

Simons, R.F. (1982) Physical anhedonia and future psychopathology: an electrocortical continuity? *Psychophysiology*, **19**, 433–41.

Sponh, H.E. and Patterson, T. (1979) Recent studies of psychophysiology in schizophrenia. *Schizophr. Bull.*, **5**, 581–611.

Spring, B. and Coons, H. (1982) Stress as a precursor of schizophrenia. In *Psychological Stress and Psychopathology.* R.W.J. Neufeld (ed), McGraw-Hill, New York, pp. 13–54.

Steinhauer, S., Gruzelier, J.H. and Zubin, J. (in press) (eds), *Handbook of Schizophrenia, 4: Experimental Psychopathology, Neuropsychology and Psychophysiology.* Elsevier, Amsterdam.

Straube, E.R. (1979) On the meaning of electrodermal nonresponding in schizophrenia. *J. Nerv. Ment. Dis.*, **167**, 601–11.

Straube, E., Wagner, W., Foerster, K. and Heimann, H. (1989) Findings significant with respect to short- and medium-term outcome in schizophrenia: A preliminary report. *Prog. Neuropsychopharm. Biol. Psychiatry*, **13**, 185–97.

Sturgeon, D., Turpin, G., Kuipers, L., Berkowitz, R.

and Leff, J. (1984) Psychophysiological responses of schizophrenic patients to high and low expressed emotion relatives: a follow-up study. *Br. J. Psychiatry*, **145**, 62–9.

Subotnik, K.L. and Nuechterlein, K.H. (1988) Prodromal signs and symptoms of schizophrenic relapse. *J. Abnorm. Psychol.*, **97**, 405–12.

Tarrier, N. (1989a) Arousal level and relatives' expressed emotion in remitted schizophrenic patients. *Br. J. Clin. Psychol.*, **28**, 177–80.

Tarrier, N. (1989b) Electrodermal activity, expressed emotion and outcome in schizophrenia. *Br. J. Psychiatry*, **155** (Suppl. 5), 51–6.

Tarrier, N. and Barrowclough, C. (1984) Psychophysiological assessment of expressed emotion in schizophrenia: A case example. *Br. J. Psychiatry*, **145**, 197–203.

Tarrier, N. and Barrowclough, C. (1987) A longitudinal psychophysiological assessment of a schizophrenic patient in relation to the expressed emotion of his relative. *Behav. Psychother.*, **15**, 45–57.

Tarrier, N., Vaughn, C.E., Lader, M.H. and Leff, J.P. (1978) Bodily reactions to people and events in schizophrenia. *Arch. Gen. Psychiatry*, **36**, 311–15.

Tarrier, N. and Turpin, G. (in press) Psychosocial factors, arousal and schizophrenic relapse: a review of the psychophysiological data. *Br. J. Psychiatry.*

Turpin, G. (1983) Unconditional reflexes and autonomic neurons system. In *Orienting and Habituation: Perspectives in Human Research*, D. Siddle (ed), Wiley, Chichester, pp. 1–70.

Turpin, G. (1985) Ambulatory psychophysiological monitoring: techniques and applications. In *Clinical and Experimental Neuropsychophysiology.* D. Papakostopolous, S. Butler and I. Martin (eds), Croom Helm, London, pp. 695–728.

Turpin, G. (1989) An overview of clinical psychophysiological techiques: tools or theories? In *Handbook of Clinical Psychophysiology.* G. Turpin (ed), Chichester, Wiley, pp. 3–44.

Turpin, G. (1990) Ambulatory clinical psychophysiological monitoring: an introduction to techniques and methodological issues. *J. Psychophysiol.*, **4**, 299–304.

Turpin, G. (1991) Psychophysiology and behavioural assessment: is there scope for theoretical frameworks? In *Handbook of*

Behavior Therapy and Psychological Science: An Integrative Approach, P. Martin (ed), Pergamon, New York, pp. 348–82.

Turpin, G. and Lader, M. (1986) Life events and mental disorder: biological theories of their mode of action. In *Life Events and Psychiatric Disorders: Controversial Issues*. H. Katschnig (ed), Cambridge University Press, Cambridge, pp. 33–62.

Turpin, G., Tarrier, N. and Sturgeon, D. (1988) Social psychophysiology and the study of biopsychosocial models of schizophrenia. In *Social Psychophysiology: Theory and Clinical Applications*. H.L. Wagner (ed), Wiley, Chichester, pp. 251–72.

Venables, P.H. (1978) Psychophysiology and Psychometrics. *Psychophysiol.*, **15**, 302–15.

Venables, P.H. (1984) Arousal: An examination of its status as a concept. In *Psychophysiological Perspectives: Festschrift for Beatrice and John Lacey*. M.G.H. Coles, J.R. Jennings and J.A. Stern (eds), Van Rostrand Reinhold, New York.

Venables, P.H. and Bernstein, A.S. (1983) The orienting response and psychopathology: Schizophrenia. In *Orienting and Habituation: Perspec tives in Human Research*. D. Siddle (ed), Wiley, Chichester, pp. 475–504.

Watt, N.F., Anthony, E.J., Wynne, L.C. and Rolf, J.E. (1984) *Children at Risk for Schizophrenia: A Longitudinal Perspective*. Cambridge University Press, Cambridge.

Weiner, H. (1977) *Psychobiology and Human Disease*. Elsevier, New York.

Wenger, M.A. (1966) Studies of autonomic balance. *Psychophysiol*, **2**, 173–86.

Wing, J.K., Cooper, J.E. and Sartorius, N. (1974) *The Measurement and Classification of Psychiatric Symptoms*. Cambridge University Press, Cambridge.

Zahn, T.P. (1986) Psychophysiological approaches to psychopathology. In *Psychophysiology: Systems, Processes and Applications*. M.G.H. Coles, E. Donchin and S.W. Porges (eds), Guilford Press, New York.

Zubin, J. and Spring, B. (1977) Vulnerability: a new view of schizophrenia. *J. Abnorm. Psychol.*, **86**, 260–6.

Zubin, J. and Steinhauer, S. (1981) How to break the logjam in schizophrenia: a look beyond genetics. *J. Nerv. Ment. Dis.*, **169**, 477–92.

Chapter 5

Biochemistry of schizophrenia

F. OWEN and A.J. CROSS

Schizophrenia is a common mental disorder with a life-time prevalence of approximately 1% (Gottesmann, 1982). It is generally accepted that genetic factors play a significant role in the aetiology of the disease although the mode of inheritance remains obscure (Matthysse and Kidd, 1976; McGue *et al.*, 1983; Karlsson, 1988). If a component of schizophrenia is genetically transmitted then it follows that a biochemical basis for the disease should be detectable. The theory that the primary disturbance in schizophrenia has a neurochemical basis is plausible because there has been a widely held view that there are no gross structural changes in the brains of schizophrenics. However in recent years there seems to be a consensus of opinion that there are some, albeit subtle, abnormalities in brain structure (e.g. Brown *et al.*, 1986). The major investigations of a neurochemical basis for schizophrenia have focused on:

1. Impairment of serotonergic function;
2. Impairment of noradrenergic function;
3. Excessive dopaminergic function;
4. A deficiency in monoamine oxidase activity;
5. an impairment of gamma-amino butyric acid (GABA) system function;
6. Impairment of excitatory amino acid systems;
7. Impairment of neuroactive peptide systems.

5.1 SEROTONERGIC FUNCTION IN SCHIZOPHRENIA

The possibility that a deficit in central serotonergic function was associated with schizophrenia was proposed by Wooley and Shaw (1954) following the observation that the administration of compounds such as yohimbine, bufotenin, harmine and lysergic acid diethylamide (LSD), which had structural similarities with serotonin (5–HT) and were active at 5–HT receptors, caused behavioural changes in animals and mental disturbances in man. However, initial reports of a reduction in central 5–HT metabolism in schizophrenia, assessed by lumbar cerebrospinal fluid (CSF) concentrations of 5-hydroxyindoleacetic acid (5–HIAA) – the major end product of 5–HT metabolism (Ashcroft *et al.*, 1966; Bowers, 1969; Post *et al.*, 1975) were not confirmed using the more refined technique employing probenecid to block the egress of 5–HIAA from CSF. Reduced plasma concentrations of tryptophan, the precursor of 5–HT, have been reported in acute schizophrenics (Manowitz *et al.*, 1973; Domino and Krause, 1974) but the therapeutic effectiveness of the administration of oral doses of tryptophan to correct this apparent deficit has produced equivocal results (Bowers, 1970; Wyatt *et al.*, 1972; Gillin *et al.*, 1976).

The work of Pollin *et al.* (1961) suggested that schizophrenia may be associated with an increase rather than a decrease in central serotonergic function since the administration of tryptophan together with a monoamine oxidase inhibitor (MAOI) to schizophrenics exacerbated the psychosis. Support for this suggestion came later from the observations that LSD appears to act as a 5–HT agonist in the central nervous system (Aghajanian *et al.*, 1970) and that some neuroleptic drugs which are effective in the treatment of schizophrenia are also potent 5–HT antagonists (Leyson *et al.*, 1978). However clinical trials of the 5–HT antagonist, cinanserin, have shown the drug to be ineffective in the treatment of schizophrenia (Gallant and Bishop, 1968; Holden *et al.*, 1971).

A direct investigation of central 5–HT metabolism in schizophrenia was carried out by Joseph *et al.* (1979), who measured the concentrations of 5–HT, 5–HIAA and their precursor, tryptophan, in three regions of post-mortem brain tissue from 23 controls and 15 schizophrenics. An analysis of the influence of drug treatment, cause of death, age and the time from autopsy to deep-freezing the brain material on the results showed that there was no generalized change in 5–HT metabolism in the brains of schizophrenics.

Serotonin receptor subtypes have been studied in brains of schizophrenics by several groups. [^{3}H]–LSD, which labels both 5–HT$_1$ and 5–HT$_2$ receptors (Cross, 1982), binds to an equal number of sites in the frontal cortex of controls and schizophrenics (Whitaker *et al.*, 1981). The binding of ligands selective for either 5–HT$_1$ or 5–HT$_2$ receptors are also unchanged in schizophrenics, although in one study a reduction in [^{3}H]–LSD binding with no change in [^{3}H]–5–HT binding was noted (Bennett *et al.*, 1979; Owen *et al.*, 1981). It would seem reasonable to conclude that changes in serotonin receptors are not a general finding in schizophrenia, and taken in conjunction with studies on serotonin metabolism it would seem that serotonergic mechanisms remain intact in schizophrenia.

Recent experimental data have implicated a role of the 5–HT$_3$ receptor in the schizophrenic process. 5–HT$_3$ receptor density is extremely low in the human brain, and it remains to be determined if 5–HT$_3$ receptors are altered in schizophrenia, and indeed if 5–HT$_3$ receptor antagonists possess antipsychotic activity in the clinic.

5.2 NORADRENERGIC FUNCTION IN SCHIZOPHRENIA

Stein and Wise (1971) postulated that a degeneration of the cortical noradrenergic reward system could account for the lack of goal-directed behaviour observed in schizophrenics. They strengthened this hypothesis by reporting a significant reduction in the activity of dopamine-β-hydroxylase (DBH) activity in post-mortem brain samples from schizophrenics (Wise and Stein, 1973). DBH catalyses the conversion of dopamine to noradrenaline and is a marker enzyme for noradrenergic neurones. However, Wyatt *et al.* (1975) failed to replicate the finding of Wise and Stein (1973) although if paranoid patients were excluded from their results DBH activity in samples from the remaining patients tended to be reduced compared with controls. Hartmann (1976) and Hartmann and Keller-Teschke (1977) elaborated on the hypothesis of Stein and Wise (1971) by suggesting that a deficit in cortical DBH activity could lead to an increased concentration of dopamine and a decreased concentration of noradrenaline in cortical regions and that this imbalance in dopamine and noradrenaline may be involved in the pathogenesis of schizophrenia. However, the evidence for a central noradrenergic deficit in schizophrenics is not strong. Cross *et al.* (1978) assessed DBH activity in 6 brain regions from 12 controls and 12 schizophrenics. The results of this investigation are presented in Table 5.1. There was no significant difference in DBH activity

Table 5.1 DBH activity in post-mortem brain of schizophrenics and controls

Brain area	(DBH activity)	
	Controls (n = 12)	Schizophrenics (n = 12)
Hypothalamus	*131.0 ± 41*	156.4 ± 55
Hippocampus	24.1 ± 8	24.8 ± 9
Parietal cortex	25.2 ± 7	21.2 ± 8
Frontal cortex	24.1 ± 7	26.8 ± 9
Occipital cortex	26.9 ± 8	23.9 ± 7
Temporal cortex	24.2 ± 6	25.2 ± 6

Results (mean ± s.d.) expressed as nmol product formed/g tissue/h.

between controls and schizophrenics in any brain region. It is noteworthy that when DBH activity was compared in neuroleptic-treated and neuroleptic-free patients a reduction in enzyme activity was observed in treated patients which reached statistical significance in the hippocampus, the brain region with the greatest DBH reduction in the initial study of Wise and Stein (1973). Cross *et al.* (1978), therefore, suggested that the adverse effect of neuroleptic medication on DBH activity together with the lability of the enzyme in post-mortem tissue might account for the reductions reported by Wise and Stein (1973). In addition, although Wise *et al.* (1974) suggested that a degeneration of noradrenergic neurones was reflected in reductions in catechol-O-methyltransferase (COMT) activity, Cross *et al.* (1978) found COMT activity to be similar in controls and schizophrenics in all 12 brain regions studied.

Joseph *et al.* (1976) attempted to assess central noradrenergic function in schizophrenia by comparing the urinary excretion of the conjugates of 3-methoxy-4-hydroxyphenylglycol (MHPG; the major end-product of noradrenaline metabolism in the brain) in chronic schizophrenics. Maas and Landis (1968) and Maas *et al.* (1973) reported that a substantial proportion of urinary MHPG was derived from the brain in the dog and in the monkey. Moreover, Bond and Howlett (1974), and Bond *et al.* (1975) suggested that the sulphate conjugate of MHPG in urine originated in the brain

whereas MHPG-glucuronide originated in the periphery. Using a specific glucuronidase to selectively hydrolyse the MHPG-glucuronide component of total urinary MHPG, Joseph *et al.* (1976) were able to compare total MHPG, MHPG-sulphate and MHPG-glucuronide excreted by controls and schizophrenics. The only significant finding was an inverse correlation between the severity of the illness and the daily excretion of MHPG-sulphate in chronic unmedicated schizophrenics. This could be interpreted as reflecting low brain noradrenaline turnover in those patients who developed a more severe illness. Since there was no difference between controls and schizophrenics in the daily excretion of MHPG-sulphate, Joseph *et al.* (1976) concluded that reduced brain noradrenaline turnover is neither necessary nor sufficient for schizophrenia to occur. Indeed in a subsequent study, Joseph *et al.* (1979) were unable to replicate an inverse correlation between MHPG-sulphate excretion and severity of schizophrenic symptoms.

There have been several other attempts to assess central noradrenergic function in schizophrenia using peripheral body fluids and tissues such as plasma, serum, platelets and lymphocytes. The results, in general, have been equivocal and often of dubious relevance to central noradrenergic function. The topic has been admirably reviewed by Van Kammen and Antelman (1984).

Adrenergic receptors have been studied using ligands selective for β-receptors and both α_1- and α_2- receptor sub-types in the basal ganglia and cortical regions. In all these studies receptor binding has been unchanged in schizophrenics (Owen *et al.*, 1981; Bennett *et al.*, 1979).

5.3 DOPAMINERGIC FUNCTION IN SCHIZOPHRENIA

The dopamine hypothesis of schizophrenia evolved from two convergent lines of evidence; (1) antipsychotic drugs are effective dopamine antagonists and (2) dopamine releasing drugs can induce a psychosis in mentally normal subjects that closely resembles paranoid schizophrenia.

5.3.1 ANTIPSYCHOTIC DRUGS

With the advent of an assay for dopamine-sensitive adenylate cyclase it became clear that the potency of a range of phenothiazine and thioxanthene drugs in this system correlated well with their clinical potency (Miller *et al.*, 1974; Clement-Cormier *et al.*, 1974). A striking discrepancy in this system was that butyrophenones, such as haloperidol, were much less effective at inhibiting dopamine-sensitive adenylate cyclase activity than their clinical potency suggested. This discrepancy was resolved when it became clear that there were at least two classes of dopamine receptors, designated D_1 and D_2 by Kebabian and Calne (1979). The potency in displacing the high affinity binding to the D_2 receptor of antipsychotic drugs, including the butyrophenones, is closely correlated with their clinical efficacy (Seeman *et al.*, 1976).

5.3.2 DOPAMINE RELEASING DRUGS

The second line of evidence suggesting that excessive central dopaminergic activity is associated with schizophrenia comes from the observation that the amphetamine psychosis closely resembles paranoid schizophrenia (Connell, 1958). In addition Randrup and Munkvad (1965, 1966) have reported that the behavioural changes induced in rats by amphetamine administration could be selectively reversed by neuroleptic drugs.

From these two lines of evidence came the suggestion (Randrup and Munkvad, 1972) that schizophrenia was associated with excessive dopaminergic function in the central nervous system.

Pharmacological evidence to support the dopamine hypothesis of schizophrenia was provided by the results of a clinical trial of the therapeutic efficacy of the optical isomers of flupenthixol. Flupenthixol exists in a cis (or α) and trans (or β) form that have many properties in common except that α-flupenthixol has much greater anti-dopaminergic potency than the β-isomer. Over a four-week trial period of patients with acute episodes of schizophrenia α-flupenthixol possessed significant therapeutic activity compared with β-flupenthixol or a placebo (Johnstone *et al.*, 1978). This result is consistent with the hypothesis of excessive central dopaminergic function in schizophrenic patients.

Investigations of the concentration of homovanillic acid (HVA – the major end-product of dopamine metabolism) in CSF have produced no evidence of increased brain turn-over of dopamine in schizophrenia (Bowers, 1974; Post *et al.*, 1975; Berger *et al.*, 1980). Similarly measurements of the concentration of dopamine and its end-products 3,4-dihydroxy-phenylacetic acid (DOPAC) and HVA in post-mortem brain tissue from schizophrenics have produced no evidence of increased dopamine turnover associated with the disease. Table 5.2 summarizes the results of a collaborative study between the Division of Psychiatry, Clinical Research Centre, Harrow, England and the MRC Neurochemical Pharmacology Unit, Cambridge, England (Bird *et al.*, 1979). Although dopamine concentrations were increased in samples of nucleus accumbens of schizophrenics in the Cambridge study and in the caudate nucleus of schizophrenics in the CRC study, in neither study were the increases associated with dopamine release since there were no corresponding increases in DOPAC or HVA. These findings do not support the hypothesis of an association between excessive dopaminergic function and schizophrenia.

Dopamine receptors have been studied extensively in the brains of schizophrenics, and in general there is a concensus that D_2 receptors are increased in the basal ganglia. Initial studies employed [3H]-spiperone or [3H]-haloperidol

Table 5.2 Dopamine and its metabolites in post-mortem brain samples from controls and schizophrenics[1]

CRC study	Controls (n=19)	Schizophrenics (n=18)
Caudate		
Dopamine	1.6 ± 0.3	2.5 ± 0.3*
HVA	5.4 ± 0.3	3.8 ± 0.5**
DOPAC	1.3 ± 0.2	0.8 ± 0.1
Accumbens		
Dopamine	0.9 ± 0.3	0.7 ± 0.1
HVA	4.7 ± 0.5	5.5 ± 0.5
DOPAC	1.5 ± 0.02	1.1 ± 0.2

Cambridge study	Controls (n=25)	Schizophrenics (n=25)
Caudate		
Dopamine	1.7 ± 0.2	2.0 ± 0.2
HVA	4.3 ± 0.4	5.6 ± 0.8
DOPAC	0.8 ± 0.1	0.5 ± 0.1
Accumbens		
Dopamine	1.4 ± 0.1	2.0 ± 0.2***
HVA	4.4 ± 0.3	4.9 ± 0.6
DOPAC	0.4 ± 0.04	0.4 ± 0.1

[1]Values are means ± SEM; μg/g tissue
* $p < 0.05$; ** $p < 0.02$; *** $p < 0.01$

to label D_2 receptors (Owen *et al.*, 1978; Lee *et al.*, 1978) and in both cases an increase in ligand binding was observed in basal ganglia. This finding has subsequently been confirmed by many other groups (Mackay *et al.*, 1980; Reynolds *et al.*, 1980; Hess *et al.*, 1987). In the initial study of Owen *et al.* (1978) it was suggested that the increase in D_2 receptors could not be attributed entirely to the neuro-leptic treatment which most of the patients had received. In subsequent studies (Table 5.3), involving a group of patients who had never received neuroleptic medication, an increase in D_2 receptor binding was apparent when compared with controls (Crow *et al.*, 1982). Whilst it is clear that chronic treatment of experimental animals with high doses of neuroleptics results in an elevation of D_2 receptors (Burt *et al.*, 1982), the increase observed in some schizophrenic patients is considerably greater than that observed experimentally.

Several studies have been performed on brain samples from patients who had received neuroleptic treatment but were not schizophrenic (Cross *et al.*, 1985). In patients with either Alzheimer-type dementia or Huntington's disease, those patients who had received neuroleptic treatment had similar D_2 receptor binding to drug-free patients (Table 5.3). Striatal degeneration occurs in Huntington's disease, and in Alzheimer-type dementia D_2 receptors are reduced compared with controls. However it has been shown in experimental animals that kainic acid-induced striatal degeneration does not affect the development of D_2 receptor supersensitivity in response to chronic neuroleptic treatment (Owen *et al.*, 1981). These results could suggest that the increase in D_2 receptors observed in schizophrenics is not entirely due to prior neuroleptic intake. Seeman and colleagues (1984) have observed a bimodal distribution

Table 5.3 Dopamine D_2 receptor binding in schizophrenia

		Controls	Drug-free patients	Drug-treated patients
Schizophrenia	Putamen	208 ± 11 (39)	324 ± 75 (7)**	419 ± 34 (23)**
	Accumbens	181 ± 15 (33)	305 ± 76 (5)*	318 ± 36 (16)**
Huntington's chorea	Caudate	—	73 ± 8 (8)	87 ± 10 (15)
Sentile dementia	Putamen	—	90 ± 9 (10)	89 ± 12 (10)

D_2 receptors assessed using [³H]-spiperone binding. For schizophrenia, maximum binding values are quoted. For Huntingtons chorea and senile dementia, binding was determined using 0.8nM ligand. Values are fmol ligand bound/mg protein, mean ± SEM, number of samples in parentheses.
* $p < 0.05$; ** $p < 0.02$

distribution of D_2 receptor binding and drug-free patients were found to be distributed equally between groups of patients with high or low D_2 receptors. Despite these observations the relationship between increased D_2 receptor binding in brains from schizophrenics and prior neuroleptic treatment remains controversial.

Dopamine D_1 receptors have also been studied in brains from schizophrenic patients (Cross *et al.*, 1981). Ligand binding studies have consistently shown that D_1 receptors are not increased in schizophrenics, and may even be decreased (Hess *et al.*, 1987; Czudek and Reynolds, 1988). Although Memo *et al.* (1983) reported an increase in dopamine-stimulated adenylate cyclase activity in the caudate nucleus and nucleus accumbens of schizophrenic patients, other studies have failed to confirm this finding (Carenzi *et al.*, 1975). In experimental animals, chronic neuroleptic treatment results in increased D_1 receptor binding. That D_1 receptors are not increased in the brains of schizophrenics may suggest that any effects of chronic neuroleptic treatment are not as important as previously supposed.

5.4 MONOAMINE OXIDASE ACTIVITY IN SCHIZOPHRENIA

Monoamine oxidase (MAO) inactivates brain catecholamines and serotonin by oxidative deamination to form the corresponding aldehyde. The enzyme has been classified as MAO-A and MAO-B on the basis of its sensitivity to inhibition by specific inhibitors. MAO-A is relatively sensitive to inhibition by clorgyline (Johnston, 1968) and MAO-B by deprenyl (Knoll and Magyar, 1972). Serotonin is a specific substrate for MAO-A (Johnston, 1968) and benzylamine for MAO-B (Christmas *et al.*, 1972).

The interest in MAO activity in schizophrenia arose from the observation that the administration of an MAOI with or without methyl donors exacerbated the symptoms of schizophrenia. (For a review see Brune, 1965.) In 1972, Murphy and Wyatt reported a significant reduction in platelet MAO activity in chronic schizophrenia. A year later Wyatt *et al.* (1973) reported that both monozygotic twins discordant for schizophrenia had significantly reduced platelet MAO activity compared with controls and hence reduced MAO activity might prove to be a genetic marker for vulnerability to schizophrenia. In a subsequent study, however, the same group (Murphy *et al.*, 1974) did not find reduced platelet MAO activity in acute schizophrenics. Several investigations confirmed the initial finding of Murphy and Wyatt (1972) of reduced platelet MAO activity in chronic schizophrenia (Domino and Khanna, 1976; Murphy *et al.*, 1976; Berrettini *et al.*, 1978; Gruen *et al.*, 1982) whereas other studies found no difference in enzyme activity between controls and schizophrenics (Owen *et al.*, 1976; Mann *et al.*, 1981).

Since platelet MAO activity has been reported to be normal in some studies of neuroleptic-free patients (Friedman *et al.*, 1974; Takahashi *et al.*, 1975; Owen *et al.*, 1976; Mann and Thomas, 1979) and particularly since it has also been reported that platelet MAO activity decreases progressively with neuroleptic medication (Takahashi *et al.*, 1975; Friedhoff *et al.*, 1978; Delisi *et al.*, 1981; Owen *et al.*, 1981) it seems increasingly likely that the reduction in platelet MAO activity in schizophrenia reported by some groups of workers is a consequence of drug treatment.

Robinson *et al.* (1968) reported that platelet MAO had some characteristics in common with the enzyme in liver and brain. Thus a possible implication of a reduction in platelet MAO activity in schizophrenia was that it was reflecting reduced MAO activity in the brain. Studies on post-mortem brain tissues from schizophrenics, however, do not support this possibility. Most studies have reported MAO activity in post-mortem brains from schizophrenics to be no different from controls

(Vogel *et al.*, 1969; Domino *et al.*, 1973; Wise *et al.*, 1974; Schwartz *et al.*, 1974; Cross *et al.*, 1977; Crow *et al.*, 1979; Revely *et al.*, 1981). In a very early study, Birkhäuser (1941) actually reported increased MAO activity in the pallidum of schizophrenics. There has been one report of an altered regional distribution of MAO activity in the brains of schizophrenics (Utena *et al.*, 1968) and more recently Fowler *et al.* (1981) reported an increased MAO-B: MAO-A ratio in the pons of patients with chronic schizophrenic and non-schizophrenic psychoses. Fowler and colleagues suggest that the increased MAO-BMAO-A ratio resulted from glial proliferation due to neuronal loss. In this respect MAO-B but not MAO-A has been shown to be increased in brains from patients dying with Alzheimer's disease (Adolfsson *et al.*, 1980) and also after hemitransection of the brain in the rat (Oreland *et al.*, 1980), in both instances there was a proliferation of glia in the degenerating regions of the brain.

Owen *et al.* (1987) assessed MAO-A and MAO-B activities in seven regions of post-mortem brains from 39 patients with schizo-phrenia and 44 control subjects. A modest decrease in MAO-B activity was observed in frontal and temporal cortex and in the amygdala. The decrease could not be accounted for by such variables as neuroleptic medication, age, sex, death to autopsy time, or the length of time the samples were stored deep-frozen prior to assay. Further analysis revealed that the reductions in MAO-B activity were specific-ally associated with negative symptoms (flattening of affect and poverty of speech) – i.e. the type II syndrome descibed by Crow (1980). However, the magnitude of the MAO-B reductions, most marked in the frontal cortex (approximately 25% decrease in MAO activity compared with controls), was insufficient to support the suggestion that low MAO activity might lead to the development of schizophrenia. Green and Grahame-Smith (1978) have demon-strated that MAO is not a rate limiting enzyme

and a large (in excess of 70%) reduction in activity is required to significantly affect monamine turnover in the brain. Owen *et al.* (1987) suggested that the decreased MAO-B activity observed in some brain regions of type II schizophrenics either reflects changes in monoamine function, as earlier suggested by Gottfries *et al.* (1974) to explain the generalized decrease in brain MAO activity found in suicide victims, or is part of the biochemical pathology in these particular brain regions.

Overall there is no convincing evidence to support the notion that reduced MAO activity in the brain plays a significant role in the aetiology of schizophrenia.

5.5 γ-AMINOBUTYRIC ACID IN SCHIZOPHRENIA

Roberts (1972) postulated that γ-amino butyric acid (GABA) systems were defective in individuals who were susceptible to schizophrenia and suggested that his postulate could be readily verified by measuring the activity of glutamate decarboxylase (GAD), the enzyme that catalyses the decarboxylation of glutamate to form GABA and is a marker for GABA-ergic neurones. Subsequently, Bird *et al.* (1977) reported a significant reduction in GAD activity in post-mortem brain samples from schizophrenics in all four brain regions examined – i.e. the nucleus accumbens, putamen, amygdala and hippocampus. How-ever, other groups failed to detect any significant difference in GAD activity in brain samples from controls and schizophrenics (Crow *et al.*, 1978; McGeer and McGeer, 1977; Roberts, 1977; Perry *et al.*, 1979; Cross and Owen, 1979). This discrepancy was resolved when Bird and colleagues re-examined necroscopy reports and it became clear that in their initial study death with bronchopneumonia was over-represented in the schizophrenic group with the terminal hypoxia adversely affecting post-mortem GAD activity (Bird *et al.*, 1978).

Perry *et al.* (1979) reported that the concentration of GABA was reduced in samples of nucleus accumbens and thalamus from schizophrenics with the degree of reduction (approximately 40%) being similar to that previously reported in Huntington's chorea (Perry *et al.*, 1973; Bird *et al.*, 1974). However Cross *et al.* (1979) found the concentrations of GABA in the same brain regions to be similar in controls and schizophrenics. Moreover the well-established deficit in GABA-ergic mechanisms in Huntington's chorea is reflected in a reduction in the concentrations of GABA in the CSF (Glaeser *et al.*, 1975), whereas CSF GABA concentrations in schizophrenics are no different from controls (Lichtenstein *et al.*, 1978).

Ligand binding to the $GABA_A$ receptor complex has been studied by several groups (Bennett *et al.*, 1979; Reisine *et al.*, 1980; Owen *et al.*, 1981), and in all investigations it has been found to be unchanged in schizophrenics compared to controls. To date, $GABA_B$ receptors have not been studied in schizophrenics.

Pharmacological evidence does not support a significant reduction in GABA-ergic function in schizophrenia. Baclofen, a GABA agonist, believed at one time to have a therapeutic effect in the treatment of schizophrenia (Frederiksen, 1975) has since been demonstrated to be ineffective or even detrimental in the treatment of schizophrenia (Simpson *et al.*, 1975). In addition, the administration of muscimol, another potent GABA agonist, does not ameliorate the symptoms of schizophrenia (Tamminga *et al.*, 1978).

Thus the evidence for the involvement of a GABA-ergic deficit in the aetiology of schizophrenia is very weak.

5.6 EXCITATORY AMINO ACIDS AND SCHIZOPHRENIA

The initial report (Nishikawa *et al.*, 1983) of increased [3H]-kainic acid binding in the frontal cortex of schizophrenics has been confirmed in a recent study (Deakin *et al.*, 1989), which also demonstrated an increase in [3H]-TCP (thienylcyclonexylpiperidine) binding to the N-methyl-D-aspartate (NMDA) receptor. These increases in post-synaptic glutamate receptor sub-types are paralleled by an increase in [3H]-D-aspartic acid binding to the presynaptic high-affinity glutamate uptake site and have been interpreted as reflecting a dysplasia of glutamatergic neurones (Deakin *et al.*, 1989). Lateralized changes in glutamate uptake sites have also been observed in other brain regions including the amygdala (Deakin, 1990).

Whilst it is possible that these changes in excitatory amino acid synapses may be related to the structural changes observed in the brains of schizophrenics, it is also possible that these changes may have broader implications. Phencyclidine has long been recognized as a psychotomimetic drug which produces a 'model psychosis' with some similarities to schizophrenia (Snyder, 1980). The realization that phencyclidine is a potent NMDA receptor antagonist and that other NMDA antagonists may also be psychotomimetic, suggests that excitatory amino acids may be more generally involved in the schizophrenic process. The NMDA receptor complex has been shown to possess several 'modulatory' sites. While direct-acting NMDA receptor agonists may be neurotoxic and proconvulsant, compounds acting at the modulatory sites on the receptor may lack these properties and may have some potential as neuroleptic agents.

Of related interest is the so-called 'sigma' receptor binding site. This was originally described as a binding site with high affinity for phencyclidine (and related dissociative anaesthetics) and some psychotomimetic opiates. The high affinity of some neuroleptic drugs (i.e. haloperidol) for this binding site raised the possibility that it might represent a receptor which mediates the psychotomimetic effects of these compounds, and that some neuroleptics might be 'sigma' antagonists. (For a review see Chavkin, 1990.) However it is clear that many chemically unrelated drugs with a wide range of pharmacological effects bind to the sigma site. Moreover, antipsychotic potency of neuroleptics does not correlate with activity at sigma sites, and any relationship with schizophrenia remains dubious. A recent post-mortem study has reported a marked reduction in the density of sigma binding sites in the hippocampus, frontal cortex and amygdala of schizophrenics (Simpson *et al.*, 1990). It was suggested that the most likely explanation of this finding was that neuroleptics present in the brain samples interfered with the binding assay. This suggests that at therapeutic doses some neuroleptics are present in the brain in sufficient concentration to interact with sigma sites.

5.7 NEUROACTIVE PEPTIDES AND SCHIZOPHRENIA

The role of neuropeptides in the aetiology of neuropsychiatric diseases has been the focus of considerable research effort. In particular, the possibility that altered levels, or abnormal metabolism of brain opioids, might be associated with schizophrenia has been extensively studied. There have been two opposing hypotheses concerning central opioid function in schizophrenia. Bloom *et al.* (1976) observed that intraventricular injections of endorphins in the rat produced a marked catatonia and suggested that schizophrenia, therefore, may be associated with an increased production of opioid peptides. On the other hand, Jacquet and Marks (1976) injected endorphins into the periaqueductal grey matter of rats and reported that the effects of the injection were similar to those produced by antipsychotic drugs and proposed that schizophrenia may result from an underactivity of opioid function.

An early study (Terenius *et al.*, 1976) reported that some opioid fractions in CSF were elevated in samples from medicated schizo-phrenics and that these levels decreased after neuroleptic medication. This was subsequently confirmed by some groups (Lindström *et al.*, 1978; Domschke *et al.*, 1979; Rimon *et al.*, 1980). However, Naber *et al.* (1981) reported significant reductions in CSF opioid activity using a radioreceptor assay in male schizo-phrenics and that ß-endorphin immunoreactivity in a sub-sample of the same patients was no different from control values.

There have been several studies of the effects of opioid receptor antagonists on schizophrenic symptoms. The initial report of a beneficial effect of naloxone administration to schizo-phrenics (Gunne *et al.*, 1977) was confirmed to some extent by some workers (Davis *et al.*, 1977; Emrich *et al.*, 1977) but not by others (Volovka *et al.*, 1977; Janowsky *et al.*, 1977). The topic has been reviewed by Mackay (1979) who concluded that the evidence for or against the efficacy of naloxone in ameliorating the symptoms of schizophrenia was evenly matched. However, a later World Health Organization collaborative study of short-term naloxone administration to schizophrenic and manic patients concluded that in their study (Pickar *et al.*, 1982) there was a significant naloxone-associated amelioration of auditory hallucinations.

The proposal that schizophrenia may be associated with an underactivity of opioid systems has also proved difficult to substantiate clinically. The administration of β-endorphins to schizophrenic patients has produced incon-clusive results (Kline *et al.*, 1977; Berger *et al.*, 1980) or no significant change in the severity of psychotic symptoms (Gerner *et al.*, 1980; Pickar *et al.*, 1981) although the administration of des-tyrosine-gamma endor-phine (DTγE) has been reported to have definite therapeutic effects in some cases of schizo-phrenia (Verhoeven *et al.*, 1979; Van Ree, 1980; Emrich *et al.*, 1980; Van Pragg, 1982). Van Ree and De Wied (1981) have suggested that in those patients in whom DTγE admini-stration was clinically effective there may be aberrant cleavage of the β-endorphin fragment from its polypeptide precursor.

The initial report by Wagemaker and Cade (1977) that renal dialysis produced a significant amelioration of schizophrenic symptoms, with the intriguing possibility that this beneficial effect resulted from the removal of excess or aberrant opioid compounds, was followed by the results of several investigations reporting that renal dialysis was ineffective as a treatment for schizophrenia (Weddington, 1977; Ferris, 1977; Levy, 1977; Begleiter *et al.*, 1981; Harisprasad *et al.*, 1981).

Neurochemical studies on post-mortem brain material from schizophrenic patients have also yielded inconclusive results. A significant reduction in the concentration of methionine-encephalin in the caudate nucleus of chronic paranoid patients has been reported by one group (Kleinman *et al.*, 1983) whereas Lightman *et al.* (1979) found the distribution of ß-endorphin in the brains of schizophrenics to be similar to controls.

In one report the binding of [³H]-naloxone, which labels all the major subtypes of opioid receptors, was found to be reduced in the basal ganglia of schizophrenics (Reisine *et al.*, 1980). However in a subsequent investigation which studied separately *mu* and *delta* plus *kappa* receptor sub-types, no changes were observed in schizophrenics (Owen *et al.*, 1985).

Neuropeptides other than opioids have been less extensively studied in relation to schizophrenia and the reports so far published are on the whole inconclusive. In post-mortem brain studies cholecystokinin-like immunoreactivity (CCK-LI) has been reported to be decreased in the temporal cortex of schizophrenics and in the hippocampus and amygdala where the reduction was selective to those patients with negative symptoms (Ferrier *et al.*, 1983; Roberts *et al.*, 1983). Conversely, CCK-LI has been reported to be unchanged in the entorhinal cortex of chronic schizophrenics and to be no different from control values in several brain regions including the amygdala and hippocampus (Kleinman *et al.*, 1983).

CCK receptors, assessed by the binding of radio-labelled CCK_{33} were found to be reduced in the frontal cortex and hippocampus of a group of schizophrenic patients (Farmery *et al.*, 1985). This is unlikely to be due to the effects of neuroleptic administration, which tends to elevate brain CCK receptors (Farmery *et al.*, 1985).

It is clear that several sub-types of CCK receptors are present in experimental animals, and that these can be differentiated with newly developed selective non-peptide antagonists. At present it is not clear how CCK receptors in the human brain are related to those of experimental animals. It would, however, seem worthwhile to examine human brain receptors in schizophrenia using selective non-peptide ligands.

Apart from the post-mortem brain investigations of CCK there have been several reports of the effects of CCK administration to schizophrenic patients with conflicting results due largely to inadequate trial design. These trials have been reviewed by Nair *et al.* (1985).

Vasoactive intestinal polypeptide-like immunoreactivity (VIP-LI) has been reported to be similar to control values in cerebrospinal fluid (Gjerris *et al.*, 1981) and post-mortem entorhinal cortex samples from schizophrenics (Perry *et al.*, 1981). Roberts *et al.* (1983) reported a significant increase in VIP-LI in the amygdala of schizophrenics with positive symptoms, but Carruthers *et al.* (1984) found VIP-LI in the amygdala to be similar in controls and schizophrenics.

Somatostatin-like immunoreactivity (SRIF-LI) in the CSF of schizophrenics has been reported to be similar to control values (Meltzer 1987). Post-mortem brain studies have, however, demonstrated some significant differences between controls and schizophrenics although the findings are not robust. Nemeroff *et al.* (1983) reported reduced SRIF-LI in frontal cortex samples from schizophrenics whereas Ferrier *et al.* (1983) found SRIF-LI to be unchanged in cortical regions but did observe increased SRIF-LI in thalamus samples from the schizophrenic group as a whole and reduced SRIF-LI in the hippocampus in a small group of patients with predominantly negative symptoms.

Neurotensin-like immunoreactivity (NT-LI) has been reported to be decreased in the CSF of some schizophrenics whose CSF level returned to normal after neuroleptic treatment (Widerlöv et al., 1982), and in post-mortem frontal cortex samples (Nemeroff et al., 1983). However there have been other reports of NT-LI being no different from control values in several brain regions (Biggins et al., 1983; Roberts et al., 1983).

Neurotensin binding sites were found to be increased by almost 100% in the substantia nigra of schizophrenics compared with controls (Uhl and Kuhar, 1984). Moreover, a similar increase in binding sites was observed in rat substantia nigra following chronic neuroleptic treatment. It was suggested that this change in neurotensin receptors may be more closely associated with the development of tardive dyskinesia rather than with the schizophrenic psychosis. In a separate study, the increase in neurotensin receptors in the substantia nigra was confirmed (Farmery et al., 1986). In addition it was demonstrated that this change is regionally specific and limited to the substantia nigra.

Both neurotensin and CCK are known to interact with dopaminergic systems in the brain. Whilst abnormalities in these neuropeptide systems may merely be secondary to changes in dopaminergic function or to neuroleptic treatment, it is also possible that these changes may be of more direct importance. It is certainly worth considering that brain-penetrating drugs with selectivity for these neuropeptide receptor sub-types may be of therapeutic potential in schizophrenia.

5.7 CONCLUSIONS

It is clear that post-mortem studies have been extremely useful in critically evaluating neurochemical hypotheses and uncovering changes in the brains of schizophrenics which may be relevant to the pathophysiology of the disease. However, the value of these studies is severely limited by the problems associated with studying primarily chronically ill patients at the end stage of the disease. In particular it is extremely difficult to exclude the possibility that supposedly drug-free patients did not receive active medication.

Most of the problems with post-mortem studies can be overcome using in vivo scanning techniques to investigate neurotransmitter receptor function in schizophrenia. To date three independent studies have been performed investigating D_2 receptors in schizophrenics. While two studies (Wong et al., 1986; Owen and Cross, 1989) demonstrated an increase in ligand binding to D_2 receptors in acute and chronically ill patients, one study demonstrated no change in D_2 receptors in acutely ill patients (Farde et al., 1986). Clearly careful selection of patient groups will resolve this issue. These studies highlight the great potential of scanning techniques in the study of human brain function in disease states, and it is in this area that future research into the biological basis of schizophrenia may prove to be rewarding.

REFERENCES

Adolfsson, R., Gottfries, C.G., Oreland, L. et al. (1980) Increased activity of brain and platelet monoamine oxidase in dementia of Alzheimer type. Life Sci., 27, 1029–34.

Aghajanian, G.K., Foote, W.E. and Sheard, M.H. (1970) Action of psychotogenic drugs on single mid-brain raphe neurones. J. Pharmacol. Exp. Ther., 171, 178–87.

Ashcroft, G.W., Crawford, T.B.B., Elleston, D. et al. (1966) 5-Hydroxyindole compounds in the cerebrospinal fluid of patients with psychiatric or neurological disease. Lancet, ii, 1049–52.

Begleiter, H., Porjesz, B. and Chou, C.L. (1981) Dialysis in schizophrenia: a double-blind evaluation. *Science*, **211**, 1066–8.

Bennett, J.P., Enna, S.J., Bylund, D.B. *et al.* (1979) Neurotransmitter receptors in frontal cortex in schizophrenia. *Arch. Gen. Psychiatry*, **36**, 927–34.

Berger, P.A., Faull, K.F., Killowski, J. *et al.* (1980) Cerebrospinal fluid monoamine metabolites in depression and schizophrenia. *Am. J. Psychiatry*, **137**, 174–80.

Berger, P.A., Watson, S.J., Akil, H. *et al.* (1980) Beta-endorphin and schizophrenia. *Arch. Gen. Psychiatry*, **37**, 635–40.

Berrettini, W.H., Prozialeck, W. and Vogel, W.H. (1978) Decreased platelet monamine oxidase activity in chronic schizophrenia shown with novel substrates. *Arch. Gen. Psychiatry*, **35**, 600–5.

Biggins, J.A., Perry, E.K., McDermott, J.R. *et al.* (1983) Post-mortem levels of thyrotropin-releasing hormone and neurotensin in the amygdala in Alzheimer's disease, schizophrenia and depression. *J. Neurol. Sci.*, **58**, 117–22.

Bird, E.D., Crow, T.J., Iversen, L.L. *et al.* (1979) Dopamine and homovanillic acid concentrations in the post-mortem brain in schizophrenia. *J. Physiol.*, **293**, 36–7.

Bird, E.D. and Iversen, L.L. (1974) Huntington's chorea: post-mortem measurement of glutamatic acid decarboxylase, choline acetyltransferase and dopamine in basal ganglia. *Brain*, **97**, 457–72.

Bird, E.D., Spokes, E.G., Barnes, J. *et al.* (1977) Increased brain dopamine and reduced glutamatic acid decarboxylase and choline acetyltransferase activity in schizophrenia and related psychoses. *Lancet*, **ii**, 1157–9.

Bird, E.D., Spokes, E.G., Barnes, J. *et al.* (1978) Glutamic-acid decarboxylase in schizophrenia. *Lancet*, **i**, 156.

Birkhäuser, H. (1941) Cholinesterase and monoaminoxylase in zentralen neurensystem. *Schweiz. Med. Wochenschrift*, **71**, 750–2.

Bloom, F.E., Segal, D., Ling, N. and Guillieman, R. (1976) Endorphins: profound behavioural effects in rats suggest new etiological factors in mental illness. *Science*, **194**, 630–2.

Bond, P.A., Dimitrakoudi, M., Howlett, D.R. and Jenner, F.A. (1975) Urinary excretion of the sulphate and glucuronide of 3-methoxy-4-hydroxyphenylglycol in a manic-depressive patient. *Psychol. Med.*, **5**, 279–85.

Bond, P.A. and Howlett, D.R. (1974) Measurements of the two conjugates of 3-methoxy-4-hydroxyphenylglycol in urine. *Biochem. Med.*, **10**, 219–28.

Bowers, M.B. (1974) Central dopamine turnover in schizophrenic syndromes. *Arch. Gen. Psychiatry*, **31**, 50–4.

Bowers, M.B., Heninger, G.R. and Gerbode, F.A. (1969) Cerebrospinal fluid 5-hydroxyindole-acetic acid and homovanilla acid in psychiatric patients. *Int. J. Neuropharmacol.*, **8**, 225–62.

Bowers, M.B. Jr (1974) Central dopamine turnover in schizophrenic syndromes. *Arch. Gen. Psychiatry*, **31**, 50–7.

Bowers, M.B. Jr (1970) Cerebrospinal fluid 5-hydroxyindoles and behaviour after L-trytophan and pyridoxine administration to psychiatric patients. *Neuropharmacology*, **9**, 599–604.

Brown, R., Colter, N., Corsellis, J.A.N. *et al.* (1986) Post-mortem evidence of structural brain changes in schizophrenia: differences in brain weight, temporal brain area, and parahippocampal gyrus compared with affective disorder. *Arch. Gen. Psychiatry*, **43**, 36–42.

Brune, G.G. (1965) Metabolism of biogenic amines and psychotropic drug effects in schizophrenic patients. *Prog. Brain. Res.*, **16**, 81–96.

Burt, D.R., Creese, I. and Snyder, S.M. (1982) Antischizophrenic drugs: chronic treatment elevates dopamine receptor binding in brain. *Science*, **196**, 326–8.

Carenzi, A., Gillin, J.C., Guidotti, A. *et al.* (1975) Dopamine-sensitive adenylyl cyclase in human caudate nucleus. *Arch. Gen. Psychiatry*, **32**, 1056–9.

Carruthers, B., Dawbarn, D., DeQuidt, M. *et al.* (1984) Changes of the neuropeptide content of the amygdala in schizophrenia. *Br. J. Pharmacol.*, **81**, 190P.

Chavkin, C. (1990) The sigma enigma: biochemical and functional correlates emerge for the haloperidol-sensitive sigma site. *Trends Pharm. Sci.*, **11**, 213–5.

Christmas, A.J., Coulson, C.J., Maxwell, D.R. and Riddell, D. (1972) A comparison of the pharmacological and biochemical properties of substrate-selective monoamine oxidase inhibitors. *Br. J. Pharmacol.*, **45**, 490–503.

Clement-Cormier, Y.C., Kebabian, J.W., Petzold, G.L. and Greengard, P. (1974) Dopamine-sensitive adenylate cyclase in mammalian brain: a possible site of action of antipsychotic drugs. *Proc. Nat. Acad. Sci. USA*, **71**, 1113–7.

Connell, P.H. (1958) *Amphetamine Psychosis.* Maudsley Monograph No. 5. Chapman and Hall, London.

Cross, A.J. (1982) Interaction of [³H]-LSD with serotonin receptors in human brain. *Eur. J. Pharmacol.*, **82**, 77–80.

Cross, A.J., Crow, T.J., Ferrier, I.N. *et al.* (1985) Chemical and structural changes in the brain in patients with movement disorder. In *Dyskinesia — Research and Treatment* D. Casey (ed), Springer-Verlag, Berlin, pp. 104–10.

Cross, A.J., Crow, T.J., Glover, V. *et al.* (1977) Monoamine oxidase activity in post-mortem brains of schizophrenics and controls. *Br. J. Clin. Pharmacol.*, **4**, 719P.

Cross, A.J., Crow, T.J., Killpack, W.S. *et al.* (1978) The activities of brain dopamine β-hydroxylase and catechol-O-methyltransferase in schizophrenics and controls. *Psychopharmacology* **59**, 117–21.

Cross, A.J., Crow, T.J. and Owen, F. (1981) ³H-Flupenthixol binding in post-mortem brains of schizophrenics: evidence for a selective increase in dopamine D_2 receptors. *Psychopharmacology*, **74**, 122–4.

Cross, A.J. and Owen, F. (1979) The activities of glutamatic acid decarboxylase and choline acetyltransferase in post-mortem brains of schizophrenics and controls. *Biochem. Soc. Trans.*, **7**, 145–6.

Cross, A.J., Owen, F. and Crow, T.J. (1979) Gamma-aminobutyric acid in the brain in schizophrenia. *Lancet*, **i**, 560–1.

Crow, T.J. (1980) Molecular pathology of schizophrenia: more than one disease process? *Br. Med. J.*, **280**, 66–8.

Crow, T.J., Baker, H.F., Cross, A.J. *et al.* (1979) Monoamine mechanisms in chronic schizophrenia: post-mortem neurochemical findings. *Br. J. Psychiatry*, **134**, 249–56.

Crow, T.J., Cross, A.J., Johnstone, E.C. *et al.* (1982) Changes in D_2 dopamine receptor numbers in post-mortem brain in schizophrenia in relation to the presence of the type I syndrome and movement disorder. In *Brain peptides and hormones*. R. Collin (ed), Raven Press, New York, pp. 43–53.

Crow, T.J., Owen, F., Cross, A.J. and Longden, A. (1978) Brain biochemistry in schizophrenia. *Lancet*, **i**, 36–7.

Czydek, C. and Reynolds, G.P. (1988) Binding of [³H]-SCH 23390 to post-mortem brain tissue in schizophrenia. *Br. J. Pharmacol.*, **95**, 282.

Davis, G.C., Bunney, W.E. Jr., DeFraites, E.G. *et al.* (1977) Intravenous naloxone administration in schizophrenic and affective illness. *Science*, **197**, 74–7.

Deakin, J.F.W. (1990) The neurochemistry of schizophrenia. In *Schizophrenia: the major issues*. P. Bebbington and P. McGuffin (eds), Heinemann, England, pp. 56–72.

Deakin, J.F.W., Slater, P., Simpson, M.D.C. *et al.* (1989) Frontal cortical and left temporal glutamatergic dysfunction in schizophrenia. *J. Neurochem.*, **52**, 1781–6.

Delisi, L.E., Wise, C.D., Bridge, T.D. *et al.* (1981) A probable effect of neuroleptic medication on platelet monoamine oxidase activity. *Psychiatry Res.*, **2**, 179–86.

Domino, E.F. and Khanna, S.S. (1976) Decreased blood platelet MAO activity in unmedicated chronic schizophrenic patients. *Am. J. Psychiatry*, **133**, 323–6.

Domino, E.F. and Krause, R.R. (1974) Free and bound serum tryptophan in drug free normal controls and chronic schizophrenic patients. *Biol. Psychiatry*, **8**, 265–79.

Domino, E.F., Krause, Q.R. and Bowers, J. (1973) Various enzymes involved with putative neurotransmitters. *Arch. Gen. Psychiatry*, **29**, 195–201.

Domschke, W., Dickschas, A. and Mitznegg, P. (1979) CSF β-endorphin in schizophrenia. *Lancet*, **i**, 1024.

Emrich, H.M., Cording, C., Piree, S., *et al.* (1977) Indication of antipsychotic action of the opiate antagonist naloxone. *Pharmacopsychiatria*, **10**, 265–70.

Emrich, H.M., Zaudig, M., Serssen, D.V., *et al.* (1980) Des-tyr-gamma-endorphin in schizophrenia. *Lancet*, **ii**, 1364–5.

Farde, L., Hall, M., Ehrin, E. and Sedvall, G. (1986) Quantitative analysis of dopamine receptor binding in the living human brain by PET. *Science*, **231**, 258–61.

Farmery, S.M., Owen, F., Poulter, M. and Crow,

T.J. (1985) Reduced high affinity cholecyst-okinin binding in hippocampus and frontal cortex of schizophrenic patients. *Life Sci.*, **36**, 473–7.

Farmery, S.M. Crow, T.J. and Owen, F. (1986) ^{125}I-iodotyrosyl neurotensin binding in post-mortem brain: comparison of controls and schizophrenic patients. *Br. J. Pharmacol.*, **88**, 380P.

Ferrier, I.N., Roberts, G.W., Crow, T.J. *et al.* (1983) Reduced CCK-LI and SST-LI in the limbic lobe is associated with negative symptoms in schizophrenia. *Life Sci.*, **33**, 475–82.

Ferris, G.N. (1977) Can dialysis help the chronic schizophrenic? *Am. J. Psychiatry*, **134**, 1310.

Fowler, C.J., Carlsson, A. and Winblad, B. (1981) Monoamine oxidase-A and -B activities in the brain stem of schizophrenics and non-schizophrenic psychotics. *J. Neural Transm.*, **52**, 23–32.

Frederiksen, P.K. (1975) Baclofen in the treatment of schizophrenia. *Lancet*, **i**, 702–3.

Friedhoff, A.J., Miller, J.C. and Weissefeund, J. (1978) Human platelet MAO in drug-free and medicated schizophrenic patients. *Am. J. Psychiatry*, **135**, 952–5.

Friedman, E., Shopsin, B., Salthananthan, G. and Gershon, S. (1974) Blood platelet monoamine oxidase activity in psychiatric patients. *Am. J. Psychiatry*, **135**, 952–5.

Gallant, D.M. and Bishop, M.P. (1968) Cinanserin (SQ 10, 643): a preliminary evaluation in chronic schizophrenic patients. *Curr. Ther. Res.*, **10**, 461–3.

Gerner, R.H., Catlin, D.H., Gorelick, D.A. *et al.* (1980) Beta-endorphin: Intravenous infusion causes behavioural changes in psychiatric inpatients. *Arch. Gen. Psychiatry*, **37**, 642–7.

Gillin, J.C., Kaplan, J.A. and Wyatt, R.J. (1976) Clinical effects of tryptophan in chronic schizophrenia. *Biol. Psychiatry*, **11**, 635–9.

Gjerris, A., Fahrenkrug, J., Bukholm, S. and Rafaelson, O.J. (1981) Vasoactive intestinal polypeptide (VIP) in cerebrospinal fluid in psychiatric disorders. *Biol. Psychiatry*, **16**, 359–62.

Glaeser, B.S., Vogel, W.H., Oleweiler, D.B. and Hare, T.A. (1975) GABA levels in cerebro-spinal fluid of patients with Huntington's chorea: a preliminary report. *Biochem. Med.*, **12**, 380–5.

Gottesmann, I.I. (1982) *Schizophrenia: the Epigenetic Puzzle*. Cambridge University Press, New York.

Gottfries, C.G., Oreland, L., Wiberg, A. and Winblad, B. (1974) Brain levels of mono-amine oxidase in depression. *Lancet*, **ii**, 360–1.

Green, A.R. and Grahame-Smith, D.G. (1978) Process regulating the functional activity of brain 5-hydroxytryptamine: results of animal experiments and their relevance to the understanding and treatment of depression. *Pharmacopsychiatrica.*, **11**, 3–16.

Gruen, R., Baron, M., Levitt, M. and Asnis, L. (1982) Platelet MAO activity and schizo-phrenic prognosis. *Am. J. Psychiatry*, **139**, 240–1.

Gunne, L., Lindstrom, L. and Terenius, L.M. (1977) Naloxone-induced reversal of schizo-phrenic hallucinations. *J. Neural Transm.*, **40**, 13–9.

Hariprasad, M.K., Nadler, I.M. and Eisinger, R.P. (1981) Hemodialysis for manic schizophrenics: No psychiatric improvements. *J. Clin. Psychiatry*, **42**, 215–6.

Hartmann, E. (1976) Schizophrenia: a theory. *Psychopharmacology*, **49**, 1–15.

Hartmann, E. and Keller-Teschke, M. (1977) Biology of schizophrenia: mental effects of dopamine-ß-hydroxylase inhibition in normal man. *Lancet*, **1**, 37–8.

Hess, E.J., Bracma, M.S., Kleinman, J.E. and Creese, I. (1987) Dopamine receptor subtype imbalance in schizophrenia. *Life Sci.*, **40**, 1487–97.

Holden, J.M.C., Keskiner, A. and Gannon, P. (1971) A clinical trial of an antiserotonin compound, cinanserin, in chronic schizophrenia. *J. Clin. Pharmacol.*, **11**, 220–6.

Jacquet, Y.F. and Marks, N. (1976) The C-fragment of β-lipoprotein: an endogenous neuroleptic or antipsychotic. *Science*, **194**, 632–5.

Janowsky, D.S., Segal, D.S., Bloom, F. *et al.* (1977) Lack of effect of naloxone on schizophrenic symptoms. *Am. J. Psychiatry*, **134**, 926–7.

Johnston, J.P. (1968) Some observations on a new inhibitor of monoamine oxidase in brain tissue. *Biochem. Pharmacol.*, **17**, 1285–97.

Johnstone, E.C., Crow, T.J., Frith, C.D. *et al.* (1978) Mechanism of the antipsychotic effect in the treatment of acute schizophrenia. *Lancet*, **1**, 848–51.

Joseph, M.H., Baker, H.F., Crow, T.J. *et al.* (1979) Brain tryptophan metabolism in schizophrenia: a post-mortem study of metabolites of the serotonin and kynurenine pathways in schizophrenic and control subjects. *Psychopharmacology*, **62**, 279–85.

Joseph, M.H., Baker, H.F., Johnstone, E.C. and Crow, T.J. (1979) 3-Methoxy-4-hydroxyphenylglycol excretion in acutely schizophrenic patients during a controlled clinical trial of the isomers of flupenthixol. *Psychopharmacology*, **64**, 35–40.

Joseph, M.H., Baker, H.F., Johnstone, E.C. and Crow, T.J. (1976) Determination of 3-methoxy-4-hydroxyphenylglycol conjugates in urine. Application to the study of central noradrenaline metabolism in unmedicated chronic schizophrenic patients. *Psychopharmacology*, **51**, 47–51.

Karlsson, J.L. (1988) Partly dominant transmission of schizophrenia in Ireland. *Br. J. Psychiatry* **152**, 324–9.

Kebabian, J.W. and Calne, D.B. (1979) Multiple receptors for dopamine. *Nature*, **271**, 93–6.

Kleinman, J.E., Iadorola, M., Govoni, S. *et al.* (1983) Post-mortem measurements of neuropeptides in human brain. *Psychopharmacol.*, **87**, 292–7.

Kline, N.S., Li, C.H. Lehmann, H.E. *et al.* (1977) Beta-endorphin-induced changes in schizophrenia and depressed patients. *Arch. Gen. Psychiatry*, **34**, 111–3.

Knoll, J. and Magyar, K. (1972) Some puzzling pharmacological effects of monoamine oxidase inhibitors. *Adv. Biochem. Psychopharmacol.*, **5**, 393–408.

Lee, T., Seeman, P., Tourtellotte, W.W. *et al.* (1978) Binding of ^{3}H-neuroleptics and ^{3}H-apomorphine in schizophrenic brains. *Nature*, **274**, 897–900.

Levy, N.B. (1977) Can dialysis help the chronic schizophrenic? *Am. J. Psychiatry*, **134**, 1310.

Leysen, J.E, Niemegeers, C.J.E., Tollenwaere, J.P. and Laduron, P.M. (1978) Serotonergic component of neuroleptic receptors. *Nature*, **272**, 168–71.

Lichtenstein, D., Dobkin, J., Ebstein, R.P. *et al.* (1978) Gamma-aminobutyric acid (GABA) in the CSF of schizophrenic patients before and after neuroleptic treatment. *Br. J. Psychiatry*, **132**, 145–8.

Lightman, S.L., Spokes, E.G., Sagnella, G.A. *et al.* (1979) Distribution of ß-endorphin in normal and schizophrenic human brains. *Eur. J. Clin. Invest.* **9**, 377–9.

Lindström, L.H., Widerlöv, E., Gunne, L.M. Wahlström, A. and Terenius, L. (1978) Endorphins in human cerebrospinal fluid: Clinical correlations of some psychotic states. *Acta Psychiatr. Scand.*, **57**, 153–64.

Maas, J.W., and Landis, D.H. (1968) In vivo studies of the metabolism of norepinephrine in the central nervous system. *J. Pharmacol. Exp. Ther.*, **163**, 147–62.

Maas, J.W., Dekirmenjian, H., Garver, D. *et al.* (1973) Excretion of catecholamine metabolites following intraventricular injection of 6-hydroxydopamine in the macaca speciosa. *Eur. J. Pharmacol.*, **23**, 121–30.

Mackay, A.V.P. (1979) Psychiatric implications of endorphin research. *Br. J. Psychiatry*, **135**, 470–3.

Mackay, A.V.P., Bird, E.D., Spokes, E.G. *et al.* (1980) Dopamine receptors in schizophrenia: drug effect or illness. *Lancet*, **ii**, 915–6.

Mann, J.J., Kaplan, R.D., Georgotas, A. *et al.* (1981) Monamine oxidase activity and enzyme kinetics in three subpopulations of density-fractionated platelets in chronic paranoid schizophrenics. *Psychopharmacology*, **74**, 344–8.

Mann, J. and Thomas, J.M. (1979) Platelet monoamine oxidase activity in schizophrenia. *Br. J. Psychiatry*, **134**, 366–71.

Manowitz, P., Gilmour, D.G. and Raceuskis, J. (1973) Low plasma tryptophan levels in recently hospitalized schizophrenics. *Biol. Psychiatry*, **6**, 109–18.

Matthysse, S.W. and Kidd, K.K. (1976) Estimating the genetic contribution to schizophrenia. *Am. J. Psychiatry*, **133**, 185–91.

McGeer, P.L. and McGeer, E.G. (1977) Possible changes in striatal and limbic cholinergic systems in schizophrenia. *Arch. Gen. Psychiatry*, **34**, 1319–23.

McGue, M., Gottesman, I.I., and Rao, D.C. (1983) The transmission of schizophrenia under a multifactorial threshold model. *Am. J. Hum. Genet.*, **35**, 1161–78.

Meltzer, H.Y. (1987) Biological studies in schizophrenia. *Schizophr. Bull.*, **13**, 77–111.

Memo, M., Kleinman, T.E. and Hanbauer, I. (1983) Coupling of dopamine D_1 recognition sites with adenylate cyclase in nuclei accubens and caudates of schizophrenics. *Science*, **221**, 1302–4.

Miller, R.J., Horn, A.S. and Iversen, L.L. (1974) The action of neuroleptic drugs on dopamine stimulated-3,5-monophosphate production in neostriatum and limbic forebrain. *Mol. Pharmacol.*, **10**, 759–66.

Murphy, D.L. and Wyatt, R.J. (1972) Reduced platelet monoamine oxidase activity in chronic schizophrenia. *Nature*, **238**, 225–6.

Murphy, D.L., Belmaker, R. and Wyatt, R.J. (1974) Monoamine oxidase in schizophrenia and other behaviour disorders. *J. Psychiatr. Res.*, **11**, 221–47.

Naber, D., Pickar, D., Post, R.M. *et al.* (1981) Endogenous opioid activity and β-endorphin immunoreactivity in CSF of psychiatric patients and normal volunteers. *Am. J. Psychiatry*, **138**, 1457–1462.

Nair, N.P.V., Lal, S. and Bloom, D.M. (1985) Cholecystokinin peptides, dopamine and schizophrenia – a review. *Prog. Neuropsychopharmacol. Biol. Psychiatry*, **9**, 515–24.

Nemeroff, C.B., Mawberg, P.J., Widerlöv, E. *et al.* (1983) Neuropeptides in cerebrospinal fluid and post-mortem brain tissue of schizophrenics, Huntington's choreics and normal controls. *Psychopharmacol. Bull.*, **19**, 369–74.

Nishikawa, T., Takashima, M. and Toru, M. (1983) Increased [³H]-kainic acid binding in the prefrontal cortex in schizophrenia. *Neurosci. Letts.*, **40**, 245–50.

Owen, F., Bourne, R.C., Crow, T.J. *et al.* (1981) Platelet monoamine oxidase activity in acute schizophrenia: relationship to symptomatology and neuroleptic medication. *Br. J. Psychiatry*, **139**, 16–22.

Owen, F., Bourne, R.C., Crow, T.J. *et al.* (1976) Platelet monoamine oxidase in schizophrenia: an investigation in drug-free chronic hospitalized patients. *Arch. Gen. Psychiatry*, **33**, 1370–3.

Owen, F., Bourne, R.C., Poulter, M. *et al.* (1985) Tritiated etorphine and naloxone binding to opioid receptors in caudate nucleus in schizophrenics. *Br. J. Psychiatry*, **21**, 507–9.

Owen, F. and Cross, A.J. (1989) Schizophrenia. In *Neurotransmitter Drugs and Disease*. R.A. Webster and C.C. Jordan (eds), Blackwell, Oxford, pp. 336–53.

Owen, F., Cross, A.J., Crow, T.J., Lofthouse, R. and Poulter, M. (1981) Neurotransmitter receptors in brain in schizophrenia. *Acta Psychiatr. Scand.* 63, Suppl. 291, 20–6.

Owen, F., Cross, A.J., Crow, T.J. *et al.* (1978) Increased dopamine receptor sensitivity in schizophrenia. *Lancet*, **ii**, 223–6.

Owen, F., Cross, A.J., Crow, T.J. *et al.* (1981) Increased dopamine receptors in schizophrenia: specificity and relationship to drugs and symptomatology. In *Biological Psychiatry*. C. Perris (ed), Elsevier, Amsterdam, pp. 699–706.

Owen, F., Crow, T.J., Frith, C.D. *et al.* (1987) Selective decreases in MAO-B activity in post-mortem brains from schizophrenic patients with Type II syndrome. *Br. J. Psychiatry*, **151**, 514–9.

Oreland, L., Fowler, C.J., Carlsson, A. and Magnusson, T. (1980) Monoamine oxidase-A and -B activity in the rat brain after hemi-transection. *Life Sci.*, **26**, 139–46.

Perry, R.H., Dockray, G.J., Dimaline, R., Perry, E.K., Blessed, G. and Tomlinson, B.E. (1981) Neuropeptides in Alzheimer's disease, depression and schizophrenia. *J. Neurol. Sci.*, **51**, 465–72.

Perry, T.L., Hanson, S. and Kloster, M. (1973) Huntington's chorea: deficiency of γ-aminobutyric acid in brain. *N. Engl. J. Med.*, **288**, 337–42.

Perry, T.L., Kish, S.J., Buchanan, J. and Hansen, S. (1979) γ-Aminobutyric-acid deficiency in brain of schizophrenic patients. *Lancet*. **i**, 237–9.

Pickar, D., Davis, G.C., Schulz, S.C. *et al.* (1981) Behavioural and biological effects of acute beta-endorphin injection in schizophrenic and depressed patients. *Am. J. Psychiatry*, **138**, 160–6.

Pickar, D., Vartanian, F., Bunney, W.E.J. *et al.* (1982) Short-term naloxone administration in schizophrenic and manic patients. *Arch. Gen. Psychiatry*, **39**, 313–9.

Pollin, W., Cardin, P.V. and Kety, S.S. (1961) Effects of amino acid feedings in schizophrenic patients treated with isoniazid. *Science*, **133**, 104–5.

Post, R.M., Fink, E., Carpentier, W.T. and Goodwin, F.K. (1975) Cerebro-spinal fluid amine metabolites in acute schizophrenia. *Arch. Gen. Psychiatry*, **32**, 1063–9.

Randrup, A. and Munkvad, I. (1965) Special antagonism of amphetamine-induced abnormal behaviour: inhibition of sterotyped activity with increase of some normal activities. *Psychopharmacologia*, **7**, 416–22.

Randrup, A. and Munkvad, I. (1966) On the role of dopamine in the amphetamine excitatory response. *Nature*, **211**, 540.

Randrup, A. and Munkvad, I. (1967) Stereotyped activities produced by amphetamine in several animal species and man. *Psychopharmacologia*, **11**, 300–10.

Randrup, A. and Munkvad, I. (1972) Evidence indicating an association between schizophrenia and dopaminergic hyperactivity in the brain. *Orthomol. Psychiatry*, **1**, 2–7.

Reisine, T.D., Rossor, M., Spokes, E. *et al.* (1980) Opiate and neuroleptic receptor alterations in human schizophrenic brain tissue. *Adv. Biochem. Psychopharmacol.*, **21**, 443–50.

Reveley, M.A., Glover, V., Sandler, M. and Spokes, E.G. (1981) Brain monoamine oxidase activity in schizophrenics and controls. *Arch. Gen. Psychiatry*, **38**, 663–5.

Reynolds, G.P., Reynolds, L.M., Riederer, P. *et al.* (1980) Dopamine receptors and schizophrenia: drug effect or illness. *Lancet*, **ii**, 1251.

Rimon, R., Terenius, L. and Kampman, R. (1980) Cerebrospinal fluid endorphins in schizophrenia. *Acta. Psychiatr. Scand.*, **61**, 395–403.

Roberts, E. (1972) An hypothesis suggesting that there is a defect in the GABA system in schizophrenia. *Neurosci. Res. Prog. Bull.*, **10**, 468–82.

Roberts, E. (1977) The γ-Aminobutyric Acid System and Schizophrenia in *Neuroregulators and Psychiatric Disorders*. E. Usdin and J.D. Barchas (eds), Oxford University Press, Oxford, pp. 347–57.

Roberts, G.W., Ferrier, I.N., Lee, Y. *et al.* (1983) Peptides, the limbic lobe and schizophrenia. *Brain Res.*, **288**, 199–211.

Robinson, D.S., Lovenberg, W., Keiser, H. and Sjoerdsma, A. (1968) Effects of drugs on human blood platelet and plasma amine oxidase activity *in vitro* and *in vivo*. *Biochem. Pharmacol.*, **17**, 109–19.

Schwartz, M.A., Aikens, A.N. and Wyatt, R.J. (1974) Monoamine oxidase activity in brains from schizophrenics and mentally normal individuals. *Psychopharmacologia*, **38**, 319–28.

Seeman, P., Lee, T., Chau-Wong, M. and Wong, K. (1976) Antipsychotic drug doses and neuroleptic/dopamine receptors. *Nature*, **261**, 717–29.

Seeman, P., Ulpian, C., Bergeron, C. *et al.* (1984) Bimodal distribution of dopamine receptor densities in brains of schizophrenics. *Science*, **225**, 728–31.

Simpson, G.M., Lee, J.H., Shrivastava, R.K. and Branchey, M.M. (1975) Baclofen in schizophrenia. *Lancet*, **i**, 966–7.

Simpson, M.D.C., Royston, M.C., Slater, P. and Deakin J.F.W. (1990) Phencyclidine and sigma receptor abnormalities in schizophrenic postmortem brain. *Schizophr. Res.*, **3**, 34.

Snyder, S.H. (1980) Phencyclidine. *Science*, **285**, 355–6.

Stein, L. and Wise, C.D. (1971) Possible etiology of schizophrenia: progressive damage to the noradrenergic reward system by 6-hydroxy-dopamine. *Science*, **171**, 1032–6.

Takahashi, S., Yamane, H. and Naosuke, T. (1975) Reduction of blood platelets monoamine oxidase in schizophrenic patients on phenothiazines. *Fol. Psychiatr. Neurol. Japan*, **29**, 207–14.

Tamminga, C.A., Crayton, J.W. and Chase, T.N. (1978) Muscimol; GABA agonist therapy in schizophrenia. *Am. J. Psychiatr.*, **135**, 746–7.

Terenius, L., Wahlström, A., Lindström, C. and Widerlöv, E. (1976) Increased CSF levels of endorphins in chronic psychosis. *Neurosci. Lett.*, **3**, 157–62.

Uhl, G.R. and Kuhar, M.J. (1984) Chronic neuroleptic treatment enhances neurotensin receptor binding in humans and rat substantia nigra. *Nature*, **309**, 350–2.

Utena, H., Kanamura, H., Suda, S. *et al.*, (1968) Studies on the regional distribution of the monoamine oxidase activity in the brains of schizophrenic patients. *Proc. Jap. Acad.*, **44**, 1078–83.

Van Kammen, D.P. and Antelman, S. (1984) Impaired noradrenergic transmission in schizophrenia. *Life Sci.*, **34**, 1403–13.

Van Praag, H.M., Verhoeven, W.M.A., Van Ree, J.M. and De Wied, D. (1982) The treatment of schizophrenic psychoses with gamma-tyr-endorphins. *Biol. Psychiatry*, **17**, 83–98.

Van Ree, J.M., De Weid, D., Verhoeven, W.M.A. and Van Praag, H. (1980) Antipsychotic effect of gamma-tyr endorphins in schizophrenia. *Lancet*, **ii**, 1363–4.

Van Ree, J.M. and De Wied, D. (1981) Endorphins in schizophrenia. *Neuropharmacology*, **20**, 1271–7.

Verhoeven, W.M.A. , Van Praag, H.M., Van Ree, J.M. and De Wied, D. (1979) Improvement of schizophrenic patients treated with (des-tyr)-gamma-endorphin (DT γE). *Arch. Gen. Psychiatry*, **36**, 294–8.

Vogel, W.H., Orfei, V. and Century, B. (1969) Activities of enzymes involved in the formation and destruction of biogenic amines in various areas of human brain. *J. Pharmacol. Exp. Ther.*, **165**, 196–203.

Volovka, J., Mallya, A., Baig, S. and Perez-Cruet, J. (1977) Naloxone in chronic schizophrenia. *Science*, **196**, 1227–8.

Wagemaker, H.J. and Cade, R. (1977) The use of hemodialysis in chronic schizophrenia. *Am. J. Psychiatry*, **134**, 684–5.

Weddington, W.W. Jr. (1977) Can dialysis help the chronic schizophrenic? *Am. J. Psychiatry*, **134**, 1310.

Whitaker, D.M., Crow, T.J. and Ferrier, I.N. (1981) Tritiated LSD binding in frontal cortex in schizophrenic. *Arch. Gen. Psychiatry*, **38**, 278–80.

Widerlöv, E., Lindstrom, L.H., Besev, G. *et al.* (1982) Subnormal CSF levels of neurotensin in a subgroup of schizophrenic patients: normalization after neuroleptic treatment. *Am. J. Psychiatry*, **139**, 1122–6.

Wise, C.D., Baden, M.M. and Stein, L. (1974) Post-mortem measurement of enzymes in human brain: evidence of a central noradrenergic deficit in schizophrenia. *J. Psychiatr. Res.*, **11**, 185–98.

Wise, C.D. and Stein, L. (1973) Dopamine-β-hydroxylase deficits in the brains of schizophrenic patients. *Science*, **181**, 344–7.

Wooley, D.W. and Shaw, E. (1954) A biochemical and pharmacological suggestion about certain mental disorders. *Proc. Nat. Acad. Sci. USA*. **40**, 228–31.

Wong, D.F., Wagner, H.N., Tune, L.E. *et al.* (1986) Positron emission tomography reveals elevated D_2 dopamine receptors in drug-naive schizophrenics. *Science*, **234**, 1558–63.

Wyatt, R.J., Murphy, D.L., Belmaker, R. *et al.* (1973) Reduced monoamine oxidase activity in platelets. A possible genetic marker for vulnerability to schizophrenia. *Science*, **179**, 916–18.

Wyatt, R.J., Schwarz, M.A., Erdelyi, E. and Barchas, J.D. (1975) Dopamine-β-hydroxylase activity in brains of chronic schizophrenic patients. *Science*, **187**, 368–70.

Wyatt, R.J., Vaughan, T., Galanter, M. *et al.* (1972) Behavioural changes of chronic schizophrenic patients given L-5-hydroxytryptophan. *Science*, **177**, 1124–6.

Chapter 6

Neuroanatomical factors in schizophrenia

TERRY L. JERNIGAN

Attempts to find neuroanatomical bases for schizophrenia began soon after the first descriptions of the syndrome. Since that time, brain structure in chronic schizophrenic patients has been examined using a variety of histopathological techniques; and more recently, medical imaging methods have been used to visualize the brain in living patients. The gross structure of the brain is remarkably normal in most schizophrenic patients, and no consistent structural aberration, at any level of anatomical analysis, has been found to be present in the brains of all patients with schizophrenia. Nevertheless, some consistency does exist regarding the increased prevalence in schizophrenia of certain anatomical features. Thus, hopes are raised that while no single abnormality may prove to be specific to schizophrenia, perhaps some pattern of anatomical factors may be; and that if this pattern were known, useful neurobehavioural models might be developed to explain the symptoms of the disorder. This chapter will not attempt an exhaustive review of anatomical studies in schizophrenia. Rather, the review will focus on those studies particularly relevant to the dominant themes that arise in the discussions that go on in the field today: namely, whether the abnormalities cluster in certain functional systems, whether they are present before the onset of the disorder, and whether they are static or progressive.

6.1 STUDIES OF AUTOPSY MATERIAL

Neuropathological studies of schizophrenia have yielded numerous, often conflicting, results (for review see Weinberger *et al.*, 1983; Jellinger, 1985; Roberts and Bruton, 1990). The earliest studies suffered from the lack of objective methods and incomplete understanding of the effects on the tissues of agonal process (i.e. the physiological effects due to the patient's terminal illness and death) and fixation procedures. More recently, however, abnormalities such as disorganization of the normal pattern of cell positions (Scheibel and Kovelman, 1981; Kovelman and Scheibel, 1984) and other cytoarchitectonic (i.e. cell structural) irregularities (Jakob and Beckmann, 1986; Benes *et al.*, 1986; Benes and Bird, 1987; Benes *et al.*, 1987), and increased gliosis (Nieto and Escobar, 1972; Fisman, 1975; Stevens, 1982), have been reported, most often in midline grey matter of the diencephalon or other deep structures, particularly those of the limbic system.

The limbic system consists of a series of

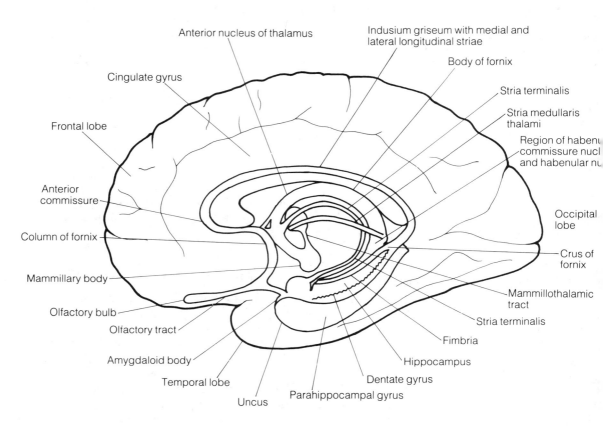

Figure 6.1 Medial aspect of right cerebral hemisphere, showing structures that form the limbic system. Modified reproduction with permission from Snell, R.S. (1980) *Clinical Neuroanatomy for Medical Students*, Little, Brown and Company, Boston, p. 276.

related structures, shown in Figure 6.1, that lie along the mesial surfaces of the cerebral hemispheres, and in the deep subcortical regions. Though still not well understood, these structures clearly play important roles in emotion, attention, and memory. They receive information from and project to widespread polymodal cortical and subcortical areas. It is, therefore, possible that they are involved in the integration of internally and externally generated information in support of abstract conceptual, social, and emotional processes. Gliosis is the focal proliferation of glial cells, a phenomenon usually associated with damage to and death of proximal neurons. Not all studies have confirmed these observations of cell disorganization or limbic gliosis in schizophrenic patients (Roberts *et al.*, 1986,

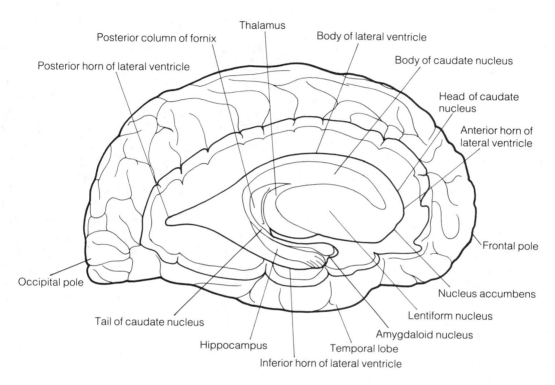

Figure 6.2 Lateral view of right cerebral hemisphere dissected to show the position of the lentiform nucleus, the caudate nucleus, the thalamus and the hippocampus. Modified reproduction with permission from Snell, R.S. (1980) *Clinical Neuroanatomy for Medical Students*, Little, Brown and Company, Boston, p. 243.

1987; Benes *et al.*, 1986; Altshuler *et al.*, 1987; Falkai *et al.*, 1988; Christison *et al.*, 1989). Questions remain, however, about whether the disparity of results may reflect differences in the methods used in the different studies (Altshuler *et al.*, 1987; Stevens and Casanova, 1988; Christison *et al.*, 1989).

Recently, several investigators have measured reduced volumes of, and/or decreased cell numbers in, mesial temporal lobe (limbic) structures including amygdala, hippocampus, parahippocampal gyrus, and entorhinal cortex

(Bogerts *et al.*, 1985; Brown *et al.*, 1986; Falkai and Bogerts, 1986; Colter *et al.*, 1987; Jeste and Lohr, 1989). Although the specific structures implicated vary from study to study, most careful histopathological investigations of these structures have revealed significant abnormalities.

Limbic structures outside of the temporal lobes have also been implicated. Benes and colleagues (Benes *et al.*, 1987; Benes and Bird, 1987) found smaller, more widely-spaced neurones, and excessive vertical axons, in the cingulate cortex of schizophrenic patients. Abnormalities of basal forebrain nuclei of the substantial innominata were also found in several studies (Nieto and Escobar, 1972; Averbach, 1981; Stevens, 1982). This region has received much attention because it is very importantly involved in the cholinergic neuro-transmitter system of the cerebral cortex.

In one study (Bogerts *et al.*, 1985), a reduction in the volume of the internal globus pallidus, as well as mesial temporal lobe reductions, was reported. This structure is a sub-part of the lenticular nucleus, which consists of the putamen and globus pallidus, and is part of a system referred to as the basal ganglia. The positions of the basal ganglia, underlying the cerebral cortex, particularly the frontal lobe, are illustrated in Figure 6.2. This system is strongly dopaminergic and has received much scrutiny due to the 'dopamine' hypothesis of schizophrenia, which is based in the ameliorative effects of drugs that block dopamine in the brain. Although excessive mineralization in the globus pallidus had been noted in neuropathological examination of some schizophrenic brains (Stevens, 1982), a recent study revealed no significant increase in iron deposition in the internal segment (Casanova *et al.*, 1990). Another basal ganglia structure that has received scrutiny, partly because of its strong connection with the limbic system, is the nucleus accumbens, in which some neurones were found to have decreased diameter (Dom *et al.*, 1981). However, the volume of this structure was unaltered in a recent study that used computer-assisted methods for estimating structural volumes (Bogerts *et al.*, 1985).

Not surprisingly, given the volume reductions noted in the studies summarized above, a slight overall reduction in brain weight and volume in schizophrenic patients has also been noted in some neuropathological studies (Brown *et al.*, 1986; Pakkenberg, 1987; Roberts and Bruton, 1990). In other studies, however, brain size in schizophrenics was equivalent to that in controls (Rosenthal and Bigelow, 1972).

Although cerebral structures have been the focus of most investigations, some have examined infratentorial structures (those in and around the cerebellum). These have yielded conflicting results. Some suggest increased prevalence of atrophy of the midline cerebellar structure called the vermis; but others do not find evidence of such atrophy. These studies were reviewed by Lohr and Jeste (1986), who themselves found no evidence for cerebellar pathology in post-mortem material from the Yakovlev Collection (Armed Forces Institute of Pathology, Washington DC).

Finally, increased corpus callosum width in schizophrenic patients has been observed (Rosenthal and Bigelow, 1972; Bigelow *et al.*, 1983).

Taken together, these findings suggest that brain structures, especially those within the limbic system, may be affected in many schizophrenic patients, but considerable variability may exist in the regional extent and severity of the abnormality within this system, and in the form of the abnormality itself (e.g. cell loss, axonal excess, failure of cells to migrate to their normal positions during development).

6.2 STRUCTURAL BRAIN IMAGING STUDIES

In vivo studies with x-ray computed tomography (CT) have focused on the sizes of CSF spaces, and less frequently on tissue CT values from within the grey or white matter of the brain. This literature has been summarized in several recent critical reviews (Weinberger, 1984; Jernigan, 1986; Shelton and Weinberger, 1986; Smith *et al.*, 1988; Miller, 1989). Results of increased ventricular size and cortical sulcal widening in schizophrenic patients relative to controls, are common; but the prevalence of such abnormalities (or the diagnostic 'effect size') varies dramatically from sample to sample. Some of this variability may be related to the selection criteria for control subjects. Several authors have noted that mean ventriculo-brain ratios (VBR) in control samples vary considerably, even when the mean ages of the subjects are comparable (Smith and Iacono, 1986; Smith *et al.*, 1988). Unfortunately, comparisons of mean VBR across studies are probably not justified given the variability in measurement technique from one research group to the next (Jernigan *et al.*, 1982a,b). Still, there is some suggestion that the use of medical controls (who presumably have undergone neurological screening) leads to an underestimate of the degree of variability in ventricular size which is actually present in the population of healthy, non-schizophrenic controls. This may lead to exaggeration of 'schizophrenia' effects in some studies. Another factor that is likely to contribute to disparities in the findings is the nature of the treatment setting from which the patients are recruited. There is some evidence that long-term, chronically hospitalized patients may be more likely to show signs of cerbral atrophy than patients with less severely disabling illnesses.

In addition to cerebral atrophy, increases in cerebellar atrophy (Heath *et al.*, 1982; Weinberger *et al.*, 1982; Lippman *et al.*, 1982; Dewan *et al.*, 1983a,b) and reversals in the typical pattern of cranial asymmetry (Luchins *et al.*, 1979a,b) have also been observed in schizophrenics, but these results have been less consistent (Coffman *et al.*, 1981; Tanaka *et al.*, 1981; Boronow *et al.*, 1985; Jernigan *et al.*, 1982b; Luchins and Meltzer, 1983). The results obtained from measurements of brain CT values have also been conflicting. Brain CT values are subject to substantial variation due to inadvertent voluming of non-brain areas within the volume elements (voxels), artefacts related to the effects of the cranium on x-ray attentuation (i.e. the spurious elevation of signal values near bony structures), and scanner calibration drift over time. The results of these studies are therefore quite difficult to interpret (see Jernigan, 1986, for review).

In summary, the CT findings suggest that in at least some schizophrenics the CSF spaces are enlarged. These findings have been taken by most to signal the presence of tissue damage in these patients, and indeed CT studies have done much to stimulate recent neuropathological studies; however, *in vivo* localization of such damage is severely limited with CT.

Magnetic resonance (MR) imaging provides a considerable increase in sensitivity and anatomical specificity over CT. This technique has been applied in a number of recent studies of schizophrenia. Several results are supportive of the neuropathological findings. In addition to CSF increases (Kelsoe *et al.*, 1988; Andreasen *et al.*, 1990; Jernigan *et al.*, 1991b), other anomalies have been observed, such as reduced cerebral size (Andreasen *et al.*, 1986; Johnstone *et al.*, 1989a; Dupont *et al.*, 1989), temporal horn abnormalities (Johnstone *et al.*, 1989b), corpus callosum and adjacent septum pellucidum abnormalities (Mathew *et al.*, 1985; Nasrallah *et al.*, 1986; Uematsu and Kaiya, 1989), and volume reductions in the thalamus (Andreasen *et al.*, 1990) and in the temporal lobe (Suddath *et al.*, 1989). Already, however, there have been inconsistent reports. No ventricular increase was found in two studies (Smith *et al.*, 1987; Rossi *et al.*, 1990), and Kelsoe *et al.* (1988) were unable to detect differences in limbic volumes or corpus callosum measurements. The results from corpus callosum measurements by Mathew *et al.* (1985) did not confirm a width increase, but their results did suggest increased size of the septum pellucidum, which was correlated with the duration of illness, and longer callosa in schizophrenic patients. The septum was increased in size in a second study by Uematsu and Kaiya (1989), but the increases were not associated with duration of illness, although they were associated with a family history of the disorder. Hauser *et al.* (1989) could not confirm any differences in corpus callosum morphology between schizophrenics and controls. Jernigan *et al.* (1991b) recently reported increased size of the lenticular nucleus and reduced volume of mesial temporal lobe structures in schizophrenic patients. Finally, decreased brain size

101

could not be confirmed in several studies (Weinberger *et al.*, 1987; Delisi and Goldin, 1987; Stevens and Waldmon, 1987; Reveley and Reveley, 1987; Kelsoe *et al.*, 1988; Andreasen *et al.*, 1990).

The explanation for disparate findings most frequently invoked in the reviews of this literature is population heterogeneity: the inclusion within the schizophrenia spectrum of patients very different in the nature and severity of their illnesses. Thus it is argued, patients with different anatomical abnormalities, possibly related to different aetiologies, will be present in different proportions from one study to the next, despite the fact that all patients meet consensus diagnostic criteria for the disorder. Unfortunately few consistent 'sub-type' effects have emerged from anatomical studies, with the possible exception that more globally dysfunctional patients seem to have more dramatic abnormalities.

Some of the inconsistency in the MR reports probably reflects the complexity of this new technique. Unlike CT, MR imaging can be accomplished in different planes of section, and can yield highly variable levels of spatial resolution and tissue contrast (depending on the protocol used for obtaining the images). In general, increases in contrast, resolution, and number of views all require additional imaging time during which the subject must be completely still. Thus, every MR image examination represents a compromise between image quality and practical considerations. Furthermore, there is very little consensus about the way to design an optimal MR imaging protocol for studies of schizophrenia, and even less about the best way to quantify the results once they are obtained. An investigator interested in the temporal lobes, for example, may choose a protocol with high spatial resolution in that region, which, however, images only part of the cerebrum. He or she may, therefore, be forced to settle for a less accurate estimate of whole brain or ventricular volume in order to obtain more sensitive measures of limbic

structures. It is, or course, a statistical fact that when two abnormalities are of equal magnitude, but one's methods are more sensitive to one abnormality than the other, one has a greater chance of detecting the abnormality for which the methods are more sensitive. Similarly, even if both are detected, the degree of abnormality will appear to be unequal. Obvious though this is, it is often ignored when interpreting results. In the hypothetical study described above, a failure to observe overall brain volume reduction, while measuring significant temporal lobe decreases, may be interpreted by the author as a demonstration of focal changes. In reality, the result may simply be due to the fact that the temporal lobe measures are more accurate. In order to avoid such errors one would need to know the relative accuracy of all of the measurement techniques used in the literature. However, this information is almost never available, even for the measures used in a single study. Under these circumstances one must be careful not to infer that knowledge resides only in those corners into which one has cast the strongest light.

Notwithstanding these problems, it is clear that the speed and quality of MR imaging is constantly improving; and that as experience with the technique grows, investigators are evolving a set of more-or-less standard measurement approaches that will find general acceptance. This should permit better method validation throughout the field. These factors should serve generally to increase the sensitivity of MR morphometrics and to promote greater consistency of the findings from different research groups.

6.3 INTERPRETIVE ISSUES

There is little consistent evidence regarding the relationship of the anatomic abnormalities described above to aetiological, treatment, or phenomenological factors. Some reviewers have concluded that structural damage to the brain probably occurs before the onset of the illness and may interact with genetic factors in the pathogenesis of the syndrome (Weinberger, 1984). Evidence for this view comes from reports of structural abnormalities in young, recent-onset patients (Schulz *et al.*, 1982, 1983a,b); association of perinatal risk factors with ventricular enlargement in schizophrenic patients (Schulsinger *et al.*, 1984; Owen *et al.*, 1988); and the presence of more structural abnormality in affected than in non-affected monozygotic twins (Reveley *et al.*, 1982; Suddath *et al.*, 1990).

Some of the evidence from anatomical studies suggests that the damage occurs before maturation of the nervous system is complete. Reduced brain size and focally decreased volumes of limbic structures, in the absence of associated gliosis, has been taken as indicative of hypoplasia, or reduced tissue growth (Colter *et al.*, 1987; Roberts *et al.*, 1987; Falkai *et al.*, 1988; Roberts and Bruton, 1990). Kovelman and Scheibel (1984) speculated that the cell disorganization they observed in the limbic system may be due to defective cell migration.

An important point made by several authors is that if such early changes lead to schizophrenia, it is unclear why the symptoms seldom emerge before adolescence (Weinberger, 1987). In 1982, Feinberg (1982/83; 1982) advanced the hypothesis that the typical peripubertal onset of the disorder may be due to the role of late brain maturation in its pathogenesis. He pointed to psychophysiological evidence for dramatic functional changes at this point in development, and the reports of a reduction of cortical synaptic density in human post-mortem material at about the same age (Huttenlocher, 1979); and argued that a perturbation of these events may result in the behavioural aberrations characteristic of major psychiatric disorders. According to this model, programmed synaptic elimination in early adolescence may be affected in schizophrenia, perhaps through an interaction between dopaminergic function and the endocrine system. It is of interest in this regard that Benes *et al.* (1987) report excessive vertical axons in anterior cingulate cortex of schizophrenics, a condition that could be due to an interruption of the normal process by which supernumerary axons are eliminated in development.

Jernigan and associates (Jernigan and Tallal, 1990; Jernigan *et al.*, 1991a) recently reported morphological changes in the cortex during adolescence on MR images. Volume reductions appeared to be particularly great in cortical regions which include the cingulate, as well as superior frontal and parietal cortices. Using the same methods, Jernigan *et al.* (1991b) noted volume reductions in limbic structures and volume increases in the lenticular nucleus in schizophrenic patients. This led to speculation that early damage to the brain leads to a failure to eliminate inappropriate neuronal constituents in critical lenticular structures at a time in late childhood when such 'pruning' is occurring in other brain structures. Thus, an imbalance between brain systems emerges at this time.

Hoffman and Dobscha (1989) recently explored the idea that a disorder of cortical 'pruning' might produce schizophrenia-like symptoms with a computer simulation. They concluded that information processing alterations in an *overpruned* neural net could resemble schizophrenia. Such exercises must be interpreted with caution, however, given current uncertainty about how cortical neuronal interactions support abstract thought and emotion.

Other investigators have proposed that at least some schizophrenics have a neurodegenerative disorder, and that this results in a deteriorating clinical course and progressive cerebral atrophy (Crow, 1980, 1983a,b). Woods and Wolf (1983) noted, after a re-analysis of the results of a study of discordant monozygotic twins (Reveley *et al.*, 1982), that an association between duration of illness and ventricular size was present within both affected and nonaffected sibling groups. Thus, it was argued, all of the subjects may have inherited a slowly progressive disorder producing cerebral atrophy. As the affected twins had larger ventricles than their co-twins, presumably an environmental insult had been an additive factor with the progressive disorder in the pathogenesis of frank psychosis in the ill siblings. Recently, Woods *et al.* (1990) reported the results of a retrospective longitudinal study of patients requiring repeated hospitalizations. CT measures suggested that increases in ventricular volume occurred over several years in many patients with affective disorder. These authors raised questions about the possible role of excitotoxic effects (Schwarz and Meldrum, 1985) in producing the progressive brain damage they observed. Excitotoxicity refers to a recently observed phenomenon in which excessive excitatory amino acids in the cellular medium is associated with cell death. Although the results of one other longitudinal CT study in schizophrenics is supportive of Woods *et al.* (1990) (Kemali *et al.*, 1989), several others using CT have failed to demonstrate progressive changes (Nasrallah *et al.*, 1986; Illowsky *et al.*, 1988; Vita *et al.*, 1988). Furthermore, many investigators have noted an absence of any association between duration of illness and structural abnormalities in their patient samples, a finding which also refutes the notion that the changes are related to chronic treatment.

A recently advanced hypothesis (Miller, 1989), invoking both neurodevelopmental and neurodegenerative factors is that anomalous connectivity within the nervous system may cause hyperactivity in limbic circuits, which in turn leads to excitotoxic cell loss. This hypothesis predicts that while anatomic disturbances may be present early in the development (and may cause abnormal neuronal interaction), additional structural damage occurs in association with episodes of symptom exacerbation. The disorder is, therefore, progressive until the aberrant hyperactivity abates due to excitotoxic loss of target cells in the limbic system. The poor association of duration of illness with the degree of cerebral atrophy challenges this hypothesis. However, since the degenerative process, as described, is likely to be self-limiting in both time and regional extent, and because it could occur within a relatively short time early in the course of the illness, a strong association between years of illness and atrophy, within groups of chronic patients, may not occur.

It is clear that much more work is necessary to resolve some of the issues raised in the preceding discussion. More accurate and more detailed information about the fine structure of the brain, and especially its synapses, in both normal and schizophrenic patients, will undoubtedly contribute much. However, some of the answers are unlikely to come from post-mortem material. MR imaging provides the first method with which it may be possible to test some of the clinico-anatomical hypotheses *in vivo*. For example, the hypothesis that damage to specific structures occurs as a concomitant of the psychosis itself may be testable (prospectively) with MR in longitudinal studies of first-break schizophrenic patients, or even youngsters 'at-risk' for developing schizophrenia. It is possible, of course, that both progressive schizophreniform neurological illnesses and stable, but chronic, psychoses with neurodevelopmental aetiologies exist within the schizophrenia spectrum. If so, longitudinal imaging studies may make a particularly important contribution in the on-going struggle to define the relevant dimensions of this heterogeneity. It is a reassuring fact that the yield from such studies will undoubtedly increase in association with the rapid technological improvements now occurring in the field of medical imaging.

REFERENCES

Altshuler, L.L., Conrad, A., Kovelman, J.A. and Scheibel, A. (1987) Hippocampal pyramidal cell orientation in schizophrenia. *Arch. Gen. Psychiatry*, **44**, 1094–8.

Andreasen, N.C., Ehrhardt, J.C., Swayze, V.W.

et al. (1990) Magnetic resonance imaging of the brain in schizophrenia. *Arch. Gen. Psychiatry*, **47**, 35–44.

Andreasen, N., Nasrallah, H.A., Dunn, V. *et al.* (1986) Structural abnormalities in the frontal system in schizophrenia: A magnetic resonance imaging study. *Arch. Gen. Psychiatry*, **43**, 136–44.

Averbach, P. (1981) Lesions of the nucleus ansae peduncularis in neuropsychiatric disease. *Arch. Neurol.*, **38**, 230–5.

Benes, F.M. and Bird, E.D. (1987) An analysis of the arrangement of neurons in the cingulate cortex of schizophrenic patients. *Arch. Gen. Psychiatry*, **44**, 608–16.

Benes, F., Davidson, J. and Bird, E.D. (1986) Quantitative cytoarchitectural studies of the cerebral cortex of schizophrenia. *Arch. Gen. Psychiatry*, **43**, 31–5.

Benes, F.M., Majocha, R., Bird, E.D. and Marotta, C.A. (1987) Increased vertical axon numbers in cingulate cortex of schizophrenics. *Arch. Gen. Psychiatry*, **44**, 1017–21.

Bigelow, L.B., Nasrallah, H.A. and Rausher, F.P. (1983) Corpus callosum thickness in chronic schizophrenia. *Br. J. Psychiatry*, **142**, 284–7.

Bogerts, B., Meertz, E. and Schönfeldt-Bausch, R. (1985) Basal ganglia and limbic system pathology in schizophrenia: A morphometric study of brain volume and shrinkage. *Arch. Gen. Psychiatry*, **42**, 784–91.

Boronow, J., Pickar, D., Ninan, P.T. *et al.* (1985) Atrophy limited to the third ventricle in chronic schizophrenia patients: Report of a controlled series. *Arch. Gen. Psychiatry*, **42**, 266–71.

Brown, R., Colter, N., Corsellis, J.A.N. *et al.* (1986) Postmortem evidence of structural brain changes in schizophrenia. Differences in brain weight, temporal horn area, and parahippocampal gyrus compared with affective disorder. *Arch. Gen. Psychiatry*, **43**, 36–42.

Casanova, M.F., Waldman, I.N. and Kleinman, J.E. (1990) A postmortem quantitative study of iron in the globus pallidus of schizophrenic patients. *Biol. Psychiatry*, **27**, 143–9.

Christison, G.W., Casanova, M.F., Weinberger, D.R. *et al.* (1989) A quantitative investigation of hippocampal pyramidal cell size, shape, and variability of orientation in schizophrenia. *Arch. Gen. Psychiatry*, **46**, 1027–32.

Coffman, J.A,. Mefferd, J., Golden, C.J. *et al.* (1981) Cerebellar atrophy in chronic schizophrenia. *Lancet*, **1**, 666.

Colter, N., Battal, S., Crow, T.J. *et al.* (1987) White matter reduction in the parahippocampal gyrus of patients with schizophrenia. *Arch. Gen. Psychiatry*, **44**, 1023.

Crow, T.J. (1980) Molecular pathology of schizophrenia: More than one disease process? *Br. Med. J.*, **280**, 66–8.

Crow, T.J. (1983a) Is schizophrenia an infectious disease? *Lancet*, **1**, 173–5.

Crow, T.J. (1983b) Schizophrenia as an infection. *Lancet*, **1**, 819–20.

Delisi, L.E. and Goldin, L.R. (1987) Hat size in schizophrenia. *Arch. Gen. Psychiatry*, **44**, 672–3.

Dewan, M.J., Pandurangi, A.K., Lee, S.H. *et al.* (1983a) Cerebellar morphology in chronic schizophrenic patients: A controlled computed tomography study. *Psychiatry Res.*, **10**, 97–103.

Dewan, M.J., Pandurangi, A.K., Lee, S.H. *et al.* (1983b) Central brain morphology in chronic schizophrenic patients: A controlled CT study. *Biol. Psychiatry*, **18**, 1133–40.

Dom, R., DeSaedeleer, J., Bogerts, J. and Hopf, A. (1981) Quantitative cytometric analysis of basal ganglia in catatonic schizophrenia. In *Biological Psychiatry*. C. Perris, G. Strewe and B. Jansson (eds), Elsevier/North-Holland Biomedical Press, Amsterdam, pp. 723–6.

Dupont, R.M., Jernigan, T.L., Gillin, J.C. *et al.* (1989 December) *Brain morphometric changes in schizophrenia and bipolar illness.* Paper presented at the Annual Meeting of ACNP, Maui, Hawaii.

Falkai, P. and Bogerts, B. (1986) Cell loss in the hippocampus of schizophrenics. *Eur. Arch. Psychiatry Neurol. Sci.*, **236**, 154–61.

Falkai, P., Bogerts, B. and Rozumek, M. (1988) Limbic pathology in schizophrenia: The entorhinal region – A morphometric study. *Biol. Psychiatry*, **24**, 515–21.

Feinberg, I. (1982) Schizophrenia and late maturational brain changes in man. *Psychopharmacol. Bull.*, **18**, 29–31.

Feinberg, I. (1982/83) Schizophrenia: Caused by a fault in programmed synaptic elimination during adolescence? *J. Psychiatr. Res.*, **17**, 319–34.

Fisman, M. (1975) The brain stem in psychosis. *Br. J. Psychiatry*, **126**, 414–22.

Hauser, P., Dauphinais, I.D. Berrettini, W., *et al.* (1989) Corpus callosum dimensions measured by magnetic resonance imaging in bipolar affective disorder and schizophrenia. *Biol. Psychiatry*, **26**, 659–68.

Heath, R.G., Franklin, D.E., Walker, C.F. and Keating, J.W. (1982) Cerebellar vermal atrophy in psychiatric patients. *Biol. Psychiatry*, **17**, 569–83.

Hoffman, R.E. and Dobscha, S.K. (1989) Cortical pruning and the development of schizophrenia: A computer model. *Schizophr. Bull.*, **15**, 477–89.

Huttenlocher, P.R. (1979) Synaptic density in human frontal cortex – Developmental changes and effects of aging. *Brain Res.*, **163**, 195–205.

Illowsky, B.P., Juliano, D.M., Bigelow, L.B. and Weinberger, D.R. (1988) Stability of CT scan findings in schizophrenia: Results of an 8 year follow-up study. *J. Neurol. Neurosurg. Psychiatry*, **51**, 209–13.

Jakob, H. and Beckmann, H. (1986) Prenatal-developmental disturbances in the limbic allocortex in schizophrenia. *J. Neural Transm.*, **65**, 303–26.

Jellinger, K. (1985) Neuromorphological background of pathochemical studies in major psychoses. In *Pathochemical Markers in Major Psychoses*. H. Beckmann and P. Riederer (eds), Springer-Verlag, Berlin, pp. 1–23.

Jernigan, T.L. (1986) Anatomical and CT scan studies of psychiatric disorders. In *American Handbook of Psychiatry*. Volume VIII, P.A. Berger and H.K.H. Brodie (eds), Basic Books Inc., New York, pp. 213–3.

Jernigan, T.L. and Tallal, P. (1990) Late childhood changes in brain morphology observable with MRI. *Dev. Med. Child Neurol.*, **32**, 379–85.

Jernigan, T.L., Trauner, D.A. Hesselink, J.R. and Tallal, P.A. (1991a) Maturation of human cerebrum observed *in vivo* during adolescence. *Brain*, **114**, 2037–49.

Jernigan, T.L., Zisook, S., Heaton, R.K. *et al.* (1991b) MR abnormalities in lenticular nuclei and cerebral cortex in schizophrenia. *Archives of General Psychiatry*, **48**, 881–90.

Jernigan, T.L., Zatz, L.M., Moses, J.A. and Berger, P.A. (1982a) Computed tomography in schizophrenics and normal volunteers: I. Fluid volume. *Arch. Gen. Psychiatry*, **39**, 765–70.

Jernigan, T.L., Zatz, L.M., Moses, J.A. and Cardellino, J.P. (1982b) Computed tomography in schizophrenics and normal volunteers: II. Cranial asymmetry. *Arch. Gen. Psychiatry*, **39**, 771–3.

Jeste, D.V. and Lohr, J.B. (1989) Hippocampal pathologic findings in schizophrenia. A morphometric study. *Arch. Gen. Psychiatry*, **46**, 1019–24.

Johnstone, E.C., Owens, D.G.C., Bydder, G.M., *et al.* (1989a) The spectrum of structural brain changes in schizophrenia: Age of onset as a predictor of cognitive and clinical impairments and their cerebral correlates. *Psychol. Med.*, **19**, 91–103.

Johnstone, E.C., Owens, D.G.C., Crow, T.J., *et al.* (1989b) Temporal lobe structure as determined by nuclear magnetic resonance in schizophrenia and bipolar affective disorder. *J. Neurol. Neurosurg. Psychiatry*, **52**, 736–41.

Kelsoe, J.R., Cadet, J.L., Pickar, D. and Weinberger, D.R. (1988) Quantitative neuroanatomy in schizophrenia: A controlled magnetic resonance imaging study. *Arch. Gen. Psychiatry*, **45**, 533–41.

Kemali, D., Maj, M., Galderisi, S. *et al.* (1989) Ventricle-to-brain ratio in schizophrenia: A controlled follow-up study. *Biol. Psychiatry*, **26**, 753–6.

Kovelman, J.A. and Scheibel, A.B. (1984) A neuro-histological correlate of schizophrenia. *Biol. Psychiatry*, **19**, 1601–21.

Lippmann, S., Manshadi, M., Baldwin, H. *et al.* (1982) Cerebellar vermis dimensions on computerized tomographic scans of schizophrenic and bipolar patients. *Am. J. Psychiatry*, **139**, 667–8.

Lohr, J.B. and Jeste, D.V. (1986) Cerebellar pathology in schizophrenia? A neuronometric study. *Biol. Psychiatry*, **21**, 865–75.

Luchins, D.J. and Meltzer, H.Y. (1983) A blind controlled study of occipital cerebral asymmetry in schizophrenia. *Psychiatry Res.*, **10**, 87–95.

Luchins, D.J., Weinberger, D.R. and Wyatt, R.J. (1979a) Anomalous lateralization associated with a milder form of schizophrenia. *Am. J. Psychiatry*, **136**, 1598–9.

Luchins, D.J., Weinberger, D.R. and Wyatt, R.J. (1979b) Schizophrenia: Evidence of a subgroup with reversed cerebral asymmetry. *Arch. Gen. Psychiatry*, **36**, 1309–11.

Mathew, R.J., Partain, C.L., Prakash, R. *et al.* (1985) A study of the septum pellucidum and corpus callosum in schizophrenia with MR imaging. *Acta Psychiatr. Scand.*, **72**, 414–21.

Miller, R. (1989) Schizophrenia as a progressive disorder: Relations to EEG, CT, neuropathological and other evidence. *Prog. Neurobiol.*, **33**, 17–44.

Nasrallah, H.A., Olson, S.C., McCalley-Whitters, M. *et al.* (1986) Cerebral ventricular enlargement in schizophrenia: A preliminary follow-up study. *Arch. Gen. Psychiatry*, **43**, 157–9.

Nieto, D. and Escobar, A. (1972) Major psychoses. In *Pathology of the Nervous System*. J. Minkler (ed), McGraw-Hill, New York, pp. 2654–5.

Owen, M.J., Lewis, S.W. and Murray, R.M. (1988) Obstetric complications and schizophrenia: A computed tomographic study. *Psychol. Med.*, **18**, 331–9.

Pakkenberg, B. (1987) Post-mortem study of chronic schizophrenic brains. *Br. J. Psychiatry*, **151**, 744–52.

Reveley, A.M., Reveley, M.A., Clifford, C.A. and Murray, R.M. (1982) Cerebral ventricular size in twins discordant for schizophrenia. *Lancet*, **1**, 540–1.

Reveley, M.A. and Reveley, A.M. (1987) Hat size in schizophrenia. *Arch. Gen. Psychiatry*, **44**, 673–4.

Roberts, G.W. and Bruton, C.J. (1990) Notes from the graveyard: Neuropathology and schizophrenia. *Neuropathol. Appl. Neurobiol.*, **16**, 3–16.

Roberts, G.W., Colter, N., Lofthouse, R., Bogerts, B., Zech, M. and Crow, T.J. (1986) Gliosis in schizophrenia: A survey. *Biol. Psychiatry*, **21**, 1043–50.

Roberts, G.W. Colter, N., Lofthouse, R. *et al.* (1987) Is there gliosis in schizophrenia? Investigation of the temporal lobe. *Biol. Psychiatry*, **22**, 1459–68.

Rosenthal, R. and Bigelow, L.B. (1972) Quantitative brain measurements in chronic schizophrenia. *Br. J. Psychiatry*, **121**, 259–64.

Rossi, A., Stratta, P., D'Albenzio, L. *et al.* (1990) Reduced temporal lobe areas in schizophrenia: Preliminary evidence from a controlled multiplanar magnetic resonance imaging study. *Biol. Psychiatry*, **27**, 61–8.

Scheibel, A.B. and Kovelman, J.A. (1981) Disorientation of the hippocampal pyramidal cell and its processes in the schizophrenic patient. *Biol. Psychiatry*, **16**, 101–2.

Schulsinger, F., Parnas, J., Petersen, E.T. *et al.* (1984) Cerebral ventricular size in the offspring of schizophrenic mothers: A preliminary study. *Arch. Gen. Psychiatry*, **41**, 602–6.

Schulz, S.C., Koller, M., Kishore, P.R. *et al.* (1982) Abnormal scans in young schizophrenics. *Psychopharmacol. Bull.*, **18**, 163–4.

Schulz, S.C., Koller, M.M., Kishore, P.R. *et al.* (1983a) Ventricular enlargement in teenage patients with schizophrenia spectrum disorder. *Am. J. Psychiatry*, **140**, 1592–5.

Schulz, S.C., Siniocrope, P., Kishore, P. and Friedel, R.O. (1983b) Treatment response and ventricular brain enlargement in young schizophrenic patients. *Psychopharmacol. Bull.*, **19**, 510–12.

Schwarcz, R. and Meldrum, B. (1985) Excitatory aminoacid antagonists provide a therapeutic approach to neurological disorders. *Lancet*, **2**, 140–3.

Shelton, R.C. and Weinberger, D.R. (1986) X-ray computerized tomography studies in schizophrenia: A review and synthesis. In *Handbook of Schizophrenia. Volume 1: The Neurology of Schizophrenia*. H.A. Nasrallah and D.R. Weinberger (eds), Elsevier, Amsterdam, pp. 207–50.

Smith, G.N. and Iacono, W.G. (1986) Lateral ventricular size in schizophrenia and choice of control group. *Lancet*, **1**, 1450.

Smith, G.N., Iacono, W.G., Moreau, M. *et al.* (1988) Choice of comparison group and findings of computerised tomography in schizophrenia. *Br. J. Psychiatry*, **153**, 667–74.

Smith, R.C., Baumgartner, R., Ravichandran, G.K. *et al.* (1987) Cortical atrophy and white matter density in the brains of schizophrenics and clinical response to neuroleptics. *Acta Psychiatr. Scand.*, **75**, 11–19.

Stevens, J.R. (1982) Neuropathology of schizophrenia. *Arch. Gen. Psychiatry*, **39**, 1131–9.

Stevens, J.R. and Casanova, M.F. (1988) Is there a neuropathology of schizophrenia? *Biol. Psychiatry*, **24**, 123–8.

Stevens, J.R. and Waldmon, I.N. (1987) Hat size in schizophrenia. *Arch. Gen. Psychiatry*, **44**, 673.

Suddath, R.L., Casanova, M.F., Goldberg, T.E.,

et al. (1989) Temporal lobe pathology in schizophrenia: A quantitative magnetic resonance imaging study. *Am. J. Psychiatry*, **146**, 464–72.

Suddath, R.L., Christison, G.W., Torrey, E.F. *et al.* (1990) Anatomical abnormalities in the brains of monozygotic twins discordant for schizophrenia. *N. Eng. J. Med.*, **322**(12), 789–94.

Tanaka, Y., Hazama, H., Kawahara, R. and Kobayashi, K. (1981) Computerized tomography of the brain in schizophrenic patients: A controlled study. *Acta Psychiatr. Scand.*, **63**, 191–7.

Uematsu, M. and Kaiya, H. (1989) Midsagittal cortical pathomorphology of schizophrenia: A magnetic resonance imaging study. *Psychiatry Res.*, **30**, 11–20.

Vita, A., Sacchetti, E., Valvassori, G. and Cazzullo, C.L. (1988) Brain morphology in schizophrenia: A 2- to 5-year CT scan follow-up study. *Acta Psychiatr. Scand.*, **78**, 618–21.

Weinberger, D.R. (1984) Computed tomography (CT) findings in schizophrenia: Speculation on the meaning of it all. *J. Psychiatr. Res.*, **18**, 477–90.

Weinberger, D.R. (1987) Implications of normal brain development for the pathogenesis of schizophrenia. *Arch. Gen. Psychiatry*, **44**, 660–9.

Weinberger, D.R., DeLisi, L.E., Perman, G.P. *et al.* (1982) Computed tomography in schizophreniform disorder and other acute psychiatric disorders. *Arch. Gen. Psychiatry*, **39**, 778–83.

Weinberger, D.R., Wagner, R.L. and Wyatt, R.J. (1983) Neuropathological studies of schizophrenia: A selective review. *Schizophr. Bull.*, **9**, 193–212.

Weinberger, D.R., Berman, K.F., Iadarola, M. *et al.* (1987) Hat size in schizophrenia. *Arch. Gen. Psychiatry*, **44**, 672.

Woods, B.T. and Wolf, J. (1983) A reconsideration of the relation of ventricular enlargement to duration of illness in schizophrenia. *Am. J. Psychiatry*, **140**, 1564–70.

Woods, B.T., Yurgelun-Todd, D., Benes, F.M. *et al.* (1990) Progressive ventricular enlargement in schizophrenia: Comparison to bipolar affective disorder and correlation with clinical course. *Biol. Psychiatry*, **27**, 341–52.

Chapter 7

The genetics of schizophrenia

T. READ, M. POTTER and H.M.D. GURLING

7.1 INTRODUCTION

Schizophrenia has traditionally tended to occupy a special position in the nature versus nurture debate. The suggestion that genes could influence a disorder such as schizophrenia has aroused apprehension in some quarters (Rose *et al.*, 1984): perhaps this has been because of the idea that if a disease is substantially 'genetic' then there is the implication that it is untreatable. Perhaps apprehension has also arisen because a genetic hypothesis for schizophrenia conflicts with ideologically attractive notions of self determination of the mind. However, not all political commentators on schizophrenia have chosen to view schizophrenia as a product of the environment: for example, Sedgwick (1976) argues strongly in favour of a medical model and that better resources for the mentally ill and better psychiatry are needed. Foucault argues that we may not be able to define 'normality' of the mind without first understanding and defining madnesses such as schizophrenia (Foucault, 1976).

The fact that schizophrenia tends to recur in families is one of the most prominent findings in schizophrenia research. This observation is simply evidence that familial factors must be involved in the development of schizophrenia. Such factors may be genetic or environmental.

Genetic methods for analysing human behavioural characteristics that have usually been thought to have a polygenic multifactorial (i.e. complex) origin have traditionally consisted of family, twin, adoption and half sib studies. These approaches can be subsumed under the title of **variance component or path analysis** (Fulke, 1973, 1978; Wright, 1983). Such analyses must always incorporate various assumptions for which there may not be a good justification (Henderson, 1982) and as a result there are limitations as to how accurately the proportions of genetic and environmental variance that contribute to a disease can be measured (Feldman and Cavalli-Sforza, 1977, 1979; Henderson, 1982). However a general impression of the relative contributions of genetic and environmental effects can be gained if all the traditional behavioural genetic methods are used in a variety of different environments at different points in time.

The principle methods for identifying a mode of transmission are known as **segregation analysis** and **genetic linkage analysis**. Segregation analysis can attempt to identify whether there may be many or a few genes (polygenic or oligogenic transmission) conferring liability to the disease. A third possibility that can be tested by segregation analysis is that there is a single abnormal gene which is providing most of the genetic effect and this is known as transmission by a single major locus (Morton *et al.*, 1983). Such an effect may be be recessive when two disease alleles, one from each parent, must be inherited, or dominant when only one disease allele is transmitted to an affected person. Morton and Maclean (1974) have proposed a 'mixed' model that combine a single major locus, a polygenic background and environmental effects.

All the above methods suffer from sources of error that may not be adequately controlled. These include reduced penetrance (the incomplete manifestation of a trait in individuals who carry the pathogenic genotype), phenocopies (cases which do not carry the genotype but who nevertheless manifest the disorder), genetic heterogeneity, diagnostic difficulties, sampling bias, ascertainment bias, mortality and variable age of onset. Despite these difficulties, recent quantitative estimates of the genetic component in the susceptibility to develop schizophrenia derived from both twin and family studies is consistent in finding that between 70% to 80% of the variance is purely genetic (Fulker, 1973; Kendler, 1983). These early family, twin and adoption studies provided important evidence for a genetic mechanism in schizophrenia but have now been superseded by the recent advances in molecular genetics using recombinant DNA technology. The recombinant DNA approach is beginning to transform schizophrenia research and may eventually lead to the identification of specific genetic mutations in terms of DNA sequence and the characterization of the abnormal brain proteins involved. This in turn should pave the way for new models of aetiology, transmission and nosology of the schizophrenias with improved methods of treatment and prophylaxis.

7.1 FAMILY STUDIES

Family studies can provide clues as to whether genetic factors might be involved in producing an illness. However this method alone does not distinguish between genetic and environmental factors. Most studies have usually observed the lifetime incidence of the illness in the relatives of schizophrenic patients and compared this with the incidence in control families and the general population. The first such study performed by Rudin in Munich (Rudin, 1916) showed an increased incidence of schizophrenia in the relatives of schizophrenics and this was confirmed by many other workers. Table 7.1 shows the combined data from almost all family studies of schizophrenia and shows that the risk increases with the degree of genetic relatedness within a family.

Table 7.1 Mean lifetime expectancy of schizophrenia in relatives of schizophrenics from previous family studies (Gottesman and Shields, 1982)

Relationship	% Schizophrenic
Parent	5.6
Sibling	10.1
Sibling (1 parent also affected)	16.7
Children	12.8
Children (both parents affected)	46.3
Uncles, aunts, nephews, nieces	2.8
Grandchildren	3.7
Unrelated	0.86

A valid criticism of these earlier studies was that they did not use a standardized diagnostic criteria or controls. Furthermore the probands as well as relatives were often not diagnosed blindly. The absence of age correction may have meant that the recurrence risk for schizophrenia was underestimated because some apparently normal individuals had yet to live through the age of maximum risk. When more narrowly defined research criteria for schizophrenia were used, the number of people diagnosed as having the illness decreased but the relative risk of developing the disorder for relatives of the index schizophrenics compared with relatives of controls remained fairly constant. The largest recent study which met modern research standards (Kendler *et al.*, 1985) showed that the morbid risk in the first-degree relatives of 253 DSM–III cases of schizophrenia was 18 times that of controls.

7.2 TWIN STUDIES

The most important assumption of the twin method is that monozygotic twins have the same genotype while dizygotic twins have on average only 50% of their genes in common with constant environmental factors. In fact the special case of twinning may make the assumption of equal environmental effects in families of MZ and DZ twin pairs questionable.

However, if the assumption is valid then for disorders with a genetic component there should be greater concordance in monozygotic twins than in dizygotic pairs. This has generally been found to be true in twin studies of schizophrenia and the MZ:DZ concordance ratio is consistently in excess of 3:1. It is true to say, however, that some of the earlier twin studies suffered from methodological deficiencies, the most important being selection bias, poor zygosity determination, lack of operational criteria and age correction.

Gottesman and Shields (1972) used systematic ascertainment by selecting their probands from the Maudsley twin register where all patients who were twins were consecutively listed. They found an MZ:DZ concordance ratio of 58:12 and taking a weighted average from their own and four other methodologically similar studies (Gottesman and Schields, 1976) found a concordance ratio of 46:14. The disconcordance rate of over 50% in monozygotic twins tends to support the importance of non-genetic biological or environmental factors. However incomplete penetrance *per se* does not necessarily mean that environmental factors are of the greatest importance because the genetic compensatory mechanisms at other loci acting stochastically could make good the defect caused by the primary mutation. Similar ratios were found by other workers using the narrow RDC, DSM–III and Feighner criteria (McGuffin *et al.*, 1984;

Farmer *et al.*, 1987).

As mentioned above, twin studies may not give accurate information about the effects of the shared family environment. Exposure to the same environmental factors may cause a similar clinical picture in twins. This could be particularly powerful in monozygotic twins because of shared placental circulation, greater psychological identification with each other and perhaps by their capacity to evoke similar responses by their similarity. Gottesman and Shields (1982) sought to clarify this by reporting 12 monozygotic twins who have been separated early in life and reared apart. Seven of these (58%) were concordant for schizophrenia and this has been interpreted as being highly suggestive of a genetic influence.

If it is accepted that the twin method is a valid approach for the investigation of schizophrenia then estimates made by Fulker (1973) by combining all the available twin study data suggests that the variance contributed by the family environment in the susceptibility to develop schizophrenia is less than 1.00%. This implies that the role of mothering and fathering in schizophrenia is virtually nil. This does not preclude a role for the family in causing readmission and affecting overall prognosis as described in theories concerning expressed emotion in schizophrenia families (see Chapter 8). Fulker's estimate of the effect of unique environmental variance that afflicts one member of a twin pair and not the other is about 20%. This proportion of the variance also includes any random effects and error but it may indicate that the non-familial environment has some role to play, perhaps in triggering episodes of illness by such factors as head injuries, birth trauma, viruses, and childbirth.

7.3 ADOPTION STUDIES

Adoption and cross fostering studies seek to further clarify the respective contributions of the genetic endowment and the environment because with this approach genes and environment are more clearly separated than in the twin method. A potential drawback is that the biological parents of adopted children are known to be more deviant with a higher rate of psychiatric disorder, alcoholism and criminality than ordinary parents (Bohman, 1978). Adopting parents are usually carefully screened and it is possible that there is a process of selective placement so that children offered for adoption are placed in homes where the adoptive parents have similar problems to those occurring in the biological parents (Rose *et al.*, 1984). In addition one might expect to find a generalized increase in psychiatric disorder in adopted children who are used as controls.

The best designed studies came from a large Danish–American collaboration which use the excellent Danish National Adoption register. The adopted-away children of schizophrenics had a significantly higher risk (18.8%) of developing schizophrenia or related conditions than the adopted-away children of controls (10.1%; Rosenthal *et al.*, 1975). Most of the children were born before the first episode of illness in the parent and about a third of the schizophrenic parents were male, thus weakening arguments that the schizophrenia may have been caused by early mother–child interaction or by an intrauterine event.

Taking a different approach to the same issue, Kety *et al.* (1975) found an increased incidence of schizophrenia and related disorders in the biological relatives of schizophrenics who had been adopted (20.3%) compared with the incidence in adoptive relatives and relatives of controls (5.8%). The same data were reanalysed using DSM–III criteria by Kendler and Gruenberg (1984). They found a 13.5% incidence of schizophrenia or schizotypal personality in the biological relatives of schizophrenics compared with 1.5% in the controls.

That genes are probably more 'schizophrenogenic' than parenting was illustrated by Wender *et al.* (1974) who found a significantly higher rate of schizophrenia spectrum disorder in the offspring of schizophrenics raised by normal adopting parents than in the offspring of psychiatrically normal adults raised by parents who subsequently became schizophrenic.

7.4 SEGREGATION ANALYSIS, VULNERABILITY MARKERS AND GENETIC LINKAGE ANALYSIS

7.4.1 SEGREGATION ANALYSIS

Taking into account all the family, twin and adoption studies described above it seems that the evidence for a genetic contribution to the aetiology of schizophrenia is strong. On the basis that such a contribution has been established there have been a number of attempts to determine a mode of genetic transmission for schizophrenia by using segregation analysis.

As described above segregation analysis is a statistical method of observing the frequency of a disorder in different generations of a series of families and inferring whether the observed patterns are compatible with certain models of genetic and environmental transmission (Morton and McLean, 1974; Morton *et al.*, 1983). In practice this means employing likelihood methods to test specific models and to determine the model that fits best. Values for parameters that vary such as disease gene frequency, penetrance, Mendelian (single major locus) transmission and polygenic/multifactorial transmission are entered into the equations and compared with one another. Of major interest to those who wish to employ molecular genetic methods is the question as to whether it is likely that there are single major locus (SML) effects involved. If these could be shown then the argument for using genetic linkage analysis would be very strong. In addition it is of interest to know the relative strengths of SML effects as part of a mixed model (Morton and Maclean, 1974; Reich *et al.*, 1975; Lalouel *et al.*, 1983). However it should be understood that segregation analysis will often not detect single major locus effects if the disease gene has low or intermediate penetrance, if there is low fertility associated with the abnormal gene and if there is underlying genetic heterogeneity with different modes of transmission operating in subtypes of schizophrenia (Kendler, 1983).

Baron (1986) has comprehensively reviewed past studies (e.g. Risch and Baron, 1984) of segregation analysis applied to schizophrenic family data. Considerable variation was evident between studies and conflicting results reported. The SML model was compatible with the data in seven of the twelve analyses but was rejected by five. In contrast the multifactorial polygenic model was rejected in one of only five studies while two studies rejected both the SML and multifactorial polygenic models. Finally the two studies that examined a model of SML with polygenic background concluded that this model was compatible with the data.

Population differences may have contributed to the conflicting results but it is clear that schizophrenia is a complex trait which does not always show simple Mendelian inheritance. This is perhaps not surprising considering its association with reduced fertility, social isolation and greater than expected familial incidence of non-schizophrenic psychiatric disorder (Gurling *et al.*, 1989). Other potential sources of error include reduced penetrance, false positive cases, genetic heterogeneity, diagnostic difficulties, sampling bias, ascertainment bias, mortality and variable age of onset.

Despite the fact that it has not been possible to define a mode of genetic transmission very precisely there have been attempts to localize mutant alleles predisposing to schizophrenia. Polygenic/threshold models do not exclude the possibility of a major gene contributing to the liability for developing special subtypes of schizophrenia (McGue *et al.*, 1985). Reviewers of this topic (Sturt and McGuffin, 1985; McGuffin and Sturt, 1986; Kendler, 1986) have therefore supported the search for genetic susceptibilities through the study of

biological vulnerability traits and genetic markers.

7.4.2 VULNERABILITY MARKERS

Vulnerability traits are biological characteristics that are connected with a genetic susceptibilty to a disorder. They may be biological, neurophysiological or morphological. The traits are presumed to be part of the pathway from the genotype to phenotype and their proximity to the original gene defect may vary. Baron (1986) has reviewed the uses and limitations of vulnerability traits in the study of schizophrenia and summarized current findings. Of the measures surveyed five potential susceptibility traits: platelet monoamine oxidase (MAO), plasma amine oxidase (PAO), catechol-O-methyl transferase (COMT), brain serum globulin binding and brain ventricular volume have been studied systematically. Reduced MAO and PAO did not appear to be a major risk factor in the development of schizophrenia (Baron *et al.*, 1983, 1984). COMT activity showed no evidence as a potential vulnerability trait (Baron *et al.*, 1984; Baron, 1986). Brain serum globulin binding was associated with an increased likelihood of the disorder in families but this was not statistically significant (Baron, 1977). The data relating to increased brain ventricular size and familial transmission is conflicting (Owen *et al.*, 1988).

Vulnerability traits provide a useful avenue of investigation but their use in determining underlying genetic aetiology is restricted because there has never been any strong *a priori* evidence for their involvement and because, in most cases, the genetics of the traits themselves are unclear. The use of genetic linkage markers provides a more robust investigation.

7.4.3 GENETIC LINKAGE AND ASSOCIATION ANALYSIS

Gene markers correspond to genetic loci with known chromosomal assignments and have simple Mendelian models of inheritance; that is, the markers are directly determined or directly reflect alleles or variant DNA sequences at specific loci. Such allelic variation is known as polymorphism and can be reliably detected independently of phases of the illness or recovery. In general the more polymorphic or variable a locus is found to be, the more useful it becomes in linkage studies. There are two approaches for the study of disorders using genetic linkage markers. Studies of association can be undertaken between markers and the disorder and then compared with a general population control group. In this instance the phenomenon of allelic association or linkage disequilibrium refers to the evolutionary tendency for DNA segments that are close enough together to remain linked in successive generations despite the presence of genetic recombination between loci. In fact, DNA sequences that are less than a distance of 1% recombination (1 million base pairs) tend to stay linked during evolution. In the case of a disease there may be marker polymorphisms that tend to be co-inherited due to linkage disequilibrium. These polymorphisms are referred to as being allele specific and are indicators that the polymorphic marker is less than approximately 1 million base pairs from the disease mutation.

Linkage analysis consists of finding polymorphic genetic markers that are sufficiently close on a chromosome so that they are inherited together with the disease mutation from one generation to the next. In such cases the marker and disease are said to be linked. The distance between illness gene and the marker locus can be calculated by observing the number of recombinations that occur (recombination is the rearrangement of alleles following exchange of material between pairs of homologous chromosomes during meiosis). The closer the disease locus is to the marker, the less likely recombination is to occur. Recombination is measured by the recombination fraction theta $(0.0 < \theta < 0.5)$. This is the proportion of instances within a pedigree that the disease

and the marker are not inherited together. A value of 0.5 indicates random segregagation of the disease and marker alleles, a value less than 0.5 indicates that linkage may be present.

The main statistical method used to analyse the observation of co-segregation of marker and disease through families is called the *lod* method (Morton, 1956). It is usually expressed as the lod score which is the logarithm to the base 10 of the odds ratio of linkage at a specified recombination fraction as opposed to linkage at 50% recombination. In practice likelihood methods are used and penetrance as well as gene frequencies are incorporated into computations. At any specific value of theta a lod score exceeding 3.0 is said to confirm linkage and a value less than -2.0 rejects linkage. A comprehensive account of linkage analysis has been given by Ott (1985) and its application to schizophrenia has been discussed by Baron (1986) and Gurling (1986, 1988).

Early attempts at linkage studies in schizophrenia were hampered by the small number of potential markers available (usually protein markers) and their relatively low degree of polymorphism. This made most studies largely uninformative. There have been nine linkage studies of schizophrenia (Elston *et al.*, 1973; Turner, 1979; McGuffin *et al.*, 1983; Andrew *et al.*, 1987; Gurling *et al.*, 1988; Sherrington *et al.*, 1988; Kennedy *et al.*, 1988; St. Clair *et al.*, 1988, 1989; Detera-Wadleigh *et al.*, 1989). Positive lod scores have been reported for the immunoglobin proteins, Gm and Bc (Elston *et al.*, 1973) and phosphoglucomutase (Andrew *et al.*, 1987). Gc has also been shown to be associated (rather than linked) with schizophrenia (Lange, 1982; Papiha 1982). Extensive association and some linkage studies between the HLA genes and schizophrenia have not produced consistent results (Kendler, 1986).

The use of linkage markers in the investigation of psychiatric genetics has been revolutionized by the use of restriction fragment length polymorphisms (RFLPs) and other DNA markers. Restriction enzymes are bacterial proteins that cut double-stranded DNA at specific sequences of nucleotide base pairs. At any one locus DNA variation can only occur between homologous chromosomes and some of these variations may create or destroy a restriction enzyme cutting site. This produces variation in the fragment lengths produced by specific enzymes. The variation in fragment lengths is observed by transferring restricted DNA fragments to a suitable membrane (Southern, 1975) and hybridizing those fragments to a cloned radioactive gene or DNA segment (known as a probe) so that any fragments containing the same sequence as the probe will become visible (Gurling, 1986). The discovery of those RFLPs and their subsequent use as linkage markers has provided a method of systematically screening chromosomes.

With the increasing numbers of RFLPs it has become possible to cover the entire genome. However, this may involve in excess of 200 markers (Lange and Boehnke, 1982) and thus 'blind' linkage studies require formidable resources. A more manageable strategy is to concentrate on areas where there is an *a priori* reason for suspecting involvement between marker and disease. Investigation at loci implicated by cytogenetic abnormalities offers one such approach.

Cytogenetic abnormalities reported in combination with schizophrenic psychoses include fragile sites (Ruddock *et al.*, 1983; Chodirker *et al.*, 1987), deletions, pericentric inversions (Axelsson and Wahlstrom 1983; Hong, 1986) trisomies (Turner, 1961; Sperber, 1975) acentric fragments (Kaplan, 1970; Dasgupta *et al.*, 1973), translocations or sex chromosome abnormalities (Kaplan, 1970; Crow, 1988). Although more common than in the general population these lesions are found only in a small proportion of those suffering from schizophrenia. However, they may be indicative of a sub-type of illness normally caused by other abnormalities at the same genomic site. The first positive, although unconfirmed,

evidence for a genetic basis to schizophrenia using linkage markers has been obtained using the strategy outlined above.

A report from Canada of a chromosomal abnormality in a Chinese man and his nephew both suffering from schizophrenia, facial dysmorphism and other abnormalities implicated an area of trisomy on chromosome 5 worthy of further investigation (Bassett *et al.*, 1988, 1989).

Linkage studies using probes localized to the chromosomal area 5q11-5q13 were undertaken in five Icelandic and two British families. The results were analysed using a variety of diagnostic classifications for schizophrenia and its associated disorders. The lod scores obtained ranged from 2.45 to 6.45 depending on the model used and provided strong evidence for the segregation of a dominant schizophrenia susceptibility allele on chromosome 5 (Sherrington *et al.*, 1988). The highest concordance for linkage was with the broadest definition of psychiatric disorder. It is therefore possible that the schizophrenia genotype may predispose to other *forme fruste* conditions that mimic other some non-schizophrenia conditions (Gurling *et al.*, 1988, 1989). This is however a preliminary finding which requires further investigation.

The findings of Sherrington (1988) and colleagues was based on the following selection criteria.

1. Only medium- to large-sized pedigrees with schizophrenia in at least three generations were sampled. This permitted computation of lod scores suggestive of linkage within single families.

2. High density pedigrees allowed suggestive lod scores to be computed by considering affected schizophrenics alone. This circumvented some of the problems of incomplete penetrance.

3. Families without manic depression present were selected. This was made possible by extensive pedigree tracing work and was

115

designed to avoid the problem of including false positive cases with schizoaffective diagnoses.

4. Families were obtained with *only one possible source for a schizophrenic allele* entering (segregating) in the kindred.
5. A population which has the *characteristics of a genetic isolate* was chosen for five out of the seven families in order to increase the chance of obtaining a genetically homogeneous sample.

The proportion of the schizophrenia that is related to the chromosome 5q11-q13 in many other populations is as yet unknown. However other studies (Kennedy *et al.*, 1988; St Clair *et al.*, 1989, 1990; Detera-Wadleigh *et al.*, 1989; McGuffin *et al.*, 1987, 1990) have failed to demonstrate chromosome 5 linkage.

However the negative results reported for chromosome 5 markers and schizophrenia need to be interpreted with some caution. The study by Kennedy *et al.* (1988) was the most comparable with the Iceland/UK sample in terms of the sample studies. These workers used a large multiplex Swedish pedigree but excluded from the sample all but definite cases of schizophrenia. Thus schizophrenia spectrum disorders of schizophrenia 'fringe' type phenotypes were not used in the analysis. The sample is thus not comparable on clinical grounds with the UK/Icelandic study for rates and types of the non-psychotic schizophrenia related disorders.

The studies of St. Clair *et al.* (1989) and Detera-Wadleigh *et al.* (1989) used some families containing both bipolar disorder and schizophrenia. A substantial proportion of the cases for genetic analysis were bipolar or schizoaffective rather than schizophrenic and such a number of false positive cases could obscure a positive linkage result. However in both cases, an analysis excluding the pedigrees containing bipolar disorder also failed to confirm linkage. Taking all the studies together, and assuming the chromosome 5 result is valid,

the evidence shows that there is heterogeneity of linkage for the susceptibility to schizophrenia with some families being chromosome 5 linked and others not. The difficulty that genetic heterogeneity presents for future linkage studies is considerable because the available statistical tests (Ott, 1985) require large family sizes in order to distinguish linked sub-groups of schizophrenia.

7.5 SCHIZOPHRENIA SPECTRUM DISORDERS

The classification of the schizophrenia spectrum disorders is a topic which is actively being investigated. Modern diagnostic criteria use narrow definitions. However, genetic studies can validate and advance existing diagnostic systems by providing some external criteria that a given genetic defect can predispose to a specific range of disorders that can be considered *forme frustes* of schizophrenia. This has useful research implications because exclusion of subjects with schizophrenia related illness such as schizotypal disorder from pedigree studies leads to an underestimation of morbidity risks and will decrease the power of statistical analysis. From a clinical point of view the under-recognition of some spectrum disorders may mean that the diagnosis and treatment of some low grade schizophrenic cases may be overlooked. So what constitutes a case?

Kety *et al.* (1968, 1975) reported increased rates of borderline schizophrenia among biological relatives in the Danish adoption studies diagnosed by clinical judgement. Spitzer *et al.* (1979) developed the concept of spectrum disorders and operational criteria were incorporated into DSM–III and DSM–III–R). The majority of family studies (e.g. Kendler *et al.*, 1984; Baron *et al.*, 1985; Frangos *et al.*, 1985) have since shown a significant increase in schizotypal personality disorder in the relatives of schizophrenics compared with the relatives of normal controls. Adoption studies (Lowing *et al.*, 1983; Kendler and Gruenberg,

1984) have strengthened the evidence that schizotypal personality is a non-psychotic manifestation of the same genotype predisposing to schizophrenia. In a multivariate analysis Baron and Risch (1987) found statistical evidence that schizophrenia and schizotypal personality were part of a single disorder and not transmitted independently.

There is some evidence that paranoid personality may be aetiologically related to schizophrenia while delusional disorder may be genetically distinct. Kendler *et al.* (1981, 1984) reanalysed the Danish data and found evidence of an increase in paranoid and schizotypal personality disorders in biological relatives of schizophrenics, but not in the relatives of patients with delusional disorder. Further research that showed delusional disorder to be a separate genetic entity was found in a family study (Kendler and Hays, 1981) where the incidence of schizophrenia was significantly less in the first-degree relatives of patients with delusional disorder than in relatives of schizophrenics.

Kety (1983) reported that Danish adoption data indicated that schizophrenia was not genetically associated with anxiety disorder, major depression, paranoid states and acute schizophrenic reaction. The status of the latter, redefined in DSM--III as schizophreniform disorder, is not clear. Tsuang *et al.* (1976) suggested that many so-called acute schizophrenic reactions were actually misdiagnosed manic illnesses.

In an exploratory study of the Maudsley twin series Farmer *et al.* (1987) found that the maximum difference in MZ/DZ concordance (i.e. the highest index for heritability) was for a definition of affection to include all psychoses that exhibited mood incongruent delusions, schizotypal personality and atypical psychosis, suggesting a common genetic origin for this spectrum of disorders. The effect of including delusional disorder and all other affective disorders was a reduction in the concordance ratio implying that they were not genetically related to schizophrenia.

In the UK/Icelandic study (Sherrington *et al.*, 1988), the highest concordance for linkage was with the broadest definition of psychiatric disorder, i.e. including the fringe phenotypes. Some patients who, for example, appeared chronically and atypically depressed may have been suffering from the effect of a schizophrenia genotype which had manifested in blunted effect, withdrawal, anhedonia and poverty of speech, as found in the negative or type 2 schizophrenic (Crow, 1980). Further evidence that these fringe phenotypes are indeed variant expressions of the same underlying mutation is required as elevation of the lod that occurred when they were included as 'cases' for linkage analysis was only about 2.00. The same study also found that all the traditional subtypes of schizophrenia — paranoid, hebephrenic, catatonic, undifferentiated and unspecified psychosis — were present in the same families within the sample. This shows that within a family a single disease genotype can give rise to clinical diversity. In other words, clinical heterogeneity does not imply underlying genetic heterogeneity. This finding is supported by family and twin studies (Delisi *et al.*, 1987; Kendler *et al.*, 1988) in which no evidence for the proband subtype to breed true was found. Other work has suggested a mild tendency towards homotypia in families with the paranoid and hebephrenic subtypes (Tsuang *et al.*, 1974; Scharfetter and Nusperli, 1980; McGuffin *et al.*, 1987). Others have put forward the idea that the hebephrenic form of schizophrenia may be more heritable than the paranoid variety (Winokur *et al.*, 1974; McGuffin *et al.*, 1984) which lends support to Tsuang and Winokur's (1974) concept of a hebephrenic-paranoid continuum of illness with the hebephrenic type being the most advanced and severe form.

Keefe *et al.*, (1987) who carried out a family study compared severely disabled 'Kraepelinian' schizophrenics with other chronic, but intermittently exacerbating, schizophrenics. They found a higher incidence of schizophrenia spectrum disorders in the relatives of the former group (19.3%) compared with the relatives of the latter group (10.7%). The Kraepelinian group were also characterized by asymmetry of the lateral ventricles and a lack of response to neuroleptics. Kane *et al.* (1988) found that 30% of neuroleptic non-responders showed some improvement with the drug clozapine which has relatively low dopaminergic activity. Again the question remains whether this group is aetiologically distinct or merely the severe end of a continuum.

There is a great potential for further linkage work using large samples to further delineate and clarify the nature of schizophrenia. Is it a single disease with marked clinical variation or is it a number of diseases with overlapping phenotypic manifestations? Traits such as social isolation, forms of unusual speech, magical thinking, suspiciousness and illusions all appear to be related to schizophrenia. These have yet to be investigated in family linkage studies. It seems that the current concept of schizotypy as defined in DSM–III-R is probably still too narrow and will need to evolve further.

7.5.1 SCHIZOAFFECTIVE DISORDER

There have been proposals (Crow, 1986) for a unitary concept of psychoses where schizophrenia and manic depression lie at opposite ends of the same spectrum. The validity of this concept for the whole of psychosis now looks increasingly inappropriate because X-chromosome linkage in manic depression has been confirmed (Winokur *et al.*, 1969; Winokur and Tanna, 1969). Initial studies reported the possibility of close linkage between colour blindness, which is an X-linked trait, and the manic depressive phenotype. Subsequently research using colour blindness and other X-chromosome markers also produced results suggestive of X linkage in a proportion of families (Baron *et al.*, 1977; Reading, 1979; Mendlewicz *et al.*, 1974, 1979, 1987; Del

Zompo *et al.*, 1984; Baron *et al.*, 1987). Other investigations have failed to show linkage to colour blindness and the glucose-6-phosphate dehydrogenase (G6PD) gene which is localized near the colour blindness gene (Goetzl *et al.*, 1974; Gershon *et al.*, 1979; Holmes *et al.*, 1989). Taking into account the earlier family genetic studies as well as the recent linkage studies of both schizophrenia and manic depression the evidence appears to show that the two disorders generally 'breed true' and segregate independently.

However schizoaffective disorder presents a challenge to this dichotomy. There are indeed reports (Walinder, 1972) of schizoaffective disorders breeding true in individual families, but epidemiological studies of schizophrenia and manic depression probands generally show an excess of both schizophrenia and affective disorders in first degree relatives. Baron *et al.* (1982) used family study data and concluded that schizoaffective disorder can be split into two genetically distinct syndromes namely schizoaffective-'schizophrenic-like' (SA-S) and schizoaffective-'affective-like' (SA-A). Kendler *et al.* (1986) found a similar pattern with an excess of schizophrenia in the relatives of SA-S patients and an excess of bipolar illness in the relatives of SA-A patients. The dual genetic vulnerability hypothesis has also been supported by Scharfetter and Nuspereli (1980) who found that the two types of schizoaffective patient (SA-S or SA-A) had an excess of relatives with either schizophrenia or affective disorders, respectively. It can be concluded that schizoaffective disorder is almost certainly heterogeneous representing either an atypical form of schizophrenia or of bipolar disorder. Those families in which both schizophrenia and bipolar affective disorder are present probably arise as a result of assortative mating for schizophrenia and bipolar disorder or 'marrying in' of independent disease alleles within a kindred.

7.6 PENETRANCE AND EXPRESSIVITY

Fischer (1971) showed that MZ twins discordant for schizophrenia had the same incidence of the illness, i.e. 16%, among their respective offspring. This illustrates that the schizophrenia genotype is not always expressed phenotypically. Fischer calculated a penetrance of 32% for the probability that a carrier would be affected. Other authors have calculated 25% (Karlsson, 1988) and 20% (Slater and Cowie, 1972). In the UK/Icelandic study (Sherrington *et al.*, 1988) the best estimate of penetrance was 71% for schizophrenia rising to 76% when including the spectrum disorders and 86% when the fringe diagnoses were included as cases. In other words, 14% of those with the disease genotypes were clinically normal and 29% did not develop the full syndrome. The Icelandic and UK families were selected for a high frequency of recurrence and were also mainly from a genetic isolate. They may not therefore be representative of schizophrenia as a whole.

The factors that affect the penetrance of schizophrenia are unknown. On *a priori* grounds there will be effects on penetrance both from allelic variation at a single disease locus as well from the involvement of distinct loci in sub-types of schizophrenia. The factors influencing penetrance are likely to be a productive research area in the future with implications for preventive psychiatry. The effects of interaction between the genotype and life events, expressed emotion and organic variables such as head injury, obstetric complications or substance abuse may be relevant. If high-risk individuals in genetically vulnerable families can be identified by genetic testing, research can focus on which interventions can minimize the development of psychiatric morbidity.

New understanding of schizophrenia may also arise from comparing aetiological subtypes with clinical variables, especially those which also seem to have a genetic basis. Brain ventricular size is also known to be abnormal in some schizophrenics (Johnstone *et al.*, 1976; Turner *et al.*, 1986). Although there is no firm consensus, this may be a marker for a less genetic form of the illness (Reveley *et al.*, 1984) especially when associated with perinatal complications (Turner *et al.*, 1986; Owen *et al.*, 1988). This relationship also seems to hold for some familial cases suggesting that the two aetiological factors can operate in a cumulative manner (Murray *et al.*, 1988) and providing an example of how penetrance might be affected by environmental factors. Negative features and lack of response to neuroleptics are also said to be characteristic of the more genetic forms of schizophrenia (Dworkin and Lenzenweger, 1984; Silverman *et al.*, 1987; Keefe *et al.*, 1987).

Smooth pursuit eye movements (SPEM) are known to be abnormal in some 60% of schizophrenics and in 45–55% of their first degree relatives (Holzmann, 1985). This may be an example of variable expressivity showing that the underlying genetic abnormality can produce both schizophrenia, spectrum disorders, 'fringe' disorders and abnormal SPEM. Further evidence (Holzman *et al.*, 1988) has suggested that SPEM and the clinical phenotypes of schizophrenia are expressions of a single trait transmitted by an autosomal dominant gene. Thus abnormal SPEM may be a marker for genetic vulnerability in psychiatrically normal individuals. Such a marker could increase the power of linkage analysis by providing more apparent cases for statistical analysis.

The search for other biological markers or endophenotypes has been disappointing. Platelet monoamine oxidase was much studied but the results were inconclusive (Reveley *et al.*, 1986). The role of EEG and evoked potentials is unclear although it has been claimed (Blackwood *et al.*, 1987) that the auditory evoked potential P300 is characteristically abnormal in schizophrenia and manic depression. It should be possible to determine whether all of the abnormalities described above are found in the chromosome 5-linked sub-type of schizophrenia. This should lead to an enhanced ability for psychiatric researchers to pursue separate sub-types of schizophrenia in their own right. However if these measures turn out to be only weakly specific to genetic sub-types of schizophrenia and present in other psychiatric disorders then they will have to be regarded as epiphenomena of whole groups of mental illness without any specificity.

7.6 GENETIC COUNSELLING

Genetic counselling for psychiatric disorders is little practised by psychiatrists and tends to arouse controversy perhaps due to memories of fascism in Nazi Germany where there were appallingly crude attempts to sanitize the so-called Aryan gene pool. However, the recent increase in public interest in psychiatric genetics has highlighted the potential demand for genetic counselling. It is a subject that the clinician should deal with sensitively because it involves personal decisions about reproduction involving whole families.

Today counselling involves the careful investigation of morbidity within a family and making sure the clinical diagnoses are as accurate as possible. After considering the emotional state of the client the present practice is simply limited to giving risk estimates according to the empirically derived values mentioned earlier in this chapter (Table 7.1). Little is known about the effects of genetic counselling for psychiatric disorders on families. Eventually information from DNA markers could enable more accurate predictions of the risk to relatives of schizophrenics for developing the illness. The problems of incomplete penetrance and the probable existence of non-genetic 'phenocopies' mean that risk prediction will always be an inexact science. On the other hand there are relatives of schizophrenics who refrain from having children for fear that they may be carriers.

Marker studies may eventually be able to reassure them that they are at low risk of transmitting the disease. An apparently negative family history does not preclude genetic vulnerability as an illness, since a penetrance of around 20% could often miss out a few generations. On the other hand, schizophrenia arising in the context of brain damage or epilepsy is not associated with an increased familial risk.

To maximize the accuracy and usefulness of genetic counselling it will be essential to know much more about the issues of heterogeneity of linkage and penetrance. In a family where a significant lod score (>3.00) has been obtained between linkage markers and schizophrenia there is a high probability that unaffected family members who have inherited the linked marker will also have inherited the schizophrenia susceptibility allele. In this situation antenatal counselling may be feasible.

7.7 FUTURE DIRECTIONS

Schizophrenia is probably best conceptualized as a multifactorial disorder in which a variety of single major gene susceptibilities as well as other subtypes of the disorder exist. Perhaps it is similar to the genetic aetiology of diabetes in which there are sub-types caused by mutant insulins, HLA gene-induced susceptibility, and defects in the insulin receptor. There is also a late onset obesity-associated genetic sub-type which may have single major gene susceptibility. Medical disorders such as multiple endocrine neoplasia for which single mutant gene loci have been found show as much incomplete penetrance and apparent 'polygenicity' as schizophrenia (Ponder *et al.*, 1988). Future linkage studies of schizophrenia should first look for chromosome 5 linkage and if negative should proceed to test other hypotheses.

There are three further ways of trying to find a linkage. The most productive method is likely to be the systematic investigation of loci that have some *a priori* reason to contain a genetic locus that is involved in schizophrenia (Gurling, 1986). This strategy has already proven sucessful and there are many more loci at which cytogenetic abnormalities have been reported in association with schizophrenia (see above). The most promising at present appears to be the genetic loci associated with albinism (Baron, 1976). A second method is the candidate gene approach using genes encoding proteins such as the D_2 receptor which has recently been cloned (Bunzow *et al.*, 1988).

Finally, because linkage markers to map the complete human genome are available (Donis-Keller *et al.*, 1987), every part of the genome can now be searched in suitably sized families and samples. When linkage to specific chromosomal loci is unequivocally established, the real work of molecular genetics is just beginning. For example, the putative chromosome 5 schizophrenia locus at 5q11-5q13 is in a region which contains over 30 million base pairs and thousands of genes. The next task will be to 'walk' or 'jump' along a chromosome using cloning techniques and methods to physically map closely linked markers, such as pulse field gel electrophoresis (Rommenns *et al.*, 1989). Fortunately the technology in this field is advancing in leaps and bounds and it should soon be possible to hone down on all the genes in a specific area and then to pick out some interesting ones that are expressed in the brain and which might cause schizophrenia.

The problem at the present time for this approach is the lack of a confirmed linkage in schizophrenia. When this has been achieved then we should be optimistic about eventually finding the cause for sub-types of schizophrenia. Once a few of the genes causing susceptibility to schizophrenia have been cloned and sequenced we should be in a position not only to develop new treatments and prevention strategies but also, paradoxically, to learn much more about the effects of the environment.

REFERENCES

Andrew, B., Watt, D.C., Gillespie, C. and Chapel, H. (1987) A study of genetic linkage in schizophrenia. *Psychol. Med.*, **17**, 363–70.

Axelsson, R. and Wahlstrom, J. (1981) Mental Disorder and Inversion on Chromosome 9. *Hereditas*, **95**, 337.

Baron, M. (1976) Albinism and Schizophreniform Psychosis, a Pedigree Study. *Am. J. Psychiatry*, **133**, 1070–2.

Baron, M. (1977) Linkage Between an Chromosome Marker (Deuxan Colour Blindness) and Affective Illness. *Arch. Gen. Psychiatry*, **24**, 721–7.

Baron, M. (1986) Genetics of schizophrenia: II. Vulnerability Traits and Gene Markers. *Biol. Psychiatry*, **21**, 1189–211.

Baron, M., Gruen, R., Asnis, L. and Kane, J. (1982) Schizoaffective Illness, Schizophrenia and Affective Disorders, Morbidity Risks and Genetic Transmission. *Acta Psychiatr. Scand.*, **65**, 253–62.

Baron, M., Asnis, L., Gruen, R. and Levitt, M. (1983) Plasma Amine Oxidase and Genetic Vulnerability to Schizophrenia. *Arch. Gen. Psychiatry*, **40**, 275–9.

Baron, M., Gruen, R., Levitt, M. *et al.* (1984) Erythrocyte Catechol O-Methyltransferase Activity in Schizophrenia: Analysis of Family Data. *Am. J. Psychiatry*, **1418**, 29–32.

Baron, M., Gruen, R., Rainer, J.D. *et al.* (1985) A Family Study of Schizophrenic and Normal Control Probands. *Am. J. Psychiatry*, **142**, 447–55.

Baron, M., and Risch, N. (1987) The Spectrum Concept of Schizophrenia, Evidence for a Genetic-Environmental Continuum. *J. Psychiatr. Res.*, **21**, 257–68.

Baron, M., Risch, N., Hamburger, R. *et al.* (1987) Genetic Linkage between X. Chromosome Markers and Bipolar Affective Disorder, *Nature*, **326**, 289–92.

Bassett, A.S. (1989) Chromosome 5 and Schizophrenia: Implications for Genetic Linkage Studies, *Schizophr. Bull.*, **15**, 393–402.

Bassett, A.S., McGillivray, B.C., Jones, B. *et al.* (1988) Partial trisomy chromosome 5 co-segregating with schizophrenia. *Lancet*, **8589**, 799–801.

References

Blackwood, D.H.R., Whalley, L.J. and Christie, J.E. (1987) Changes in P3 Auditory Evoked Potential in Schizophrenia and Depression. *Br. J. Psychiatry*, **150**, 154–60.

Bohman, M. (1978) Some genetic aspects of alcoholism and criminality. *Arch. Gen. Psychiatry*, **35**, 269–76.

Bunzow, J.R., Van Tol, H.H.M., Grandy, D.K. *et al.* (1988) Cloning and Expression of a Rat D2 Dopamine Receptor cDNA. *Nature*, **336**, 783–5.

Chodirker, B., Chudley, A., Ray, M. *et al.* (1987) Fragile 19p13 in a Family with Mental Illness. *Clin. Genet.* **31**, 1–6.

Crow, T.J. (1980) Molecular Pathology of Schizophrenia; More than One Disease Process. *Br. Med. J.*, **1**, 66–8.

Crow, T.J. (1986) The Continuum of Psychosis and its Implication for the Structure of the Gene. *Br. J. Psychiatry*, **149**, 419–29.

Crow, T.J. (1988) Sex Chromosomes and Psychosis. *Br. J. Psychiatry*, **153**, 675–83.

Dasgupta, J., Dasgupta, D. and Balasubrahmanyan, M. (1973) XXY Syndrome XY/XO Mosaicisms and Acentric Chromosomal Fragments in Male Schizophrenics. *Ind. J. Med. Res.*, **61**, 62–70.

Delisi, L.E., Goldin, L.R., Maxwell, L.W. *et al.* (1987) Clinical Features of Illness in Siblings with Schizophrenia or Schizoaffective Disorder. *Arch. Gen. Psychiatry*, **44**, 891–7.

Del Zompo, M., Brochetta, A., Goldin, L.R. and Corsini, G.U. (1984) Linkage Between X Chromosome Markers and Manic Depressive Illness: Two Sardinian Pedigrees. *Acta Psychiatr. Scand.*, **70**, 282–7.

Detera-Wadleigh, S.D., Goldin, L.R., Sherrington, R. *et al.* (1989) Exclusion of Linkage to 5q11-13 in Families with Schizophrenia and Other Psychiatric Disorders. *Nature*, **340**, 391–3.

Donis-Keller, H., Green, P., Helms, C. and Cartinhour, S. (1987) A Genetic Linkage Map of the Human Genome. *Cell*, **51**, 319–37.

Dworkin, R.H. and Lenzenweger, M.F. (1984) Symptoms and Genetics of Schizophrenia, Implications for Diagnosis. *Am. J. Psychiatry*, **141**, 1541–5.

Elston, R.C., Kringlen, E. and Namboodiri, K.K. (1973) Possible Linkage Relationship between Certain Blood Groups and Schizophrenia. *Behav. Genet.*, **3**, 101–6.

Farmer, A.E., McGuffin, P. and Gottesman, I.I. (1987) Twin Concordance for DSM-111 Schizophrenia. *Arch. Gen. Psychiatry*, **44**, 634.

Feldman, M.W. and Cavalli-Sforza, L.L. (1977) The evolution of continuous variation. II. Complex transmission and assortative mating. *Theor. Popul. Biol.*, **11**, 161–81.

Feldman, M.W. and Cavalli-Sforza, L.L. (1979) Aspects of variance and covariance analysis with cultural inheritance. *Theor. Popul. Biol.*, **15**, 276–307.

Fischer, M. (1971) Psychoses in the Offspring of Schizophrenic Monozygotic Twins and their Normal Co-twins. *Br. J. Psychiatry*, **118**, 43–52.

Foucault, M. (1976) *Mental Illness and Psychology.* Harper Colophon, New York.

Frangos, E. and Athenassenas, G. (1985) Prevalence of DSM III Schizophrenia Among First Degree Relatives of Schizophrenic Probands. *Acta Psychiatr. Scand.*, **72**, 382–6.

Fulker, D.W. (1973) A Biometrical Genetic Approach to Intelligence and Schizophrenia. *Soc. Biol.*, **20**, 266–75.

Gershon, E.S., Targum, S.D., Matthyse, S. and Bunney, W.E. (1979) Color blindness not Closely Linked to Bipolar Illness. *Arch. Gen. Psychiatry*, **36**, 1423.

Goetzl, V., Green, R., Whybrown, P. and Jackson, L. (1974) X linkage revisited, a further study of manic depression. *Arch. Gen. Psychiatry*, **31**, 665–72.

Gottesman, I.I. and Bertlesen, A. (1988) Personal Communication, Cold Spring Harbor Meeting on the Genetics of Schizophrenia.

Gottesman, I.I. and Shields, J. (1972) *Schizophrenia and Genetics, A Twin Study Vantage Point.* Academic Press, London.

Gottesman, I.I., and Shields, J. (1976) Critical Review of Recent Adoption, Twin and Family Studies. *Schizophr. Bull.*, **21**, 360–364.

Gottesman, I.I. and Shields, J. (1982) *Schizophrenia, The Epigenetic Puzzle.* Cambridge University Press, Cambridge.

Gurling, H.M.D. (1986) Candidate Genes and Favoured Loci. *Psychiatr. Dev.*, **4**, 289–309.

Gurling, H.M.D., Read, T., Sherrington, R. *et al.* (1989) Recent and Future Molecular Genetic Research into Schizophrenia. *Schizophr. Bull.*, **15**, 373–82.

Gurling, H.M.D., Sherrington, R., Brynjolfsson,

J. *et al.* (1988) Genetic Linkage Studies of Schizophrenia Using the M13, 33.15 and 33.6 Hypervariable DNA Polymorphisms. In: *A Genetic Perspective for Schizophrenia and Related Disorders*, E. Smeraldi and K. Kidd, (eds), Edi-Hermes, Milan, pp. 43-8.

Henderson, N. (1982) Behaviour genetics. *Ann. Rev. Psychol.*, **33**, 403-40.

Hodgkinson, S., Sherrington, R., Gurling, H.M.D. *et al.* (1987) Molecular Genetic Evidence for Heterogeneity in Manic Depression. *Nature*, **325**, 805-6.

Holmes, D., Sherrington, R.P., Hodgkinson, S. *et al.* (1989) Linkage Analysis in Manic Depression Families Identifies a Non 11p/nonX Type. *Am. J. Hum. Genet.* **45**, A195.

Holzman, P.S. (1985) Eye Movement Dysfunction and Psychosis. *Int. Rev. Neurobiol.* **27**, 179-205.

Holzman, P.S., Kringlen, E., Mattysse, S. *et al.* (1988) A Single Dominant Gene Can Account for Eye Tracking Dysfunctions and Schizophrenia in Offspring of Discordant Twins. *Arch. Gen. Psychiatry*, **45**, 641-7.

Hong, M.L. (1986) Pericentric Inversions of Chromosome 9 in Patients and Controls, *Chin. J. Neurol. Psychiatry*, **19**, 188-91.

Johnstone, E.C., Crow, T.J., Frith, C.D. *et al.* (1976) Cerebral Ventricle Size and Cognitive Impairment in Chronic Schizophrenia. *Lancet*, **ii**, 924-6.

Kane, J.M., Honigfeld, G., Singer, J. and Meltzer, H. (1988) Clozapine in Treatment Resistant Schizophrenics. *Arch. Gen. Psychiatry*, **15**, 789-96.

Kaplan, A. (1970) Chromosomal Mosaicisms and Occasional Acentric Chromosomal Fragments in Schizophrenic Patients. *Biol. Psychiatry*, **2**, 89-94.

Karlsson, J.L. (1988) Partly Dominant Transmission of Schizophrenia in Iceland. *Br. J. Psychiatry*, **152**, 324-9.

Keefe, R.S.E, Mohs, R.C., Losonczy, M.F. *et al.* (1987) Characteristics of Very Poor Outcome Schizophrenia. *Am. J. Psychiatry*, **144**, 889-94.

Kendler, K.S. (1983) Overview: A Current Perspective on Twin Studies of Schizophrenia. *Am. J. Psychiatry*, **140**, 1413-25.

Kendler, K. (1986) The Feasibility of Linkage Studies in Schizophrenia. *Dahlem Konferenzen, Biological Perspectives in Schizophrenia.*

Dahlem Foundation-Wallostr., 10, 1000 Berlin 33.

Kendler, K.S. and Hays, P. (1981) Paranoid Psychosis and Schizophrenia. *Arch. Gen. Psychiatry*, **38**, 547-51.

Kendler, K.S. and Greunberg, A.M. (1984) An Independent Analysis of the Danish Adoption Study of Schizophrenia. *Arch. Gen. Psychiatry*, **41**, 982-4.

Kendler, K.S. Gruenberg, A.M. and Strauss, J.S. (1984) An Independent Analysis of the Copenagen Sample of the Danish Adoption Study of Schizophrenia. *Arch. Gen. psychiatry*, **38**, 392-9.

Kendler, K.S, Gruenberg, A.M. and Tsuang, M.T. (1985) Psychiatric Illness in First Degree Relatives of Schizophrenic and Surgical Control Patients. *Arch. Gen. Psychiatry*, **42**, 770-9.

Kendler, K.S., Gruenberg, A.M. and Tsuang, M.T. (1986) A DSM-III Family Study of Non Schizophrenic Psychotic Disorders. *Am. J. Psychiatry*, **143**, 1098-105.

Kendler, K.S., Gruenberg, A.M. and Tsuang, M.T. (1988) A Family Study of the Subtypes of Schizophrenia. *Am. J. Psychiatry*, **45**, 57 -62.

Kennedy, J.L., Giuffa, L.A., Moises, H.W. *et al.* (1988) Evidence Against Linkage of Schizophrenia to Markers on Chromosome 5 in a Northern Swedish Pedigree. *Nature*, **336**, 167-70.

Kety, S.S. (1983) Mental Illness in the Biological and Adoptive Relatives of Schizophrenic Adoptees. *Am. J. Psychiatry*, **140**, 720-7.

Kety, S.S., Rosenthal, D. and Wender, P.H. (1968) Mental Illness in the Biological and Adoptive Relatives of Adopted Schizophrenics. *J. Psychiatr. Res.*, **6**, 345-62.

Kety, S.S., Rosenthal, D. and Wender, P.H. (1975) Mental Illness in the Biological and Adoptive Families of Adopted Individuals who have become Schizophrenic. In *Genetic Research in Psychiatry*. R.R. Fieve, N. Rosenthal and H. Brill (eds), Johns Hopkins University Press, Baltimore, pp. 95-105.

Lalouel, J.M., Rao, D.C., Morton, N.E. and Elston, R.C. (1983) A Unified Model of Complex Segregation Analysis. *Am. J. Hum. Genet.*, **35**, 816-26.

Lange, K. (1982) Genetic Markers for Schizophrenia Subgroups. *Psychiatr. Clin.*, **15**, 133-44.

Lange, K. and Boehnke, M. (1982) How Many Polymorphic Genes will it Take to Span the Human Genome? *Am. J. Hum. Genet.*, **34**, 842–5.

Lowing, P.A., Mirsky, A.F. and Pereira, R. (1983) The Inheritance of Schizophrenia Spectrum Disorders. Reanalysis of the Danish Adoptee Study Data. *Am. J. Psychiatry*, **140**, 1167–71.

McGue, M., Gottesman, I.I. and Rao, D.C. (1985) Resolving Genetic Models for the Transmission of Schizophrenia. *Genet. Epidemiol.*, **46**, 44–55.

McGuffin, P. (1989) oral communication. First World Congress in Psychiatric Genetics, Cambridge. UK.

McGuffin, P. and Sturt, E. (1986) Genetic Markers in Schizophrenia. *Hum. Hered.*, **36**, 65–8.

McGuffin, P., Festenstein, H. and Murray, R. (1983) A Family Study of HLA Antigens and Other Genetic Markers in Schizophrenia. *Psychol. Med.*, **13**, 31–43.

McGuffin, P., Farmer, A.E., Gottesman, I.I. *et al.* (1984) Twin Concordance for Operationally Defined Schizophrenia. *Arch. Gen. Psychiatry*, **41**, 541–7.

McGuffin, P., Farmer, A.E. and Gottesman, I.I. (1987) Is There Really a Split in Schizophrenia? The Genetic Evidence. *Br. J. Psychiatry*, **150**, 581–92.

McGuffin, P., Sargeant, M., Hetti, G. *et al.* (1990) Exclusion of susceptibility gene from the chromosome 5q11–q13 region: New Data and a reanalysis of previous reports. *Am. J. Hum. Genet.*, **47**, 524–35.

Mendlewicz, J. and Fleiss, J.L. (1974) Linkage studies with X chromosome markers in bipolar (manic-depressive) and unipolar (depressive) illness. *Biol. Psychiatry*, **9**, 261–4.

Mendlewicz, J., Fleiss, J.L. and Gieve, R.R. (1972) Evidence for X Linkage in the Tranmission of Manic Depressive Illness. *J. Am. Med. Assoc.*, **222**, 1624–7.

Mendlewicz, J., Linkowski, P., Guroff, J.J. and Van Praag, H.M. (1979) Color Blindness Linkage to Bipolar Manic Depressive Illness. *Arch. Gen. Psychiatry*, **36**, 1442–7.

Mendlewicz, J., Linkowski, P. and Wilmotte J. (1980) Linkage Between 6-Phosphate Dehydrogenase Deficiency and Manic Depressive Psychosis. *Br. J. Psychiatry*, **134**, 337–42.

Mendlewicz, J., Simon, P., Sevy, S. *et al.* (1987) Polymorphic Marker on X chromosome and manic depression. *Lancet*, **8544**, 1230–1.

Morton, N.E. (1956) The Detection and Estimation of Linkage between the Genes for Rh Bloodtype. *Am. J. Hum. Genet.*, **8**, 80–96.

Morton, N.E. and Maclean, C.J. (1974) Analysis of Family Resemblance III. Complex Segregation Analysis. *Am. J. Hum. Genet.*, **26**, 489–503.

Morton, N.E., Rao, D.C. and Lalouel, J.M. (1983) *Methods in Genetic Epidemiology*. Karger, Basel.

Murray, R.M., Lewis, S.W., Owen, M.J. and Foerster, A. (1988) The Neurodevelopmental Origins of Dementia Praecox. In *Schizophrenia: the Major Issues*, P. Bebbington and P. McGuffin (eds), Heinemann, London, pp. 90–107.

Ott, J. (1985) *Analysis of Human Genetic Linkage*. Johns Hopkins University Press, Baltimore.

Ott, J. (1986) The Number of Families Required to Detect or Exclude Linkage Heterogeneity. *Am. J. Hum. Genet.*, **39**, 159–65.

Owen, M.J., Lewis, S.W. and Murray, R.M. (1988) Obstetric Complications of Schizophrenia, A CT study. *Psychol. Med.*, **18**, 331–40.

Papiha, C.S., Roberts, D.F. and McLeigh, L. (1982) Group Specific Component (Gc) Subtypes and Schizophrenia. *Clin. Genet.*, **22**, 321–6.

Ponder, B.A.J., Coffey, R., Gagel, R.F. *et al.* (1988) Risk Estimation and Screening in Families of Patients with Medullary Thyroid Carcinoma. *Lancet*, **1**, 397–400.

Reading, C.M. (1979) X Linked Dominant Manic Depressive Illness: Linkage with Xg Blood Group, Red Green Color Blindness and Vitamin B12 Deficiency. *Orthomol. Psychiatry*, **8**, 68–77.

Reich, T., Clininger, C.R. and Guze, S.B. (1975) The multifactorial model of disease transmission. *Br. J. Psychiatry*, **127**, 1–10.

Reveley, A.M., Reveley, M.A. and Murray, R.M. (1984) Cerebral Ventricular Enlargement in Non Genetic Schizophrenia: A Controlled Twin Study. *Br. J. Psychiatry*, **144**, 89–93.

Reveley, M.A., Reveley, A.M., Clifford, C. and Murray, R.M. (1986) Platelet MAO and Schizophrenia. In *Contemporary Issues in Schizophrenia*. A. Kerr and P. Snaith (eds), Gaskell Press, Ashford, Kent, pp. 310–26.

124

Risch, N. and Baron, M. (1984) Segregation Analysis of Schizophrenia and Related Disorders. *Am. J. Hum. Genet.*, **36**, 1039–59.

Rommens, J.H., Tannuzzi, J.C.,. Karem, B.S. *et al.* (1989) Identification of the Cystic Fibrosis Gene: Chromosome Walking and Jumping. *Science*, **245**, 1059–65.

Rose, S., Kamin, L.J. and Lewontin, R.C. (1984) *Not in our Genes, Biology, Ideology and Human Nature*. Pelican Books, Harmondsworth, Middx.

Rosenthal, D., Wender, P.H., Kety, S.S. *et al.* (1975) Parent Child Relationships and Psychopathological Disorder in the Child. *Arch. Gen Psychiatry*, **32**, 466–73.

Rudduck, C. and Franzen, G. (1983) A New Heritable Fragile Site on Human Chromosome 3. *Hereditas*, **98**, 297–9.

Rudin, E. (1916) *Zur Vererbung und Neuentstehung der Dementia Praecox*. Springer. Verlag, Berlin and New York.

St. Clair, D., Blackwood, D., Muir, W. *et al.* (1989) No Linkage to Chromosome 5q11-q13 Markers to Schizophrenia in Scottish Families. *Nature*, **339**, 305–9.

St. Clair, D., Blackwood, D., Muir, W. *et al.* (1990) Association of a Balanced Autosomal Translocation with Major Mental Illness. *Lancet*, **336**, 13–6.

Scharfetter, C. (1981) Subdividing the Functional Psychoses: a Family Hereditary Approach. *Psychol. Med.*, **11**, 637–40.

Scharfetter, C. and Nusperli, M. (1980) The Group of Schizophrenias, Schizo-affective Psychoses and Affective Disorders. *Schizophr. Bull.*, **6**, 586–91.

Scharfetter, C.(1981) Subdividing the Functional Psychoses; a Family Hereditary Approach. *Psychol. Med.*, **11**, 637–40.

Sedgwick, P. (1976) *Psychopolitics*. Pluto Press, London.

Sherrington, R., Brynjolfsson, J., Petursson, H. *et al.* (1988) The Localization of a Susceptibility Locus for Schizophrenia on Chromosome 5. *Nature*, **336**, 164–7.

Silverman, J.M., Mohs, R.C., Davidson, M. and Losonczy. M.F. (1987) Familial Schizophrenia and Treatment Response. *Am. J. Psychiatry*, **144**, 1271–6.

Slater, E. and Cowie, V. (1972) *The Genetics of Mental Disorders*. Oxford University Press, London.

Southern, E.M. (1975) Detection of Specific Sequences Among DNA Fragments Separated by Gel Electrophoresis. *J. Mol. Biol.*, **98**, 503–17.

Sperber, M.A. (1975) Schizophrenia and Organic Brain Syndrome with Trisomy 8 (group c – trisomy 8[47,xx,8+]), *Biol. Psychiatry*, **10**, 27–43.

Spitzer, R.L., Endicott, J. and Gibbon, M. (1979) Crossing the Border into Borderline Personality and Borderline Schizophrenia. *Arch. Gen. Psychiatry*, **36**, 17–24.

Sturt, E. and McGuffin, P. (1985) Can Linkage and Marker Association Resolve the Genetic Aetiology of Psychiatric Disorders? Review and Argument. *Psychol. Med.*, **15**, 455–62.

Tsuang, M.T. and Winokur, G. (1974) Criteria for Subtyping Schiozophrenia. Clinical Differentiation of Hebephrenic and Paranoid Schizophrenia. *Arch. Gen. Psychiatry*, **31**, 43–7.

Tsuang, M.T., Dempsey, G.M. and Rauscher, F. (1976) A study of atypical schizophrenia. *Arch. Gen. Psychiatry*, **33**, 1157–60.

Tsuang, M.T., Fowler, R.C., Cadoret, R.J. and Monnelly, E. (1974) Schizophrenia among Relatives of Paranoid and Non Paranoid Schizophrenics. *Compr. Psychiatry*, **15**, 295–302.

Turner, B. and Jennings, A.N. (1961) Trisomy for Chromosome 22, *Lancet*. **2**, 49–50.

Turner, S.W., Toone, B.K. and Brett-Jones, J.R. (1986) Computerized tomography Scan Changes in Early Schizophrenia Preliminary Findings. *Psychol. Med.*, **16**, 219–25.

Turner, W.J. (1979) Genetic markers for schizotaxia. *Biol. Psychiatry*, **14**, 177–206.

Walinder, J. (1972) Recurrent Familial Psychosis of the Schizoaffective Type. *Acta Psychiatr. Scand.*, **48**, 274–9.

Wender, P.H., Rosenthal, D., Kety, S. *et al.* (1974) Cross Fostering, A Research Strategy for Clarifying the Role of Genetic and Experiential Factors in the Aetiology of Schizophrenia. *Arch. Gen. Psychiatry*, **30**, 121–8.

Winokur, G. and Tanna, V.L. (1969) Possible Role of X Linked Dominant Factor in Manic Depressive Disease. *Dis. Nerv. Sys.*, **30**, 89–93.

Winokur, G., Morrison, J., Clancy, J. and Crowe, R. (1974) The Iowa 500. The Clinical and Genetic Distinction of Hebephrenic and Paranoid Schizophrenia. *J. Nerv. Ment. Dis.*, **15**, 12–9.

Winokur, G., Clayton, P.J. and Reich, T. (1969) *Manic Depressive Illness*. C.V. Mosby, St. Louis.

Wright, S. (1983) On 'Path Analysis in Genetic Epidemiology': A critique. *Am. J. Hum. Genet.*, **35**, 757–68.

125

Chapter 8

Life events and social factors

PAUL BEBBINGTON and LIZ KUIPERS

We now have a considerable knowledge of the factors that affect the positive and negative symptoms of schizophrenia. In this chapter we will describe the particular social circumstances that are associated with the emergence and re-emergence of positive symptoms.

8.1 EARLY SOCIAL THEORIES OF SCHIZOPHRENIA

In the 1950s, a number of theories were put forward linking social factors with the onset of schizophrenia. They had ambitious aims, as they attempted to provide a virtually complete explanation of the emergence of the disease. They were also primarily cognitive theories: early experience was held to result in ways of perceiving (and therefore of interacting with) the social world that correspond to the observed symptoms of schizophrenia.

So schizophrenia was held to be the result of the family's 'double bind' communication (Bateson *et al.*, 1956), or a 'fragmented' or 'amorphous' parental style of communication (Wynne and Singer, 1963, 1965). Lidz and his colleagues (1957) claimed that such parents showed 'schism' or 'skew' in their marriages, together with a narcissistic egocentricity. Finally, Laing and Esterson (1964) held that schizophrenia was an understandable response to pressures in the family and in society at large.

For good reasons, these theories are now unfashionable. Hirsch and Leff (1975) reviewed the experimental evidence for them, and concluded that the oddities of the parents were not marked, and almost certainly not the cause of the condition. They thought there was reasonable support for a few rather modest relationships, including an increase in conflict and disharmony between the parents of schizophrenic patients, and in concern and protectiveness of their mothers, both in their current situation and before they fell ill. These seem likely to be mere reactions to offspring showing abnormalities that may have pre-dated the development of obvious schizophrenia, but nevertheless formed part of the same process. Hirsch and Leff (1975) were in any case unable to replicate the findings of Wynne and Singer (1963, 1965). This has been the only independent attempt to test out these 'grand' social theories of the origins of schizophrenia.

Causal direction is impossible to establish from retrospective studies like these. However, prospective studies are expensive, as most of the people laboriously followed up will never develop schizophrenia. A less costly approach involves following up families with children who may be at 'high risk' of developing schizophrenia (e.g. Venables, 1977; Goldstein, 1985). They, however, have their own problems, such as high drop out rates, the length of time required to complete the study, and the ethics of not intervening (Shakow, 1973).

One such study has actually been reported by Doane and her colleagues (1981; Goldstein, 1987). They followed up adolescents thought to be at increased risk of developing schizophrenia, namely those attending a psychiatric out-patient department for disturbed behaviour. They have now reported results available after a 15-year interval. Only four adolescents developed definite schizophrenia in this time, but parental abnormalities of communication and affective style, and a measure of family atmosphere, all rated at induction, were clearly associated with the later emergence of schizophrenic spectrum disorders.

However it is not clear what these findings actually say about the causes of schizophrenia, particularly if a narrower and more usual definition is used. It is possible that the more disturbed adolescents drew extreme reactions from their parents, and happened also to be those who went on to develop the disease.

These interesting studies did at least have the effect of obtaining acceptance for a social dimension to the disorder, opening the door for more refined hypotheses. They also seem to have been responsible for the tendency of some professionals to blame families for the state of the patient. This is inappropriate: apart from any other consideration, the evidence for major genetic and physical environmental components cannot sustain a belief that relatives by their behaviour actually 'cause' schizophrenia.

8.2 SOCIAL INFLUENCES ON THE TIMING AND COURSE OF SCHIZOPHRENIA

Modern social theories of schizophrenia have more modest aims. They start from the sensible proposition that social influences act together with factors at other levels to determine at least the timing, and possibly the fact, of schizophrenic breakdown. They rely on the concept of psychosocial stress, measured in terms of 'life events' and 'expressed emotion'. They thus reflect the widely held clinical opinion that people with schizophrenia are very responsive to their social environment despite the social withdrawal seen in many cases.

8.2.1 LIFE EVENTS

Several sources of evidence suggest that *changes* in the social environment may lead to the emergence of schizophrenic symptoms in susceptible individuals. So, for instance, acute florid symptoms may reappear in patients subjected to too much pressure in rehabilitation programmes, or discharged before they are ready (Wing *et al.*, 1964; Stevens, 1973; Goldberg *et al.*, 1977).

The evidence from specific life event studies that stress has some part in precipitating episodes of schizophrenia has so far appeared rather fragile. The requirements that should be met before concluding that life events have a definite role in engendering episodes of schizophrenia are listed in Table 8.1. No study so far published meets all of them, and we must therefore depend upon an integrated evaluation of several flawed studies.

Two complementary strategies have been used to assess the role of life events. The first relies on the demonstration of differences between cases and controls in the frequencies of events. The second depends on using cases as their own controls by breaking down events according to their timing and showing that their frequency peaks significantly before onset.

Case control studies carry the assumption that people with schizophrenia are influenced by life events that would have an impact on anyone, although their response is obviously idiosyncratic. If, however, schizophrenic subjects were hypersensitive to the social environment, this would be much more difficult to demonstrate and must rely on the less powerful technique of using subjects as their own controls in order to reveal a relative excess

Table 8.1 Requirements for life event studies in schizophrenia

Standardized method of symptomatic assessment
Standardized method of case definition
Limitation to cases where it is possible to date onset accurately
Onset defined as move from effectively symptom-free period before onset
Precise dating of events to identify the salient period of effect
Objective ratings of the impact of events
Objective rating of the degree to which events are independent of actions of the subject that might have been due to emerging illness
An appropriate control group

of pre-onset events, possibly of a minor significance. There is some evidence that people with schizophrenia view events in ways that might make them more susceptible to their impact (Ventura, personal communication). Hirsch *et al.* (1975) have obtained findings suggesting that patients without the protection of medication may be particularly likely to break down in the face of stressful events.

The first study of life events and schizophrenia was that of Brown and Birley (1968). They used fairly sophisticated methods for the time, and found an increase in events of various degrees of impact, limited to the 3-week period before onset. Even so, only 45 of their 50 cases had received clinical diagnoses of schizophrenia, and in only 29 cases was onset from a state of normality to the emergence of schizophrenic symptoms. Jacobs and Myers (1976) also used sophisticated methods, but their inconclusive findings cannot be interpreted easily as they chose to examine events in the 6-month antecedent interval. They may have thereby obscured a real increase in frequency limited to the weeks immediately before onset. This might also have accounted for the negative results in the study of Malzacher *et al.* (1981), although they did give results for the three-month period before onset. Al Khani *et al.* (1986) used reasonably adequate methods in a Saudi Arabian study, but with complicated

results, showing an effect of life events restricted to certain groups. Canton and Fraccon (1988) included events that could have occurred after onset, thus disqualifying them from consideration as causal agents. Those studies attempting to link events to onset are so few in number they can be readily summarized in tabular form (Table 8.2).

The literature has recently been considerably expanded by the publication of a large WHO collaborative study (Day *et al.*, 1987). Although limited by the lack of control groups, it is important. It was conducted in nine catchment areas from around the world. The selection of cases was deliberately broad and included an appreciable minority of doubtful diagnosis. All told, the study included 386 cases out of the 435 screened and in scope. 'Onset' could be from a state without symptoms, from one with only minor neurotic symptoms, or from one with minor psychotic symptoms. Cases were only included when onset had occurred within six months of screening and was capable of being dated to within a one-week period. Events were recorded for the 3-month period preceding onset.

As it was not possible to establish control groups, the value of the findings comes from the patterning of life events before onset. Although this could be artefactual, for instance, due to recall effects, or the 'search after meaning' (Brown, 1974), the results are suggestive. In all the centres, events tended to cluster in the three weeks before onset, and perhaps, to a lesser extent, in the three-week period before that. When all events were considered together, these findings were significant in six of the nine centres. The remaining three centres either had small numbers of cases or a low event rate, and this might be the reason for non-significant results. When independent events were considered on their own, the results from one more centre became non-significant. The trend was, however, clear.

Two papers with a novel prospective design have recently added considerably to the evidence

Table 8.2 Life event studies in schizophrenia

Author	Location	No. of subjects	Case selection	Definition of episode onset	Life event measure	Period of analysis	Control group
Brown and Birley (1968)	S. London	50	Kraepelinian criteria based on PSE. First admissions and readmissions	Normal to psychotic Neurotic to psychotic or minor to major psychotic onset within 3 months of admission, datable to within 1 week.	Semistructured interview (early version of LEDS — Brown and Harris, 1978)	3 months prior to onset in 3-week sub-divisions	325 selected from local firms (i.e. imperfectly random)
Jacobs and Myers (1976)	New Haven	62	Schizophrenia 'broadly defined': first admissions	Onset dated to within days based on emergence of exacerbation of symptoms and changes in social functioning	Modified version of Holmes and Rahe (1967) inventory given at interview	1 year prior to onset in 6-month sub-divisions	62 matched for age, sex, social class, ethnicity, from random population sample
Malzacher et al. (1981)	Zurich	33	Clinical definition cf. Brown and Birley 1968: first admissions	Emergence of psychotic symptoms	Life event inventory based on Tennant and Andrews (1976)	6 months prior to onset in 3-month sub-divisions	33 matched for age, sex marital status from random population sample
Canton and Fracon (1985)	Venice	54	DSM–III criteria: not all first admissions	Not defined	Life event inventory based on Paykel (1971) given at interview	6 months before admission or interview	54 normal normotensive subjects from hypertensive screening clinic matched for age, sex, social class marital status
Al Khani et al. (1986)	Riyadh	48	Narrow operational definition: 92% CATEGO S+: not all first admissions	Exactly as Brown and Birley (1968)	WHO life events schedule given at interview	6 months prior to onset in 3-month sub-divisions, 3 months in 3-week sub-divisions	62 members of local community: imperfectly random sample
Chung et al. (1986)	Sydney	15	DSM–III criteria: not all first admissions	Onset within 12 months: 'accurately' datable. Normal to psychotic, normal, to prodromal, minor to major psychotic	LEDS (Brown and Harris 1978)	6 months, 13 weeks, 4 weeks prior to onset	Matched for age, sex, partly from local population, partly surgical patients
Day et al. (1987)	Multicentre	386 from 9 centres	Broad range of psychotic cases, classified by local clinical diagnosis and CATEGO. Discrepant classifications in up to 28% of cases.	Onset within 6 months, datable to within 1 week. Normal to psychotic; minor neurotic to psychotic; minor psychotic to major psychotic	WHO life events schedule given at interview	3 months prior to onset in 3-week sub-divisions	No controls

for a causal role of life events. Ventura *et al.* (1989) have carried out a prospective study in which life events were recorded at monthly intervals for 12 months in a group of schizophrenic patients. They found that the frequency of events in the month preceding onset was significantly greater than in analogous months not followed by onset in the same patient. It was also greater than the mean monthly rate in non-relapsing patients. Jolley, Cramer and Hirsch (personal communication) have conducted a study with a very similar design. Fifty-six patients have been analysed to date; life events were rated at two-monthly intervals and there was a significant increase in event frequency in the four-week period immediately preceding onset, compared with the three preceding four-week periods, and with any of the four-week periods in the non-relapsed patients. It also appeared that the risk of relapse following an event was increased tenfold in those not receiving medication.

Partly on the basis of the data from their schizophrenia study described above, Brown and his colleagues (Brown *et al.*, 1973; Brown and Harris, 1978) have argued that life events are related in different ways to the onset of schizophrenia and of depression. They claim that in depression events play a 'formative' role, that is, they are of fundamental aetiological significance, being more important in the causation of the condition than dispositional factors. In schizophrenia they merely have a 'triggering' role: dispositional factors play the larger part, and life events merely aggravate a strong pre-existing tendency. Others have suggested (e.g. Tennant *et al.*, 1981) that the findings merely indicate a greater association between life events and depression than between life events and schizophrenia. Paykel (1979) has calculated that in the six months following the occurrence of a major event, the risk of developing schizophrenia is increased three- or fourfold over the general population rate, while the risk of developing depression is increased sixfold.

It is plain from reviewing these studies that the role of life events in schizophrenia is still somewhat conjectural. The proposition that schizophrenia is a condition significantly affected by social circumstances is however considerably strengthened by the literature on expressed emotion.

8.3.2. EXPRESSED EMOTION

Expressed emotion (EE) is now a long established concept, which has been reviewed at length elsewhere (Kuipers, 1979; Hooley, 1985; Leff and Vaughn, 1985; Koenigsberg and Handley, 1986; Kuipers and Bebbington, 1988, 1990; Vaughn, 1989). It was based on an unexpected finding, which was then seized upon, leading first to a series of increasingly sophisticated corroborative studies, and ultimately to planned interventions with families and prescriptions for routine clinical practice.

The original finding was reported in a study by Brown and his colleagues of the prognosis of male mental patients with a variety of discharge arrangements (Brown *et al.*, 1958; Brown, 1959). Against expectation, patients who went back to live with parents or spouses did surprisingly badly; moreover, this effect seemed to be dose-related: it depended on the amount of contact between relative and patient. The authors tentatively concluded that certain intense relationships might increase the risk of relapse.

Brown *et al.* (1962) subsequently developed a semi-structured interview to assess the emotional atmosphere in the home with the aim of predicting relapse. The interview was refined and validated, and became the Camberwell Family Interview (CFI) (Brown and Rutter, 1966; Rutter and Brown, 1966). Ratings of relatives in terms of the number of critical comments they made, and their overall hostility and emotional over-involvement were used to construct a composite score of expressed emotion. This was found to predict relapse rates in a follow-up study of schizophrenic patients returning to their homes (Brown *et al.*, 1972). Fifty-eight

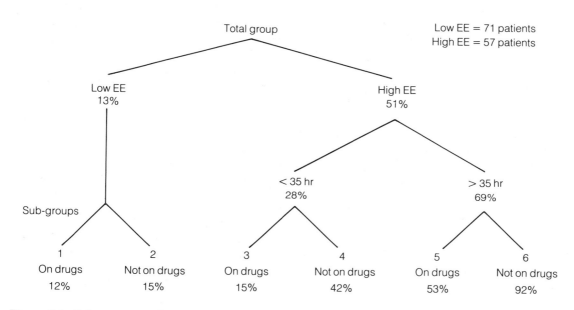

Figure 8.1 Relapse rates at 9 months in the study by Vaughn and Leff (1976).

per cent of patients returning to high EE homes relapsed, compared with 16% of those living with low EE relatives. The dose effect was again apparent: face-to-face contact of more than 35 hours per week increased the relapse rate in those patients living with high EE relatives.

This result was impressive, but might have been due to initial differences in the patients that in time brought out different responses from the relatives. The authors did consider this, but the difference in outcome persisted after controlling for the patients' previous work impairment and behavioural disturbance.

The findings were almost exactly replicated by Vaughn and Leff (1976a) in a smaller study comparing groups of neurotically depressed and schizophrenic patients. As they used methods identical to the 1972 study, they were able to combine their data on schizophrenia to give a larger sample (128). This allowed them to explore whether medication modified relapse rates by providing protection against the effects of the family environment.

These results are shown in Figure 8.1. The implications are: first, relapse in schizophrenia does indeed appear to be influenced by social circumstances; second, patients with a high risk of relapse can be identified; and third, since factors associated with relapse were pinpointed, so too were the targets of a possible intervention programme. These targets comprise the effective provision of medication, a reduction of face-to-face contact, and a lowering of EE in the family.

How secure are these findings? The EE measure was originally developed in Britain, but has now been used in an increasing number of countries, both in the developed and in the developing world. These studies are summarized in Table 8.3.

Of all these studies, only four show no predictive value of EE (Köttgen *et al.*, 1984; Parker *et al.*, 1988; McCreadie and Phillips, 1988; Ferrera *et al.*, 1989). The first of these has major methodological flaws that may reduce the credence given to its findings (Vaughn, 1986). The most crucial defects are that not all the patients were actually living at home and an unknown number of patients counted as relapsing had not recovered in the first place.

Idiosyncrasies and flaws are also apparent in the other three studies, but it seems inappropriate to make too much of these — after all, none of the studies reporting positive findings are without blemish. There are several failings in the Australian study of Parker *et al.* (1988), but they anticipate criticism by providing analyses that consider most of them. They did have very high rates of relapse in their low EE patients, and it is just possible that they were an unusual and chaotic group — they often changed residence and their very inconsistency may have taken them out of close contact with their relatives.

The study by McCreadie and Phillips (1988) of patients in remission living in a rural community reported an extremely low overall relapse rate (17%). Studying good prognosis cases makes it harder to demonstrate the effect of factors influencing course, and the effect itself may be less, relative to unknown intrinsic factors. The frequency of high EE (42%) is also the lowest reported in any Western population (Table 8.4).

The predictive studies of EE should be evaluated overall: although the importance of the time relatives spend together has only shown up in studies carried out by the original group of British workers, they add up to quite an impressive consensus for the value of the measure.

Hogarty (1985) raised the possibility that EE only predicts relapse in men, not women: this

seems to have some support from the available evidence (e.g. Vaughn *et al.*, 1984). Brown *et al.* (1972) did claim that EE was equally predictive for male and female sufferers, but, even so, EE may be of less clinical significance in women because the prognosis is relatively better for other reasons (Salokangas, 1983). The question of the role of EE in female patients remains open.

If EE is a robust predictor of relapse, the relapse rate of schizophrenia should be affected by anything that affects EE. One example is the different organization of family life in many Third World countries in comparison with the industrialized West. In particular, extended families are the norm in the former. It is clear from Table 8.4 that the proportion of families rated high in EE is at its greatest in Western industrialized societies.

The better course and outcome of schizophrenia in developing countries is well established (WHO, 1979): could it be the result of different family characteristics as reflected by the EE measure? Wig *et al.* (1987a) carried out an EE study in the area around the Indian city of Chandigarh. As expected, relapse rates were low, particularly in the rural areas. Despite this, there was still an association between hostility expressed by relatives and subsequent relapse a year later. This suggests that the good outcome of schizophrenia in this culture might indeed be the result of beneficial family structures and traditions (Leff *et al.*, 1987). In other words, both in Chandigarh and in London the relapse rate appears to be related to EE, but relapses are less frequent in India. This could therefore have been due to lower levels of EE. Using the pooled Indian and London results (Leff and Vaughn, 1976; Leff *et al.*, 1987), loglinear analysis suggested that the better outcome in India can be entirely explained by lower levels of EE and that the effect is of considerable strength (Kuipers and Bebbington, 1988). So, not only does EE have predictive value across very different cultures, it may also serve to explain differences in

Table 8.3 Results of prospective studies of expressed emotion (EE)

Author	Location	No. of subjects	Episode	Follow-up	Relapse rate high EE	Relapse rate Low EE
Brown et al. (1962)[1]	S. London	97 (male)	All	1 year	56%	21%
Brown et al. (1962)	S. London	101	All	9 months	58%	16%
Vaughn and Leff (1976)	S. London	37	All	9 months	50%	12%
Leff and Vaughn (1981)[2]	S. London	36	All	2 years	62%	20%
Vaughn et al. (1984)	Los Angeles	54	All	9 months	56%	28%
Moline et al. (1985)[3]	Chicago	24	All	1 year	91%	31%
Dulz and Hand (1986)[4]	Hamburg	46	All	9 months	58%	65%
Macmillan et al. (1986)	N. London	67	First	2 years	63%	39%
Nuechterlein et al. (1986)[5]	Los Angeles	26	All	1 year	37%	0%
Karno et al. (1987)	S. California	44	All	9 months	59%	26%
Leff et al. (1987)	Chandigargh India	76	First	1 year	33%	14%
Tarrier et al. (1988)[6]	Salford England	48	All	9 months	48%	21%
Parker et al. (1988)[7]	Sydney Australia	57	All	9 months	48%	60%
McCreadie and Phillips (1988)	Nithsdale Scotland	59	NA	6 months / 12 months	13% / 17%	11% / 20%
Budzyna-Dawidowski et al. (1989)	Cracow Poland	36	All	1 year / 2 years	32% / 72%	9% / 18%
Ivanović and Vuletić (1989)	Belgrade Yugoslavia	60	All	9 months	64%	7%
Možný (1989)	Rural Czechoslovkia	68	All	1 year	60%	29%
Cazzullo et al. (1989)	Milan Italy	45	All	9 months	58%	21%
Stricker et al. (1989)	Munster W. Germany	99	All	9 months	'Significantly higher'	38%
Ferrera et al. (1989)	Madrid Spain	31	All	9 months	44%	
Barrelet et al. (1990)	Geneva Switzerland	41	First	9 months	32%	0%
Vaughn (pers. comm.)	Sydney Australia	87	All	9 months	52%	23%

1. Their measure of 'emotional overinvolvement' was the prototype of EE.
2. Follow-up of same patients as Vaughn and Leff (1976).
3. Non-standard criteria for high EE.
4. An unknown number of subjects were not living with their EE rated relatives.
5. All patients on fixed dose fluphenazine.
6. Patients receiving standard care with or without education in the authors' intervention.
7. All relatives were parents. An unknown number of subjects were not living with parents at the time of readmission or reassessment.

Table 8.4 The applicability of EE measures

Author	Location	Proportion of relatives rated high on EE (in %)	Proportion of households rated high on EE (in %)
Brown *et al.* (1962)	S. London	NA	52
Brown *et al.* (1972)	S. London	NA	45
Vaughn and Leff (1976)	S. London	NA	49
Vaughn *et al.* (1984)	Los Angeles	NA	67
Moline *et al.* (1985)	Chicago	NA	70
MacMillan *et al.* (1986)	N. London	53	NA
Karno *et al.* (1987)	Los Angeles (Mexican–American)	28	41
Wig *et al.* (1987)	Aarhus	NA	54
Leff *et al.* (1987)	Chandigarh	23 30 urban 8 rural	23
McCreadie and Robinson (1987)	Nithsdale Scotland	43	42
Tarrier *et al.* (1988)	Salford	73	77
Parker *et al.* (1988)	Sydney Australia	NA	74
Barrelet *et al.* (1990)	Geneva Switzerland	NA	66
Vaughan (personal communication)	Sydney Australia	NA	53
Rostworoska (personal communication)	Cracow Poland	NA	70

outcome of schizophrenia in those cultures.

However, the explanation of these findings cannot lie in the overt structural differences between families in India and the West. Although there were fewer high EE families in the rural than in the urban areas studied in Chandigarh, there appeared to be no relationship between EE levels and the type of gross family structure (i.e. extended vs. nuclear). The uniformly low EE levels in Indian families must therefore arise from other family attributes.

8.2.3 HOW DOES AN ADVERSE HOME ENVIRONMENT LEAD TO RELAPSE?

It has always been assumed, not unreasonably, that the home environment characterized by high EE represents a form of psychosocial stress. How then is relapse mediated? One possibility is that it operates via physiological arousal.

There is now considerable evidence from psychophysiological studies in line with this suggestion. Patients seem to be physiologically aroused with high EE relatives, but not with low EE relatives (Tarrier *et al.*, 1979, 1988b; Sturgeon *et al.*, 1984). Indeed, Tarrier and Barrowclough (1987) demonstrated a differential psychophysiological effect in a man living with one high and one low EE parent, depending on which was present. The arousal provoked by critical relatives seems to be non-specific, and has been observed in non-schizophrenic disturbed adolescents (Valone *et al.*, 1984).

However, despite changes in EE due to a successful social intervention programme (Leff *et al.*, 1982), there were no concomitant changes in psychophysiological ratings of patients, which turned out to be independently related to relapse. In other words, the benefit from changes in EE does not appear to work through changes in levels of arousal. This research has been reviewed in more detail elsewhere (Kuipers and Bebbington, 1988; Turpin *et al.*, 1988).

Leff *et al.* (1983) have incorporated these ideas about arousal into an overall model of relapse in schizophrenia, using material from their intervention study to strengthen their argument. They concluded that patients unprotected by medication might relapse in response to **either** a life event **or** living with a high EE relative, but that patients taking medication required exposure to both factors before they would relapse. In this model, medication operates generally to raise the threshold for the psychosocial provocation of relapse, suggesting that life events and EE might perhaps have a common mechanism.

8.2.4. THE DISTINCTION BETWEEN CRITICISM AND OVER-INVOLVEMENT

For historical reasons, the expressed emotion measure is something of a mixture. It covers two attributes of relatives that at first sight seem distinctly different. It would seem reasonable to regard criticism and hostility as similar, and to distinguish them from the other attribute of EE, that is, emotional over-involvement. Criticism is seen frequently in both spouses and parents of those with schizophrenia, whereas spouses are less likely to be over-involved than parents. Can these two aspects of EE be regarded as inherently different, and if so in what sense?

Some authors (e.g. Koenigsberg and Handley, 1986) are very keen on the principle of keeping them distinct. There may well be differences in their associations: for instance, emotional over-involvement may be particularly associated with poor premorbid social functioning (Brown *et al.*, 1972; Miklowitz *et al.*, 1983). However, Tarrier *et al.* (1988b) failed to distinguish between the two patterns of behaviour from the patients' psychophysiological responses to the presence of a relative. Moreover, where studies have presented results separately for criticism and emotional over-involvement each shows a similar ability: to predict relapse, although it is relatively rare for the latter to be present alone (Brown *et al.*, 1972; Vaughn *et al.*, 1984; Leff *et al.*, 1987). Thus, although the attitudes look very different and may have different origins, they may actually work in the same way. Hooley (1985) argues that both criticism and over-involvement are strategies reflecting a need to control situations. Is emphasizing these similarities useful? It is probably worth retaining some separation of the two ideas for clinical reasons: emotional over-involvement and criticism may require different therapeutic strategies (Kuipers and Bebbington, 1990).

8.2.5. WHAT DOES EE INDICATE ABOUT FAMILY RELATIONSHIPS?

EE uses an individual relative's behaviour at a single time to predict the likelihood of a subsequent relapse in the schizophrenic patient with whom that relative lives. What does EE actually mean in terms of the interplay between members of the patient's family?

It has always been presumed that the measure is predictive because it indicates either some continuing feature of the interaction between the relatives, or their capacity to deal with crises (Kuipers, 1979). Certainly, relatives who made frequent critical comments when interviewed alone behave similarly in the presence of the patient, albeit more restrained in the second setting (Rutter and Brown, 1966; Brown and Rutter, 1966). There is now further evidence for the generalization of relatives' behaviour. Miklowitz *et al.* (1984, 1989) and Strachan *et al.* (1986) have used the Affective Style coding system developed by Doane *et al.* (1981) to assess families taking part in a standardized task designed to recreate interaction in a laboratory setting (Goldstein *et al.*, 1968). Negative affective style in these direct interactions is consistently highly correlated with EE measured in the usual way. Hubschmid and Zemp (1989) have shown that high EE relatives engender a more negative emotional climate, a conflict prone structure, and more rigid patterns of interaction.

Kuipers *et al.* (1983) also found it possible to distinguish between high and low EE relatives in family interviews. During discussions that included the patient, high EE relatives talked longer and were poorer listeners than low EE relatives. MacCarthy *et al.* (1986) have recently found that highly critical relatives appear to provide an unpredictable home environment for schizophrenic patients. Greenley (1986) has shown that high EE is associated with fears and anxieties by relatives, particularly when they did not attribute the patient's behaviour to illness. Preliminary results of a study of attribution in the relatives of schizophrenic patients suggest that causal beliefs are systematically related to the relatives' emotional characteristics. The more critical and hostile relatives tended to attribute negative outcomes to causes that were more idiosyncratic to and controllable by the patient (Brewin *et al.*, 1991).

A study of depressed spouses throws incidental light in the behavioural counterparts of EE. Hooley and Hahlweg (1986) reported sequential analyses of interaction patterns between 44 couples where one partner was depressed. They found that high EE couples had a varied but largely negative style of interaction. Low EE spouses typically provided a continuous positive exchange. It was also possible to distinguish between the high and low EE samples on levels of warmth and marital satisfaction.

There is now evidence that high EE is associated with less effective coping responses (Kuipers *et al.*, 1983; Bledin *et al.*, 1990; MacCarthy, personal communication). High EE carers of demented elderly people used strategies such as distraction, avoidance, overeating and denial, rather than more positive approaches like problem-solving and seeking social support (Bledin *et al.*, 1990).

Birchwood and Smith (1987) have been primarily interested in describing and quantifying families' coping behaviour and coping styles. They investigated the relationship between these characteristics of relatives and the outcome of disorder in terms of relapse, social adjustment and psychopathology. Although overlapping with the previous EE research, their work provides new data on family behaviour in this situation. Clearly the link between relatives' ability to cope with the problems of living with someone suffering from schizophrenia and the affective style of their interaction with them is a crucial issue: the causal direction is unknown, but probably complex. It is a pity that these studies (Birchwood and Smith, 1987) have been developed independently of any EE assessment, although the authors' current research does include it. Indirectly, their examples add to the evidence that poor coping in relatives overlaps with high levels of EE.

Interestingly, when the patients' own responses are examined, those living with low

EE relatives give vent to significantly fewer critical statements and more autonomous statements than those from high EE families. In other words, criticism is reciprocated. This finding is independent of the level of symptoms experienced by the patients (Strachan *et al.*, 1989).

Finally, it is clear that the attitudes and behaviours represented by EE seem to characterize the relatives of those who suffer from a number of other conditions in addition to schizophrenia. These include depression (Vaughn and Leff, 1976a; Hooley *et al.*, 1986), bipolar disorder (Miklowitz *et al.*, 1988) anorexia (Szmukler *et al.*, 1987), mental handicap (Greedharry, 1987), Parkinson's disease (MacCarthy, personal communication), inflammatory bowel disease (Vaughn, personal communication) and senile dementia (Bledin *et al.*, 1990). While much theoretical and clinical interest remains in the use of EE in schizophrenia, the measure itself appears to tap difficulties common to the care of many disabling problems. High EE ratings have also been noted in the key workers of long-term patients with schizophrenia (Watts, 1988).

8.2.6 THE ORIGINS OF FAMILY ATTITUDES TOWARDS A MENTALLY ILL RELATIVE

The EE measure therefore probably reflects a variety of attitudes and behaviours characterizing the family's response to chronically disturbed relatives. What is the origin of these characteristics?

Birchwood and Smith (1987) have argued that the original workers were wrong in thinking that the EE reflects some enduring trait of relatives, and that the measure actually picks up an emerging attribute. In other words, high EE is something that develops as the response of some relatives to the burdens of living with someone who has schizophrenia. They based their argument on the fact that high EE is less apparent in relatives of those experiencing first rather than subsequent admissions for schizophrenia. There is certainly a lower relapse rate in first admission patients (33%) than in those subsequently admitted (69%) (Leff and Brown, 1977), although there are alternative explanations for this. Moreover, recent work has suggested that at least some components of high EE are associated with abnormalities of various sorts in the patient (Miklowitz *et al.*, 1983; Mavreas *et al.*, 1992). However, the causal direction is as usual unclear.

Birchwood and Smith (1987) therefore present a feedback or adjustment model, whereby families' coping efficacy and coping style, along with other predictors such as the quality of family relationships, will develop over time. In a sense, they have attacked something of a straw man. It must be virtually axiomatic that the characteristics of high EE arise from an interaction between the attributes of relative and patient.

One obvious way of examining this interaction is to relate levels of EE to the 'burden' experienced by relatives. Researchers have hardly ever done this, although the literature on burden is now substantial (Fadden *et al.*, 1987). It seems likely that relatives with high levels of EE will find the same behaviour much more burdensome than those who are low on EE. This is also probably related to coping styles. Bledin *et al.* (1990) have recently shown that high levels of strain, EE, and maladaptive coping strategies tended to be associated in those caring for demented elderly persons.

The data on social contact from the British studies are open to more than one interpretation. They may indicate that greater social contact with a high EE relative is more stressful, but the schizophrenic patients most vulnerable to stress may be precisely those who are least able to control and manage their social relationships — unable to process information effectively because of their cognitive defects, they allow themselves to become overloaded (Hemsley, 1987). Those with over-involved relatives are often the most impaired socially (Brown *et al.*, 1972; Miklowitz *et al.*, 1983) and may be most at risk, either because of their intrinsic problems or because an over-involved relative is harder to get away from. Mavreas *et al.* (1989) make an interesting claim in this context: that behavioural abnormalities are more common in schizophrenic patients when none of the relatives in the household is rated low in EE — that is, where *no* domestic relationships are 'safe'.

8.2.7 THE STABILITY OF EE RATINGS

The value of EE assessment may be crucially related to the fact that the relative is dealing with the upheaval surrounding the patient's admission to hospital. In time the disturbance settles, and at least some high EE relatives become less critical (Brown *et al.*, 1972; Dulz and Hand, 1986; Hogarty *et al.*, 1986; Tarrier *et al.*, 1988a; Favre *et al.*, 1989). Initial assessments have therefore focused on the admission period. Low EE relatives tend to stay low, although Tarrier and his colleagues (1988a) did report a minority who changed to high levels. There is relatively little other evidence as to the stability of EE measures over time. In the studies of Leff and his colleagues (1982, 1985), the high EE control group showed no significant overall changes in EE over the intervention of nine months, although two of the twelve relatives did spontaneously become low EE.

It seems possible that there are three groups of relatives: at one extreme, there are the very low EE relatives who cope well whatever the circumstances. At the other extreme are very high EE relatives who have multiple problems, which they cope with badly. In between seems to be a variable group who may change category spontaneously or through the intervention of others, depending on their ability to learn new coping skills and to use them in surmounting crises. If the new skills are insufficient, they may display reduced EE at one assessment, but revert back when there is a crisis which they are unable to manage

(Figure 8.2). This idea has recently received some confirmation in a study of the stability of EE over a nine-month period in 35 relatives of 22 patients with schizophrenia (Favre *et al.*, 1989). They found stable high- and low-EE relatives, but also a proportion of unstable relatives who typically displayed fewer critical comments (6–10) than the stable high EE group. The authors noted that the relatively few changes observed in EE levels seemed to depend on factors other than the clinical state of the patients.

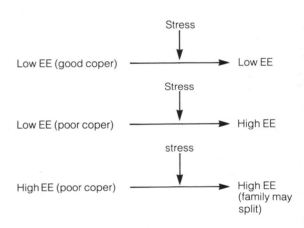

Figure 8.2 Patterns of EE over time.

8.2.8 INTERVENTION STUDIES

Several reports of social intervention with the relatives of patients with schizophrenia have now been published, and others are nearing completion. Such studies are important both clinically and theoretically. Critics of EE research must contend with their generally positive results. Successful interventions have almost always managed to reduce EE, contact or negative affective style (Leff *et al.*, 1982; Falloon *et al.*, 1982), whereas less successful interventions (Köttgen *et al.*, 1982; McCreadie *et al.*, 1990) did not manage to reduce EE. We have reviewed these in detail elsewhere (Kuipers and Bebbington, 1988, 1990; see also Chapter 23).

8.3 CONCLUSION

The very extensive literature that we have reviewed here is consistent in supporting a major effect of the social environment on the course and outcome of schizophrenia, and social influences probably have an effect on the first emergence of the condition, at least in its timing. In our view the implications of this finding should shape the clinical management of schizophrenia, which should be based on a proper attention to the social environment, particularly for patients with a history of several relapses.

REFERENCES

Al Khani, M.A.F., Bebbington, P.E., Watson, J.P. and House, F. (1986) Life events and schizophrenia: a Saudi Arabian study. *Br. J. Psychiatry*, **148**, 12–22.

Barrelet, L., Ferrero, F., Szigethy, L., Giddey, C. and Pellizzer, G. (1990) Expressed Emotion and first admission schizophrenia: a replication in a French cultural environment. *Br. J. Psychiatry*, **156**, 357–62.

Bateson, G., Jackson, D.D., Hally, J. and Weakland, J.H. (1956) Towards a theory of schizophrenia. *Behav. Sci.*, **1**, 251–64.

Birchwood, M. and Smith, J. (1987) Schizophrenia in the family. In *Coping with Disorder in the Family*. J. Orford (ed), Croom Helm, London.

Bledin, K., MacCarthy, B. Kuipers, L., and Woods, R. (1990) EE in the daughters of the demented elderly. *Br. J. Psychiatry*, in press.

Brewin, C.R., McCarthy, D., Duda, K. and Vaughn, C.E. (1991) Attribution and expressed emotion in the relatives of patients with schizophrenia. *J. Abnorm. Psychol.*, **100**, 546–54.

Brown, G.W. (1959) Experiences of discharged chronic schizophrenic mental hospital patients in various types of living group. *Millbank Mem. Fund Q.*, **37**, 105–31.

Brown, G.W. (1974) Meaning, measurement and stress of life events. In *Stressful Life Events: Their Nature and Effects*. B.S. Dohrenwend and B.P. Dohrenwend (eds), John Wiley, New York, pp. 217–44.

Brown, G.W. and Harris, T.O. (1978) *Social Origins of Depression*. London, Tavistock.

Brown, G.W. and Rutter, M.L. (1966) The measurement of family activities and relationships. *Hum. Relations*, **19**, 241–63.

Brown, G.W., Carstairs, G.M. and Topping, G.C. (1958) The post hospital adjustment of chronic mental patients. *Lancet*, **ii**, 685–9.

Brown, G.W., Monck, E.M., Carstairs, G.M. and Wing, J.K. (1962) Influence of family life on the course of schizophrenic illness. *Br. J. Prev. Soc. Med.*, **16**, 55–68.

Brown, G.W. and Birley, J.L.T. (1968) Crises and life changes and the onset of schizophrenia. *J. Health Soc. Behav.*, **9**, 203–14.

Brown, G.W., Birley, J.L.T. and Wing, J.K. (1972) Influence of family life on the course of schizophrenic disorders: A replication. *Br. J. Psychiatry*, **121**, 241–58.

Brown, G.W., Harris, T.O. and Peto, J. (1973) Life events and psychiatric disorders. Part 2: Nature of causal link. *Psychol. Med.* **3**, 159–76.

Budzyna-Dawidowski, P., Rostworowska, M. and de Barbaro, B. (1989) *Stability of Expressed Emotion. A 3 year follow-up study of schizophrenic patients*. Paper presented at the 19th. Annual Congress of the European Association of Behaviour Therapy, Vienna, Sept 10–24.

Canton, G. and Fraccon, I.G. (1985) Life events and schizophrenia: a replication. *Acta Psychiatr. Scand.*, **71**, 211–6.

Cazzullo, C.L., Bertrando, P., Bressi, C., Clerici, M., Beltz, J. and Invernizzi, G. (1989) *Expressed Emotion in Italian families: A comparison between schizophrenics and other patients*. Paper presented at the 19th. Annual Congress of the European Association of Behaviour Therapy, Vienna, Sept 20–24.

Day, R., Neilsen, J.A, Korten, A. *et al.* (1987) Stressful life events preceding the acute onset of schizophrenia: a cross-national study from the World Health Organization. *Cult. Med. Psychiatry*, **11**, 123–206.

Doane, J.A., West, K.L., Goldstein, M.J., Rodnick, E.H. and Jones, J.E. (1981) Parental communication deviance and affective style: predictors of subsequent schizophrenia spectrum disorders in vulnerable adolescents. *Arch. Gen. Psychiatry*, **38**, 679–85.

Dulz, B. and Hand, I. (1986) Short-term relapse in young schizophrenics: Can it be predicted and affected by family (CFI), patient, and treatment variables? An experimental study. In *Treatment of Schizophrenia: Family Assessment and Intervention*. M.J. Goldstein, I. Hand and K. Hahlweg (eds), Springer-Verlag, Berlin, pp. 59–75.

Fadden, G.B., Bebbington, P.E. and Kuipers, L. (1987) The burden of care: the impact of functional psychiatric illness on the patient's family. *Br. J. Psychiatry*, **150**, 285–92.

Falloon, I.R.H., Boyd, J.L., McGill, C.W., Razani, J., Moss, H.B. and Gilderman, A.M. (1982) Family management in the prevention of exacerbations of schizophrenia. A controlled study. *N. Engl. J. Med.*, **306**, 1437–40.

Favre, S., Gonzales, C., Lendais, G. *et al.* (1989) *Expressed Emotion (EE) of schizophrenic relatives*. Poster presented at VIII World Congress of Psychiatry, Athens, 12th–19th October.

Ferrera, J.A. and Vizarro, C. (1989) *Expressed Emotion and course of schizophrenia in a Spanish sample*. Paper presented at the 19th Annual Congress of the European Association of Behaviour Therapy. Vienna, Sept 20–24.

Goldberg, S.C., Schooler, N.R., Hogarty, G.E. and Roper, M. (1977) Prediction of relapse in schizophrenic outpatients treated by drug and sociotherapy. *Arch. Gen. Psychiatry*, **34**, 171–84.

Goldstein, M. (1985) Family factors that antedate the onset of schizophrenia and related disorders: the results of a 15 year prospective longitudinal study. *Acta Psychiatr. Scand.*, **71**, Suppl 319, 7–18.

Goldstein, M. (1987) The UCLA high-risk project. *Schizophr. Bull.*, **13**, 505–14.

Goldstein, M., Judd, L.L., Rodnick, E.H., Alkire, A. and Gould, E. (1968) A method for studying social influence and coping patterns within families of disturbed adolescents. *J. Nerv. Ment. Dis.*, **147**, 233–51.

Greenley, J.R. (1986) Social control and Expressed Emotion. *J. Nerv. Ment. Dis.*, **174**, 24–30.

Greedharry, D. (1987) Expressed Emotion in the families of the mentally handicapped: A pilot study. *Br. J. Psychiatry*, **150**, 400–2.

Hemsley, D.R. (1987) Psychological models of schizophrenia. In *Textbook of Abnormal Psychology*. E. Miller and P. Cooper (eds), Churchill Livingstone, Edinburgh.

Hirsch S.R. and Leff J.P. (1975) *Abnormalities in the Parents of Schizophrenics*. Maudsley Monograph No. 22. Oxford University Press, Oxford.

Hogarty, G.E. (1985) Expressed Emotion and schizophrenic relapse: Implications from the Pittsburgh Study. In *Controversies in Schizophrenia*. M. Alpert (ed), Guilford Press, New York.

Hogarty, G.E., Anderson, C.M., Reiss, D.J. *et al.* (1986) Family psycho-education, social skills training and maintenance chemotherapy in the aftercare treatment of schizophrenia. I. One year effects of a controlled study on relapse and Expressed Emotion. *Arch. Gen. Psychiatry* **43**, 633–42.

Hooley, J.M. (1985) Expressed Emotion: a review of the critical literature. *Clin. Psychol. Rev.*, **5**, 119–39.

Hooley, J.M. and Hahlweg, K. (1986) The marriages and interaction patterns of depressed patients and their spouses: Comparison of high and low EE dyads. In *Treatment of Schizophrenia: Family Assessment and Intervention*. M.J. Goldstein, I. Hand and K. Hahlweg (eds), Springer-Verlag, Berlin, pp. 85–96.

Hooley, J.M., Orley, J. and Teasdale, J. (1986) Levels of Expressed Emotion and relapse in depressed patients. *Br. J. Psychiatry*, **148**, 642–7.

Hubschmid, T. and Zemp, M. (1989) Interactions in high- and low-EE families. *Soc. Psychiatry Psychiatr. Epidemiol.*, **24**, 113–19.

Ivanović, M. and Vuletić, Z. (1989) *Expressed Emotion in the families of patients with a frequent type of schizophrenia and its influence on the course of illness*. Paper presented at the 19th Annual Congress of the European Association of Behaviour Therapy. Vienna, Sept 20–24.

Jacobs, S. and Myers, J. (1976) Recent life events

and acute schizophrenic psychosis: a controlled study. *J. Nerv. and Ment. Dis.*, **162**, 75–87.

Karno, M., Jenkins, J.H., de la Selva, A. *et al.* (1987) Expressed Emotion and schizophrenic outcome among Mexican-American families. *J. Nerv. Ment. Dis.*, **175**, 143–51.

Koenigsberg, H.W. and Handley, R. (1986) Expressed Emotion: From predictive index to clinical construct. *Am. J. Psychiatry*, **143**, 1361–73.

Köttgen, C. Sonnichsen, I., Mollenhauer, K. and Jurth, R. (1984) Group therapy with the families of schizophrenic patients: results of the Hamburg Camberwell Family Interview Study III. *Int. J. Fam. Psychiatry*, **5**, 84–94.

Kuipers, L. (1979) Expressed Emotion: a review. *Br. J. Soc. Clin. Psychol.*, **18**, 237–43.

Kuipers, L. (1983) *Family factors in schizophrenia: an intervention study.* Ph.D. Thesis. University of London.

Kuipers, L., Sturgeon D., Berkowitz, R. and Leff, J.P. (1983) Characteristics of Expressed Emotion: its relationship to speech and looking in schizophrenic patients and their relatives. *Br. J. Soc. Clin. Psychol.*, **22**, 257–64.

Kuipers, L. and Bebbington, P.E. (1988) Expressed Emotion research in schizophrenia: theoretical and clinical implications. *Psychol. Med.*, **18**, 893–910.

Kuipers, L., MacCarthy, B., Hurry, J. and Harper, R. (1989) Counselling the relatives of the long-term mentally ill. II. A low-cost supportive model. *Br. J. Psychiatry*, **154**, 775–82.

Kuipers, L. and Bebbington, P.E. (1990) *Working in Partnership: Clinicians and Carers in the Management of Longstanding Mental Illness.* Heinemann Medical, Oxford.

Laing, R.D. and Esterson, A. (1964) *Sanity, Madness and the Family*, Penguin, Harmondsworth, Middlesex.

Leff, J.P. and Brown, G.W. (1977) Family and social factors in the course of schizophrenia, *Br. J. Psychiatry*, **130**, 417–20.

Leff, J.P. and Vaughn, C.E. (1981) The role of maintenance therapy and relatives' Expressed Emotion in relapse of schizophrenia: a two year follow up. *Br. J. Psychiatry*, **139**, 102–4.

Leff, J.P. and Vaughn, C. (1985) *Expressed Emotion in Families.* Guilford Press, New York.

Leff, J.P., Kuipers, L., Berkowitz, R., Eberlein-Fries, R. and Sturgeon, D. (1982) A controlled trial of social intervention in schizophrenic families. *Br. J. Psychiatry*, **141**, 121–34.

Leff, J.P., Kuipers, L., Berkowitz, R., Vaughn, C.E. and Sturgeon, D. (1983) Life events, relatives' Expressed Emotion and maintenance neuroleptics in schizophrenic relapse. *Psychol. Med.*, **13**, 799–806.

Leff, J.P., Kuipers, L., Berkowitz, R. and Sturgeon, D. (1985) A controlled trial of social intervention in the families of schizophrenic patients: Two year follow up. *Br. J. Psychiatry*, **146**, 594–600.

Leff, J.P., Wig, N., Ghosh, A. *et al.* (1987) Influence of relatives' Expressed Emotion on the course of schizophrenia in Chandigarh. *Br. J. Psychiatry*, **151**, 166–73.

Leff, J., Berkowitz, R., Sharit, N., Strachan, A., Glass, I. and Vaughn, C. (1989) A trial of family therapy v. a relatives' group for schizophrenia. *Br. J. Psychiatry*, **154**, 58–66.

Lidz, T., Cornelison, A.R., Fleck, S. and Terry, D. (1957) The intrafamilial environment of the schizophrenic patient. I. *Psychiatry*, **20**, 329–42.

MacCarthy, B. (1988) The Role of Relatives in *Community Care and Practice* eds. A. Lavender and F. Holloway, Wiley & Sons, Chichester, pp. 207–27.

MacCarthy, B., Hemsley, D., Schrank-Fernandez, C., Kuipers, L. and Katz, R. (1986) Unpredictabilty as a correlate of Expressed Emotion in the relatives of schizophrenics. *Br. J. Psychiatry*, **148**, 727–30.

McCreadie, R.G. and Robinson, A.T.D. (1987) The Nithsdale Schizophrenia Survey: VI. Relatives' Expressed Emotion: prevalence, patterns and clinical assessment. *Br. J. Psychiatry*, **150**, 640–4.

McCreadie, R.G. and Phillips, K. (1988) The Nithsdale Schizophrenia Survey: VII. Does relatives' high Expressed Emotion predict relapse? *Br. J. Psychiatry*, **152**, 477–81.

McCreadie, R.G., Phillips, K., Harvey, J.A., Waldron, G., Stewart, M. and Baird, D. (1991) The Nithsdale Schizophrenia Surveys VIII. Do relatives want family intervention and does it help? *Br. J. Psychiatry*, **158**, 110–13.

MacMillan, J.F., Gold, A., Crow, T.J., Johnson, A.L. and Johnstone, E.C. (1986) The Northwick Park Study of First Episodes of Schizophrenia. IV. Expressed Emotion and relapse. *Br. J. Psychiatry*, **148**, 133–43.

MacMillan, J.F., Crow, T.J., Johnson, A.L. and Johnstone, E.C. (1987) Expressed Emotion and relapse in first episodes of schizophrenia. *Br. J. Psychiatry*, **151**, 320–3.

Malzacher, M., Merz, J. and Ebnother, D. (1981) Einschneidende Lebensereignisse im Vorfeld akuter schizophrener Episoden: Erstmals erkrankte Patienten im Vergleich mit einer Normalstichprobe. *Arch. Psychr. Nerv.*, **230**, 227–42.

Mavreas, V., Tomaros, Carydi, N. *et al.* (1992) Expressed Emotion in families of chronic schizophrenics and its association with clinical measures. *Soc. Psychiatry Psychiatr. Epidemiol.*, (in press).

Miklowitz, D.J., Goldstein, M.J. and Fallon, R.H. (1983) Premorbid and symptomatic characteristics of schizophrenics from families with high and low levels of Expressed Emotion. *J. Abnorm. Psychol.*, **92**, 359–67.

Miklowitz, D.J., Goldstein, M.J., Fallon, R.H. and Doane, J.A. (1984) Interactional correlates of Expressed Emotion in the families of schizophrenics. *Br. J. Psychiatry*, **144**, 482–7.

Miklowitz, D.J., Goldstein, M.J., Nuechterlein, K.H., Snyder, K.S., and Mintz, J., (1988) Family factors and the course of bipolar affective disorder. *Arch. Gen. Psychiatry*, **45**, 225–31.

Miklowitz, D.J., Goldstein, M.J., Doane, J.A. *et al.* (1989) Is Expressed Emotion an index of a transactional process. I. Parent's Affective Style. *Fam. Process*, **28**, 153–67.

Moline, R.A., Singh, S., Morris, A. and Meltzer, H.Y. (1985) Family Expressed Emotion and relapse in schizophrenia in 24 urban American patients. *Am. J. Psychiatry*, **142**, 178–81.

Možný, P. (1989) *Expressed Emotion and rehospitalization rates of schizophrenics in the psychiatric hospital Kromeriz, CSSR.* Paper presented at the 19th Annual Congress of the European Association of Behaviour Therapy, Vienna, Sept 20–24.

Nuechterlein, K.H., Snyder, K.S., Dawson, M.E.,

Rappe, S., Gitlin, M. and Fogelson, D. (1986) Expressed Emotion, fixed-dose fluphenazine decanoate maintenance, and relapse in recent onset schizophrenia. *Psychopharm. Bull.*, **22**, 633–9.

Parker, G., Johnston, P., and Hayward, L. (1988) Parental 'Expressed Emotion' as a predictor of schizophrenic relapse. *Arch. Gen. Psychiatry*, **45**, 806–13.

Paykel, E.S. (1979) Recent life events in the developments of the depressive disorders. In *The Psychobiology of the Depressive Disorders: Implications for the Effects of Stress.* R.A. Depue (ed), Academic Press, New York, 245–62.

Rutter, M.L. and Brown, G.W. (1966) The reliability and validity of measures of family life and relationships in families containing a psychiatric patient. *Soc. Psychiatry*, **1**, 38–53.

Salokangas, R.K.R. (1983) Prognostic implications of the sex of schizophrenic patients. *Br. J. Psychiatry*, **142**, 145–51.

Shakow, D. (1973) Some thoughts about schizophrenic research in the context of high-risk studies. *Psychiatry*, **36**, 353–65.

Stevens, B.C. (1973) Evaluation of rehabilitation for psychotic patients in the community. *Acta Psychiatr. Scand.*, **46**, 136–40.

Strachan, A.M. (1986) Family intervention for the rehabilitation of schizophrenia. *Schizophr. Bull.*, **12**, 678–98.

Strachan, A.M., Leff, J.P., Goldstein M.J., Doane, A. and Burt, C. (1986) Emotional attitudes and direct communication in the families of schizophrenics: A cross-national replication. *Br. J. Psychiatry*, **149**, 279–87.

Strachan, A.M., Feingold, D., Goldstein, M.J., Miklowitz, D.J., and Nuechterlein, K.H. (1989) Is Expressed Emotion an index of a transactional process II. Patient's coping style. *Fam. Process*, **28**, 169–81.

Stricker, K., Rook, A. and Buchkremer, G. (1989) *Expressed Emotion and course of disease in schizophrenic outpatients: Results of a two year follow-up in a German study.* Paper presented at the 19th. Annual Congress of the European Association of Behaviour Therapy, Vienna, Sept 20–24.

Sturgeon, D., Turpin, D., Kuipers, L., Berkowitz, R. and Leff, J. (1984) Psychophysiological responses of schizophrenic patients to high and low Expressed Emotion relatives: a follow-up study. *Br. J. Psychiatry*, **145**, 62–9.

Szmukler, G.I., Berkowitz, R., Eisler, I., Leff, J. and Dare, C. (1987) Expressed Emotion in individual and family settings: a comparative study. *Br. J. Psychiatry*, **151**, 174–8.

Tarrier, N. and Barrowclough, C. (1987) A longitudinal psychophysiological assessment of a schizophrenic patient in relation to the Expressed Emotion of his relatives. *Behav. Psychother.*, **15**, 45–57.

Tarrier, N., Vaughn, C.E., Lader, M.H. and Leff, J.P. (1979) Bodily reactions to people and events in schizophrenics. *Arch. Gen. Psychiatry*, **36**, 311–5.

Tarrier, N., Barrowclough, C., Porceddu, K. and Watts, S. (1988a) The assessment of psychophysiological reactivity to the Expressed Emotion of the relatives of schizophrenic patients. *Br. J. Psychiatry*, **152**, 618–24.

Tarrier, N., Barrowclough, C., Vaughn, C. et al, (1988b) The community management of schizophrenia: a controlled trial of a behavioural intervention with families to reduce relapse. *Br. J. Psychiatry*, **153**, 532–42.

Tennant, C., Bebbington, P.E. and Hurry, J. (1981) The role of life events in depressive illness: is there a substantial causal relation? *Psychol. Med.*, **11**, 379–89.

Tidmarsh, D. and Wood, S. (1972) Psychiatric aspects of destitution. In *Evaluating a Community Psychiatric Service*. J.K. Wing and A.M. Hailey (eds), Oxford University Press, London.

Tomaros, V., Valachonikolis, I.G., Stefanis, C.N. and Madianos, M. (1988) The effect of individual psychosocial treatment on the family atmosphere of schizophrenic patients. *Soc. Psychiatry*, **23**, 256–61.

Turpin, G., Tarrier, N. and Sturgeon, D. (1988) Social psychophysiology and the study of biopsychosocial modesl of schizophrenia. In *Social Psychophysiology: Theory and Clinical Applications*. H. Wagner (ed), Wiley, Chichester.

Valone, K., Goldstein, M.G. and Morton, J.P. (1984) Parental Expressed Emotion and psychophysiological reactivity in an adolescent sample at risk for schizophrenic spectrum disorders. *J. Abnorm. Psychol.*, **93**, 448–57.

Vaughn, C. (1986) Patterns of emotional response in the families of schizophrenic patients. In *Treatment of Schizophrenia: Family Assessment and Intervention*. M.J. Goldstein, I. Hand and K. Hahlweg (eds), Springer-Verlag, Berlin.

Vaughn, C.E. (1989) Annotation: Expressed Emotion in family relationships. *J. Child Psychol.*, **30**, 13–22.

Vaughn, C. and Leff, J.P. (1976a) The influence of family and social factors on the course of psychiatric illness: a comparison of schizophrenic and depressed neurotic patients. *Br. J. Psychiatry*, **129**, 125–37.

Vaughn, C.E. and Leff, J.P. (1976b) The measurement of Expressed Emotion in the families of psychiatric patients. *Br. J. Clin. Soc. Psychol.*, **15**, 157–65.

Vaughan, C.E., Snyder, K.S., Jones. S. *et al.* (1984) Family factors in schizophrenic relapse. Replication in California of British research in Expressed Emotion. *Arch. Gen. Psychiatry*, **41**, 1169–77.

Venables, P. (1977) *Psychophysiological high risk strategy with Mauritian children: Methodological issues*. Paper read at the Psychophysiological Conference, London.

Ventura, J., Nuechterlein, K.H., Lukoff, D. and Hardesty, J.P. (1989) A prospective study of stressful life events and schizophrenic relapse. *J. Abnorm. Psychol.*, **98**, 407–11.

Wallace, C.J. and Liberman, R.P. (1985) Social skills training for patients with schizophrenia: a controlled clinical trial. *Psychiatry Res.*, **15**, 239–47.

Watts, S. (1988) *A Descriptive Investigation of the Incidence of High EE in Staff working with Schizophrenic Patients in a Hospital Setting*. Unpublished dissertation. Diploma in Clinical Psychology, British Psychological Society.

Wig, N.N., Menon, D.K., Bedi, H. *et al.* (1987a) The cross-cultural transfer of ratings of relatives' Expressed Emotion. *Br. J. Psychiatry*, **151**, 156–60.

Wig, N.N., Menon, D.K., Bedi, H. *et al.* (1987b) The distribution of Expressed Emotion components among relatives of schizophrenic patients in Aarhus and Chandigarh. *Br. J. Psychiatry*, **151**, 160–5.

143

Wing, J.K., Bennett, D.H. and Denham, J. (1964) *The Industrial Rehabilitation of Long Stay Schizophrenic Patients*. Medical Research Council Memo No. 42, HMSO, London.

World Health Organization (1979) *Schizophrenia: An International Follow-up Study*. John Wiley and Sons, Chichester.

Wynne, L.C. and Singer, M. (1963) Thought disorder and family relations of schizophrenics. I. *Arch. Gen. Psychiatry*, **9**, 191–206.

Wynne, L.C. and Singer, M. (1965) Thought disorder and family relations of schizophrenics. II. *Arch. Gen. Psychiatry*, **12**, 187–212.

Chapter 9

Criminality, dangerousness and schizophrenia

PAUL E. MULLEN

9.1 INTRODUCTION

This chapter will examine the relationship between suffering a schizophrenic illness and an increased propensity to act in a criminal, and in particular a violent manner. This is an emotive issue, because in part to argue for such a connection is to risk reawakening in our community the fear of the mad with its attendant demands for containment, and in part, because if accepted it could indiscriminately stigmatize all those who come into contact with the mental health services. The demystifying of madness and the refuting of popular and professional prejudices about the violent proclivities of the mentally disordered, particularly those with schizophrenic conditions, was important in the change in emphasis from control and containment toward management and normalization. Those of us committed to further progress along this particular road have every reason to be wary of the use that will be made by those who favour a return of asylum incarceration, any suggestion that those with schizophrenic disorders are prone to criminality and violence.

In addressing questions of dangerousness it is necessary to clarify the context in which the question is posed and the purpose for which the answer is required. The potential dangerousness of sufferers of chronic schizophrenic disorders, posed in the context of the threat to the community presented by the closure of the large mental hospitals, requires one approach. A different approach to the available evidence is required when the same question is posed in terms of the measures, if any, a clinical service should introduce to minimize aggressive outbursts among patients in their care. Not only are different studies relevant to these two contexts, but different levels of relative risk are appropriate to guide action. The possibility, albeit distant, of violence in a particular patient living in the community may well justify more frequent monitoring of their clinical and social state. The same relative risk would not however justify placing restrictions on this individual or provide reasons for opting for custodial care.

The notion that in our present state of knowledge it is possible to provide a single answer to the question of the potential violence of those suffering from schizophrenia which transcends the contingencies of context has led to considerable confusion and sterile debate. This chapter will review a number of studies of violence and criminality among the mentally disordered with particular attention to schizophrenia. These studies be employed in discussing the clinically relevant questions.

9.2 WHOSE DANGEROUSNESS, WHOSE CRIMINALITY?

Violence and dangerousness are qualities which may be ascribed to actions, but they are not abiding attributes the individuals themselves. Dangerous actions occur within contexts which, for the individual, have particular meanings. Violence is rarely, if ever, the product of a non-specific reaction, rather it is the result of responses to situations which, however, mistakenly, are believed to be sufficiently threatening or provocative to justify aggression. Some of us are predisposed to cope with stress in a belligerent manner, but this does not inevitably involve violence. These points may seem too obvious to be worth mentioning, but they can all too easily be lost sight of and dangerousness become reified into a thing attributed to a class such as that of schizophrenics.

Integral to the ordinary person's view of mental illness is a loss of self control and disturbed, if not frankly violent, behaviour (Nunally, 1961). In the popular imagination violence and madness walk hand-in-hand. Though public attitudes are becoming less negative, the fear of the unpredictability and potential for violence of the mentally ill remains (Rubkin, 1974). Sadly, such prejudices are also apparent in studies of the attitudes of medical and nursing personnel (Viukari *et al.*, 1979). These fears are fed by the media. A study of television in the USA revealed that mental illness was depicted in some 17% of drama programmes with 73% of the mentally disordered portrayed as violent and no less than 23% as homicidal maniacs (Gerbner *et al.*, 1981). Fear, as Gunn (1982) has argued, is at least as important in the attribution of dangerousness as any statistical calculation of actual risk. Because the mad are objects of fear they will be viewed as dangerous by many, irrespective

of actual behaviour. Such pre-existing fear will also look for justification in any suggestion that the mentally ill have been responsible for acts of violence. It is against this background that the public debate takes place on the dangerousness of the mentally disordered.

The realities of life in the community for many disabled by schizophrenic disorders places them at high risk of coming into conflict with the law. For those to whom inadequate community support is given or for those who lose contact with such services, there is a risk of social dislocation and eventual vagrancy. The homeless and drifting, particularly when also evincing odd behaviours, become not only objects of fear for their fellow citizens, but often find themselves arrested on a range of public nuisance offences. Poverty is the lot of many disabled by schizophrenia and this, combined with dependence on various pensions and social security payments, can lead to temptations to indulge in petty thefts and minor benefit frauds. Those disabled by schizophrenia have difficulties coping with the demands of urban living: they may as a result withdraw and give up or they may become frustrated and angry. The angry outbursts and occasionally associated damage to property can lead to them appearing before the courts. It is this criminality of the disabled and disadvantaged which contributes disproportionately to the offending rate of the mentally disordered.

In assessing the criminality of those with a history of mental disorder the frequency of criminal convictions among the general population needs to be taken into consideration. In western societies nearly half of the male population will appear before the courts on charges other than traffic related offences at some time in their lives (Farrington, 1981; Blumstein and Cohen, 1987). Those at highest risk of arrest are the economically and socially deprived (Reiss and Tonry, 1986) and it is into the socially disadvantaged that the disabled schizophrenics are so often recruited. Once an individual has been convicted of an offence the chances of reappearing before the courts is greatly increased; statistics from the USA for serious crime suggest recidivism rates as high as 90% (Blumstein and Cohen, 1979). Thus those with schizophrenic disorders in the community all too often find themselves in social contexts conducive to offending and once launched into a criminal career they are likely to reoffend. Such offending is often only tangentially related to the primary symptoms of schizophrenia, but centrally related to the quality of treatment and care provided.

The majority of studies concentrate on violent offending. Not only does that leave us ill informed about most of the criminal acts committed by those with schizophrenia, but it creates a misleading emphasis on violence.

9.3 WHOSE SCHIZOPHRENIA?

The literature on mental disorder and offending often treats the mentally disordered as a single entity. Even when distinctions are made between different diagnostic groups, the basis for such distinctions is often unclear or unconvincing. The standards of diagnostic practice now considered mandatory in other areas of research concerning schizophrenia have yet to penetrate this field. Case definition varies from the use of standardized instruments such as the full PSE, as in Taylor and Gunn's (1984) study, to approaches such as that of Teplin (1985) who classified her cases in the basis of the opinions of clinical psychology students derived from their observations of the subject's behaviour during encounters with the police.

9.4 OFFENDING AMONG PATIENTS WITH SCHIZOPHRENIC DISORDERS

9.4.1 PRIOR TO ADMISSION

Johnstone *et al.* (1986) as part of their study of schizophrenia, collected data on disturbed and threatening behaviour prior to a patient's

first admission. Nineteen per cent of this sample had, in the month prior to admission, behaved in a manner which put the safety of others at risk and nearly a third had damaged property. Despite this level of criminal behaviour and the fact that in 22% the police had been involved at some stage in the events leading up to admission, less than 5% had been charged with any offence. A study on a cohort of 1033 patients found 11% to have had acts of violence noted on their admission record and though they were diagnostically heterogeneous many would have received a diagnosis of schizophrenia (Craig, 1982). The largest study comes from New York where Tardiff and Sweillain (1982) examined the admission records of 9365 patients and found 8% to have been noted as assaultative. Thirty percent of this sample received a diagnosis of schizophrenia, but accounted for 40% of the violent incidents. A study from Rossi *et al.* (1986) on aggressive behaviour associated with admission, distinguished between fear-inducing behaviours such as verbal abuse and damage to property, and assaultative behaviour which included not only actual attacks, but threats to attack others. Within the assaultative group there were significantly more patients with a diagnosis of paranoid schizophrenia. Non-paranoid schizophrenia did not differ significantly from affective disorders. Patients prior to second or subsequent admissions were more likely to be both aggressive and fear-inducing than first admission patients.

The only studies which specifically detail aggressive behaviour in patients with schizophrenic disorders in the weeks prior to their first admission are those from the UK by Johnstone *et al.* (1986) and from the USA by Rossi *et al.* (1986). There are considerable difficulties interpreting even these results in terms of the potential dangerousness of those with schizophrenic disorders. The period prior to admission is often disturbed and distressing for the patient and their family. Conflicts are likely to arise, not only as a direct result of the patient's symptoms, but also from the actions of those around him who intrude and place pressure upon the patient, albeit from the best of motives. There is a considerable difference in how a violent act should be regarded between one motivated by delusional preoccupations and one committed in an attempt to resist physical removal to hospital. The level of aggression noted in the patients also has to be placed against the background of the levels of aggressive behaviour prevailing in the environment. In short, these studies, though suggestive of increased levels of disturbed and disturbing behaviour prior to admission, do not demonstrate that it is the schizophrenia itself which is responsible.

9.4.2 STUDIES ON INPATIENTS

The early studies on the levels of assaultative behaviour among inpatients tended to rely on retrospective analysis of incident reports (Kalogerakis, 1971; Evenson *et al.*, 1974). The problem with such studies was underlined by Lion *et al.* (1981) who demonstrated that incidents formally reported constituted less than 20% of the violent outbursts noted in the ward records. An attempt to systematically gather information from a large cohort of general psychiatric inpatients suggested that 7% were involved in assaults during a three-month period (Tardiff, 1982). Schizophrenic patients were over-represented among the assaultative, but interestingly it was those with non-paranoid rather than paranoid disorders who accounted for the increased rates. Fottrell (1980), in a prospective study from three English hospitals, concluded that there were many incidents of petty violence, but serious assaults were fortunately rare. Those committing assaults were most frequently schizophrenic, young, and in contrast to studies of patients in the community, female. A prospective study of physical assaults from a British General Hospital psychiatric unit reported lower levels of violence than usually found in North American studies (Edwards *et al.*, 1988). Less

than 5% of patients were involved in assaults over a period of a year. There was, as in most studies, an over-representation of patients with schizophrenia among the assaultative group.

An interesting study from Binder and McNeil (1988) looked at aggressive behaviour both prior to admission and during the index admission for both schizophrenic and non-schizophrenic patients. They noted that schizophrenic patients were more likely to commit assaults prior to admission, 26% having made attacks on people and a further 36% to have indulged in fear-inducing behaviour. Though the patients with schizophrenia remained at higher risk of committing assaults in hospital than the general run of patients, they were significantly less prone to attacks in the hospital context than the manic patients.

Studies specifically concerned with inpatients receiving treatment for schizophrenia are limited. Shader and his group (1977) reported that over a six-month admission period 43 of 99 patients with schizophrenia committed some violent act, which was a significantly higher rate than for non-schizophrenic patients. A retrospective study by Karson and Bigelow (1987) of a highly selected group of patients in the research wards of the National Institute of Mental Health noted that during the year of the study 41 of 97 inpatients with schizophrenia became assaultative in contrast to only 4 of 43 patients with other diagnoses. The patients in these two studies suffered intractable disorders and caution is required in extrapolating these high levels of violence to the general run of patients with schizophrenia.

9.4.3 DISCHARGED PATIENTS IN THE COMMUNITY

A number of studies have attempted to calculate the rates of criminality and violence in patients following discharge from hospital. Studies prior to the mid-1960s suggested that patients post-discharge had subsequent conviction rates lower than or similar to that of the general population

(Ashley, 1922; Pollock, 1938; Cohen and Freeman, 1945). More recent studies have however, raised the spectre of significantly higher levels of offending in the ex-patient group (Giovanni and Gurel, 1967; Zitrin *et al.*, 1976; Durbin *et al.*, 1977; Sosowsky, 1978; Grunberg *et al.*, 1978). The publications suggesting discharged mental patients may be more likely to offend have been criticized for methodological flaws including failure to control for relevant demographic variables, sample size and previous arrest records (Cohen, 1980; Teplin, 1985; Monahan and Steadman, 1983; Krakowski *et al.*, 1986). Monahan (1981) argued: 'The higher rate of violent crime committed by released mental patients can be accounted for entirely by those with records, particularly an extensive record, of criminal activity that pre-dated their hospitalization'. Sosowsky (1980), however, specifically denied that the increased rate among ex-patients could simply be explained away by a group with previous arrest records, for in his study those with no previous arrests still had a subsequent rate of offending three times higher than expected.

Chuang *et al.* (1987) compared a group of schizophrenic outpatients with matched controls drawn from medical outpatients. They interviewed subjects to explore a wider range of dangerous and criminal behaviour than that captured in statistics on convictions. No significant differences emerged between schizophrenics and controls for a range of criminal behaviour, except in traffic offences where the controls reported more infringements, possibly due to greater access to motor vehicles. This study's design demands respect, but unfortunately the number of subjects, 42 schizophrenics and 42 non-psychiatric controls, is too small for confident extrapolation from their comforting results. Studies employing similar designs, but with larger samples, are urgently required.

Phillips and his group (1988) linked data from police records, court reports and clinical files for 2735 psychiatric referrals from the criminal justice system of Alaska between 1977 and 1981. One hundred and eighteen persons with schizophrenic disorders were referred by the courts for evaluation following being charged with a violent crime during the period of study. If this represented all of those with this disorder appearing before the courts on charges involving violence, then the authors calculate this to be about twice the expected rate of 0.6 per 100. The authors acknowledge that if not all those with schizophrenia appearing before the court are recognized at the time, they may not be referred for psychiatric evaluation and will be missed. Assuming only 50% are in fact ascertained the percentage of violent offending accounted for by schizophrenics would double to 2.3%. The authors conclude that even if this second figure is closer to the truth that: 'Schizophrenic patients are not to any appreciable extent responsible for the high level of violence in our society'. This is clearly correct given that schizophrenics constitute less than 1% of the population, but a rate of violent offending twice or four times that expected does raise questions of its explanation, if not some anxiety.

A 10-year follow-up of 644 patients discharged following treatment for schizophrenia compared their offending using a population based register of criminal offences with that for the general population of Stockholm (Lindqvist and Allenbeck, 1990). The schizophrenic group committed almost four times as many violent offences as the general population, though there was no increase in property crimes. This study did not control for socioeconomic status nor for prior arrest records. It also relies exclusively on offences coming to the attention of the police and there is evidence to suggest that the mentally ill are more liable to detection and arrest when they offend than their healthier compatriots (Robertson, 1988). The linking of data from patient registers with registers of criminal offending offers a potentially useful technique for monitoring criminality amongst those who have, or have had mental disorders, but such data will need to be interpreted with caution.

9.5 MENTAL DISORDER AMONG OFFENDERS

9.5.1 AT THE POINT OF ARREST

The vast majority of criminal acts go undetected and even when the offender is apprehended by the police there are a wide variety of selective factors operating at each stage of the male-factor's journey from arrest to imprisonment. For example, even when the police become involved at the scene of a crime informal dispositions predominate and arrest is a relatively infrequent outcome (Black, 1980). The discretion of the police officer is central in deciding whether or not to proceed and their assessment of the offender's mental state is an accepted element in that decision (Campbell, 1988). Some of these factors will tend to militate against the chances of such individuals ending up in jail, while some may operate to enhance the chances of such individuals being incarcerated. Monahan and Steadman (1983) have argued that the earlier in this process studies are undertaken the closer we will be to the matching of true rates of crime to mental disorder. In their own study of police perceptions of those apprehended for criminal behaviour they reported that only 2% were des-cribed as seriously mentally ill, though a further 28% had some degree of disturbance. On this basis they argue that only 2% of offenders at this stage in the criminal justice system are psychotic, which is close to the proportion to be expected from the level of such mental disorder in the community.

The most detailed study of the level of mental disorder among citizens whose behaviour attracts police attention is Teplin's (1985) study from Chicago. She used a team of five clinical psycho-logy students who accompanied police and observed the police-offender interactions. These observations were collected over 14 months,

involved 2200 hours and captured 1072 inter-actions involving 2122 citizens. The largest category of offences by far, were to public order with violent personal crime constituting less than 4%. Based on the observers' judgement of the mental state of those involved with the police it was estimated that less than 5% of them were mentally disordered. This figure is for all who were in contact with the police be they witnesses, complainant, or suspects, and for suspects alone the figure is slightly higher at 6%. On the basis of these figures Teplin states: 'Contact by police with mentally disordered citizens make up less than 5% of the persons involved with the police; this figure is within the expected range indicated by epidemiological studies of the true prevalence of serious mental disorder'. The author's position is made clear in the title chosen for the paper. 'The Criminality of the Mentally Ill: a Dangerous Misconcep-tion'. Sadly, this extensive and criminologically sophisticated study is vitiated by the naivety of the approach to psychiatric diagnosis.

9.5.2 REMAND POPULATIONS

A proportion of those who appear before the courts are remanded in custody prior to trial or final disposal. The homeless and the socially isolated are over-represented together with those charged with more serious crimes. In an important study Taylor and Gunn (1984) examined the psychiatric status of a cohort of 1241 men remanded to a London prison. They found evidence of psychiatric illness in over 8% of the sample with the majority of the disorders being in the schizophrenic spectrum. Nine percent of those subsequently convicted of non-fatal violence and 11% of homicides were diagnosed as having a schizophrenic disorder. Given the annual prevalence of between 0.4% and 0.6% for the population served by this prison, it suggests a clear over-representation of schizophrenia among violent offenders. Though this association for violent offenders in general could be accounted for by any bias towards preferentially remanding the mentally disordered, it would not explain the high rates among homicide offenders nearly all of whom are remanded in custody.

Coid (1988a), relying on retrospective analysis of prison records, identified 253 (2.5%) men as having schizophrenic disorders out of a total remand population of nearly 10 000. Schizophrenics were over-represented among the violent offenders, but Coid noted that although the violence covered the full spectrum, the majority was minor in nature. The picture of the schizophrenics offending which emerges from his study is predominantly that of disorganized and vagrant men committing trivial thefts, public nuisances and occasionally becoming violent, particularly when apprehended or restrained. Coid's (1988a, b) methodology would not have the accuracy in ascertainment of mental disorder of Taylor and Gunn's (1984) work and the population he studied does not have the high concentration of offences involving serious violence, but his large sample enables a picture to be obtained of how the bulk of those with schizophrenia present in remand prisons.

9.5.3 SENTENCED PRISONERS

The level of mental disorder, including schizophrenia, in prison populations has been examined on a number of occasions though the varying methodologies and case identification procedures make comparisons difficult. The studies of Guze (1976) in the USA and Gunn *et al.* (1978) in the UK suggested that less than 1% of sentenced prisoners have a schizophrenic illness. In special prison facilities, particularly those dealing with habitually violent offenders, significantly higher rates of psychosis have been reported (Bach-y-Rita and Veno, 1974; Roth and Ervin, 1971). Taylor (1986) examined 175 men serving life sentences and ascertained 17 (9.9%) as having schizophrenia, and in a further 20 there was evidence for significant disorder which could have been the product of

a developing or quiescent schizophrenic process. A study on a similar population by Heather (1977) of 42 'lifers' also suggested higher rates of disorder, 10% being of a schizophrenic type. These levels of schizophrenic disorders are both surprising, as it would be hoped that those with such illnesses would have been screened out and directed to hospitals rather than prison, and distressing given the likely effects of a prison environment on someone rendered vulnerable by schizophrenia. Taylor had no doubt from her study that the vast majority of the schizophrenic illnesses were present at the time the offenders were tried and sentenced to life in prison.

9.6 REOFFENCE RATES IN MENTALLY DISORDERED OFFENDERS

An important practical question is whether knowing that an offender has a mental disorder is a guide to the likelihood of them reoffending. Early studies suggested that the reoffence rate for mentally ill offenders was low (Rappeport and Lassen, 1965) or much the same as for offenders without mental disorder (Morrow and Petersen, 1966). There was some suggestion that mentally abnormal offenders on release might be reconvicted more frequently for minor offences of the social nuisance type (Rollin, 1969). A comparison of mentally abnormal offenders with a group of mentally normal ex-prisoners who had committed similar offences revealed a higher rate of subsequent offending among the mentally normal (Butler, 1975). The reconviction rate for property offences was 32%, as against 54% for the control group, though for violent or sexual offences a 6% rate was found in both groups. The possibility that habitual offenders are more likely to be mentally disturbed has been examined on a number of occasions (Morris, 1951; Hammond and Chayen, 1961). The recidivist population does contain a number of mentally disturbed individuals, but no clear association between mental disorder and repeat offending has been demonstrated.

9.7 SPECIFIC OFFENCES

9.7.1 HOMICIDE

To discuss the possible contribution of those with schizophrenia to homicide offences is to risk sensationalizing. In our societies killing is fortunately still a rare offence and for that reason extreme caution needs to be practised in extrapolating from this offence to the commoner forms of interpersonal violence. Homicides are, however, a particularly important group for study, as unlike other forms of violent crime, the majority of offenders are known, are effectively all charged and most are psychiatrically assessed in considerable detail.

For many years in the UK between 40 and 50% of those charged with murder have been found either unfit to plead, insane or of diminished responsibility on the grounds of mental disorder (Bowden, 1990; Tidmarsh, 1990). To the 'abnormal murders' must be added 5–10% of those who commit suicide after killing their victim. In a number of studies of these so-called abnormal murderers, schizophrenic disorders have been claimed to account for 50% or more of the mental disorders (Gibbens, 1958; McKnight *et al.*, 1966; Schiphowensky, Wong and Singer, 1973). A more precise picture can be obtained from studies such as those of Petersen and Gudjonson (1981, 1982) from Iceland who examined all the records of those charged with murder over an 80-year period, revealing 15% as likely to have been schizophrenic. The study of Hafner and Boker (1982) studied the relationship between serious crimes of violence and mental disorder in Western Germany over the period 1955 to 1964. This impressive study investigated 655 homicides committed by 533 offenders of whom 7.7% of the men and 6.4% of the women were considered to have had a schizophrenic illness. This constituted 53% of those offenders deemed

mentally disordered, with mental defect (13%) being the next most common diagnosis.

The victims of killings perpetrated by those with schizophrenic disorders are even more likely to be members of their immediate family than with mentally competent offenders (Gibson, 1975; Hafner and Boker, 1982).

9.8 THE RELATIONSHIP BETWEEN THE OFFENDING AND THE ILLNESS

The offending which occurs in those with schizophrenia could in theory relate to the illness in a number of ways:

1. In conjunction with active symptoms where the disordered state of mind was the necessary and sufficient cause of the offending; or more usually where some relatively trivial event triggers the offending by interaction with the patient's disordered world view. The first is illustrated by the situation where a patient damages telephone or power lines around their house, labouring under the conviction that they are responsible for their experience of being controlled by outside forces. The more usual situation is where someone inadvertently does or says something which resonates with the patient's disordered experiences to produce an angry or aggressive outburst.
2. Where the schizophrenic process has led to an impairment in, for example motivation, self control or awareness of the rights and needs of others. These predominantly negative symptoms can be risk factors in certain situations for offending.
3. The offending of the mental disorder may be entirely unrelated.
4. The offending and the consequences of its detection may precipitate the emergence of mental disorder.

A number of studies have attempted to delineate the relationship between the patient's disordered state of mind and the actual offending. Lanzkron (1963), in a study of violent offenders with major mental disorders, predominantly schizophrenic, reported that offending arose in 40% as a direct consequence of hallucinatory or delusional experiences. In a similar study employing court reports, Virkkunen (1974) identified just under 40% of violent acts committed by those with schizophrenia as consequent on active symptoms. In a study of violent incidents among hospital inpatients it was found, perhaps not surprisingly, that virtually all the patients were symptomatic at the time (Planasky and Johnson, 1977). Hafner and Boker's (1982) study points to the vast majority of serious violence in schizophrenia arising in close relationship to delusional and hallucinatory experiences. The outstanding study to date in this area is that of Taylor (1985) who supplemented case report analysis with direct interviews carried out within a short time of offending. She concluded that virtually all of her 121 psychotic subjects had positive symptoms at the time of their offence.

Delusions, particularly the systematized variety of the paranoid schizophrenias, usually preoccupy the patients and not surprisingly may lead to actions motivated by the pathological beliefs. Delusions of infidelity in pathological jealousy deserve their sinister reputation for predisposing to violence (Mullen, 1990), though it should be remembered that schizophrenia only accounts for between 5% and 10% of most samples of pathological jealousy (Shepherd, 1961; Langfeldt, 1961; Mullen and Maack, 1985). Other delusional syndromes occasionally encountered in schizophrenia such as erotomania and mis-identification syndromes are reported to be associated with aggressive outbursts (Taylor *et al.*, 1983; De Pauw and Szulecka, 1988). Minor nuisance crimes are on occasion motivated by the patients' beliefs about their rights and prerogatives. One of my patients entered a Royal Palace to the consternation of those responsible for security, acting on his belief that he was heir to the throne. Another created a number of disturbances by acting on his belief that he was commissioner for police. Acts of vandalism may also be committed by those labouring under delusions and acts of desecration and the criminal damage of churches may arise from religious delusions.

Auditory hallucinations, and in particular command hallucinations, have been claimed to play a role in aggressive outbursts (Yesavage, 1983). Those studies that have attempted to study hallucinatory experiences in violent offending have not been able to confirm the claimed association (Hafner and Boker, 1982; Taylor, 1985). Hellerstein *et al.*, (1987) studied a cohort of 789 patients including 159 with schizophrenia. Command hallucinations were surprisingly common with 18% of the schizophrenic cohort reporting them. No association was found of such voices with assaultativeness and the authors concluded that the command hallucinations alone may not imply a greater risk for acute life threatening behaviour. That being said, it is worth remembering that patients may report both violent impulses and voices commanding them to harm themselves or others as a way of alerting care givers to their own fears of impending loss of control. In this context it would be cavalier to ignore the patient's warning.

In long-standing schizophrenic disorders there may occur profound changes in the patient's personality. Increasing social withdrawal, a loss of interpersonal sensitivity, emotional detachment and the development of odd preoccupations and rigid beliefs and behaviours may all engender conflict between the patient and those around them. The total disregard for convention can create not just distress for family and friends, but lead to police involvement. One of my patients who was afflicted with beliefs about changes in his body and sexual identity was repeatedly arrested because of his habit of dressing in bizarre approximations to female attire and making inept sexual advances to young men. Though no studies have directly addressed the question there is a clinical impression that some offending may arise from the patient's gross insensitivity to the feelings of others.

Those with schizophrenia who commit acts of violence have nearly always had the disorder for some considerable time. Serious offending is rare in the first illness and seems to be more likely to arise in those who have been ill for years rather than weeks (Hafner and Boker, 1982). The available studies highlight the central importance of continuing supervision and care in the community (Bowden, 1981), for the majority of serious offending occurs in established schizophrenics who have drifted out of any ongoing care and supervision (Mullen, 1989).

9.9 ASSESSING THE EVIDENCE

Though there is a considerable body of empirical evidence bearing on the question of the propensity of those with schizophrenia to offend, the assessment of that literature is fraught with difficulties. Well-informed reviewers can come to diametrically opposed conclusions using essentially the same database. Monahan and Steadman (1983), two of the most impressive workers in this field concluded: 'There is no consistent evidence that the true prevalence rate of criminal behaviour among former mental patients exceeds the true prevalence rate of criminal behaviour among the general population matched for demographic factors and prior criminal history'. Hafner and Boker (1982) concluded from their own monumental study that: 'If we define dangerousness of the mentally abnormal as the relative probability of their committing a violent crime, then our findings show that this does not exceed the dangerousness of the legally responsible adult population as a whole'. In stark contrast is the conclusion of Tidmarsh (1990), an experienced clinician who has spent many years working with some of the most violent and disturbed offenders. He noted in this review of the subject: 'It is the author's belief that schizophrenics are more likely than non-schizo-

phrenics to commit certain offences and that their over-representation in the statistics reflects this rather than being an artefact of the selection process which operates at every level of the criminal justice system'. Wessely and Taylor (1990), in a review which provided an exemplary account of the methodological problems concluded: 'No single study will ever be able to overcome all the methodological problems', but 'despite these caveats it is still possible to draw some practical conclusions . . . certain groups of the mentally ill (specifically those with schizophrenia) do present an increased risk of both criminality and violent behaviour'.

The current evidence is still so finely balanced that it is possible to draw, and sustain, diametrically opposed conclusions. In the final analysis it is our personal experience and prior ideological committments which tip that balance. As a practising clinician I find myself coming down on the side of Tidmarsh, Wessely and Taylor, though this probably reflects primarily our common backgrounds in forensic psychiatry.

If having schizophrenia is an independent risk factor for criminal behaviour then there should be differences in the profiles of offenders with these disorders from those not so afflicted. This appears to be so. The criminal careers of those with mental disorders tend to start at a later stage than in the mentally competent (Gibbens and Robertson, 1983; Wessely and Taylor, 1990). The mentally ill tend to continue offending to a more advanced age and they form an increasing proportion of the violent offenders among the older age groups. The offending in those with schizophrenia tends to occur most frequently during periods when they are symptomatic rather than in periods of remission (Hafner and Boker, 1982; Taylor, 1985). In many cases of offending, particularly violent offending, a direct relationship is demonstrable to the nature and content of the disturbances (Taylor, 1985). Though far from conclusive, these differences in the profiles of offenders with schizophrenia do speak to the illness being a contributory factor.

9.10 CONCLUSION

The association of schizophrenia with criminal behaviour, even if accepted, has to be interpreted within the context of clinical realities. Relative risks of from two to five appear to emerge from certain studies, but before such figures become clinically meaningful they have to be translated into estimates of the frequency with which those with schizophrenia are likely to actually commit offences. Fortunately serious violence, though more frequent than one would wish, is rare. The annual rates of violent offending in Australasian communities are in the region of two to four per 1000. Even in the worst case scenario this would still imply that only 2% of those with schizophrenia are likely to be involved in such criminal behaviour and using the more modest and probably more reliable estimates this falls to a fraction of 1%. Hafner and Boker (1982) attempted a quantification of the risks presented by those with schizophrenia and estimated the risks of a homicidal attack to be 0.05%. These figures, though giving some comfort, have to be placed alongside studies of community samples reviewed earlier which suggest that aggressive behaviour is not uncommon. Such aggression usually results in little, if any, serious damage to persons or property, but it is not trivial in that it can occasion considerable fear and distress in relatives and neighbours. The frequency of such behaviour among those with schizophrenic disorders living in the community has still not been adequately documented.

In conclusion, an attempt will be made to give the author's best guess at the answers to a number of central clinical questions.

(1). Does the knowledge that someone suffers a schizophrenic disorder enable you to predict an increased likelihood of future criminal or dangerous behaviour? The answer is, for practical purposes, no. The problems of prediction in these circumstances are such that no meaningful statements are possible for individual cases on the information only of their diagnosis (Mullen, 1989).

(2). Is the fact of having a schizophrenic disorder irrelevant to criminal behaviour? The answer to this is also no. The apparent paradox is due to the need to integrate the information as to diagnosis with information about past behaviour and current circumstances. A patient with a schizophrenic illness who has a history of assaultative behaviour in the context of delusional preoccupations and who is suffering a recurrence of those delusions may well be at risk for repeating the violence, particularly if the context is again conducive to conflict, real or imagined. To ignore the history of mental disorder in such a case would be absurd.

(3). Does the current evidence on the criminal behaviour of those with schizophrenia justify a return to more custodial methods of care? The answer is surely no. Even those who advocate preventive detention in some circumstances insist that it should only apply where there is a high probability (at least 75%) of future offending (Walker, 1982). Those with schizophrenia, even by the most gloomy of prognostications, are nowhere near presenting such a risk.

(4). Are there any messages from this literature relevant to the management of schizophrenia? Yes, it would appear that serious violence is associated with active symptoms usually in those with long-standing illnesses who have drifted out of care and supervision. The message is clear, that more adequate community care and support for those at risk and a policy of active follow-up of patients with schizophrenic disorders are required. The response to the knowledge that schizophrenia may bring with it an increased risk of criminal behaviour is not to abandon community care, but to make it a reality, particularly for the most disabled and disadvantaged amongst those with schizophrenia.

REFERENCES

Ashley, M. (1922) Outcome of 1000 cases paroled

from the Middletown State Homeopathic Hospital. *New York State Q.*, **8**, 64–70.

Bach-y-Rita, G. and Veno, A. (1974) Habitual violence: a profile of 62 men. *Am. J. Psychiatry*, **131**, 1015–17.

Binder, R.L. and McNeil, D.E. (1988) Effects of diagnosis and context on dangerousness. *Am. J. Psychiatry*, **145**, 728–32.

Black, D. (1980) *The Manners and Customs of the Police*. Academic Press, New York.

Blumstein, A. and Cohen, J. (1987) Estimation of individual crime rates from arrest records. *J. Crim. Law Criminol.*, **70**, 561–85.

Bowden, P. (1981) What happened to patients released from special hospitals. *Br. J. Psychiatry*, 143, 362–75.

Bowden, P. (1990) Homicide. In *Principles and Practice of Forensic Psychiatry*. R. Bluglass and P. Bowden (ed), Churchill Livingstone, London, pp. 507–22.

Butler, R.A. (1975) *Report of the Committee on Mentally Abnormal Offenders*. HMSO, London.

Campbell, I.G. (1989) *Mental Disorder and Criminal Law in Australia and New Zealand*. Butterworths, Sydney.

Chuang, H., Williams, R. and Dalby, T. (1987) Criminal behaviour among schizophrenics. *Can. J. Psychiatry*, **32**, 255–8.

Cohen, C.I. (1980) Crime among mental patients – a critical analysis. *Psychiat. Q.*, **52**, 100–7.

Cohen, L. and Freeman, J. (1945) How dangerous to the community are State hospital patients? *Conn. State Med. J.*, **9**, 697–700.

Coid, N. (1988a) Mentally abnormal remands I: rejected or accepted by the National Health Service. *Br. Med. J.*, **296**, 1779–82.

Coid, J. (1988b) Mentally abnormal prisoners on remand II — comparison of services provided by Oxford and Wessex regions. *Br. Med. J.*, **296**, 1783–4.

Craig, T.J. (1982) An epidemiological study of problems associated with violence among psychiatric inpatients. *Am. J. Psychiatry*, **139**, 1262–6.

De Pauw, K. and Szulecka, T.K. (1988) Dangerous delusions: violence and misidentification syndromes. *Br. J. Psychiatry*, **132**, 91–6.

Durbin, J., Paseward, R. and Albers, D. (1977) Criminality and mental illness. *Am. J. Psychiatry*, **135**, 80–3.

Edwards, J., Jones, D., Reid, W. and Chu, C. (1988) Physical assaults in a psychiatric unit of a general hospital. *Am. J. Psychiatry*, **145**, 1568–71.

Evenson, R.C., Sletten, I.W., Altman, H. and Brown, M.L. (1974) Disturbing behaviour: a study of incident reports. *Psychiat. Q.*, **48**, 266–75.

Farrington, D. (1981) The prevalence of convictions. *Br. J. Criminol.*, **21**, 173–5.

Fottrell, E. (1980) A study of violent behaviour among patients in psychiatric hospitals. *Br. J. Psychiatry*, **136**, 216–21.

Gerbner, G., Gross, L., Morgan, M. and Signorielli, N. (1981) Health and medicine on television. *N. Engl. J. Med.*, **305**, 901–4.

Gibbens, T. (1958) Sane and insane homicide. *J. Crim. Law Criminol. Police Sci.*, **49**, 110–15.

Gibbens, I.C.N. and Robertson, G. (1983) A survey of the criminal careers of restriction order patients. *Br. J. Psychiatry*, **143**, 362–75.

Gibson, E. (1975) *Homicide in England and Wales 1967–1971*. Home Office Research Studies No. 31. HMSO, London.

Giovannoni, J. and Gurel, L. (1967) Socially disruptive behaviour of ex-mental patients. *Arch. Gen. Psychiatry*, **17**, 146–53.

Grunberg, F. Klinger, B.I. and Grumet, B. (1978) Homicide and deinstitutionalization of the mentally ill. *Am. J. Psychiatry*, **134**, 685–7.

Gunn, J. (1982) An English psychiatrist looks at dangerousness. *Bull. AAPL*, **10**, 143–54.

Gunn, J., Dell, S. and Way, S. (1978) *Psychiatric Aspects of Imprisonment*. Academic Press, London.

Guze, S. (1976) *Criminality and Psychiatric Disorders*. Oxford University Press, London.

Hafner, H. and Boker, W. (1982) *Crimes of Violence by Mentally Abnormal Offenders*. (trans. by H. Marshall), Cambridge University Press, Cambridge.

Hammond, W.H. and Chayen, E. (1961) *Persistent Criminals*. HMSO, London.

Heather, N. (1977) Personal illness in lifers and the effects of long-term indeterminate sentences. *Br. J. Criminol.*, **17**, 378–86.

Hellerstein, D., Frosch, W. and Koenigsberg, H.W. (1987) The clinical significance of command hallucinations. *Am. J. Psychiatry*, **144**, 219–21.

Johnstone, E., Crow, T., Johnston, A. and MacMillan F. (1986) The Northwick Park Study of first episodes of schizophrenia. 1: presentation of the illness and problems relating to admission. *Br. J. Psychiatry*, **149**, 51–6.

Kalogerakis, M.G. (1971) The assaultive psychiatric patient. *Psychiatr. Q.*, **45**, 372–81.

Karson, C. and Bigelow, L.B. (1987) Violent behaviour in schizophrenic patients. *J. Nerv. Ment. Dis.*, **175**, 161–4.

Krakowski, M., Volavka, J. and Brizer, D. (1986) Psychopathology and violence: a review of the literature. *Compr. Psychiatry*, **27**, 131–48.

Langfeldt, G. (1961) The erotic jealousy syndrome: a clinical study. *Acta Psychiatr. Scand.*, Suppl. 151.

Lanzkron, J. (1963) Murder and insanity: a survey. *Am. J. Psychiatry*, **119**, 754–58.

Lindqvist, P. and Allenbeck, P. (1990) Schizophrenia and crime. A longitudinal follow-up of 644 schizophrenics in Stockholm. *Br. J. Psychiatry*, **157**, 345–50.

Lion, J., Snyder, W. and Merrill, G. (1981) Underreporting of assaults on staff in a state hospital. *Hosp. Community Psychiatry*, **32**, 497–8.

McKnight, G., Mohr, J., Quinsey, R. and Erochko, J. (1966) Mental illness and homicide. *Can. Psychiatr. Assoc. J.*, **11**, 91–8.

Monahan, J. (1981) *The Clinical Prediction of Violent Behaviour*. Maryland, United States Department of Health and Human Service.

Monahan, J. and Steadman, H. (1983) Crime and mental illness: an epidemiological approach. In *Crime and Justice, Vol. 4*. N. Morris and M. Tonry (eds), University of Chicago Press, Chicago, pp. 145–89.

Morris, N. (1951) *The Habitual Criminal*. Londman Green, London.

Morrow, W.R. and Petersen, D.B. (1966) Follow-up of discharged psychiatric offenders. *J. Crim. Law Criminol. Police Sci.*, **57**, 31–4.

Mullen, P.E. (1989) Violence and Mental Disorder. *Br. J. Hosp. Med.*, **44**, 460–3.

Mullen, P.E. (1990) Morbid jealousy and delusions of infidelity. In *Principles and Practice of Forensic Psychiatry*. R. Bluglass and P. Bowden (eds), Churchill Livingstone, London, pp. 823–35.

Mullen, P.E. and Maack, L.H. (1985) Jealousy, Pathological Jealousy and Aggression. In *Aggression and Dangerousness*. D.P. Farrington and J. Gunn (eds), Wiley, London, pp. 103–26.

Nunally, J.C. (1961) *Popular Conceptions of Mental Health*. Holt, Rinehart and Winston, New York.

Petersen, H. and Gudjonson, G.H. (1981) Psychiatric aspects of homicide. *Acta Psychiatr. Scand.*, **64**, 363–72.

Phillips, M., Wolf, A. and Coons, D. (1988) Psychiatry and the criminal justice system: testing the myths. *Am. J. Psychiatry*, **145**, 605–10.

Planansky, K. and Johnson, R. (1977) Homicidal aggression in schizophrenic men. *Acta Psychiatr. Scand.*, **55**, 65–73.

Pollock, H.M. (1938) Is the paroled patient a menace to the community? *Psychiatr. Q.*, **12**, 236–44.

Rabkin, J. (1974) Attitudes Towards Mental Illness. *Schizophr. Bull.*, **10**, 7–33.

Rappeport, J.R. and Lassen, G. (1965) Dangerousness — arrest rate comparison of discharged patients and the general population. *Am. J. Psychiatry*, **121**, 776–83.

Robertson, G. (1988) Arrest patterns among mentally disordered offenders. *Br. J. Psychiatry*, **153**, 313–16.

Rollin, H.R. (1969) *The Mentally Abnormal Offender and the Law*. Pergamon, Oxford.

Rossi, A.M., Jacobs, M., Monteleone, M. *et al.* (1986) Characteristics of psychiatric patients who engage in assaultive or other fear-inducing behaviours. *J. Nerv. Ment. Dis.*, **174**, 154–60.

Roth, L.J. and Ervin, F.R. (1971) Psychiatric care of federal prisoners. *Am. J. Psychiatry*, **128**, 56–62.

Schipkowensky, N. (1973) Epidemiological Aspects of Homicide. In *World Biennial of Psychiatry and Psychotherapy*. S. Arieti (ed), Basic Books, New York, pp. 192–215.

Shader, R., Jackson, A., Harmatz, J. and Appelbaum, P. (1977) Patterns of violent behaviour in schizophrenic inpatients. *Dis. Nerv. System*, **38**, 13–6.

Shepherd, M. (1961) Morbid jealousy: some clinical and social aspects of a psychiatric syndrome. *J. Ment. Sci.*, **107**, 687–753.

Sosowsky, L. (1978) Crime and violence among mental patients reconsidered in view of the new legal relationship between the state and the mentally ill. *Am. J. Psychiatry*, **135**, 33–42.

Sosowsky, L. (1980) Explaining the increased arrest rate among mental patients: a cautionary note. *Am. J. Psychiatry*, **137**, 1602–5.

Tardiff, K. (1982) A survey of five types of dangerous behaviour among chronic psychiatric patients. *Bull. AAPL*, **10**, 177–82.

Tardiff, K. and Sweillam, A. (1982) Assaultive behaviour among chronic inpatients. *Am. J. Psychiatry*, **139**, 212–5.

Taylor, P. (1985) Motives for offending among violent and psychotic men. *Br. J. Psychiatry*, **147**, 491–8.

Taylor, P. (1986) Psychiatric disorder in London's life-sentenced offenders. *Br. J. Criminol.*, **26**, 63–78.

Taylor, P. and Gunn, J. (1984) Violence and psychosis 1 — risk of violence among psychotic men. *Br. Med. J.*, **288**, 1945–9.

Taylor, P. and Parrott, J. (1988) Elderly offenders: a study of age-related factors among custodially remanded prisoners. *Br. J. Psychiatry*, **152**, 340–6.

Taylor, P. and Wessely, S. (1991) Madness and crime: criminology versus psychiatry. *Crim. Behav. Ment. Health*, **1**, 193–228.

Teplin, L. (1985) The criminality of the mentally ill: a dangerous misconception. *Am. J. Psychiatry*, **142**, 593–9.

Tidmarsh, D. (1990) Schizophrenia. In *Principles and Practice of Forensic Psychiatry*. R. Bluglass and P. Bowden (eds), Churchill Livingstone, London, pp. 321–344.

Virkkunen, M. (1974) Observations on violence in schizophrenics. *Acta Psychiatr. Scand.*, **50**, 152–60.

Viukari, M., Rimon, R. and Soderholm, S. (1979) Attitudes towards criminals and other patients. *Acta Psychiatr. Scand.*, **59**, 24–30.

Walker, N. (1982) Ethical aspects of detaining dangerous people. In *Dangerousness, Psychiatric Assessment and Managers*. J.R. Hamilton and H. Freeman (eds), Gaskell Press, London, pp. 23–9.

West, D.J. (1965) *Murder Followed by Suicide*. Heinemann, London.

Wong, M. and Singer, K. (1973) Abnormal homicide in Hong Kong. *Br. J. Psychiatry*, **123**, 295–8.

Yesavage, J. (1983) Inpatient violence and the schizophrenic patient. *Acta Psychiatr. Scand.*, **67**, 353–7.

Zitrin, A., Hardesty, A.S., Burdock, E.I. and Drossman, A.K. (1976) Crime and violence among mental patients. *Arch. Gen. Psychiatry*, **133**, 142–9.

Part Two
Assessment of Schizophrenia

Introduction

The remainder of the book is devoted to issues for clinical practice. In the current section, the main assessment domains are reviewed. Each chapter outlines some of the major issues and reviews the current status of assessment methods, with a special emphasis on approaches that the authors have been researching. Together, they offer a comprehensive coverage of the main assessment domains that are implicated in schizophrenia.

Chapter 10 reviews the challenges for diagnostic assessment of psychoses, emphasizing the danger that validity may be sacrificed in the search for high reliability. It describes recent developments in formal diagnostic assessment, and discusses the relative merits of current instruments (including a new instrument that has been developed by the authors).

Chapter 11 introduces the concepts involved in social competence and social skills, and discusses a range of strategies that are used for social skill assessment. The chapter details ways to develop reliable and valid assessments from role plays, and provides sample role play scenarios and rating scales.

Chapter 12 discusses the nature of life skills and their relationship with the course of the disorder and with the quality of life that is enjoyed by patients and their families. It reviews a number of assessment devices, including the authors' Life Skills Profile, and

discusses some of the problems that they encounter.

Chapter 13, on assessment for rehabilitation, brings together some of the issues that were introduced in the previous three chapters and describes strategies that are especially relevant for rehabilitation of people with severe disabilities. These strategies include a number of instruments that the author and her colleagues have developed.

Life events present difficult problems for assessment, particularly when we are trying to decide whether an experience is affecting the course of the disorder. Chapter 14 discusses these problems and solutions that have been advanced to them. It critically evaluates the current life event instruments and sees a need for brief measures that are applicable to clinical settings and retain the reliability and validity of an extended interview.

Interactions between family members have generated a great deal of interest since the concept of expressed emotion (EE) was developed. Chapter 8 reviewed the current status of EE as a predictor of the course of schizophrenia and a possible determinant of relapse. Chapter 15 applies Patterson's coercion theory to dysfunctional interactions within the family, and relates the interactions to the burden that members experience when they are coping with the behaviour of a person with schizophrenia.

It reviews the empirical status of the main instruments that have been used to assess family interaction, and relates the material to a case example.

Relationships outside the family may also be important. Chapter 16 discusses the impact of schizophrenia on social networks, and reviews the literature on their potential implications for prognosis. It critically evaluates the utility of current measures of networks and social support when they are applied to schizophrenia.

The section concludes with two chapters on prediction. Chapter 17 looks at the prediction of relapses by capitalizing on recurrent patterns of prodromal signs. The authors discuss the development of instruments that sufferers and their families can use to assist in detecting relapses at an early stage, by being able to institute treatment that may avert a complete episode and the disruption that this entails.

Chapter 18 builds on the material in the author's earlier chapter on the relationship between criminality and schizophrenia (Chapter 9). It examines the features that have been used in an attempt to predict violent behaviour by people with mental disorders and derives a set of predictors that can be empirically justified.

David J. Kavanagh

Chapter 10

Diagnostic and symptomatological assessment

PATRICK D. McGORRY, BRUCE S. SINGH
and DAVID L. COPOLOV

10.1 INTRODUCTION

Prior to the 1960s, psychiatric diagnosis was not only unreliable, it was also relatively unpopular. Interest in descriptive psychopathology was overshadowed by a preoccupation with the content of psychiatric phenomena on the one hand, and the social correlates on the other. However, in the face of a sustained attack upon the discipline of psychiatry, an attack which employed diagnostic unreliability as a key weapon, a dramatic revival of interest in diagnosis and psychopathological assessment has occurred (Kendell 1975, 1989), which spawned a series of methodological advances in psychopathological assessment. These new tools, principally structured interview schedules and operational definitions for symptoms and syndromes, have greatly improved the reliability of ratings and diagnoses. Unfortunately, perhaps because of the partly defensive nature of this revival process, its focus has been too narrow, and the more fundamental question of validity of the phenomena and diagnostic concepts has received inadequate attention (McGorry et al. 1989). Kendell (1989) recently used the term 'clinical validity' in contrasting the roles of clinicians with basic scientists in improving the validity of clinical concepts. This chapter adopts a similar validity-oriented perspective, and begins with a critique of the present nosology of psychotic disorders, followed by a series of principles and a description of a method for maximizing the validity of psychopathological assessment in the functional psychoses.

The phenomenological approach in psychiatry has been particularly influential in the assessment of the psychopathology of psychosis. A fundamental principle is that it 'attempts to describe phenomena avoiding prior theoretical commitment, taking nothing for granted' (Mullen, 1984). The theoretical world is 'put in brackets', and phenomena are only secondarily related to systems of classification or diagnostic concepts. Given the discouraging lack of progress in aetiological progress in functional psychosis, which may be linked to conceptual flaws and their consequences (McGorry et al., 1990c), it is timely to apply this phenomenological principle to the nosology of psychosis and conduct a 'present state examination'. In doing so we will briefly review the current concepts around which our ideas of psychosis are crystallized.

10.2 PARADIGMS OF PSYCHOSIS

The dominant paradigm is obviously the two-entity principle which was enunciated by Emil Kraepelin. It has resisted challenge for nearly a century, and has in fact been strengthened in recent years by the thrust towards greater reliability of diagnosis which has led to operational definitions (e.g. DSM–III and DSM–III-R).

A number of assumptions underpin Kraepelin's principle. These include the view that the categorical model of psychiatric disorder is correct, that there are only a small number of disorders, that each disorder is associated with a relatively stable pathognomonic clinical syndrome and that clinical boundaries separate discrete underlying pathophysiological processes.

Both before and since Kraepelin several other models have been put forward. During the 19th century Griesinger proposed the idea of a unitary psychosis, namely one in which a single disease process subsumed all psychopathological phenomena. Many influential approaches to classification during this century can be seen as expressions of the unitary view, in particular those of Adolf Meyer and Karl Menninger. In recent years Crow (1986) has been prominent in his criticism of the Kraepelinian dichotomy and has proposed instead a continuum of psychosis extending from unipolar through bipolar affective illness and schizoaffective psychosis to typical schizophrenia with increasing degrees of defect.

The dimensional model attempts to define psychopathology in terms of a small number of dimensions, differing from the unitary view in that more than one dimension is usually proposed. Claridge (1987) advanced the view of the 'schizophrenia as nervous types', assuming that the manifestations of psychosis

represent extreme forms of biologically based characteristics which were normally distributed in the population. Zubin and Spring's (1976) influential 'vulnerability model' may be seen as a similar proposition, namely that the vulnerability to develop schizophrenia is normally distributed in the population.

A more radical approach to the dichotomy between the categorical and the dimensional views of psychopathology was originally stated by Jaspers (1962). We term it the loose linkage model to highlight its fundamental feature, namely that a close or constant linkage between the symptom level and the anatomical or physiological level may not exist. Human beings may only be able to respond to distress or disruption with a finite number of symptom complexes. Such patterns may be variably linked with an aetiological factor. This perspective comes from the growing awareness that a strict localizationist approach in psychiatry has been unsuccessful. As Jaspers (1962) put it: 'The actual psychic changes are probably not specific for any particular organic cerebral process although sometimes certain changes appear with characteristic frequency'.

Two concepts are useful in further understanding of this model, namely heterogeneity and pleiotropism. Most clinical syndromes in medicine may have a number of underlying causes. The likelihood of such aetiological heterogeneity was recognized by Bleuler (1950) and was reflected in the title of his monograph 'The Group of Schizophrenias'. Davison and Bagley (1969) in their influential review highlighted the heterogeneity of the schizophrenia syndrome by pointing out that symptoms characteristic of the syndrome could arise in the course of a number of disorders. Schneider's (1959) injunction that 'coarse brain disease,' had to be excluded before schizophrenia could be considered the cause of his pathognomic symptoms of the first rank, is an explicit acknowledgement of heterogeneity.

The increasing recognition of the heterogeneity in schizophrenia does not augur well for the existence of a close relationship between syndrome and individual disease entity. Paradoxically however, many of the classical diagnoses of schizophrenia depend on the presence of so called pathognomonic symptoms which are considered essential for diagnosis. This 'core symptom assumption' reflects the belief that in the psychoses a close link exists between disease and its symptomatological expression. The most widely accepted of these has been the work of Schneider (1959) in relation to his symptoms of the 'first rank'. However it is interesting to read what Schneider himself stated about the tentative nature of the link.

> Thought-withdrawal, for instance, is at bottom not a symptom of the purely psychopathologically conceived state of schizophrenia, but it is a factor frequently found and therefore a prominent feature of it. Further, in this case we cannot conclude from a specific observation that a specific illness is present . . . If I find thought-withdrawal in a psychosis of no known somatic base, there is only an agreed convention that I then call this psychosis *a* [present authors' emphasis] schizophrenia.
>
> (Schneider, 1959, p. 131)

Conversely, the reciprocal concept of pleiotropism (McKusick, 1969) refers to the phenomenon in which a single aetiological agent or pathophysiological process can manifest as multiple clinical syndromes. Huntington's disease is a good example in which a highly specific genetic abnormality can lead to the full range of neurotic and psychotic psychopathology (Caine and Shoulson, 1983; Tobin, 1987). Acceptance of the validity of both these concepts when applied to the major psychoses leads to major reservations as to the validity of the Kraepelinian paradigm. Both heterogeneity and pleiotropism would favour what we have called the loose linkage model.

10.3 MUTABILITY OF DISEASE

Hare (1974) has used the term 'mutability of disease' to refer to the trend for a disorder to change in its manifestation in different settings over time and as a result of various pathoplastic influences. We use the term here to refer to a body of evidence supporting a loose linkage model.

10.3.1 SYNDROME CLARITY

A major problem for the clinico-pathological strategy relates to the fact that it has been difficult to define clear syndromal entities within the psychoses. As a result a range of competing operational definitions for syndromes has evolved. This evolution reflects the reality that mixed pictures are very common.

In psychiatric disorders variability and instability of the clinical picture may be simply too great for this task to be logical or fruitful. For example, Strauss *et al.* (1979) showed that while prototypical or archetypal syndromes do exist, the vast majority of actual patients fall between them, displaying characteristics from several of them. Recent genetic studies (Crow, 1986) also lend weight to the proposition that the schizophrenic and affective psychoses may be more closely related than the apparently clear-cut findings of the first generation of studies (Rosenthal and Kety, 1968) may have indicated. The assumption that a clear-cut clinical picture is linked to an underlying genetic diathesis is being steadily eroded. In addition, it has been recognized that the presence of one symptom or syndrome increases the likelihood of others being present, representing a general tendency toward co-morbidity of disorder (Sturt, 1981; Boyd, *et al.*, 1984). This phenomenon of co-morbidity is attracting increased attention (Boyd *et al.*, 1984; Barlow *et al.*, 1986; Morey, 1987; Black *et al.*, 1988; Fryer *et al.*, 1988). The existence of concurrent co-morbidity (intra-episode) and sequential co-morbidity (a possible cause of diagnostic instability *between* episodes) can be regarded as reflecting pleiotropism within individuals, though other sources of variability that are independent of a narrow disease model, could account for or contribute to it. Concurrent co-morbidity can therefore be seen as one possible source of poor cross-sectional syndrome clarity.

The traditional method for handling both concurrent and sequential co-morbidity diagnostically has been through the use of hierarchical decision rules (Jaspers, 1962; Foulds and Bedford, 1975; Morey, 1985, 1987), a strategy which tends to create a spuriously inflated impression of diagnostic clarity and stability. It represents a formal way of reinforcing the categories based upon prototypes through the exaggeration of homogeneity within groups and of heterogeneity between groups, in a sense operationalizing the disadvantages of natural categorizations (Cantor and Genero, 1986). An example of how this strategy tends to exaggerate syndrome clarity is provided by the study of Siris *et al.* (1984). In this study, 'update' diagnostic interviews were performed during the course of the acute episode in a sample of psychotic patients who were initially diagnosed as schizophrenic according to Research Diagnostic Criteria. New affective syndromes commonly emerged during this phase which could affect diagnostic assignment depending on how they were handled by the prevailing set of hierarchical decision rules. In addition to indicating the extent of intra-episode co-morbidity in psychosis, this study highlights the limitations of the single diagnostic interview and information source in truly reflecting the psychopathology of the complete episode.

10.3.2 SYNDROME STABILITY

A number of studies in the area of psychosis has demonstrated that the rate of diagnostic reassignment of patients initially admitted with one type of psychosis is high. Recently for example, Jorgensen and Mortensen (1988), in a register-based study of first-admitted patients with functional psychosis, found that over a two-year observation period half of those readmitted had their diagnosis changed. Diagnostic stability (same diagnosis at first and latest admission) was 74.6% for schizophrenia, 72.9% for manic depressive psychosis, 49.7% for reactive psychosis, and 48.3% for paranoia.

The reasons for this may be:

- The disorder is the same but gives rise to different syndromes at different phases (pleiotropism).

- Two independent disorders are present and manifest themselves sequentially.

- Misclassification has occurred, i.e. a single diagnosis is present but has been incorrectly diagnosed at one time point. In this instance the follow-up diagnosis may be seen as more valid because it corrects an earlier mistake as a result of additional information.

Psychiatric disorders also appear to change over time. A number of authors have commented that schizophrenia does not appear to present as it did early on this century: catatonic types are rarer and the concurrence of affective symptoms much more prominent (Hare, 1974; Ellard, 1985).

Other pathoplastic features (Berrios, 1989) may also influence the clinical picture: gender (Copolov *et al.*, 1990), personality, intelligence, developmental stage (Rutter, 1988) and sociocultural factors (Eisenberg, 1988). In addition, it is clear that individuals' reactions to the experience of a psychotic disturbance vary across a wide spectrum. As Zubin (1985) has commented:

If we could dissect the behaviour due to the mental disorder from the behaviour due to the premorbid personality and to their interaction, we could recognize the focal disorder in isolation from its surround and probably find this factor characteristic of all similarly affected patients. What we perceive, however, is not the effect of the focal disorder alone, but the effect of the illness, which reflects the premorbid personality, and the focal disorder, and their interaction. This is why no two schizophrenics are alike: their focal disorder may be the same but their illness is different. (p. 223)

The key issue is that the modality for expression of the core symptomatology of the core disorder is the same as for expression of the response. Bleuler (1950) was the first to try to separate these in his idea of primary and secondary symptoms in schizophrenia.

We assume the presence of a process, which directly produces the primary symptoms; the secondary symptoms are partly psychic functions operating under altered conditions and partly the results of more or less successful attempts at adaptation to the primary disturbances. (p. 461)

10.4 RELATIONSHIP BETWEEN RELIABILITY AND VALIDITY IN ASSESSING PSYCHOPATHOLOGY IN THE PSYCHOSES

The reasons for attempts to improve diagnostic reliability are well known, the most important being the generalizability of clinical and research findings made in different settings. Diagnostic reliability has been seen as critical because it was believed that it constituted a 'ceiling' for validity.

'There is no guarantee that a reliable system is valid but assuredly an unreliable system must be invalid' (Spitzer and Fleiss, 1974, p. 341). However, challenges to this view have now appeared. Blashfield (1984) argues that high level reliability is not always necessary for acceptable levels of validity, calling into question the assertion of Spitzer and Fleiss that

'an unreliable system must be invalid'. This counter-intuitive argument emphasizes that reliability must always be viewed within the broader context of validity, and that rather than being thought of as possessing any intrinsic merit of its own, it should be regarded as a 'service concept' to assess the extent to which measurement error limits validity. Carey and Gottesman (1978) pointed out that reliability could be improved either by teaching clinicians to rate symptoms better without changing the definition of the symptom or syndrome, or by changing the definition of the symptom of diagnosis in such a way that it could be more reliably rated.

Deliberate attempts to improve the psychiatric ratings by improving only their reliability may have the disastrous consequence of making the ratings less valid than they were originally. When the specificity is increased and the sensitivity decreased by the adoption of a narrower definition which approximates the 'textbook case', the attenuation of validity by increases in reliability becomes a real problem. The existence of this attenuation effect means that even if reliability were to represent something of a ceiling for validity, raising the ceiling to its maximum height would not necessarily result in a proportional increase in validity, and could paradoxically lead to a reduction. The attenuation paradox may occur where diagnostic categories became overly narrow and precise, or diagnostic interview schedules excessively rigid, through differential and inverse effects upon sensitivity and specificity. Important reservations may be expressed on the above grounds regarding instruments such as the Diagnostic Interview Schedule (DIS), designed for epidemiological use with lay interviewers, and which has a very highly structured format (Robins *et al.*, 1981). It has been used extensively in large-scale community surveys (Regier *et al.*, 1984) but the highly rigid nature of the instrument, which precludes the use of cross-examination in clarifying psychopathology, is likely to produce spuriously high reliability and reduce descriptive validity.

This potential trade-off between reliability and validity can be seen more clearly through the use of some well-known clinical illustrations. First, it is possible to measure the height of schizophrenics with a high degree of accuracy and reliability, however such a measure has little or nothing to do with the validity of the construct of schizophrenia. It has been argued that Schneider's first rank symptoms are somewhat similar in that they have been favoured because they can be reliably recognized, but are lacking in validity (Kendell *et al.*, 1979). The corollary of this approach is that other symptoms of potentially high validity which are difficult to define, may be excluded from diagnostic instruments and criteria. Vaillant (Klerman, 1984) cites autism as an example of this, and Wing acknowledges that symptoms such as *'praecox gefuhl'* (praecox feeling) were omitted from the PSE on the basis of the difficulty in defining them precisely.

A major perpetuating factor in the current preoccupation with reliability is the lack of progress in identifying direct measures of criterion validity within the psychoses. Researchers have been forced to focus upon indirect sources of validity such as family history, treatment response, outcome and a variety of relatively crude peripheral biological makers, (e.g. ventricular enlargement on CT scan) as substitutes for the elusive underlying pathophysiological correlates. The extent of this research bottleneck is indicated by the proliferation of an array of rival operational definitions for each major syndrome. These definitions, of comparable reliability, tend to be poorly concordant with one another (Brockington *et al.*, 1978; Brockington and Leff, 1979; Endicott *et al.*, 1982; Kendell, 1982; Brockington *et al.*) reflecting the degree of conceptual heterogeneity which exists.

10.5 HOW CAN THE VALIDITY OF OUR ASSESSMENTS OF PSYCHO-PATHOLOGY BE IMPROVED?

10.5.1 SELECTION OF A 'NATURAL BOUNDARY' AND COMPREHENSIVE COVER OF PHENOMENA ENCOMPASSED BY THAT BOUNDARY

In view of the unresolved problem of the comparative validity of rival operational definitions for any given diagnostic concept, it is clear that the selection of a natural boundary for research purposes is extremely problematical. In such a situation broad samples of patients should be studied and relatively robust boundaries chosen, so that premature closure does not occur. One such candidate is the boundary between psychosis and non-psychosis even though interforms do straddle this boundary. The next step is then to assess the phenomenology of the psychoses comprehensively. This requires the collection of data which are not simply the criteria necessary to come to a diagnostic decision in one or two diagnostic systems but those that might be derived from a broader array of systems. This is discussed in greater detail in 10.5.2.

10.5.2 THE MULTI-DIAGNOSTIC APPROACH

Strauss and Gift (1977) initially proposed a response to the disturbing fact that while operational definitions had been developed and could be reliably applied to the major syndrome, the level of concordance between these competing definitions was relatively poor. They suggested the concurrent collection of data relevant to several or multiple diagnostic systems. The major diagnostic instruments, apart from the PSE, have been developed after the advent of operational definitions and hence tend to be closely tied to particular systems of diagnosis. In this sense they are unidiagnostic or oliogodiagnostic, a feature which gives rise to two major deficiencies. First, they fail to comprehensively cover the range of clinical features found in the domain of funtional psychosis, since they only collect psychopathology relevant to one or a small number of diagnostic concepts. This means that content and descriptive validity are significantly reduced. In contrast, the inclusion of a broad range of diagnostic concepts from a number of cultures and historical schools increases the coverage of symptomatology and improves content and descriptive validity. A true multidiagnostic approach, defined as the simultaneous application of a range of competing and variably concordant systems of operational criteria to the same sample of patients, should fulfill both requirements as well as possessing a number of other advantages, especially related to the evaluation of comparative validity.

10.5.3 MULTIPLE INFORMATION SOURCES AND UPDATE INTERVIEWS

Luria and Guziec (1981), in a comparison of the SADS with the PSE, have pointed out that the PSE is by content and method a mental status examination despite the development of supplementary historical schedules. On the other hand, the SADS and its more recent North American relatives are by content an amalgam of mental status examination and history of the present illness. They regard neither as approximating a complete traditional clinical assessment, with its ability to draw upon multiple information sources and incorporate the full range and temporal sequence of the symptomatology.

The potential improvement in descriptive validity which could be expected from the use of multiple information sources has been examined by a number of researchers (Carpenter *et al.*, 1976; Strauss *et al.*, 1978; Downing *et al.*, 1980; Brockington and Meltzer, 1982). It is clearly relevant to the issue of the trade-off between reliability and validity already discussed. One of the ways in which

inter-rater reliability can be improved is by limiting information variance, and the standard method of achieving this is through the standardization of the assessment procedure. Many structured interviews fail to allow for the inclusion of data from sources other than the patient or fail to indicate how such information should be incorporated into the rating process, especially where it conflicts with what the patient has stated. Excluding non-patient information sources reduces information variance, but such exclusions reflect how the preoccupation with reliability can conflict with attempts to improve validity. Such exclusions are the result of the use of lay interviewers and the consequent need to rigidly structure the assessment procedure as seen with the DIS. In direct contrast, what is required is the development of a paradigm in which multiple information sources can be utilized in a standardized and reproducible way. This should be accompanied by clear ground rules for the melding of data from multiple sources, for example to handle the situation where two information sources, (e.g. patient and relative) provide conflicting data. If this latter step fails to occur (e.g. with the Structured Clinical Interview for DSM–III or SCID; Spitzer and Williams, 1984), information variance may continue to present significant problems.

In addition to including information from informants, it is also important to fully document an episode of psychiatric illness by incorporating information from sequential assessments during the episode. In this respect, the limitations of a single structured psychiatric interview need to be appreciated. In the psychoses the prerequisite that the patient needs to be capable of giving a clear account is not met in about 25% of the cases, so that the documentation of recent symptoms may not be possible. Observational data, which with training can be rated with high levels of inter-rater reliability, suffers from the limited time-frame sampled by the interview, a period poorly representative of the episode as a whole. The poor test-retest reliability found at the item level in a number of studies reflects genuine changes in the patients' clinical status over and above measurement error. This component of 'un-reliability' is known as occasion variance, and its existence is a powerful argument for multiple sampling of symptoms and behaviour during an illness episode.

A corollary, then, of the fact that the single interview is deficient, is that multiple sources of information need to be accessed in constructing an accurate picture of a psychotic episode. Brockington and Meltzer (1982) outlined how this might be done in practice through the combined use of numerical and narrative records. Multiple research interviews are proposed, supplemented by informant interviews, nurse ratings and narrative accounts, and self-report data, all of which may be combined in 'master ratings' for the episode as a whole.

Current controversy centres upon whether lay interviewers can be relied upon to elicit psychopathology and arrive at psychiatric diagnoses in a valid way. The evidence is less than encouraging and some authors have expressed grave misgivings about the use of lay interviewers and the associated requirement to rigidly structure the assessment tool. Schwartz and Wiggins (1987) highlight the fact that experienced clinicians develop a preconceptual familiarity or 'typification' which allows them to make important first steps towards diagnosis. The absence of such a skill from the repertoire of inexperienced practitioners is likely to lead to reduced validity. Other studies have focused upon the rating of symptoms by psychiatrists and nonpsychiatrists and have found that nonpsychiatrists tend to have a lower threshold for rating positively. An adequate training period, however, appears to correct this tendency. If validity is to be emphasized, variables such as level of previous clinical experience with the relevant patient group, intelligence and motivation, and the length and quality of the training period are of obvious importance. We would contend on validity grounds that experienced clinicians, specifically psychologists, psychiatric social workers, and selected psychiatric nurses, represent the minimum acceptable alternative to psychiatrists in the research assessment of clinical psycho-pathology.

10.5.4 HIERARCHY-FREE APPROACH

Hierarchical diagnostic decision rules and exclusion criteria ideally correspond with actual points of rarity between syndromes and thus represent a kind of clinical discriminant analysis. They represent one solution to the problem of co-morbidity which reflects a particular set of hypotheses about the nature of psychopathology, hypotheses which remain largely implicit because of their time-honoured status. There is also a general tendency toward the co-occurrence of psychiatric disorders, and there is additional evidence that there are other significant associations between disorders not addressed by the DSM–III exclusion rules. This indicates the need for empirical studies to examine the assumptions underlying the use of diagnostic hierarchies. Such a move is under-way in the anxiety and affective disorders, and may be overdue in the psychoses for a variety of reasons. Any method of assessment should therefore ensure it collects data relevant to all major syndromes regardless of their prominence and timing. Naturally the sequence, duration and relative prominence need to be ascertained as well. All the relevant information must be available for the evaluation of alternative hierarchical systems in addition to the dominant system as well as other non-hierarchical models.

10.5.5 TIME PERIOD CONSIDERED

The unit of time focused upon by the major diagnostic interview schedules is variable. This might be the past month, the period when symptoms were at their peak, or the subject's entire life span. It may be that separate modules or instruments with different overlapping symptom pools are required for the different phases of illness. For example, the assessment of the acute psychotic episode would require an item pool enriched with a wide range of florid or productive symptomatology, while in the recovery or prodrome greater coverage of the more subtle prodromal and residual and affective symptoms may be indicated.

10.5.6 ATTEMPT TO SEPARATE CORE SYMPTOMS FROM RESPONSE TO PSYCHOSIS

In common with anyone suffering from a major physical illness, patients with severe psychiatric illnesses will manifest a range of psychological responses to the emergence or recrudescence of their underlying disorder. The problem is that in psychiatry these responses may be difficult or impossible to distinguish from the primary disturbance. We really have very little idea of the pattern of such responses in patients experiencing and recovering from a psychotic episode, and in fact have tended to deal with the issue diagnostically through the use of hierarchies to 'explain' lower level symptomatology. The problem cannot be easily resolved, but perhaps a first step might be to attempt to define a typology of responses to an acute psychotic episode (with assistance from studies of analogous physical illnesses) and subtract such patterns from the psychopathology of the episode for individual patients. This could lead to a clarification of the 'core' symptomatology and its separation from secondary features which Berrios (1984) has termed 'pathoplastic noise'.

Of course, whether we see such features as 'noise' depends on whether we are focusing on distinguishing major syndromes or examining differences between reactions within syndromes — i.e. the 'level' of categorization involved. Clearly this issue is one of both clinical and

theoretical importance, and is one that is poorly addressed by DSM–III–R (e.g. depression in schizophrenia).

10.5.7 USE OF CONSENSUS DIAGNOSES FOR PROCEDURAL VALIDITY

In the absence of fundamental markers of validity, a strategy which has often been advocated as a substitute measure in methodological studies of diagnosis is the independent assignment of a 'consensus' diagnosis. This has been carried out by our team in the following manner. Research diagnoses based upon interviews with patients and other standardized procedures are produced by independent raters. In parallel, the clinical team with access to this body of data as well as more extensive contact with the patient would meet and review the total information base in detail. This group of psychiatrists, perhaps three as a minimum, assign a 'consensus diagnosis' to the patient using first the current DSM–III or DSM–III–R classifications, and second a more 'flexible' approach which would allow the use of alternative concepts such as cycloid psychosis. The degree of consensus achieved and the degree of certainty of the diagnosis are rated to provide a measure of 'textbookness' or prototypicality of the case. This latter concept is important in the interpretation of reliability data since the proportion of textbook vs. nontextbook cases in a sample of patients may exert a strong influence upon the level of reliability of diagnosis within that sample. Nevertheless the issue has not been adequately studied to date and current measures of reliability do not consider it. Spitzer has proposed a method to evaluate the validity of diagnostic assessment instruments which incorporates many of the principles described above. This method, termed the LEAD standard (Longitudinal Expert Diagnosis using All Data), an acronym intended to contrast the method with the more elusive 'gold' standard, relies upon consensus (expert) diagnoses as criterion measures for validation purposes.

10.6 CURRENT INSTRUMENTS FOR ASSESSING SYMPTOMATOLOGY AND DIAGNOSES IN THE PSYCHOSES

Over the past four decades a number of methods have been developed to assess psychopathology in the psychoses. From 1984 a new research programme focusing upon the psychoses was initiated at our centre and has since developed into the National Health and Medical Research Council Schizophrenia Research Unit. The need for a core diagnostic instrument for the comprehensive assessment of patients with an acute psychotic episode was recognized, and a number of existing interview schedules were examined as potential candidates. These included the PSE, the SADS, the DIS, the CIDI, the SCID, and the Landmark schedule. Difficulties were found with each of them in regard to the set of guiding principles outlined above. Several were too closely tied to a single diagnostic system or group of related systems to allow the implementation of the multi-diagnostic principle. The PSE provided excellent coverage of the symptom domain including subtle phenomenological differences, however it lacked a historical component and, unless modified, was not easily wedded to the broad range of diagnostic systems. More recently, some of these deficiencies may have been overcome in the revision of the PSE (PSE–10) and the development of the Schedules for Clinical Assessment in Neuropsychiatry (SCAN), however these clinical tools have not yet become widely available and methodological research involving them has not yet been published. Other instruments were too coarse in their assessment of psychotic symptomatology. As a result we decided to construct an assessment tool *de novo*, beginning with the selection of the range of systems to be included, a process which in turn largely defined the symptom domain based on the principles described above. This instrument we named the Royal Park Multi-Diagnostic Instrument for Psychosis (RPMIP). In this section, other assessment instruments are briefly described and then contrasted with the RPMIP (Table 10.1), and a brief description is given of the instrument itself.

10.6.1 PRESENT STATE EXAMINATION — PSE–9 (Wing *et al.*, 1974)

The Present State Examination was developed as a guide to structuring the clinical interview and was not designed around a specific set of diagnostic criteria. PSE–9 was substantially completed prior to the appearance of explicit sets of operational definitions and is intended to provide the user with a method of deriving a comprehensive picture of relevant mental functioning, including psychotic and neurotic aspects, in the previous month. It is essentially a semi-structured interview for conducting the mental status examination and scoring the findings. Historical material has been covered only in adjunctive schedules, though in PSE-10, there is a specific clinical history module. The interviewer is expected to employ a cross-examination style to discover whether certain symptoms are present and a degree of flexibility is permitted. Detailed accounts of the instrument and comparisons with other schedules are readily available.

An important issue to highlight is that the rationale for and process of development of the PSE was significantly different from interview schedules which are 'criteria-driven'. The latter have followed a reverse sequence beginning with one or more sets of operational criteria for various disorders and constructing probes to elicit material relevant to these. The PSE approach results in a sophisticated coverage of the spectrum of psychotic symptoms. Other interview schedules such as the SADS, which by method are modelled on the psychiatric history (Luria and Guziec, 1981), contrast with the PSE in their ability to utilize sources of information in addition to that provided by the patient. In contrast to both, the RPMIP attempts to combine the history of the present illness and

Table 10.1 Comparison of RPMIP with existing assessment procedures

	PSE	SADS	DIS	CIDI	SCID	Landmark	PODI	RPMIP
Epidemiological (E) vs. clinical (C)	C	C	E	E	C	C	C	C
Number of interviews	1	1	1	1	1	1	1	2+
Time period considered	Previous month	1 wk (most severe) + lifetime	Lifetime	Previous month + lifetime	Previous month + lifetime	Total period of illness	Current episode only	Current episode only
Degree of structure	+	+	+++	+++	+	+	++	+
Overview	−	+/−	−	−	+	−	+	+
Multiple information sources	−	+	−	−	+	−	+	+
Multiple diagnostic systems	−	−	+	+	−	+++	+++	+++
Coverage of disorder (psychotic + neurotic)	+++	+	+++	+++	+++	+	++	+
Coverage of psychotic + affective features	+++	++	+	+	+	+++	++++	++++
Experienced raters required	+	+	−	−	+	+	+	+
Glossary	+	+/−	−	+	+/−	+	−	+
Linkage to operational definitions	−	+	+	+	+	++	++	++
Historical (H) vs mental status (M) method	M	H	H	HM	H	HM	HM	HM
Computer algorithm	+	−	+	+	−	+	+	+

mental status methods in one procedure which seeks to approximate the traditional clinical approach.

10.6.2 THE SCHEDULE FOR AFFECTIVE DISORDERS AND SCHIZOPHRENIA — SADS (Endicott and Spitzer, 1978)

The SADS was developed specifically to record the information necessary for making RDC diagnoses. The time frame is quite different in that the SADS focuses upon the one-week period during the current episode when the particular feature under consideration was most severe. The disadvantage of this is that the time period evaluated for each symptom is thus defined independently of other symptoms, so that the SADS profile could conceivably amount to a composite of temporally unrelated symptoms instead of a syndrome. Advantages of the SADS include the use of the history of the present illness method which allows

information from multiple sources to be utilized, and the existence of a current state or change version, which allows repeat or update interviews to influence the ultimate diagnosis. Its principal disadvantages from our own perspective are its unidiagnostic basis with consequent poor coverage of the range of psychotic symptomatology and the uncoupling of individual symptoms from one another in terms of their time course.

10.6.3 THE STRUCTURED CLINICAL INTERVIEW FOR DSM–III/DSM–III-R — SCID/SCID-R (Spitzer *et al.*, 1988)

This interview schedule, intended for use by relatively experienced clinicians to elicit DSM–III/DSM–III-R diagnoses across a broad range of psychopathology, has been developed at the New York State Psychiatric Institute. The structure of the interview is such that a flexible overview is conducted, followed by a structured interview with multiple skip points. Depending upon the subject's responses, very different paths through the interview are followed, with variable areas of psychopathology being covered or omitted. This results in a data base with multiple lacunae at the symptom level. For this reason the SCID is purely a diagnostic schedule, eliciting the minimum information for DSM–III diagnoses to be made. In summary, it represents a reliable (Copolov *et al.*, 1986), efficient and probably more valid method for experienced clinicians to elicit DSM–III diagnoses in a relatively standardized way without excessive rigidity.

10.6.4 DIAGNOSTIC INTERVIEW SCHEDULE — DIS (Robins *et al.*, 1981)

The DIS is a fully structured interview developed for the Epidemiologic Catchment Area (ECA) programme. It provides fixed phrasing for questions about symptoms, and standard probes to determine whether a symptom is severe enough to meet criteria. This format is designed to reduce the amount of clinical experience required to conduct the interview and make ratings, and the DIS represents an attempt to make diagnostic interviews accessible to lay interviewers. Although cheaper and more feasible, this involves a potential sacrifice in terms of validity, an issue which has been examined in several studies. A computer algorithm is applied to the interview data and enables diagnoses to be made according to three related diagnostic systems, Feighner, RDC, and DSM–III.

The coverage of psychotic symptoms in the DIS is somewhat coarse and limited, which is quite appropriate in the context of a large epidemiological survey, but not in inpatient studies of severe psychiatric disorder. The end-product is certainly not comparable with that, for example, of a PSE interview in terms of comprehensiveness of mental status information. The use of informants

is not routine with the DIS, which tends to further reduce the validity of the data obtained.

10.6.5 THE COMPOSITE INTERNATIONAL DIAGNOSTIC INTERVIEW — CIDI (Robins *et al.*, 1988)

This interview schedule combines questions from the DIS with questions designed to elicit PSE items, thus enabling DSM–III diagnoses to be ascertained in addition to allowing a cross-cultural focus. It was intended for use as an international epidemiological tool which would allow diagnoses to be made according to multiple diagnostic systems when administered by non-clinicians and scored by computer. It will eventually allow diagnoses to be made according to ICD–10 criteria and be available in many languages. Its limitations in relation to psychotic disorder appear to be similar to those of the DIS, nevertheless it does represent an improvement on that instrument in that it can be better used cross-nationally and allows more valid coverage of psychotic phenomena.

10.6.6 LANDMARK MANUAL FOR THE ASSESSMENT OF SCHIZOPHRENIA (Landmark, 1982)

This truly multi-diagnostic schedule provided the idea and the model for the development of the RPMIP. The manual was developed in Canada by a Norwegian psychiatrist, Johan Landmark, for the purpose of reassessing the diagnoses of a sample of patients with a diagnosis of chronic schizophrenia attending an outpatient clinic. Thirteen concepts of schizophrenia and related non-affective psychoses were assembled, some of which already existed in an operationalized form. The remainder, mainly historical concepts such as Bleulerian schizophrenia, were operationalized by Landmark in close consultation with the originator of the concept or their descendants (e.g. Manfred Bleuler, Gabriel Langfeldt) wherever this was possible.

10.6.7 POLYDIAGNOSTIC INTERVIEW — PODI (Philipp and Maier, 1986)

Closer still and with similar antecedents and path of development to the RPMIP is the Polydiagnostic Interview or PODI, developed in West Germany to facilitate the emergent polydiagnostic approach in Europe. The SCID was used as a basis for constructing the PODI, however it was richly supplemented by additional questions and new sections where required to allow a very broad range of diagnoses from the psychotic and affective spectra to be ascertained. The mental status section was modelled on the PSE. Complex criteria were broken down into their component parts to improve precision, and reduce methodological distortions, and questions are generally short and clearly formulated. The interview is only administered once and concentrates upon the most severe phase of the current episode. It does allow all available information to be considered by the rater and is intended for use by expert clinicians, a feature which is used unconvincingly in our view to justify the lack of a detailed glossary. A computer program has been developed to apply the diagnostic algorithms for the various systems, which now include the research criteria for ICD–10 and the DSM–III-R criteria.

10.6.8 ROYAL PARK MULTI-DIAGNOSTIC INSTRUMENT FOR PSYCHOSIS — RPMIP (McGorry *et al.*, 1990a, 1990b)

The development of the RPMIP involved a series of steps which may be summarized as follows. The range of concepts of psychotic disorders was considered and grouped into four categories — those relating to schizophrenia, affective psychosis, schizoaffective and atypical psychosis and other concepts. In an attempt to attain maximum coverage of the spectrum of psychoses we tended to be over-inclusive in incorporating atypical and heterogeneous diagnostic systems. We accepted that in some systems we needed to include individual components that are difficult to operationalize (e.g. autism). We then recast all definitions in operational form. The details of how this was done are fully described elsewhere (McGorry *et al.*, 1990a,b).

The major components of the instrument are the main interview schedule itself, the illness duration (informant) interview, a discharge score sheet, diagnostic decision rules and a summary sheet. In addition a glossary of all terms has been produced, and a computer program to generate diagnoses developed. Three interviews are carried out, two with the patient at different phases of the illness and one with an informant. The first interview occurs early in the acute psychotic breakdown whilst the second occurs prior to discharge and allows a somewhat different reconstruction of the events, as well as performing an update function.

The main interview consists of the following components: an overview of the whole illness episode, data on the onset and duration, a section in which the use of drugs and alcohol is assessed, an affective disorders section, a psychotic symptoms section and a prodromal/residual symptoms section. The interviewer is also expected to complete a graph of the syndromal pattern over time and make observational ratings. Examples of questions used to assess possible delusions are as follows:

- Has anybody been giving you a hard time or trying to hurt you?

- What about accusing you of things?

- Who is involved in this?

- How do you know?

- Are the events/people connected in some way?

COURSE

No particular questions are required but it is essential to establish the onset and offset of the various syndromes presented below. Mark the onset and offset with a cross and connect with a horizontal line. Ensure you know whether manic or depressive syndromes preceded the psychotic symptoms. Also, were there psychotic symptoms in the absence of manic or depressive symptoms, and for how long.

COURSE FOLLOWING ADMISSION

	OTHER SYMPTOMS
	PROMINENT MANIC SYMPTOMS
	PROMINENT DEPRESSIVE SYMPTOMS
	ACTIVE PSYCHOTIC SYMPTOMS

ADMISSION   Weeks following admission

COURSE PRECEDING ADMISSION

Include fluctuations if known. Otherwise draw a st. line connecting onset & offset. Specify the type of prodrome (whether DSM III or not) above the line.

	PRODROME
	DEPRESSIVE SYNDROME
	MANIC SYNDROME
	ACTIVE PSYCHOTIC SYMPTOMS
	DRUG ABUSE (Name drugs)
	ALCOHOL ABUSE

19 18 17 16 15 14 13 12 11 10 9 8 7 6 5 4 3 2 1   ADMISSION
Weeks
preceding admission

Figure 10.1 Course of the major syndromes: assessment sheet from RPMIP.

Table 10.2 Concepts of psychotic disorder covered by the RPMIP procedure

Diagnostic concept

A. *Schizophrenia*
  Kraepelin
  E. Bleuler
  Langfeldt
  K. Schneider
  M. Bleuler
  Feighner
  WHO-IPPS
  Taylor and Abrams
  Cloninger
  RDC
  DSM–III
    Positive (Andreasen)
    Negative (Andreasen)
    Mixed (Andreasen)
    With atypical depression

B. *Schizophreniform*
  Langfeldt
  DSM–III
    With atypical depression

C. *Schizoaffective*
  Kasanin
  Welner
  Feighner
    Depressed
    Manic
  RDC
    Depressed
    Manic
  DSM–III

D. *Affective*
  Depression
  RDC
    Non-psychotic
    Psychotic
  DSM–III
    Non-psychotic
    Psychotic
      MC
      MI

D. *Affective*
  Bipolar
  RDC manic
    Non-psychotic
    Psychotic
  DSM–III bipolar
    Manic episode
      Non-psychotic
      Psychotic
        MC
        MI
    Bipolar (Mixed)
      Non-psychotic
      Psychotic
        MC
        MI

E. *Atypical*
  DSM–III brief reactive psychosis
  Dongier/acute delusional psychosis
  Bouffee delirante
  Cycloid psychosis
  RDC unspecified functional
    Psychosis
  DSM–III atypical psychosis

F. *Miscellaneous*
  DSM–III paranoid disorder
  DSM–III paranoia
  Schizophrenia spectrum disorders
    (DSM–III schizoid/schizotypal PD)
  Any DSM–III personality disorder
  Drug-related psychosis
  No psychotic diagnosis

Key: MC = Mood congruent; MI = Mood incongurent

The following series of questions are used to assess made impulses.

- Do you ever experience urges or the need to do things that are forced upon you by other people or outside forces?

- If yes, what has happened?

In the prodromal and/or residual symptoms section, probes to assess symptomatology must of necessity be more sensitive. For example to tap the dimension of social isolation or withdrawal the following questions are used.

- Did you see any members of your family on a regular basis?
- Who?
- How often?
- Did you have friends, acquaintances or workmates with whom you had regular contact?
- Who were they?
- How often did you see them?
- What did you do together?
- Did you avoid being with others?
- To what extent?
- How much time were you spending alone?
- What effect did this have on your life?

Based on the answers to these probes the interviewer makes a judgement as to whether the item described is true, false or not able to be assessed.

Interviewers are expected to gain an overview of the course of each major syndrome both prior to and following admission and are required to chart its course on a graph (Figure 10.1).

Observational ratings include items such as catatonic behaviour, posturing, autism, ambivalence, absence of rapport etc. The glossary provides detailed information on the criteria to be used to rate each of these.

Each patient interview takes approximately one to one and a half hours to complete with the second or update interview often being able to be done in half that time. The informant interview takes approximately half to three-quarters of an hour to complete and documents psychopathology prior to admission. These multiple information sources, including the nursing modification of BPRS data collected on all patients (McGorry *et al.*, 1988), are incorporated into a final score sheet of ratings for the episode. Diagnostic decision rules can then be applied both manually and via computer algorithms to the data set to give the final

diagnoses. The range of diagnoses currently covered by the instrument are detailed in Table 10.2.

10.7 CONCLUSION

This chapter began with a 'present state examination' of the nosology of psychosis, emphasizing the critical importance for nosology and psychopathological assessment strategy of the phenomena of heterogeneity and pleiotropism. Having defined some boundaries and a conceptual structure for assessment in the light of the above concepts, a number of principles designed to maximize the validity of psychopathological assessment were introduced. A method of assessment based upon these principles was described and contrasted with other approaches in relation to a range of parameters.

REFERENCES

Barlow, D.H., DiNardo, P.A., Vermilyea, B.B. *et al.* (1986) Co-Morbidity and depression among the anxiety disorders. — Issues in Diagnosis and Classification. *J. Nerv. Ment. Dis.*, **174**, 63–72.

Berrios, G.E. (1984) Descriptive psychopathology: conceptual and historical aspects. *Psychol. Med.*, **14**, 303–13.

Black, D.W., Winokur, G., Bell, S. *et al.* (1988) Complicated mania. *Arch. Gen. Psychiatry*, **45**, 232–6.

Blashfield, R.K. (1984) *The Classification of Psychopathology: Neo-Kraepelinian and Quantitative Approaches.* Plenum Press, New York.

Bleuler, E. (1950) *Dementia Praecox, on the Group of Schizophrenias.* International Universities Press, New York.

Boyd, J.H., Burke, J.D., Gruenberg, E. *et al.* (1984) Exclusion criteria of DSM–III. *Arch. Gen. Psychiatry*, **41**, 983–9.

Brockington, I.F. and Leff, J.P. (1979) Schizo-affective psychosis: definitions and incidence. *Psychol. Med.*, **9**, 91–99.

Brockington, I.F. and Meltzer, H.Y. (1982) Documenting an episode of psychiatric illness: need for multiple information sources, multiple raters, and narrative. *Schizophr. Bull*, **8**, 485–92.

Brockington, I.F., Kendell, R.E. and Leff, J.P. (1978) Definitions of schizophrenia: concordance and prediction of outcome. *Psychol. Med.*, **8**, 387–98.

Brockington, I.F., Hillier, V.F., Francis, A.F. *et al.* (1983) Definitions of mania: concordance and prediction of outcome. *Am. J. Psychiatry*, **140**, 435–9.

Brockington, I.F. and Leff, J.P. (1979) Schizo-affective psychosis: definitions and incidence. *Psychol. Med.*, **9**, 91–99.

Caine, E.D. and Shoulson, I. (1983) Psychiatric syndromes in Huntington's disease. *Am. J. Psychiatry*, **140**, 728–33.

Cantor, N. and Genero, N. (1986) Psychiatric diagnosis and natural categorization: a close analogy. In *Contemporary Directions in Psychopathology*. T. Millon and G.L. Klerman (eds), Guilford Press, New York, pp. 233–54.

Carey, G. and Gottesman, I.I. (1978) Reliability and validity in binary ratings. *Arch. Gen. Psychiatry*, **35**, 1454–9.

Carpenter, W.T., Sacks, M.H., Strauss, J.S. *et al* (1976) Evaluating signs and symptoms: comparison of structural interview and clinical approaches. *Br. J. Psychiatry*, **128**, 397–403.

Claridge, G. (1987) The Schizophrenias as nervous types revisited. *Br. J. Psychiatry*, **151**, 735–43.

Copolov, D.L., McGorry, P.O., Singh, B.S. *et al.* (1990) The influence of gender on the classification of psychotic disorders — a multidiagnostic approach., *Acta Psychiatr. Scand.*, in press.

Copolov, D.L., Rubin, R.T., Mander, A.J. *et al.* (1986) DSM–III Melancholia: Do the criteria accurately and reliably distinguish endogenous pattern depression? *J. Affective Disord.*, **10**, 191–202.

Crow, T.J. (1986) The continuum of psychosis and its implications for the structure of the gene. *Br. J. Psychiatry*, **149**, 419–29.

Davison, K. and Bagley, C.R. (1969) Schizophrenia-like psychoses associated with organic disorders of the central nervous system: a review of the literature. *Br. J. Psychiatry*, **114**, 113–84.

Downing, A.R., Francis, A.F. and Brockington, I.F. (1980) A comparison of information: sources in the study of psychiatric illness. *Br. J. Psychiatry*, **137**, 38–44.

Eisenberg, L. (1988) Editorial — The social construction of mental illness. *Psychol. Med.*, **18**, 1–9.

Ellard, J. (1985) Schizophrenia: here today, gone tomorow? *Mod. Med. Aust., January*, 9–13.

Endicott, J., Nee, J., Fleiss, J. *et al.* (1982) Diagnostic criteria for schizophrenia: reliabilities and agreement between systems. *Arch. Gen. Psychiatry*, **39**, 884–9.

Endicott, J. and Spitzer, R.L. (1978) A diagnostic interview: the schedule for affective disorders and schizophrenia. *Arch. Gen. Psychiatry*, **35**, 837–44.

Foulds, G.A. and Bedford, A. (1975) Hierarchy of classes of personal illness. *Psychol. Med.*, **5**, 181–92.

Fyer, M.R., Frances, A.J., Sullivan, T. *et al.* (1988) Comorbidity of borderline personality disorder. *Arch. Gen. Psychiatry*, **45**, 348–52.

Hare, E.H. (1974) The Changing Content of Psychiatric Illness. *J. Psychosom. Res.*, **18**, 283–9.

Jaspers, K. (1962) The patient's attitude to his illness. In *General Psychopathology*. M.W. Hamilton (ed), Manchester University Press, Manchester, pp. 414–427.

Jorgensen, P. and Mortensen, P.B. (1988) Admission pattern and diagnostic stability of patients with functional psychosis. *Acta Psychiatr. Scand.*, **78**, 361–5.

Kendell, R.E. (1989) Clinical validity. *Psychol. Med.*, **19**, 45–55.

Kendell, R.E. (1982) The choice of diagnostic criteria for biological research. *Arch. Gen. Psychiatry*, **39**, 1334–9.

Kendell, R.E., Brockington, I.F., and Leff, J.P. (1979) Prognostic implications of six alternative definitions of schizophrenia. *Arch. Gen. Psychiatry*, **36**, 25–31.

Kendell, R.E. (1975) *The Role of Diagnosis in Psychiatry 1. The Importance of Diagnosis*. Blackwell, Oxford.

Klerman, G.L., Vallant, G.E., Spitzer, R.L. *et al.* (1984) A debate on DSM–III. *Am. J. Psychiatry*, **191**, 539–53.

Landmark, J. (1982) A manual for the assessment of schizophrenia. *Acta Psychiatr. Scand.* **65**, Suppl. 298, 1–88.

Luria, R.E. and Guziec, R.J. (1981) Comparative description of the SADS and PSE. *Schizophr. Bull.*, **7**, 248–57.

McGorry, P.D., Copolov, D.L. and Singh, B.S. (1990a) The Royal Park multidiagnostic instrument for psychosis: Part I: rationale and review. *Schizophr. Bull.*, **16**, 501–15.

McGorry, P.D., Singh, B.S., Kaplan, I. *et al.* (1990b) The Royal Park multi-diagnostic instrument for psychosis: Part II. Development and structure, reliability and procedural validity. *Schizophr. Bull.*, **16**, 517–36.

McGorry, P.D., Copolov, D.L. and Singh, B.S. (1990c) Current concepts in functional psychosis: the case for a loosening of associations. *Schizophr. Res.*, **3**, 221–39.

McGorry, P.D., Copolov, D.L. and Singh, B.S. (1989) The validity of the assessment of psychopathology in the psychoses. *Aust. N.Z. J. Psychiatry*, **23**, 469–82.

McGorry, P.D., Goodwin, R.J. and Stuart, G.W. (1988) The development, use, and reliability of the brief psychiatric rating scale (nursing modification) — an assessment procedure for the nursing team in clinical and research settings. *Compr. Psychiatry*, **29**, 575–87.

McKusick, V.A. (1969) On lumpers and splitters, or the nosology of genetic disease. *Perspect. Biol. Med.*, **21**, 298–313.

Morey, L.C. (1985) A comparative validation of the Foulds and Bedford hierarchy of psychiatric symptomatology. *Br. J. Psychiatry*, **146**, 424–8.

Morey, L.C. (1987) The Foulds hierarchy of personal illness: a review of recent research. *Compr. Psychiatry*, **28**, 159–68.

Mullen, P.E. (1984) Introduction to Descriptive Psychopathology. In *The Scientific Principles of Psychopathology*. P. McGuffin, M.F. Shanks and R.J. Hodgson (eds), Academic Press, London, pp. 607–21.

Philipp, M. and Maier, W. (1986) The polydiagnostic interview: a structured interview for the polydiagnostic classification of psychiatric patients. *Psychopathology*, **19**, 175–85.

Regier, D.A., Myers, J.K., Kramer, M. *et al.* (1984) The epidemiologic catchment area programme. *Arch. Gen. Psychiatry*, **41**, 934–41.

Robins, L.N., Helzer, J.E., Croughan, J. and Ratcliff, K.S. (1981) National Institute of Mental Health diagnostic interview schedule. *Arch. Gen. Psychiatry*, **38**, 381–9.

Robins, L.N., Wing, J., Wittchen, H.U. *et al.* (1988) The composite international diagnostic interview. *Arch. Gen. Psychiatry*, **45**, 1069–77.

Rosenthal, D. and Kety, S.S. (1968) *The Transmission of Schizophrenia*. Pergamon Press, Oxford.

Rutter, M. (1988) Epidemiological approaches to developmental psychiatry, *Arch. Gen. Psychiatry*. **24**, 399–411.

Schneider, K. (1959) *Clinical Psychophathology*. Grune and Stratton, New York.

Schwartz, M.A. and Wiggins, O.P. (1987) Diagnosis and ideal types: a contribution to psychiatric classification. *Am. Psychopathol. Assoc.*, **28**, 277–91.

Siris, S.G., Rifkin, A., Reardon, G.T. *et al.* (1984) Course-related depressive syndromes in schizophrenia. *Am. J. Psychiatry*, **141**, 1254–7.

Spitzer, R. (1983) Psychiatric diagnosis: Are clinicians still necessary? *Comp. Psychiatry*, **24**, 399–411.

Spitzer, R.L., Williams, J.B.W. *et al.* (1988) *Structured Clinical Interview for DSM–III–R — Patient Version (SCID-P, 6/1/88)*. New York State Psychiatric Institute, New York.

Spitzer, R.L. and Williams, J.B.W. (1984) *Structural Clinical Interview for DSM–III (SCID 5/1/84)*. New York State Psychiatric Institute, New York.

Spitzer, R.L. and Fleiss, J.L. (1974) A re-analysis of the reliability of psychiatric diagnosis. *Br. J. Psychiatry*, **125**, 341–7.

Strauss, J.S. and Gift, T.E. (1977) Choosing an approach for diagnosing schizophrenia. *Arch. Gen. Psychiatry*, **34**, 1248–53.

Strauss, J.S., Kokes, R.F., Ritzler, B.A. *et al.* (1978) Patterns of disorder in first admission psychiatric patients. *J. Nerv. Ment. Dis.*, **166**, 611–25.

Strauss, J.S., Gabriel, R., Kokes, R.F. *et al.* (1979) Do psychiatric patients fit their diagnoses?. *J. Nerv. Ment. Dis.*, **167**, 105–13.

Sturt, E. (1981) Hierarchical patterns in the distribution of psychiatric symptoms. *Psychol. Med.*, **11**, 783–94.

Tobin, A.J. (1987) Molecular biology and schizophrenia: lessons from Huntington's disease. *Schizophr. Bull.*, **13**, 199–203.

Wing, J. (1983) Use and misuse of the PSE. *Br. J. Psychiatry*, **143**, 111–17.

Wing, J.K., Cooper, J.E. and Sartorius, N. (1974) *Measurement and Classification of Psychiatric Symptoms*. Cambridge University Press, Cambridge.

Zubin, J. (1985) Negative symptoms: are they indigenous to schizophrenia. *Schizophr. Bull.*, **11**, 461–70.

Zubin, J. and Spring, B. (1977) Vulnerability — a new view of schizophrenia. *J. Abnorm. Psychol.*, **86**, 103–26.

Chapter 11

Social skills assessment

KIM T. MUESER and MARGARET D. SAYERS

11.1 SOCIAL COMPETENCE AND SCHIZOPHRENIA

Markedly aberrant, dysfunctional social behaviour has long been recognized to be a core characteristic of schizophrenia. For example, the following description by Kraepelin (1919) illustrates his observation that the social behaviour of persons with schizophrenia is the most salient feature of the illness:

> The disease makes itself noticeable in by far the most striking way in the activities of the patients. Already in the beginning of the malady a change in their behavior invariably sets in. They become dreamy, shy of their fellow-beings, withdraw themselves, shut themselves up, do not greet their friends any more, stand about in corners, stare intently in front of them, give no answer, talk with themselves. (p. 96)

Pervasive impairments in social functioning are an integral feature of schizophrenia according to modern diagnostic criteria. The diagnosis of schizophrenia according to DSM–III-R criteria (American Psychiatric Association, 1987) requires the presence of no specific symptom (e.g. delusions or hallucinations), yet there must be evidence of a clear deterioration in functioning in the areas of social relationships, work, or self-care.

The problems in social functioning characteristic of schizophrenia are nowhere more evident than in the impoverished quality of life most patients experience (Lehman, 1983; Simpson *et al.*, 1989). Those patients in the community who do not live with relatives often reside in squalid living conditions in low income urban areas, and many are homeless (Drake *et al.*, 1989; Susser *et al.*, 1989). The difficulties patients have in social interactions impede their ability to effectively advocate for themselves thereby making it impossible to improve their living conditions, gain access to social and rehabilitative services, or resolve medication issues with the treating physician.

In addition to the inadequate living conditions persons with schizophrenia often bear as a consequence of their poor social competence, their social lives are often devoid of close, meaningful relationships. The development of schizophrenia with its inherent social impairments inevitably strains the social networks of patients (Hammer, 1986; Cohen and Kochanowicz, 1989). People with schizophrenia are often avoided by others, because of the stigma of mental illness (Mansouri and Dowell, 1989). Patients may be reluctant to re-establish old friendships, either due to lack of motivation or anxiety about how the other person will respond. Attempts to rekindle former relationships are often rebuffed because the person with schizophrenia does not seem to 'fit in' with his or her previous peer group. The peculiar behaviour of people with schizophrenia, their dull emotional responsivity, and lack of ordinary social graces act as barriers to continuing relationships and establishing new, supportive friendships. As a result, schizophrenia limits and weakens the social networks of patients, placing a heavy burden on the few persons involved, who are usually family members (Hatfield and Leafly, 1987).

It is apparent from clinical descriptions and diagnostic criteria that social functioning is impaired in schizophrenia. While positive symptoms such as delusions and hallucinations can interfere with social functioning, it has long been observed that impairments in social competence often precede the acute onset of the illness, and in some cases date back as far as childhood (Lewine *et al.*, 1978). Premorbid social competence has repeatedly been found to be an important predictor of illness outcome (Zigler and Glick, 1986) and of morbid social competence (Mueser *et al.*, 1990b). Whether premorbid social competence is an early sign of schizophrenia or is associated with a higher risk of developing the illness is not known (Pogue-Geile and Zubin, 1988). However, the extent of social contacts a patient has *after* the onset of schizophrenia is also predictive of the outcome of the illness (Rajkumar and Thara, 1989). This may reflect the role of social support systems in 'buffering' the negative effects of stress in patients, affording some protection from stress-induced relapses (Liberman and Mueser, 1989). The overriding importance of social competence to the development, course, and outcome of schizophrenia has led to efforts to assess and directly enhance patients' social functioning.

11.2 SOCIAL SKILLS: DEFINITIONS AND CONCEPTUAL ISSUES

Over the past decades the concept of social skill and the relationship between skill and social competence has been the topic of much scientific inquiry. Despite differences in scope, most definitions of social skills share the assumption that social skills are behaviours or cognitive-perceptual abilities that enable people to be 'effective' during interactions with others (i.e. to get their point across and achieve personal goals). Thus, social skills are a set of abilities that exist on a continuum of adequacy, depending upon how the goal of the interaction is defined. The overlap in conceptualizations of social skills is illustrated in the following definitions. Hersen and Bellack (1977) define social skill as the

> ability to express both positive and negative feelings in the interpersonal context without suffering consequent loss of reinforcement. Such skill is demonstrated in a large variety of interpersonal contexts and involves the coordinated delivery of appropriate verbal and non-verbal responses. In addition, the socially skilled individual is atuned to the realities of the situation and is aware when he is likely to be reinforced for his efforts. (p. 512)

Trower *et al.* (1978) also define social inadequacy or poor social skill primarily in terms of the ability of the person to favourably influence his social environment:

> A person can be regarded as socially inadequate if he is unable to affect the behaviour and feelings of others in the way that he intends and society accepts. Such a person will appear annoying, unforthcoming, uninteresting, cold, destructive, bad-tempered, isolated or inept, and will generally be unrewarding to others. (p. 2)

While Hersen and Bellack's (1977) and Trower *et al.*'s (1978) definitions convey the notion that social skill is required for effective social interactions, Liberman and Mueser's (1989) definition is tailored to the specific social problems common to schizophrenia:

Social skills can be defined as those interpersonal behaviors required to attain instrumental goals necessary for community survival and independence and to establish, maintain, and deepen supportive and socially rewarding relationships. (p. 797)

This definition clarifies the relationship between social skill and adequate social functioning in schizophrenia and suggests that such skills enable patients to function in the community.

The distinction between the instrumental and affiliative aspects of social skill introduced in Liberman and ˙Mueser's definition can be illustrated by examples of each type of situation. Instrumental social skills are relevant in discussing a possible medication side effect with the physician, seeking information regarding vocational rehabilitation programmes or asking for travel directions. Examples of affiliative goals include initiating a conversation with a new person at a day treatment/vocational programme, expressing affection, and asking someone out on a date. Naturally, some situations involve both instrumental and affiliative goals such as expressing appreciation to a relative for doing a chore (Liberman, 1982). Situations may also serve an instrumental need for one person and an affiliative need for another, such as when a person requests a friend to do an errand (Liberman, 1982). In sum, social skills can be broadly conceptualized as interpersonal abilities that promote adequate social functioning.

Defining social skills in terms of the intended and attained goals of social interactions provides a general framework for evaluating the extent of deficits in social functioning. Such a functional approach to social skills is not sufficient, however, to pinpoint specific impairments for the purposes of remediation. The topographical conceptualization of social skills focuses on the specific abilities that enable persons to achieve their interpersonal goals. While early definitions of social skill mainly emphasized overt behaviours, the importance of including perceptual and cognitive skills in the domain of social skill is now widely accepted.

Social interactions can be conceptualized as requiring three different types of skill corresponding to the perceptual, cognitive, and behavioural stages of social interaction. The first stage of social interaction requires *perceptual skills*, the ability to accurately recognize relevant social parameters, such as another person's facial expression, body language, relationship to the patient and situational factors. Persons with schizophrenia often lack the necessary perceptual skills to respond appropriately in a range of situations. In particular, they have been found to have impairments in recognizing others' emotions, particularly negative affect (Morrison *et al.*, 1988), which limits their ability to respond appropriately to others in conflict situations.

After accurately 'sizing up' the situation, *cognitive skills* are required for the person to determine the best course of action for achieving the interpersonal goal(s). The cognitive skills (also called 'information processing' or 'problem solving skills') necessary for effective interpersonal communication involve the ability to formulate a goal for the interaction, generate alternative responses, weigh the relative advantages and disadvantages of the responses, select a best response, and anticipate and plan for possible obstacles to successful implementation of the response. Abundant evidence indicates that persons with schizophrenia have impairments in cognitive skills (Nuechterlein and Dawson, 1984). Cognitive processes such as generating and evaluating different possible responses are assumed to occur in all social interactions, although the validity of this assumption has been questioned (Bellack *et al.*, 1989), and it is clear that much social interaction is spontaneous with little conscious cognitive planning.

The final stage of social interaction involves the actual implementation of the plan, the *behavioural skills* that are necessary to complete the interaction itself. Similar to the demonstrated impairments in perceptual and cognitive skills, ample evidence exists that persons with schizophrenia often have deficient interpersonal behaviours (Bellack *et al.*, 1990a,b).

A wide range of component behaviours are combined to produce effective social interactions. Behavioural skills can be sub-divided into four general categories, including speech form and content, paralinguistic features, nonverbal communication, and interactive balance. Each of these categories contains specific component behaviours which are the main targets for modification in social skills training programmes.

Speech form and content refers to what is actually said, the choice of words and the main thrust of the communication. Problems in thinking can interfere with the organization and structure of speech (Hotchkiss and Harvey, 1986). For example, a person with formal thought disorder may fail to supply adequate linkages between speech clauses (Rutter, 1985) or intermingle references to personal concerns or remote topics without explaining the connection (Harrow and Miller, 1980). Individuals with schizophrenia may also have few common experiences to talk about and little interest in such topics as current events.

Paralinguistic features are the vocal characteristics of speech, such as voice tone, loudness, and fluency that contribute to the quality and persuasiveness of communication. Voice tone is probably the most important paralinguistic feature since it conveys the speaker's affect and is often blunted or inappropriate in persons with schizophrenia.

Nonverbal communication includes everything the person does with his or her face or body, including behaviours such as facial expression and gestures. Similar to paralinguistic features, nonverbal communication plays an important role in providing the

'meaning' of a communication and may convey messages independent of verbal content. Facial expression is the most critical nonverbal behaviour for the communication of emotions, and similar to voice tone, it is frequently flattened or inappropriate in individuals with schizophrenia.

Interactive balance is necessary for maintaining the natural flow of a conversation, and it includes skills such as the timing of responses and the nature of verbal content in relation to the partner's responses. Long latencies of response are often experienced as awkward and uncomfortable for a conversational partner, whereas very brief latencies and interruptions can be annoying and interfere with the partner's train of thought and flow of speech. Table 11.1 summarizes the behavioural components of social skill.

11.2.1 ASSUMPTIONS OF THE SOCIAL SKILLS MODEL

The social skills approach to assessment and remediation of problematic interpersonal behaviour in schizophrenia involves several basic assumptions regarding the development and nature of social skill.

(1) **Social skills are learned abilities which can be taught to impaired individuals**. Skills are acquired through the combined influences of observation of appropriate role models, social reinforcement, and material reinforcement. The specific learned abilities required to interact effectively in different social situations comprise an individual's repertoire of social skills. Individuals who fail to demonstrate these skills in appropriate situations are described as having deficits in social skills. The origin of these deficits in schizophrenia is multiply determined, and may include the loss of skills through disuse or lack of motivation, the effects of positive symptoms, and changes in the environment that lead to contingencies which are less reinforcing for appropriate social behaviours (e.g. diminished social networks,

Table 11.1 Behavioural components of social skill

Behaviour		Definition and examples of appropriate and inappropriate behaviours
Content and verbal form	Appropriate	Using 'I' statements.
	Inappropriate	Calling physician by his/her first name.
Voice tone and pitch	Appropriate:	Inflection when asking a question.
	Inappropriate:	Voice tone inconsistent with affect.
Loudness	Appropriate:	Speaking at a volume which is audible and comfortable to the listener.
	Inappropriate:	Speaking softly in a noisy room.
Rate of speech	Appropriate:	Speaking more quickly than usual when excited or angry.
	Inappropriate:	Speaking very slowly with distracting pauses.
Duration of utterance	Appropriate:	Saying a complete thought and then stopping while other person(s) respond.
	Inappropriate:	Conveying too much information in one talk turn for others to respond to.
Fluency	Appropriate:	Speaking without repeating or skipping words.
	Inappropriate:	Speech dysfluencies such as stammering.
Gaze	Appropriate:	Speaker looking at listener periodically while talking.
	Inappropriate:	Staring too long.
Proximity	Appropriate	18 inches – 4 feet for an informal conversation.
	Inappropriate:	<18 inches or >4 feet for an informal conversation.
Orientation	Appropriate:	Body positioned toward the other person(s) involved in the interaction.
	Inappropriate:	Turning away from the other person(s) involved in the interaction.
Gestures	Appropriate:	Raising three fingers for emphasis while saying, ''There are three main points.''
	Inappropriate:	Hand-wringing or nail biting during a social encounter (self-oriented gestures).
Body language	Appropriate:	Slow and deliberate head nods while listening to another person.
	Inappropriate:	Shaking leg or foot to indicate impatience with another person.
Affect	Appropriate:	Affect which is consistent with verbal content such as angry affect when expressing anger.
	Inappropriate:	Affect which is inconsistent with verbal content such as smiling when expressing anger, or affect which is non-expressive, muted.
Posture	Appropriate:	Leaning forward when seated to indicate interest in what another person is saying.
	Inappropriate:	Slouching in chair or drooping head suggests disinterest.
Appearance	Appropriate:	Maintaining good hygiene and dressing neatly.
	Inappropriate:	Unkempt clothing, disheveled hair, poor hygiene.
Meshing	Appropriate:	Pausing briefly before responding to another's question or statement.
	Inappropriate:	Pausing too long before responding to another's utterance.
Balance of time	Appropriate:	Roughly equal amount of talking among all talk parties in the interaction.
	Inappropriate:	One person doing most or very little of the talking compared to the other person.
Self-disclosure	Appropriate:	High disclosure to a few close persons and medium disclosure to others.
	Inappropriate:	Either high or low disclosure to virtually everyone.
Social reinforcement	Appropriate:	Occasional head nods and saying 'I see' while another person is speaking.
	Inappropriate:	Failure to indicate interest in what another person is saying.

socially impoverished settings such as psychiatric hopsitals for the chronically mentally ill).

(2) **Social skills are situationally specific**. The appropriateness of social behaviour depends in part on the nature of the environmental context in which it occurs. Few social behaviours are appropriate in all situations. The wide range of different factors governing the rules of social behaviour include the focus of the interaction, the gender of participants, their degree of familiarity and the relationship between two people, the number of people present, the setting, time and location. While people are sometimes described as either socially 'skilled' or 'unskilled, the situational variability of social behaviour precludes being either socially skilled in all situations or unskilled in all situations. For this reason, social performance must be assessed across a variety of different situations.

(3) **Social skills facilitate but do not ensure social competence**. Social skills are defined as the specific perceptual, cognitive, and behavioural abilities that maximize an individual's ability to achieve instrumental and affiliative goals in interpersonal encounters. Social competence, on the other hand, is the actual attainment or the ability to attain these goals, and hence is the net result of the person's social skills, non-skill factors (e.g. anxiety), and the environment. For example, poor motivation is a common negative symptom of schizophrenia which may inhibit the use of social skills present in the person's behavioural repertoire, thereby resulting in poor social competence.

(4) **Social skills play a role in the social functioning and course of schizophrenia**. The surge of interest in social skills training is based on the assumption that enhanced social skills will improve the prognosis of schizophrenia. Donahoe and Driesenga (1988) provide a two-part rationale for social skills training: (a) improving the quality of life and (b) reducing the risk of symptom exacerbations (relapses). Social skills are assumed to be a critical determinant of quality of life since they enable patients to advocate for themselves and maintain interpersonal relationships. Deficits in social skills are also believed to underlie at least some of these social impairments seen in people with schizophrenia.

11.3 FUNDAMENTALS OF SOCIAL SKILLS ASSESSMENT

The assessment of social skills, like other forms of behavioural assessment, is an on-going process that occurs throughout therapy and serves to continuously guide the clinician in planning and implementing the intervention. Assessment serves three primary functions in remediating the social impairments of schizophrenia. First, rigorous assessments of social skill are necessary to identify the specific behavioural deficits and excesses that are targeted for modification in social skills training. Second, assessments conducted during and after skills training interventions are vital to evaluating the impact of training on the *acquisition* (i.e., learning) *maintenance* (i.e., durability over time), and *generalization* of social skill (i.e., transfer of skills from trained situations to untrained ones). Third, changes in social skill following training need to be assessed in order to evaluate the hypothesized functional relationship between social skill and illness, including social adjustment, negative symptoms, and risk of relapse. Changes in skill that are correlated with or predictive of improvements in any of these specific domains of functioning would support the role of social skill in mediating the social functioning and course of schizophrenia. If changes in skill are observed without improvements in the course of the illness, the clinician may need to examine factors that could account for the discrepancy, such as the functional relevance of the targeted skills, medication non-compliance, alcohol or substance abuse (Mueser *et al.*, 1990b), unmitigated negative ambient emotion (e.g., family expressed emotion), a socially unreinforcing and impoverished environment, or frequent and disruptive life events.

In this chapter we focus on the assessment of social skills *per se*, that is the perceptual cognitive, and behavioural skills necessary for effective social interactions. We do not address procedures for the assessment of a broad range of phenomena that influence and are influenced by social behaviour, such as affect, cognition, imagery, and sensations. Liberman (1982) has stressed the importance of conducting a multi-modal assessment (Lazarus, 1981) when evaluating social skill, and Shepherd (1984) has comprehensively reviewed strategies for assessing cognitions related to social situations. While a multi-modal approach to assessment is important for developing a comprehensive understanding of patients' overall psychosocial functioning, it is beyond the scope of this chapter.

The assessment of social skills can be organized around four questions.

1. **In what areas do interpersonal dysfunctions occur?** The social performance of schizophrenic patients may be impaired in a wide range of different content areas, as outlined in Table 11.2. Within each general content area, several specific skills are also identified. For example, the general content area of 'basic conversational skills' can be broken down into several specific skills, including initiating, maintaining, and ending conversations. Each specific skill can be further divided into component skills, and it is the teaching of these components that is the main focus of social skills training. Table 11.3 provides examples of the component behaviours for two skills. Naturally, any framework that categorizes the range of possible adaptive social behaviours is somewhat arbitrary. However, there is much overlap between the skill areas identified in Table 11.2 and social skills training programmes developed by other clinical researchers (Trower *et al.*, 1978; Hargie and McCartan, 1986).

Table 11.2 General content areas and specific skills for the assessment of social skills

General content area	Specific skills
Basic conversational skills	Starting, maintaining, and ending conversations Listening skills Giving opinions and information Asking questions
Intermediate/advanced conversational skills	Self-disclosure Recognizing and expressing emotions Changing topics
Positive assertion	Expressing positive feelings Making requests Making apologies
Negative assertion	Refusing unreasonable requests Resisting persuasion Expressing disapproval and annoyance
Conflict resolution	Compromise and negotiation Responding to criticisms
Medication management	Obtaining information about medication and side effects Talking with physicians about medication and side effects Negotiating medication issues (e.g. side effects)
Friendship and dating	Enhancing physical attractiveness Giving and receiving compliments Expressing affection Finding activities to do together Asking for a date Responding to a date request
Social problem solving	Defining the problem Generating possible solutions Evaluating solution(s) Choosing the best solution(s) Planning to implement the solutions
Vocational skills	Job interviewing Job maintenance

Table 11.3 Examples of component content skills

Starting a conversation
1. Choose the right time and place.
2. Introduce yourself or greet the person you wish to talk to (e.g., smile and say 'Hello *name*').
3. Make small talk (e.g., about the weather, sports, something in the immediate environment).
4. Judge whether the other person is listening or interested.

Negotiating medication issues
1. Choose an appropriate time and place.
2. Greet the doctor in a pleasant manner.
3. Describe problem with medication in specific terms.
4. Make a request about a change in the medication, such as change in dose, change in type, or change in schedule.
5. Negotiate the details of medication changes.
6. Thank doctor for his or her help.

2. **Are the interpersonal dysfunctions related to deficits in social skill?** There is no definitive test that can determine whether a social impairment is caused by poor social skill or by some other factor. In general, social skill problems are situationally specific and relatively stable over time. Hence, global impairments in social skill or deficits that spontaneously improve may reflect the influence of non-skill factors on social performance. Some of these factors primarily influence social performance but not social skill (e.g. lack of social reinforcement), while other factors influence both social skill *and* social performance (e.g. blunted affect). Evaluating the role of these factors is necessary in order to determine whether social performance can be improved through methods other than social skills training (e.g. modifying medication). In some cases, social skills training may be the most effective intervention for improving skill deficits that are secondary to other factors such as negative symptoms (Wixted *et al.*, 1988).

Environmental factors. Impoverished, socially unreinforcing environments can suppress effective social behaviours even when patients have the necessary skills in their behavioural repertoires (Wing and Freundenberg, 1961). Attending to and modifying environmental constraints may result in spontaneous improvements in social performance and is a prerequisite for effective social skills training.

Illness factors. A wide range of factors related to schizophrenia can impair social skills and social performance, including chronicity, symptom exacerbations, and symptomatology. The relationship between chronicity of the illness and social skill deficits is unclear. More chronic, 'burned out' patients are often described as having pronounced deficits in social skill. However, we have found that briefly hospitalized schizophrenic patients living in the community had slightly *better* social skills when they were older and had a longer illness duration (Mueser *et al.*, 1990b). These findings appear consistent with evidence from longitudinal studies showing gradual improvements in the severity of the illness over a patient's lifetime (Ciompi, 1980).

Symptom exacerbations can temporarily impair social skills which subsequently improve as symptoms abate. Little research has examined directly the influence of symptom relapses on social skill. A longitudinal study in which social skills were assessed during a hospitalization and one year later (Mueser *et al.*, 1991) demonstrated modest improvements in some dimensions of social skill (meshing, duration of utterance, affect), but not others (gaze, verbal content, overall social skill).

Symptoms can have a profound impact on patients' social performance and social skill. Anecdotal evidence abounds that positive symptoms can impair social performance, mainly because of incomprehensible, bizarre, or unacceptable behaviours. However, positive symptoms have *not* been found to be related to impairments in social skill (Bellack *et al.*, 1990b; Mueser *et al.*, 1990b), suggesting that delusions and hallucinations do not influence social competence *per se*, but that they may alter the nature of patient's interpersonal goals. Negative symptoms, on the other hand, are strongly related to both social performance and social skills (Bellack *et al.*, 1990). Apathy can prevent patients from using skills in their behavioural repertoires, leading to poor social performance in the absence of skill deficits. Blunted affect in particular is correlated with impairments in non-verbal measures of social skill, since the symptom is defined in terms of the ability to communicate affect through non-verbal and paralinguistic channels. Despite the overlap between negative symptoms and social skills deficits, the constructs are not isomorphic. In a cluster analysis, negative symptom patients were distinguishable from patients with deficits in social skills (Morrison *et al.*, 1990).

Medication side effects. Neuroleptic medications can cause a wide range of side effects that impair social performance and skills. Akinesia, also referred to as 'akinetic depression' (Van Puttan and May, 1978), is a poorly understood extrapyramidal side effect characterized by sedation, a 'mask-like' face, lack of gestures and voice intonation, and gait abnormalities. Akinesia is difficult to assess reliably due to differences in available rating scales, and it is hard to distinguish from negative symptoms, social skill deficits, and depression (deLeon and Simpson, 1990) Akathisia, or motor restlessness, is more readily measured, and may also impair social skill or performance due to patients' inability to sit still and their anxious appearance. Modifying the patient's medication regimen, either by altering the dose, introducing anticholinergic medication, or switching the class of neuroleptic, may be necessary to distinguish between skill deficits and social impairments that are secondary to neuroleptic side effects.

Negative affective states. Depression, anxiety, and anger can all influence social skills in the general population. In our research on schizophrenia, we have not found that patients with negative affective states have impaired

social skills (Mueser *et al.*, 1990b). However, individual changes in mood may nevertheless influence skill and should be included in any comprehensive assessment.

Demographic characteristics. Few studies have examined the relationship between demographic characteristics and social skill or performance in schizophrenia. In our research, both age and gender have been related to social skill in individuals with schizophrenia, but not in affective disorder patients or non-patient controls. Females with schizophrenia tend to have better social skills than males (Mueser *et al.*, 1990a); young males appear to have the most impaired social skills, consistent with the stereotype of the young, chronic mental patient (Pepper *et al.*, 1981).

(3) **Under what conditions does the skill deficit occur?** In order to tailor skills training to the specific deficits of the patients, the relevant situations they face must be assessed. For example, patients with schizophrenia tend to be unassertive, but this can vary depending on the gender and familiarity of the other person and whether positive or negative feelings are being expressed (Eisler *et al.*, 1975; Hersen *et al.*, 1978). Research on expressed emotion suggests that individuals with schizophrenia have difficulty dealing with criticism and anger from family members (Koenigsberg and Handley, 1986), but it is not known whether patients also have difficulty with negative affect from others.

(4) **How can the specific skills deficits best be described?** Social skill consists of a variety of different behavioural components (Table 11.1). Patients will differ in the actual pattern of deficits they display, with some showing a greater need for training in speech content, and others requiring more training in non-verbal or paralinguistic skills. Specifying the precise pattern of deficits for the individual is essential for determining which behaviours to target in skills training. Specific assessment requires direct observation of behaviour since patients and significant others are generally not able to describe these problems in sufficient detail.

11.4 PROCEDURES FOR ASSESSING SOCIAL SKILL

A variety of different strategies are available for the assessment of social skill, including interviews, self-report questionnaires, naturalistic observations and role play tests. Each method has its advantages and disadvantages, so that it is necessary to employ multiple assessment strategies in order to obtain a comprehensive picture of patients' social assets and deficits. In general, the assessment of social skills procedes from obtaining general information about areas of social dysfunction to more specific information concerning the exact nature of the skills deficit. A first step in identifying social problems might be to read medical records. Interviews with patients and significant others, as well as self-report measures can provide additional information. Finally, more specific data can be gathered through naturalistic observations and role play tests. The utility of interviews, self-reports, naturalistic observation, and role play tests for assessing social skill are discussed next.

11.4.1 INTERVIEWS

Interviews with patients and others who know the patient well yield valuable information regarding problem areas in social functioning. While some patients are unable to describe specific problems or deny that they have problems, interviews may still provide general information about social problems. The directly observable behaviour of the patient during the interview is also a useful source of data about social skills (i.e. the appropriateness of verbal content, specific non-verbal behaviours, paralinguistic features, interactive balance skills).

Information gathered from staff members, relatives, and significant others regarding patients' social behaviours is particularly important when the patient cannot provide reliable information. Structured or semi-structured interviews are useful for identifying general problem areas in social functioning: examples are the Katz Adjustment Scale (Katz and Lyerly, 1963), the Structured and Scaled Interview to Assess Maladjustment (Gurland *et al.*, 1972), the Social Adjustment Scale (Schooler *et al.*, 1978), the Social Behaviour Assessment Schedule (Platt *et al.*, 1980), and the Social Behaviour Schedule (SBS) (Wykes and Sturt, 1986). Interviewing others may also reveal whether the patient displays certain problem behaviours that suggest skill deficits, such as speaking in a monotone, poor eye contact, nagging or begging, making unreasonable demands, frequently interrupting others, rambling on with delusional or irrelevant statements, rarely expressing personal needs, frequent crying, or difficulty initiating or maintaining simple conversations.

11.4.2 SELF-REPORT

Self-report measures do not have well-established validity for assessing social skill in schizophrenia. The reliability of self-report measures is often questionable (Bellack and Hersen, 1977; Liberman, 1982) and can be influenced by characteristics of the illness such as attentional impairments, comprehension problems and symptoms. There are also psychometric problems with self-report measures. These instruments are usually standardized on the general population rather than the schizophrenic population, they often fail to adequately sample relevant domains to this population, and they may be insensitive to change following interventions. Finally, individuals with schizophrenia often find questionnaires confusing or boring, resulting in a high refusal rate or inaccurate reporting. On the other hand, self-report questionnaires have definite advantages since they are easy to administer and score. Questionnaires for the assessment of social skill have been employed with some success in patients with schizophrenia, particularly those tapping assertiveness and social anxiety, such as the Social Anxiety and Distress Scale (Watson and Friend, 1969), the Fear of Negative Evaluation Scale (Watson and Friend, 1969), the Rathus Assertiveness Schedule (Rathus, 1973), the Interpersonal Situation Inventory (Goldsmith and McFall, 1975), the Social Reaction Inventory – Revised (Curran *et al.*, 1980), and the Independent Living Skills Survey (Wallace, 1986). See Wallace (1986) for a detailed discussion of instruments for evaulating functioning in the community.

11.4.3 NATURALISTIC OBSERVATION

Once situations have been identified in which deficits in social skill may be present, more systematic behavioural assessment can be conducted through naturalistic observation and role play tests. Naturalistic observation has inherent limitations. First, a wide range of spontaneous interaction is not readily observable by an independent person, and conducting a rigorous assessment of different situations can be time-comsuming and labour-intensive. In addition, the nature of naturalistic observation precludes the ability to control extraneous situational factors that may affect skill, making it more difficult to standardize the measure and rendering the measure less sensitive to changes resulting from interventions. Last, naturalistic observations are easily obtained only in situations in which the clinician has access to patients in a variety of situations, such as inpatient or residential settings.

There are, however, many advantages to using naturalistic observations. The ecological validity of naturalistic observations is generally high, especially when relevant situations are selected. In addition, direct observation does not constrain the range of possible behaviour that can be evaluated, since extended inter-

actions may be observed. Also, naturalistic observations provide unique information about how *others* respond to the patient in a social situation, as well as the interactive balance skills of the patient (e.g. meshing, use of social reinforcers, appropriateness of self-disclosures). Finally, direct observation affords a more precise assessment of social skill, a necessary ingredient for targeting specific behaviours for modification in social skills training.

A variety of different standardized systems have been developed for the naturalistic observation of inpatient behaviour, including the Observational Record of Inpatient Behaviour (Rosen, 1988) and the Time Sample Behaviour Checklist (Paul and Lentz, 1977). Despite the high inter-rater reliabilities achieved by these systems through the use of time-sampled observations (i.e. behaviours are observed for a brief time interval, recorded on an occurrence/non-occurrence basis, and then observed again), they suffer from problems of high cost and low relevance (Bellack and Mueser, 1990). Extensive training of observers is necesssary, and the multiple observations of patients on a daily basis requires substantial staff time. The problem of low relevance of these systems stems from the lack of data pertaining to the relationships between these behavioural observations and measures of social adjustment, clinical variables, and outcome. In particular, these systems do not focus on actual social skills, but rather on discrete behaviours which may or may not reflect domains of social skill.

In most cases, some degree of naturalistic observation of patients' social skills is possible and is a useful complement to other sources of information regarding patient functioning. However, to assess skills in the relevant social situations, the observations must be tailored to the specific problem. Usually this means that clinicians must develop their own observational measures to assess the skill area targeted for modification. An example of a naturalistic observation measure designed for the assessment of social skills in severely disabled schizophrenic patients, the Social Interaction Schedule (Liberman *et al.*, 1989) is provided in Appendix 11.A.

A different approach to naturalistic observations that has been used is staged social interactions with the patient in the natural environment without the patient's prior knowledge. For example, a confederate approaches a patient at the day treatment programme and makes an unreasonable demand (negative assertion) or initiates a conversation (conversational skill). This approach has some advantages over truly naturalistic observations since the interaction can be tightly controlled by the confederate's responses, but it is fraught with ethical problems due to its deceptive nature. Hence, staged interactions in patients' natural environments are rarely employed.

11.4.4 ROLE PLAY ASSESSMENTS

The main vehicle for assessing social skills in schizophrenia is the role play, a structured simulated social interaction with a confederate in which the patient interacts as he or she ordinarily would in such a situation in the 'real world'. Because role plays allow for a more fine-grained assessment of social skills than other methods, they are usually the final step in assessment before development of individual social skills training regimens. Role playing is also used throughout the skills training process, since behavioural rehearsal is an important active ingredient in acquiring new social skills.

The main advantages of role plays over other assessment techniques are that extraneous situational factors can be controlled, the patient's behaviour can be recorded for subsequent rating of global social skills and specific component behaviours, and the assessments are cost effective. A critical feature of role plays is that the assessment can be standardized, permitting the use of multiple assessments to objectively evaluate the impact of training on social skills. Like any analogue measure, role plays have disadvantages. Patients usually perform more skillfully in role plays than when faced with comparable situations in the natural environment since role plays may not generate high levels of negative effect and do not have real consequences. Conversely the testing situation can evoke anxiety not usually present in the patient's encounters, resulting in poorer performance than would occur in the natural environment. The differences between skill in simulated situations compared to real situations may be important for differentiating *performance deficits* from *skills deficits*. Both types of problems are amenable to social skills training.

The validity of role play tests has been a topic of much debate over the past 15 years. The central issue in the debate has been the consistency between patient behaviour in role play assessments and in the natural environment. Some studies failed to find significant correlations between paralinguistic and non-verbal behaviours observed during role plays and observations made in more naturalistic settings (Bellack, 1979). Other investigations have reported that skill during role plays *is* related to social skill in natural interactions (Merluzzi and Biever, 1987), and there is an extensive literature documenting that role plays are sensitive to the effects of social skills training (Donahoe and Dreisenga, 1988). Furthermore, evidence from our laboratory indicates that role play performances among psychiatric patients is a strong predictor of a range of different social behaviours, including behaviour observed during family interactions and interview measures of social adjustment and quality of life (Bellack *et al.*, 1990a). Taken together, the data indicate that role plays provide a valid measure of patients' social skills and functioning in the natural environment.

All role plays, whether they are conducted to evaluate the effects of skills training or in a group as a part of the training process, share a set of features: (1) identifying a relevant situation for assessment; (2) informing the patient about the role play procedures; (3) providing a description of the situation and ensuring that it is plausible and understood by the patient; (4) engaging the patient in a role play with a confederate, either for a structured brief interaction or for a more open-ended interaction; and (5) evaluating the patient's social skill performance.

A number of different standarized role play tests have been developed, including the Behavioural Assertiveness Test – Revised (Eisler *et al.*, 1975), the Interpersonal Situation Inventory (Goldsmith and McFall, 1975), the Social Interaction Test (Trower *et al.*, 1978), and the Simulated Social Interaction Test (Monti *et al.*, 1980). However, these standardized tests are often not applicable to specific situations faced by patients or the problem areas that are targeted for modification. In most cases role plays must be developed by the clinician to assess the problem areas of the specific patients who will be treated. We will briefly address some of the issues involved in Designing and conducting role play assessments. The focus here is on assessments that are conducted outside of social skills training groups for the purposes of identifying suitable behavioural targets and evaluating the effects of training. We will assume that the role play interactions are video- or audiotaped for subsequent behavioural ratings. The reader is referred to Bellack (1983), and Liberman *et al.* (1989) for a more extensive description of procedures for conducting role play assessments.

11.4.4.1 Selecting relevant situations for assessment

Situations used in role plays should be as similar as possible to the real-life situations that patients frequently encounter. Different role plays, like natural social interactions, will evoke a range of different behaviours from the same person. In order to obtain a more reliable assessment of social skill it is advisable to develop several role play situations for each problem area, with minor differences between them (e.g. sex of the confederate, location, who initiates the interaction).

11.4.4.2 Instructing patients about the role play test

Patients with schizophrenia have long been observed to be sensitive to criticism (Koenigsberg and Handley 1986). For this reason it is important that efforts be made to help patients feel as relaxed as possible in the testing situation. This can be aided by ensuring their physical comfort in the testing situation (e.g. allowing rest breaks, comfortable seating arrangements, unobtrusive placing of recording devices. Procedures should be described in a relaxed manner with attention paid to patients' concerns or reservations. The assessor explains that the purpose of the assessment is not to compare the patient with others, but to identify which social situations the person does well in and which situations are more difficult. To enlist patients' cooperation, it is crucial that they understand how role play assessments will help them progress towards their personal goals.

The specific instructions depend on the purpose of the assessment. It is vital that the instructions describe the entire role play procedure, and that they allow ample opportunity for the patient to ask questions. An example of an instructional set we use for conducting role play assessments of patients' social skills in managing conflict situations is provided below. The assessment is conducted with the patient by two staff members, a narrator and a confederate. The narrator speaks:

The purpose of this procedure is to find out how you react to situations that typically occur on a day-to-day basis. We will do this by role playing these situations, in other words, by acting them out with another person — that will be Jane.

Jane will play the part of either your mother or a friend, and you should pretend you are really in the situation with her. Some of the situations will involve conflicts or disagreements and these of course are only imaginary, but you should respond as if you were actually in that situation with your mother or with a friend.

The procedure will be as follows: First, you will read the situation which is typed on a card. Be sure to read it carefully and try to imagine that you are actually in that situation. At that point, I will ask you who Jane will be acting the part of — your mother or a friend — just to make sure it is clear who she is pretending to be. Then I will read a description of that same scene; be sure to listen carefully as the situation is described.

After you have familiarized yourself with the scene by reading the card and hearing the description, you and Jane will act out the situation. Jane will say something to you and you should respond to continue the conversation. Please keep the conversation going back and forth between you and Jane until I tell you when to stop. You should respond as if you were actually in that situation with a friend or your mother — that's the part Jane will be playing. You will be playing yourself, responding as if the situation were really occurring.

Do you understand the procedure? Any questions? Let's do a couple of practice scenes first so you can see how they go.

11.4.4.3 Describing the role play situations

When role play situations have been selected, scenarios describing each situation need to be developed. Scenarios should be relatively brief, ranging from two to five sentences. Scenarios should clearly establish; (a) the location; (b) the relationship between the patient and the confederate (e.g. stranger, acquaintance, relative, therapist); (c) the patient's goal in the interaction (e.g. to start a conversation); and (d) who initiates the role play. Because patients often have difficulty attending to instructions and descriptions of situations, periodically checking on the patient's understanding can help keep him or her on task. It is also useful to evaluate the plausibility of the situation by asking whether the person can imagine himself or herself in the situation. When a scenario is difficult to imagine and seems unrealistic, minor changes can be made to create a more plausible situation. Table 11.4. contains two examples of role play scenarios.

Table 11.4 Sample scenarios for role play assessments

Conversational skills
You have been working at a new job for the past week. So far, none of your new co-workers has approached you or said anything to you. Today, as you are punching in at the time clock, a woman who works in your department arrives to punch in. She says, 'Hi, you're new here, aren't you?'

Medication issues
Your doctor has decided that it would be better for you to take injectable medication. You do not like the idea of getting shots at all, but would like to know more about the benefits of taking the medication by injection. You are determined to make an informed decision instead of simply agreeing to the change. Today, during your appointment, your doctor says, 'So from now on you'll be getting your medication through injections, right?'

11.4.4.4 Determining the length of the role plays

The most important facet of the actual interaction between the patient and confederate is determining in advance the length of the

Table 11.5 Example of standardized confederate responses for a role play test

---

Negative assertion

You are in a restaurant and have just finished your meal. The waiter brings your check and you notice he has *overcharged* you one dollar.

He says:

1. 'Thank you, please come again.'

Non-compliance

2. 'No, I don't think so.'
3. 'I usually don't make mistakes.'

Compliance

2. 'It's been a pleasure to serve you.'
3. 'You can pay the cashier on your way out.'

---

encounter. Brief and extended role plays each have their advantages and drawbacks, and choosing the length of the encounter depends in large part on the problem area to be assessed. Very brief role plays requiring only a single response from the patient have been found to have poor generalizability and should be avoided. It is easier to standardize confederate responses in brief role plays with two to four patient responses. Also, brief role plays are easier to rate, making them more convenient as research tools than longer interactions. Table 11.5 illustrates how the confederate's responses can be standardized in a brief role play so that they are contingent upon what the patient says.

The main disadvantage of brief role plays is that they have limited generalizability, since few social encounters last for only a few verbal exchanges.

In contrast to brief role plays, extended interactions offer a more realistic glimpse of the patient's social skills. Patients often respond more favourably to extended interactions which seem more natural and give more time to adjust to the situation. Longer role plays are more useful for the assessment of certain problem areas (e.g. maintaining conversations, conflict resolution) than others (e.g. starting conversations, assertiveness). On the other hand, the use of extended role play interactions also has inherent limitations. Once an interaction lasts

longer than a few exchanges, it becomes exceedingly difficult to standardize the confederate's behaviour and to replicate the role play assessment with different patients and over time. Rating longer role plays is also more difficult, since the scoring system must be sensitive to a broader range of possible behaviours.

11.4.4.5 Scoring behaviours

Which behaviours should be rated and at what level of specificity is an important issue and depends partly on the resources available to the clinician and on the nature of the planned intervention. In general, it is preferable to obtain ratings that tap the range of possible behavioural skills, including verbal content, non-verbal and paralinguistic elements, and interactive balance. Molecular ratings of specific behavioural components can usually be made reliably when multiple ratings are made over brief time intervals (e.g. 15 or 30 second intervals). While it is impractical to rate every possible kind of behaviour, a selection of the most relevant behaviours can be made based on the impairments most commonly present in schizophrenic patients. For example, we have found it useful to rate the following molecular behaviours in our assessments of social skill in schizophrenia: gaze (nonverbal), affect (nonverbal and paralinguistic behaviours rated together), length of utterance (paralinguistic), meshing (interactive balance), and appropriateness of verbal content.

The relative merits of molecular versus global ratings of social skill have been the topic of much debate (Curran, 1979; Bellack, 1983; Curran *et al.*, 1984; Becker and Heimberg, 1988). The main advantages of molecular ratings is that they are easier to rate reliably, and they provide information regarding the performance of specific behaviours. The latter advantage is especially important since social skills training focuses on improving specific behavioural competencies. On the other hand, molecular ratings are much more time-consuming than global ratings, and the validity of molecular ratings is questionable, as it is unclear which exact behaviours actually influence social skill and competence. Conversely, the advantages of global ratings are that they are easily obtained and have more face validity and external validity (Wessberg *et al.*, 1981; McNamara and Blumer, 1982). However, they provide less information regarding suitable behavioural targets for modification via social skills training. We prefer to obtain both molecular and global ratings of social skill. We have found that global ratings of social skill are highly correlated with the composite of molecular ratings, but that the latter tend to be more sensitive to minor changes in patients' role play performance (Mueser *et al.*, 1991a).

Practical considerations play a key role in the choice of a scoring format. Two general scoring formats are possible: frequency counts and Likert scale ratings. Frequency counts are too time-consuming or meaningless for many types of behaviour. However, when specific components of an interaction can be identified, particularly verbal content components, frequency counts can be made of the different components and summed to form a measure of social appropriateness. Table 11.6 illustrates

Table 11.6 Sample coding form for component behaviours

Directions: Check to indicate successful completion of the step. Leave blank if the step was omitted.

Role Play #1: Compromise and negotiation
  1. Look at the person _____
  2. Explaining your viewpoint _____
  3. Listen to the other's viewpoint and repeat it back _____
  4. Suggest a compromise _____

Role Play #2: Expressing negative feelings
  1. Look at the person _____
  2. Speak calmly and firmly _____
  3. Tell the person what upset you _____
  4. Tell how it made you feel _____
  5. Suggest how to prevent it from happening in the future _____

Table 11.8 A Likert scale used to rate assertiveness

+ --------	+ --------	+ --------	+ -------	+
1	2	3	4	5
Very unassertive	Somewhat unassertive	Neither unassertive nor assertive	Somewhat assertive	Very assertive

Definition: The ability to stand up for one's rights and achieve one's goals in social situations. The assertive individual can make requests and express feelings. He or she is not passive and compliant when treated inappropriately or imposed upon. The assertive individual can be firm and insistent but can also compromise when necessary. Assertiveness should not be confused with hostility; it employs reason and logic, not threats or anger. Appropriate assertion is usually characterized by clear statements about what one wants or does not want without apologies or disclaimers, the use of 'I' statements, and firm voice tone without dysfluencies.

---

two rating forms we use for the assessment of specific behavioural components taught in our skills module on conflict resolution (Douglas and Mueser, 1990; Mueser *et al.*, 1990c).

Likert-type rating scales ranging from three to ten points can be used for global ratings of skills such as assertiveness, overall social skill, appropriateness of voice tone, and affect. Raters can learn to use these scales reliably without extensive training, although care must be taken in research studies to ensure that the entire range of points is used. The scales are also vulnerable to 'halo' effects when several different behaviours are rated by the same judge for the same patient. While these scales are useful for describing how socially appropriate a behaviour is, they fail to adequately describe the precise nature of the skill impairment. Table 11.7 illustrates the Likert scale for the rating of assertiveness and affective tone.

Most behaviours of interest occur on a continuum, with intermediate responses being the most appropriate. For example, speech duration may be too short or too long; voice volume can be too soft or too loud; in a situation requiring negative assertion skills, the response can be meek and ineffectual or hostile and nasty. In order to measure the specific nature of social skill deficits, bidirectional scoring

Social skills assessment

methods can be used. Bidirectional ratings preserve information regarding the patient's idiosyncratic responses, while they can be collapsed to reflect overall appropriateness. The reliability of bidirectional scoring systems can be enhanced by the use of behaviourally anchored definitions (Bellack, 1983). Examples of bidirectional scales are in Table 11.8.

Table 11.8 Examples of bidirectional scoring scales

Gaze — Eye contact rated only when subject is speaking
O Normal gaze frequency and pattern.
A 1. Infrequent looking. Unrewarding.
   2. Almost no looking. Extreme avoidance. Very unrewarding.
B 1. Excessive or frequent looking. Unpleasant.
   2. Stares almost continually. Very unpleasant.

Meshing — Turn taking or flow of speech from one speaker to the other
O Normal meshing.
A 1. Response noticeably delayed. Unpleasant or uncomfortable (or one good, one delayed).
   2. Response extremely delayed. Extremely uncomfortable. Awkward.
B 1. Interruptions noticeably frequent or long. Annoying.
   2. Interruptions extremely frequent or long. Very annoying.

The question of the validity of skill ratings is at the very heart of social skills assessment. There are two general approaches to establishing the validity of social skill ratings. First, the appropriateness of social skills assessed during a role play test can be rated by untrained persons drawn from the community. These ratings can be used to evaluate the social skill of patients before and after social skills training, or to compare with ratings made by trained raters (Hansen *et al.*, 1988; Charisou *et al.*, 1989). This approach can be used to support the generalizability of social skill ratings made by trained judges to the general population of untrained persons. Of course, such ratings do not reflect whether the patients actually *use*

the skills in their natural environment or if they are related to patients' social competence. The second approach to validation is to examine the correspondence between social skills measured in the role play and measures of social functioning or behaviour in the environment (Bellack *et al.*, 1990a). Failure to identify and measure patients' social competence in their natural environment will always leave doubt as to whether the skills elicited and rated in role plays are truly relevant to patients' social functioning.

11.5 ASSESSMENT OF PERCEPTUAL AND COGNITIVE SKILLS

Although social perception and cognitive or information processing skills are widely accepted to be impaired in schizophrenia (Morrison *et al.*, 1988; Bellack *et al.*, 1989), standardized tests for the clinical assessment of these skills are not yet available. For this reason, these skills are not usually assessed during role play tests that are conducted before and after patients' participation in social skills training groups. During the course of social skills training, however, perceptual and cognitive skills can be routinely assessed and trained by asking the patient relevant questions during role plays. The social perception questions aim to evaluate whether the patient is able to attend to and accurately perceive problem situations and social cues. The cognitive skill questions tap the patient's ability to identify suitable responses in a situation and to anticipate their probable consequences. Wallace and Liberman (Wallace *et al.*, 1980; Liberman *et al.*, 1989) developed a set of questions to assess perceptual and cognitive skills during social skills training. Perceptual skills can be assessed by asking questions such as: 'What was _____ feeling?'; 'What was your short-term goal?'; and 'What was your long-term goal?' Cognitive skills can be assessed by asking questions such as 'If you did _____, what would the other person feel?'; 'Would doing _____ achieve your short/long-term goal(s)?'; 'What else could you do that might help you achieve your goal?'; and 'Would you use that alternative and why?' These questions can be asked before and after role plays, and deficits in perceptual and cognitive skills can be trained by strategies such as focusing the patient's attention, prompting correct responses, modelling, reinforcing correct answers, and engaging in problem solving exercises.

Combining the behavioural assessment of social skills with on-going assessment and training in perceptual and cognitive skills provides a comprehensive approach to the identification and remediation of deficits in social functioning.

REFERENCES

American Psychiatric Association (1987) *Diagnostic and Statistical Manual of Mental Disorders (3rd ed. revised)*. Washington, DC.

Becker, R.E. and Heimberg, R.G. (1988) Assessment of social skills. In *Behavioural Assessment: A Practical Handbook (third ed.)*. A.S. Bellack and M. Hersen (eds) Pergamon Press, New York, pp. 365–95.

Bellack, A.S. (1979) A critical appraisal of strategies for assessing social skill. *Behav. Assess.*, **1**, 157–76.

Bellack, A.S. (1983) Current problems in the behavioural assessment of social skills. *Behav. Res. Ther.*, **21**, 29–42.

Bellack, A.S. and Hersen, M. (1977) Self-report inventories in behavioral assessment. In *Behavioral Assessment*. J.D. Cone and R.P. Hawkins (eds), Brunner/Mazel, New York, pp. 52–76.

Bellack, A.S. and Mueser, K.T. (1990) Schizophrenia. In *International Handbook of Behavior Modification (2nd ed.)*. M. Hersen and A.E. Kazdin (eds), Pergamon Press, New York, pp. 353–69.

Bellack, A.S., Morrison, R.L. and Mueser, K.T. (1989) Social problem solving in schizophrenia. *Schizophr. Bull.*, **15**, 101–16.

Bellack, A.S., Morrison, R.L., Mueser, K.T. *et al*. The utility of role play for assessing the social competence of psychiatric patients. *J. Consult. Clin. Psychol. Psychol. Assess.*, in press.

Bellack, A.S., Morrison, R.L., Wixted, J.T. and Mueser, K.T. (1990) An analysis of social competence in schizophrenia. *Br. J. psychiatry*, **156**, 809–18.

Charisiou, J., Jackson, H.J., Boyle, G.J. *et al.* (1989) Which employment interview skills best predict the employability of schizophrenic patients? *Psychol. Rep.*, **64**, 683–94.

Ciompi, L. (1980) The natural history of schizophrenia in the long term. *Br. J. Psychiatry*, **136**, 413–20.

Cohen, C.I. and Kochanowicz, N. (1989) Schizophrenia and social network patterns: A survey of black inner-city outpatients. *Community Ment. Health J.*, **25**, 197–207.

Curran, J.P. (1979), Pandora's box reopened: The assessment of social skills. *J. Behav. Assess.*, **1**, 55–71.

Curran, J.P., Corriveau, D.P., Monti, P.M. and Hagerman, S.B. (1980) Social skill and social anxiety. *Behav. Mod.*, **4**, 493–512.

Curran, J.P., Farrell, A.D. and Grunberger, A.J. (1984) Social Skills training: A critique and a rapprochement. In *Radical Approaches to Social Skills Training*. P. Trower, (ed), Croom Helm, London, pp. 14–46.

deLeon, J. and Simpson, G.M. (1990) Assessment of neuroleptic-induced extrapyramidal symptoms. In *Adverse Effects of Psychotropic Drugs*. J.M. Kane and J. Lieberman (eds), The Guilford Press, New York, in press.

Donahoe, C.P. and Driesenga, S.A. (1988) A review of social skills training with chronic mental patients. In *Progress in Behaviour Modification*. M. Hersen, R.M. Eisler and P.M. Miller (eds), Sage, Newbury Park, pp. 131–64.

Douglas, M.S. and Mueser, K.T. (1990) Teaching conflict resolution skills to the chronically mentally ill: Social skills training groups for briefly hospitalized patients. *Behav. Mod.*, **14**, 519–47.

Drake, R.E., Wallach, M.A. and Hoffman, J.S. (1989) Housing instability and homelessness among aftercare patients of an urban state hospital. *Hosp. Community Psychiatry*, **40**, 46–51.

Eisler, R.M., Hersen, M., Miller, P.M. and

Blanchard, E.B. (1975) Situation determinants of assertive behaviors. *J. Consult. Clin. Psychol.*, **43**, 330–40.

Falloon, I.R.H., Boyd, J.L. and McGill, C.W. (1984), *Family Care of Schizophrenia*. Guilford Press, New York.

Goldsmith, J.B. and McFall, R.M. (1975) Development and evaluation of an interpersonal skill-training program for psychiatric inpatients. *J. Abnorm. Psychol.*, **84**, 51–8.

Gurland, B.J., Yorkston, N.J., Stone, H.R. *et al.* (1972) The Structured and Scaled Interview to Assess Maladjustment (SSIAM): description, rationale, and development. *Arch. Gen. Psychiatry*, **27**, 259–64.

Hammer, M. (1986) The role of social networks in schizophrenia. In *Handbook of Studies on Schizophrenia, Part 2*. G.D. Burrow, T.R. Norman and G. Rubinstein (eds), Elsevier Science Publishers, New York, pp. 115–128.

Hargie, O. and McCartan, P. (1986) *Social Skills Training and Psychiatric Nursing*. Croom Helm, London.

Harrow, M. and Miller, J.G. (1980) Schizophrenic thought disorders and impaired perspective. *J. Abnorm. Psychol.*, **89**, 717–27.

Hatfield, A.B. and Lefley, H.P. (eds) (1987) *Families of the Mentally Ill: Coping and Adaptation*. Guilford Press, New York.

Hersen, M. and Bellack, A.S. (1977) Assessment of social skills. In *Handbook of Behavioral Assessment*. A.R. Ciminero, K.S. Calhoun and H.E. Adams (eds), Wiley and Sons, New York, pp. 509–54.

Hersen, M., Bellack, A.S. and Turner, S.M. (1978) Assessment of assertiveness in female psychiatric patients: Motoric and physiological measures. *J. Behav. Ther. Exper. Psychiatry*, **9**, 11–6.

Hotchkiss, A.P. and Harvey, P.D. (1986) Linguistic analyses of speech disorder in psychosis. *Clin. Psychol. Rev.*, **6**, 155–75.

Katz, M. and Lyerly, S. (1963) Methods of measuring adjustment and social behavior in the community: Rationale, description, discrimination validity and scale development. *Psychol. Rep.*, **13**, 503–34.

Koenigsberg, H.W. and Handley, R. (1986) Expressed emotion: From predictive index to clinical construct. *Am. J. Psychiatry*, **143**, 1361–73.

Kraepelin, E. (1971) *Dementia Praecox and Paraphrenia*. Robert E. Krieger, Huntington.

Lazarus, A.A. (1981) *The Practice of Multimodal Therapy*. McGraw-Hill, New York.

Lehman, A. (1983) The well-being of chronic mental patients. *Arch. Gen. Psychiatry*, **40**, 369–73.

Lewine, R.R.J., Watt, N.F. and Fryer, J.H. (1978) A study of childhood social competence, adult premorbid competence, and psychiatric outcome in three schizophrenic subtypes. *J. Abnorm. Psychol.*, **87**, 294–302.

Liberman, R.P. (1982) Assessment of social skills. *Schizophr. Bull.*, **8**, 62–82.

Liberman, R.P., DeRisi, W.J. and Mueser, K.T. (1989) *Social Skills Training for Psychiatric Patients*. Pergamon Press, New York.

Liberman, R.P., Massel, H.K., Mosk, M.D. and Wong, S.E. (1985) Social skills training for chronic mental patients. *Hosp. Community Psychiatry*, **36**, 396–403.

Liberman, R.P. and Mueser, K.T. (1989) Schizophrenia: Psychosocial treatment. In *Comprehensive Textbook of Psychiatry IV*. H.I. Kaplan and B.J. Sadock (eds), Williams and Wilkins, Baltimore, pp. 792–806.

Liberman, R.P., Mueser, K.T. and Wallace, C.J. (1986a) Social skills training for schizophrenics at risk for relapse. *Am. J. Psychiatry*, **143**, 523–6.

Liberman, R.P., Mueser, K.T., Wallace, C.J. *et al.* (1986b) Training skills in the psychiatrically disabled: Learning coping and competence. *Schizophr. Bull.*, **12**, 631–47.

Mansouri, L. and Dowell, D.A. (1989) Perceptions of stigma among the long-term mentally ill. *Psychosoc. Rehab. J.*, **13**, 79–91.

McNamara, J.R. and Blumer, C.A. (1982) Role playing to assess social competence: Ecological validity considerations. *Behav. Mod.*, **6**, 519–49.

Merluzzi, T.V. and Biever, J. (1987) Role-playing procedures for the behavioral assessment of social skill: A validity study. *Behav. Assess.*, **9**, 361–77.

Monti, P.M., Curran, J.P., Corriveau, D.P. *et al.* (1980) Effects of social skills training groups and sensitivity groups with psychiatric patients. *J. Consult. Clin. Psychol.*, **48**, 241–8.

Morrison, R.L. and Bellack, A.S. (1981) The role

of social perception in social skill. *Behav. Ther.*, **12**, 69–79.

Morrison, R.L., Bellack, A.S. and Mueser, K.T. (1988) Deficits in facial-affect recognition and schizophrenia. *Schizophr. Bull.*, **14**, 67–83.

Morrison, R.L., Bellack, A.S., Wixted, J.T. and Mueser, K.T. (1990) Positive and negative symptoms in schizophrenia: A cluster-analytic approach. *J. Nerv. Ment. Dis.*, **178**, 377–84.

Mueser, K.T., Bellack, A.S., Morrison, R.L. and Wade, J.H. (1990a), Gender, social competence, and symptomatology in schizophrenia: A longitudinal analysis. *J. Abnorm. Psychol.*, **99**, 138–47.

Mueser, K.T., Bellack, A.S., Morrison, R.L. and Wixted, J.T. (1990b) Social competence in schizophrenia: Premorbid adjustment, social skill, and domains of functioning. *J. Psychiatr. Res.*, **24**, 51–63.

Mueser, L.T., Levine, S., Bellack, A.S. *et al.* Social skills training for acute psychiatric inpatients. *Hosp. Community Psychiatry*, in press.

Mueser, K.T., Bellack, A.S., Douglas, M.S. and Morrison, R.L. (1991) Prevalence and stability of social skill deficits in schizophrenia. *Schizophr. Res.*, **5**, 167–76.

Nuechterlein, K.H. and Dawson, M.E. (1984) Information processing and attentional functioning in the developmental course of schizophrenic disorders. *Schizophr. Bull.*, **10**, 160–203.

Paul, G.L. and Lentz, R.J. (1977) *Psychosocial Treatment of Chronic Mental Patients: Milieu Versus Social-Learning Programs.* Harvard University Press, Cambridge, MA.

Pepper, B., Kirshner, M.C. and Ryglewicz, H. (1981) The young adult chronic patient: overview of a population. *Hosp. Community Psychiatry*, **32**, 463–9.

Platt, S., Weyman, A., Hirsch, S. and Hewett, S. (1980) The Social Behaviour Assessment Schedule (SBAS): Rationale, contents, scoring and reliability of a new interview schedule. *Soc. Psychiatry*, **15**, 43–55.

Pogue-Geile, M.F. and Zubin, J. (1988) Negative symptomatology and schizophrenia: a conceptual and empirical review. *Int. J. Ment. Health*, **16**, 3–45.

Rajkumar, S. and Thara, R. (1989) Factors affecting relapse in schizophrenia. *Schizophr. Res.*, **2**, 403–9.

Rathus, S.A. (1973) A 30-item schedule for assessing assertive behavior. *Behav. Ther.*, **4**, 398–406.

Rosen, A.J. (1988) Observational Record of Inpatient Behavior. In *Dictionary of Behavioral Assessment Techniques.* M. Hersen and A.S. Bellack (eds), Pergamon Press, New York, pp. 320–2.

Rutter, D.R. (1985) Language in schizophrenia: The structure of monologues and conversation. *Br. J. Psychiatry*, **146**, 399–404.

Schooler, N., Hogarty, G. and Weissman, M. (1978) Social Adjustment Scale II (SAS–II). In *Resource Materials for Community Mental Health Program Evaluations.* W.A. Hargreaves, C.C. Atkisson and J.E. Sorenson (eds), Publication No. (ADM) 79328, DHEW, Rockville, Maryland.

Shepard, G. (1984) Assessment of cognitions in social skills training. In *Radical Approaches to Social Skills Training.* P. Trower (ed), Croom Helm, London, pp. 260–83.

Simpson, C.J., Hyde, C.E. and Faragher, E.B. (1989) The chronically mentally ill in community facilities: A study of quality of life. *Br. J. Psychiatry*, **154**, 77–82.

Susser, E., Struening, E.L. and Conover, S. (1989) Psychiatric problems in homeless men. *Arch. Gen. Psychiatry*, **46**, 845–50.

Trower, P., Bryant, B. and Argyle, M. (1978) *Social Skills and Mental Health.* University of Pittsburgh Press, Pittsburgh.

Van Putten, T. and May, P.R. (1978) 'Akinetic depression' in schizophrenia. *Arch. Gen. Psychiatry*, **35**, 1101–7.

Wallace, C.J. (1986) Functional assessment in rehabilitation. *Schizophr. Bull.*, **12**, 604–30.

Wallace, C.J., Nelson, C.H., Liberman, R.P. *et al.* (1980) A review and critique of social skills training with schizophrenic patients. *Schizophr. Bull.*, **6**, 42–63.

Watson, D. and Friend, R. (1969) Measure of social-evaluative anxiety. *J. Consult. Clin. Psychol.*, **33**, 448–57.

Wessberg, H.W., Curran, J.P., Monti, P.M. *et al.* (1981) Evidence for the external validity of a social simulation measure of social skills. *J. Behav. Assess.*, **3**, 209–20.

Wing, J.K. and Freudenberg, R.K., (1961) The response of severely ill chronic schizophrenic patients to social stimulation. *Am. J. Psychiatry*, **118**, 311–22.

Wixted, J.T., Morrison, R.L. and Bellack, A.S. (1988) Social skills training in the treatment of negative symptoms. *Int. J. Ment. Health*, **17**, 3–21.

Wykes, T. and Sturt, E. (1986) The measurement of social behaviour in psychiatric patients: An assessment of the reliability and validity of the SBS Schedule. *Br. J. Psychiatry*, **148**, 1–11.

Zigler, E., and Glick, M. (1986) *A Developmental Approach to Adult Psychopathology*. John Wiley & Sons, New York.

APPENDIX 11.A DEFINITIONS AND CRITERIA FOR MAKING RATINGS WITH THE SOCIAL INTERACTION SCHEDULE (adapted from Liberman, DeRisi and Mueser, 1989)

11.A.1 BEHAVIOURAL OBSERVATION

A. **Activity** Activity can be recorded as either isolate or interactive. These categories are mutually exclusive, that is, every patient will fall into one and only one category.

ISOLATE: Isolate behaviours are those behaviours that a patient engages in alone. The behaviours in this category are unrelated to phsyical proximity or eye contact with other patients. Isolate behaviour can be divided into active and inactive categories.

1. **Active**. This category includes activities engaged in by only one patient. Examples include watching TV, reading, writing, playing solitary games, performing work, exercising, grooming, or smoking.

If the patient is walking or running without simultaneously engaging in another behaviour (isolate or active), continue to observe until it can be determined whether or not the movement is goal directed. If it is goal directed, score it as active. Examples of goal-directed walking/running include behaviours such as going to the ping-pong table to play or watch a game or walking to a meal. If it cannot be determined that the walking is goal directed after 10 seconds of observation, score it inactive.

2. **Inactive**. This category covers those patients who do not appear to be engaged in any of the behaviours previously defined as isolate active, such as lying down, staring into space, and pacing.

INTERACTIVE: Two patients or a patient and staff must be clearly participating in a joint activity to be scored in this category. Interactive behaviour can be of a negative or positive nature.

1. **Positive**. At least two or more people must be engaged in an appropriate activity — that is, behaviour actively performed in the right strength and intensity for the time, place, or working constructively with at least one other individual. This includes talking, listening, playing or working with another individual.

2. **Negative**. This category includes activities that are clinically inappropriate — that is, behaviours whose strength, intensity, or content are maladaptive regardless of time, place, or circumstance, or maladaptive due to infringement on the rights of others. This category includes screaming, hitting, kicking, grabbing an object from another patient, pulling hair, and other aggressive behaviours.

If behaviours in two or more of the Activity categories are observed in the same brief observation interval, use the following priority rules to determine which one to score.

(a) If behaviours in two or more of the Activity categories are observed in the brief observation interval, always score the category of the FIRST behaviour observed. For example, if a positive interaction is observed and then the patient engages in isolate behaviour, score only the positive interaction.

(b) If interactive and isolate behaviours occur simultaneously during the brief observation interval, score only the interactive behaviour.

(c) If positive AND negative interactions occur simultaneously during the brief observation interval, score only the positive interaction.

(d) If active and inactive isolate behaviours occur simultaneously during the same observation interval, score only the active behaviour.

B. Inappropriate patient characteristics.
(These categories are NOT mutually exclusive.)

1. **Inappropriate dress/grooming** (Score if any of the following are observed):

(a) Patients without shoes. Slippers and sandals with or without socks or stockings will be considered a type of shoe, but socks or stockings alone will not.

(b) Patients with torn, dirty, excessively wrinkled, or sloppy clothing. 'Dirty' refers to visual appearance and should not be evaluated on the basis of odour. Score male patients without shirts in this category. 'Sloppy' clothing would include such things as shirt tails out, unless the shirt is designed to be worn out, shirt unbuttoned or buttoned incorrectly, extremely dishevelled clothing, dress falling off shoulders, clothes worn inside out, pants unzipped or with broken zipper, and shoes untied.

(c) Patients inappropriately dressed. This category includes bizarre dress as well as wearing clothes that are inappropriate for the temperature, setting, or time of day. For example wearing two shirts at the same time.

(d) Inappropriate grooming. Dirt or food apparent on any part of body or clothing, hair disarrayed or obviously dirty, any buttons (except collar area), snaps, zippers, laces undone, wearing excessive or bizarre make-up.

2. **On bed, couch, floor** Patients on the floor. This includes those patients who have any part of bodies except their feet in contact with the floor, or the majority of their body weight being supported by a bed or couch including those sitting upright.

3. **Talking to self** This category includes those residents who are talking or mumbling with no apparent listener. Do not record for reading aloud, single exclamations in response to an appropriate stimulus or appropriate reactions to athletic events and shows on TV or radio.

4. **Facial movement** Apparently involuntary wormlike wiggle of tongue, darting tongue, lateral jaw movement, rapid blinking, tremor of facial muscles, or grimacing.

5. **Repetitive and stereotypic body movements** The individual repeatedly moves any part of the body continually throughout the observation, or makes peculiar or bizarre gestures or other movements at any time during the observation. Examples include hand wringing and rocking in bed.

6. **Pacing** The individual walks alone without apparent destination throughout the entire observation.

7. **Awake/asleep** This category describes whether the patient is awake or asleep during the observation.

(a) *Awake*. Record if the patient's eyes are open any time during the observation. If the eyes cannot be observed, record when the individual is engaged in some activity for which the eyes would ordinarily be open.

(b) *Asleep*. Record if the patient's eyes are closed throughout the entire observation (unless it is clearly evident that the patient is engaged in an activity that is physically incompatible with sleep). If it is impossible to determine whether the yes are open or closed, check this code when the individual is *not* engaged in some activity for which the eyes would ordinarily be open.

11.A.2A CONVERSATIONAL BEHAVIOUR

A. Eye contact
  1 = No or very little eye contact; excessive staring
  2 = Some avoidance
  3 = Appropriate eye contact during the interaction

B. Amount of speech
  1 = No or very little response to questions; telegraphic speech; rambling on and on, dwelling on the same subject for most of the conversation
  2 = Minimum amount of speech necessary to participate in conversation; speaking a little too much on one subject
  3 = OK; uses enough speech for one to totally understand the topic; gives complete answers to questions and volunteers additional information when appropriate

C. Rate of speech
  1 = So slow that speech is not understandable, speech is too fast to be understood
  2 = Understandable, but obviously too fast or slow
  3 = OK

D. Voice volume
  1 = Very soft/inaudible; very loud/ screaming for no apparent reason
  2 = Soft/barely audible, loud for no apparent reason

  3 = OK — easily audible at a distance of 3 feet

E. Voice inflection
  1 = Flat, monotone, no inflection; excessive, overly forceful inflection
  2 = Infrequent or inappropriate inflection; moderate frequency or overly forceful inflection
  3 = OK; uses appropriate inflection and inflection appropriate to content of speech

F. Speech intelligibility (coherence)
  1 = Very poor; speech is obscured by distorted grammar, lack of logical connection between one part of a sentence and another or between sentences
  2 = Speech is generally understandable, but some words or phrases not clear
  3   OK; speech is clear and understandable; only occasional words or phrases are unintelligible

G. Speech appropriateness (rationality and relevance)
  1 = Very poor; delusional speech and/ or unrelated speech for conversation; ignores speech of other person. Sudden irrelevancies; grossly pedantic phrases and answering off the point; long pauses between words
  2 = Minimal delusional and/or unrelated speech; minimal wandering off topic
  3 = OK; asks and answers questions at appropriate times during the conversation; does not wander off topic or interrupt; discusses topics generally considered appropriate for social interaction among acquaintances and friends

Table 11.9 Social Interaction Schedule (SIS) Data Sheet

Patient _____ Date _____

	Time of observation or rating					
Behavioural observation of social interaction (Check only 1)						
• Isolate Active						
• Isolate Inactive						
• Interaction Positive						
• Interaction Negative						
• Inappropriate behaviours						
(Check only 1)						
• Awake						
• Asleep						
(Check all that apply)						
• Inappropriate dress/grooming						
• Talking to self						
• On bed, couch, or floor						
• Facial						
• Repetitive stereotypic movements						
• Pacing						

Conversation behaviours
   (Use 0–2–3 ratings)

• Eye contact						
• Amount of speech						
• Rate and fluency of speech						
• Voice volume						
• Voice tone						
• Coherence						
• Rationality of discourse						

Chapter 12

The relevance and use of life skills assessments

DUŠAN HADŽI-PAVLOVIĆ, ALAN ROSEN
and GORDON PARKER

The schizophrenic has grown weary of internal and external pressure; he lives out everything that is on his mind, regardless of any benefits to his existence. He cannot exist in a conventional adaptation to the real world, but struggles for the concept of a world that would adapt to him. Or, in a somewhat loose, oversimplified statement it might be said that schizophrenia is the extreme rejection of established convention. (E. Bleuler, 1978, p. 487).

12.1 OVERVIEW

The effective treatment of those with schizophrenia asks that we find for them a place in the world — one in which they are comfortable, and which in turn is comfortable with them. Whatever their relative merits, the choice of hospital or community, and more specifically, where in the community?, where in the hospital?, need to be formed by the knowledge of the patient's capacity to survive and to achieve a satisfactory quality of life in each of these settings. We suggest that this capacity can be summarized by assessing a particular range of behaviours and abilities — so-called 'life skills' — whose scope, description and measurement occupy a middle ground between that of 'living skills' and ''social skills''. For individuals with schizophrenia and their carers such assessments are intended to help them in thinking about how

the individual might fare in each of the available treatment and living options; while for the community it is meant to help by identifying the range of treatment and living options that it needs to provide or support. In describing our way of thinking about life skills we have tried to look not only at the theory, but at the nitty-gritty of making such a measure part of the clinical practice of a wide range of professionals.

12.2 DISABILITY AND DYSFUNCTION

Using the terminology of Anthony and Liberman (1986), it is convenient to see schizophrenia as a pathology (or pathological process) leading to various forms of impairment which might produce disabilities that might result in handicap. For example, the brain pathology may lead to a paranoid process and accompanying delusions, which produce behaviours in the workplace which cause friction and then result in unemployment. The way in which disability manifests as handicap is intimately related to the individual's society; in rough terms, to what that society will tolerate and the types of health services which it will fund. In a society that gracefully accepts from each according to his means, becoming unemployed would have few consequences. If it were a sufficiently benign society, then the friction would be put aside or not even occur. The work of Warner (1988) is interesting, in this regard, for the way in which he incorporates social factors; asserting a strong association between the economy — especially unemployment — and the detected rates of occurrence of schizophrenia and apparent recovery from it. However, there are no hard and fast causes, no inevitable sequelae — the potential for various positive symptoms might be primed in brain chemistry, but the likelihood of their emergence appears to be related to an additional component, as is asserted for instance by the EE research (e.g. Kuipers and Bebbington, 1988).

12.3 SURVIVAL AND ADAPTATION

The thrust of current thought is that the prognosis for schizophrenia is a more optimistic one than previously held and that as much of its course as possible should be lived in the community and not in institutions. (This optimism has encouraged many to speak of 'the person with schizophrenia' rather than, like Bleuler (1978) of 'the schizophrenic'.) While the community management of the acute stage is feasible and effective (e.g. Hoult *et al.* 1984; Chapter 25), the bulk of life with schizophrenia and the accompanying normal life, usually occurs in a less intensely managed environment. Even so, our expectation is that a large percentage of schizophrenics can, for example, have an acute episode whilst remaining in the community; retain a job; find decent stable accommodation; and receive adequate service from health professionals. This is not an expectation of survival by the skin of their teeth, but survival in the fullest sense of a reasonable level of functioning accompanied by a sense of well being and an adequate quality of life. Their failure to do so is not only a failure to survive in the community or institution, but a failure of management. The person with schizophrenia

who is not surviving can only begin to do so by adapting, which means either changing his or her habits and skills, or finding a niche in which they can survive. The main purpose of a life skills assessment is to enable carers to assist in that adaptation. A second purpose is to tell society which kinds of niches it ought to be creating, what bits of the world it ought to be adapting to fit the individual with schizophrenia who, in Bleuler's words, 'lives out everything that is on his mind'.

12.4 DEFINITION OF LIFE SKILLS

Life skills can be defined as those abilities which are components of essential functional roles; which are expressed in terms of self-care, work, leisure and relationships; and which contribute to an individual's survival in the fullest sense when she or he is attempting to live in some form of community.

Clearly then a life skills measure will need to focus around those forms of disability which may be associated with the large range of handicaps that affect survival in the community or the institution. Conversely, we can think of this as a focus on those those strengths and abilities essential to satisfactory life in the community. These handicaps are essentially those that restrict the person's access to the interpersonal, social and physical supports provided by society. Life skills, as exemplified in Rosen *et al.* (1989), are a mixture of questions about the performance of an ability A: 'Can the person do A?' and 'Does the person do A?', with the latter being more important. We are ultimately interested in the actual — 'Does the person survive?' — and not in the potential — 'In theory, could the person survive?' Many of the life skills are intertwined with each other and it is part of management to decide which deficit to address. Cooperation with medication, for example, is an item in the assessment scale of Rosen *et al.* (1989), but it will also influence the level of other life skills in that scale that are controlled by medication.

12.5 LIFE SKILLS AND SURVIVAL IN THE INSTITUTION AND THE COMMUNITY

Even if institutional care becomes briefer and less frequent the institution remains an environment which many patients will have to survive at some time. Indeed the asylum provided by an institution might well be necessary and useful for some patients at some time. There are of course grades of institution — from locked ward to half-way house, each providing less asylum and demanding more of the patient — but the crude hospital–community split will suffice.

12.5.1 IN THE INSTITUTION

Two ways in which the hospital and life skills affect each other are: (1) To what extent do a patient's life skills stop him from receiving the maximum care available? While the hospital largely ensures that the patient receives food and medication, some behaviours can stretch the tolerance of staff and affect the effort they invest, or lead to consignment to a low-input back ward, premature discharge and/or a later reluctance to admit. (2) To what extent does the institution foster/hinder life skills? Most institutions are thought to have negative effects on a patient's life skills, perhaps chiefly by providing an unrealistic model of the 'real world' into which the individual must return. This might occur when institutions make insufficient demands on life skills and so do not encourage their development and maintenance; are too tolerant of disruptive or offensive ways and habits; or provide life skills training which is not sufficiently specific to the patient's life situation and is not followed up by training in the community. In consequence it does not generalize to community living.

12.5.2 IN THE COMMUNITY

A person with schizophrenia who is surviving in the community is one who among other things:

Is less likely to relapse. Avoiding relapse is an ill-understood combination of at least maintenance on, or strategic use of, medication; and stress minimization, often including low intensity network support and meaningful activity.

Stays out of hospital. This means both being more likely to accept (or be in a position to accept) community treatment of an acute episode (where appropriate) and being less likely to need asylum or containment in a hospital during times of stress.

Obtains and continues in an appropriate type of employment. If we accept the findings of Warner (1988), then employment is a very important element in recovery and helping a patient to find it warrants considerable effort. Economic conditions and global functioning will of course place constraints upon employment prospects, but if a choice is available, then a match between the individual's life skills and some aspects of the work conditions should help in a better choice. The idea here is that we try to assess the kinds of behaviours that the particular workplace will and will not tolerate, and if there is a mismatch then either try to place the patient elsewhere or else give the relevant skill deficit priority in management.

Finds and stays in well-matched accommodation. As with employment this involves determining the patient's life skills and finding a setting where someone with those skills is likely to achieve a foothold and survive on a stable basis.

Survives in the family. We cannot go out and find a new family for a patient. So the task is to identify the areas of mismatch and then make them part of the family management of the patient, which might include helping the individual and family to live separately while retaining contact on the best terms possible.

Has an adequate support network. This can be provided by neighbours, friends, co-workers and health professionals.

12.6 GOALS OF A MEASURE

A life skills measure should do the following:

(1) Address the concepts contained in the definition of life skills.

(2) Target the broad aspect of any life skill. For example, co-operating with medication is a life skill; understanding and following a medication regime, monitoring side effects etc. are the finer components and are better examined in the context of living skills and social skills (Chapter 20).

(3) Allow for diversity of assessors. An assessment probably needs to be made by those who know the patient best. This could be a health professional, but could also be someone working in a boarding house, or a relative. For this reason the measure must be straightforward and non-technical, avoiding expressions that might elicit bias or emotions associated with being a friend or carer.

(4) Have assessment of functioning in the community as its primary goal. Given that the great majority of people with serious psychiatric disorder are in the community, and the current approaches to treatment, a focus on community functioning seems an appropriate enough emphasis, even though it might make a measure less immediately applicable to people in institutions, or elsewhere where a full range of demands is not made of them.

(5) Assess functioning in general and not that surrounding acute episodes. The great majority of patients spend their time in the community, with minimal positive symptoms, and it is how they manage in this state that determines how well they do overall.

(6) Be brief and simple to encourage use. Only researchers fill out long forms, so if the measure is to be a serious candidate for a role in decision making, it should be brief and easy to use, and require little or no training. This also makes it practical and accessible to the diversity of assessors mentioned above. This brevity must be balanced against the need for detail in a way that recognizes that it is difficult to get a broad range of people to make ratings; that these ratings cannot be too demanding of time or effort; and that in most situations many goals have to be met by a single rating scale.

(7) Allow for different targets of assessment. Earlier we said that in order for a patient to be matched to accommodation or a workplace we needed to know which behaviours were tolerated in each place. This implies that a life skills questionnaire needs to be able to be twisted around so that (for example) along with asking 'Is the patient disruptive of others? we can ask 'Can the facilities and carers at this hostel cope with disruptive residents'?

(8) Assess observed behaviours. Self-report of what one is, or is not, doing is problematic at the best of times; with a population that has a severe psychiatric disorder, the rating should be based solely on what the rater has seen and not on what the patient reports.

(9) Avoid fine detail while still distinguishing specific dimensions. A number of the above points indicate the need to have a measure that avoids global and/or complex judgements; and that can be meaningfully filled in by someone who only has a moderate

acquaintance with the patient. Nevertheless, we probably cannot just ask 'will this person make it out in the community'? Social settings require a number of dimensions to describe them and so a measure needs to be able to be split up into relevant subscales if so required. An analogy is IQ: total IQ suffices for some purposes; a split into verbal and performance IQ is needed for other purposes; while sub-test by sub-test scores are needed for some fine decisions. Note that if items and their definitions are crisp enough, then even individual items will serve a useful purpose in certain situations.

(10) Be sensitive to change. The clearest least useful indicator of deterioration in functioning is failure to survive. Though emphatic, it is slower and subtler than acute symptoms and so the task of detecting it is much harder.

(11) Be meaningful to the patient. An assessment is much more likely to be useful in treatment if its contents can be shared with the patient and if it can be seen as relevant by the patient.

12.7 MEASURES TO ASSESS LIFE SKILLS

While the Life Skills Profile (LSP) (Rosen *et al.* 1989) was our attempt to embody the ideas expressed in this chapter, there are a number of measures which should be considered for the assessment of life skills. Many of these scales are very good and a case might be made that they do the job better; or that they would do it better if some modifications were made; or that they should be preferred in some circumstances since they also fulfill other assessment goals. In all cases, they are interesting either because of their frequent use, aims and content, or methods and development. Our reservations refer to the set of goals set out above and not to the goals that the scales' devisers set

themselves. Some scales can potentially be altered to suit our goals; for example, a scale that requires a lengthy interview could be used by raters implicitly interviewing themselves and then making the global judgements.

Social Behaviour Schedule (Wykes and Sturt, 1986). The main part of this scale is a set of 21 questions (mainly rated 0–4) and covering areas such as 'conversation: incoherence', 'social mixing: proportion of social contacts which are hostile in nature' and 'socially unacceptable habits or manners'. Agreement for the individual items varies and depends on the particular comparison. For raters attending the same interview the majority of kappas are over 0.7; test-retest kappas are markedly lower (most are below 0.5), as are inter-informant and inter-setting kappas. Percentage agreement is usually very high, suggesting that there is the potential for higher agreement in this scale. While there is insufficient validity data at this stage, there is a modest association between the number of problems and the amount of supervision in the person's setting. This scale's scope is not limited to schizophrenia and so has a number of items that are not directly relevant; additionally, it would need some changes to bear more closely on community living. It requires a sophisticated or trained rater to make complex judgements about behaviours and symptoms based on an interview with an informant which limits its applicability, though such raters can do so with excellent test-retest reliability. As some of the questions confound different dimensions of behaviour and symptoms, a sufficiently fine analysis of functioning is not fully available.

Disability Assessment Scale (Schubart *et al.*, 1986). A series of questions guides the rater through an interview with the person who has had the most contact with the patient over the last month. This forms the basis for six-point ratings of 12 key sections corresponding to behaviour such as 'self-care', 'social role performance' and 'friction in interpersonal relations'. The items represent an amalgam of features which make them potentially ambiguous, and difficult for the untrained rater. For the individual items the inter-rater coefficient kappa is reported as being between 0.82 and 0.85, with a correlation of 0.79 between the global assessment from the scale and ratings by psychiatrists.

Global Assessment Scale (Endicott *et al.*, 1976). This scale gives a single 0–100 score. As might be anticipated with a global rating it is not possible to tease out the differential effects of symptoms and more general functioning, thus leaving carers with minimal information about the source of any dysfunction.

Katz Adjustment Scales (Katz and Lyerly, 1963). These scales comprise 205 questions which include both self-report and ratings made by close informants covering the broad areas of symptoms, social behaviour, free-time activity and socially expected activities. The sub-scales of the KAS have reasonable validity as shown by agreement with clinical judgement, in defining types that show differential drug response, and by having relationships with relapse and hospitalization. The scales would need to have the symptom ratings removed as well as have the questions on community living expanded beyond the current emphasis on living in a family.

Social Adjustment Scale (Weissman and Paykel, 1974). Because the scale is quite broad in its scope, it does not sufficiently emphasize a number of areas that are important for living skills, although the version designed for use with people with schizophrenia has attempted to address this difficulty (Weissman *et al.*, 1981). It requires a trained rater to make global judgements based on 48–52 questions asked during a semi-structured interview. There do not appear to be any published data on the validity and inter-rater reliability though Glazer *et al.* (1980) found high agreement between patients and raters.

Social Behaviour Assessment Scale (Platt *et al.*, 1980). This is an excellent scale that covers many areas of social performance and addresses the issue of burden. While it is very long and detailed (239 items, 45–75 minutes), it can be tailored by leaving unwanted sections out. For the three broad areas of 'behaviour', 'social performance' and 'adverse effects' the scale provides both an objective rating of their extent and a rating of their distress upon family members. The initial reliability studies showed excellent intraclass correlations for the broad subsections of the scale, and acceptable to a very good kappa coefficients of agreement for individual items. What stands against its practical implementation is that it requires a close informant to be given a semi-structured interview by a well-trained interviewer. Though the three-point rating could be thought insensitive to change, the evidence from Platt *et al.* (1981) suggests that it can detect change — certainly over the period immediately following an admission.

Morningside Rehabilitation Status Scale (Affleck and McGuire, 1984). This is a brief scale intended to be rated by someone well informed about the patient. A rating of 0–7 is made on each of four scales ('dependency', 'inactivity (occupation and leisure)', 'social integration/isolation' and 'effects of current symptoms and deviant behaviour'). The reliabilities of these are given as 0.90, 0.74, 0.68 and 0.74. There is very limited evidence of its validity in that the scales appear to differentiate patients with particular problem behaviours. It is essentially a global rating scale, whose applicability is not confined to schizophrenia and as such does not provide sufficient detail.

Scale for the Assessment of Negative Symptoms (Andreason, 1982a). The ratings on this scale follow observation of the patient and interviews with the patient and informants. Each broad area is rated on a number of individual items (range 0–5), plus a subjective rating by the patient which is usually not

211

used) and a global rating. The areas are affective flattening (7 individual items; e.g. 'paucity of expressive gestures'); alogia (4 items; e.g. 'poverty of speech'); avolition-apathy (3 items; e.g. 'grooming and apathy'); anhedonia-associality (4 items; e.g. recreational interests and activities'); and attentional impairment (2 items; e.g. 'work inattentiveness'). A number of areas that we would regard as important are well covered, though a few are too globally assessed. As many of the ratings require judgements that cover many dimensions the scale is probably not suitable for untrained raters. The inter-rater reliability is very good with intraclass coefficients greater than 0.80 for most of the ratings. Patients classed as having 'negative schizophrenia' using this scale appear to be a group with greater psychiatric morbidity and poorer adjustment (Andreasen and Olsen, 1982).

12.8 THE LIFE SKILLS PROFILE

The scale was developed to fit the criteria listed earlier and involved both considering alternatives such as those listed above and consulting with a broad range of people who deal with schizophrenia. It consists of 39 four-point items which are anchored by variants of 'not at all', 'slight', 'moderate' and 'extreme'. Our preference is to think of these items as measuring ability rather than disability, and so to score them so that high scores indicate high 'ability' (although Andrews *et al.*, 1990, scored the items reversely). For each domain the scale asks for an assessent of general functioning in the last three months (excluding crises) and the rater is only required to have moderate contact with the patient over that period of time. Sample questions (one from each of the five sub-scales below) are:

14. 'Does this person generally have an offensive smell (e.g. due to body, breath or clothes)?'
25. 'Does this person generally have problems (e.g. friction, avoidance) living with others in the household?'

20. 'Is this person generally inactive (e.g. spends most of the time sitting or standing around doing nothing?'
2. 'Does this person generally intrude or burst in on others' conversations (e.g. interrupts you when you are talking)?'
18. 'Is this person willing to take psychiatric medication when prescribed by a doctor?'

A principal component of the items indicated five main dimensions and these were used to define sub-scales that were labelled 'self-care', 'non-turbulence', 'social contact', 'communication' and 'responsibility'. The study of Andrews *et al.* (1990) using long-stay hospital patients discharged to the community suggests that these dimensions can be further reduced to two which they describe as 'general impairment' and 'the potential difficulty that patient's management could present'.

The results in Parker *et al.* (1991) have shown the inter-rater agreement for social scores and most of the sub-scales to be quite acceptable. Test-retest ratings made by case workers, residential carers and parents on two occasions four weeks apart showed intraclass correlations for the five sub-scales of 0.90, 0.84, 0.87, 0.78 and 0.84; and of 0.89 for the total score. Case workers were more reliable than residential carers and they than parents. Inter-rater agreement for mothers and fathers ranged from 0.40 to 0.75 for the sub-scales (0.80 for the total); for residential carers from 0.48 to 0.80 (0.83); and for case workers from 0.53 to 0.75 (0.77). While residential carers agreed with case workers (0.55 to 0.68) parent and case workers agreed poorly on 'responsibility' (-0.06) and 'non-turbulence' (0.19); and only moderately on the other scales (0.38–0.47) and the total (0.36).

The findings for parents are equivocal since in the development study (Rosen *et al.*, 1989) parents agreed with these other groups. Such findings indicate that either the 'objective' view which parents provide might be different — more contact with the patient, different types of contact — but that the 'subjective' effects might also differ — parents respond differently to dysfunction. Finally, we note that patients asked to rate themselves mostly tend to rate their functions higher and have almost no agreement with anyone else; this is not say that one could not use such a self-assessment as a tool in management. Other research substantiates the validity of the measure. In Rosen *et al.* (1989) we found that: (a) life skills increased with increasing age was primarily due to increased turbulence diminishing and 'responsibility' increasing and was consistent with clinical observations that violence, turbulence and irresponsibility are more likely in younger schizophrenic subjects. (b) The more changes of accommodation a person had over the preceeding year the lower their scores on all sub-scales (except 'communication'), suggesting that those with poor life skills are less stable in accommodation.

Andrews *et al.* (1990) found that: (a) 'impairment' (as measured by the LSP) was significantly associated with complaints to police, complaints by neighbours and hospital readmissions; and (b) those patients living in hospital wards were highly impaired and/or potentially diffculty to manage; those in nursing homes were more impaired than average, but clearly not difficult to manage; those in boarding houses were the reverse of those in nursing homes; those living with parents had the highest impairment, but only an average potential for difficult management. In Rosen *et al.* (1989) the associations with accommodation type were not as clear as in this study.

12.9 PROBLEMS WITH MEASURING LIFE SKILLS

12.9.1 ASSESSING UNUSED SKILLS

A commonly encountered difficulty is how to rate a life skill which the person does not have to use. One example is of patients in those institutions which make few if any demands on their patients. If the staff automatically ensure that the patient washes, eats and takes medication, how can we determine if the patient has these skills?

In some situations and with some measures this will be an unavoidable flaw, although a measure with sub-scales has a good chance of still providing a number of useful scores. An improvement would be to ignore these items and then to make some kind of statistical adjustment to obtain the final score(s). To be done with any precision this would require a large database which is usually not available — certainly early on — and so is not feasible except in a crude form. Such a data base is currently being built up for the LSP. A second possibility is to test specifically for these skills or to infer them from other assessments. Patients in an institution might well have been given a complete living and social skills assessment that would enable some estimate to be made. Finally, of course, one could design measures specific to particular settings. A corollary of this problem is that as patients are exposed to the demands of living — for example, when they leave the protected confines of hospital or home — their living skills can often appear to worsen as inabilities are exposed.

12.9.2 PATIENTS WHOM NO ONE KNOWS

For many reasons some patients will not be known especially well by anybody — their case manager might only see them during a periodic attendance at a depot phenothiazine clinic; they could be living alone or in a situation with a high turnover of staff — and it will be difficult for any individual to fill in a measure. In such situations an assessment might be impossible and nothing can be done about it. A possibility would be to have different individuals fill out any sections of the assessment that they can and thereby obtain a complete assessment. Finally, a short period of low-level hospitalization (or some community equivalent) is likely to enable some observations to be made.

More broadly this raises the issue of 'how well do we have to know the patient before we can make an assessment'? Certainly, as far as the LSP is concerned, we do not know the answer. On the one hand there are questions that would seem to be answerable by someone who, provided they had the appropriate sort of contact, need have only low contact (for example, 23. 'Can this person generally prepare (if needed) her or his own food/meals?'). On the other hand, for some — particularly those related to critical, but low frequency behaviour — it is not so certain (for example, 34. 'Is this person violent to others?'), particularly when the high visibility of behaviour can compensate for low contact. Future research could test for associations between level of contact with patient and inter-rater agreement.

12.9.3 WHEN TO ASSESS?

For the LSP patients are rated on how they are 'generally', ignoring when they are in crisis or becoming ill. While there are good reasons for so defining the rating period – most of the life of individuals with schizophrenia is 'normal' life, and not 'acute' life, it is not clear how to demarcate out the 'becoming ill' period; further, no indication is given about how to treat the 'becoming better' period.

12.9.4 SUBJECTIVITY

The utility of life skills presupposes that there is something fairly objective that is being assessed, but it is still necessary to try and reduce subjective influences. Some potential rating influences stem from 'self-defence'. A person making an assessment may believe that higher levels of disability imply that they are failing the patient or not doing their job properly. Hence the chance of them over-rating ability might be quite high. However, this might be counterbalanced by the desire to show that

you are dealing with a time consuming and difficult caseload due to the low level of functioning of your patients. Ratings may also be influenced by the level of coping by the rater. If the rater or carer is coping well with the patient's behaviours, then here is the potential for the patient to be rated as having higher ability than they actually have. The converse of this is also possible. This effect is mainly a confounding of living skills with features like burden of care and emotional involvement.

12.9.5 ETHICS OF ASSESSMENT.

Because a life skills assessment will often require one of a broad range of people in the community to make the assessment, we must respect the ethical issues that are inherent in talking to 'outsiders' about the patient and also in using their comments to guide management. This is made easier in community treatment where the 'community' is the carer and thus includes many who are not professionals or immediate family. Even so, such assessments should be made with the knowledge and permission of the patient, with a view to sharing the results with the patient.

12.10 LIFE SKILLS AND THE BURDEN OF CARE

Attending to the burden on carers is recognized as an important component of health services (Anderson, 1987) and its importance is increasing with the shift to community care. While the burden of care usually refers to family and friends, it can be extended to all health workers and others who provide services to the patient – a conscientious boarding house proprietor can be effectively a family member. This burden can affect the patient:

(1) If the social performance of the carer diminishes and the patient's environment is impoverished.

(2) If stresses emerge that can initiate relapse.

(3) If the care of the patient falls away, such as when health workers become fed up with the patient.

(4) If providers of a service withdraw that service, such as when the patient is asked to leave his boarding house accommodation.

Taking care of the carers can be as useful as taking care of the patient.

In a chronic disorder the burden due to constant strain needs to be distinguished from that due to crises — in schizophrenia these are most likely due to negative symptoms and positive symptoms respectively. The burden itself is worth dividing into worry, concern and stress and into the need to do things for the patient, with life skills impinging on both areas. Some of this can be dealt with by social services, while the rest will be part of therapeutic management.

How to translate patient disability into carer burden is not readily apparent, nor do we know if it is necessary to make use of a life skills measure at all in assessing burden. A four-point scale such as used by Falloon *et al.* (1984) might sometimes suffice. The scale showed differential response to individual and family management in their study. On the other hand carers are often willing to put up with a great deal, and their burden can easily be centred on just one or two behaviours that make all the difference. An overall disability score might not tell us a lot in these circumstances. An obvious approach is to ask how burdensome are the patient's behaviours, though how to ask this is not clear, since carers can be reluctant to acknowledge a burden lest they seem uncaring. In Rosen *et al.* (1989) we tried to get around that by asking raters to say whether each behaviour was 'hard to take' or 'not hard to take'. Platt (1985) provides a relevant review of this issue. For patient management it makes sense to use a list of potentially burdensome behaviours, since this will help the carer to identify specific difficulties.

Providing care is a skill, and the less of this skill that a family member has the greater the burden is likely to be. Given fixed social circumstances such skill will be a mixture of the family member's knowledge, life skills and social skills. If a patient's mother cannot look after her own health she is unlikely to be able to help her daughter with medication and the appraisal of professional advice; if her father is rude and interruptive he is unlikely to be able to intervene effectively with professionals; and both parents will be poor models for the patient. These are cases for the assessment and teaching of life skills to carers as aspects of care provision. An example more at the level of personality than skill, would be a mother who is strongly upset by her son's standard of cleanliness and so is continually criticizing him about it, and where we might try an intervention that deals with her unease rather than her son's behaviour. [1] Ameliorating the burden of care is one situation where working with the carer might be more important than working with the patient.

12.11 LIFE SKILLS AND THE QUALITY OF LIFE

There are enormous difficulties both in stating precisely what quality of life is and then in ascertaining whether an individual has it. The problems of homelessness and exploitation among a proportion of the mentally ill living in the community are an obvious example. More subtly the difficulty can be seen in the trade-off between the 'high satisfaction/high terror' of living alone outside an institution without support, versus the 'low satisfaction/ low terror' of living inside one. Of course, given adequate support, the community alternative becomes comparatively 'high satisfaction/low terror'. Any life skill that helps the following would seem to have a plausible association with a better quality of life in the community: (a) adequate support systems of a social (e.g. family), clinical and functional (rehabilitation) kind; (b) reduced occurrence of relapse and positive symptoms either through encouraging cooperation with treatment, ensuring the enthusiasm of carers, or reducing the incidence of stressors; (c) ability to find 'higher level' employment and retain it; (d) ability to find 'better' accommodation and continue living in it. These objectives interact with each other of course; so for example, reduced symptomatology makes the other objectives more likely, and they in turn make relapse less likely.

12.12 LIFE SKILLS AND CLINICAL COURSE

We mentioned earlier that life skills are likely to improve with age as the most turbulent phase of schizophrenia recedes. Apart from this, how might life skills reflect the course of the illness?

The exacerbation of positive symptoms is almost certain to reduce abilities, but as suggested earlier it is worth separating out acute episodes for the purposes of assessing general on-going life skills. While the functional effects of acute exacerbations might be transient, residual functioning might still be compromised and require evaluation to assist rehabilitation planning.

If the phase preceding an acute lapse is protracted, then we might expect at least some of the life skills to show signs of deterioration – provided we are assessing them regularly (say every three months). We do not know the answers to the following questions:

(a) Are measures of life skills sensitive to this kind of change, and in particular do they show up before other kinds of changes such as increased features of depression/anxiety or soft cognitive signs? This is very difficult to show and any measure which could detect such 'early warning' signs would be a most valuable clinical tool.

(b) Which life skills might deteriorate first? In the absence of data our suspicion is that this is as likely to be evident across the board as it is to be variable. If we take the early symptoms of first episode schizophrenia (Chapman, 1966) as some indicator of what might appear prodromally to any episode, and then extrapolate these to life skills, it is hard to see a clear picture of any skill being affected above others.

In the period of recovery after an acute episode, specific life skills might show improvement before others. It is tempting to think that as the psychotic phenomena recede that features of uncharacteristic turbulence and irresponsibility will go with them, unless a concomitant entrenched personality disorder is revealed following adequate treatment of the psychotic symptoms.

12.13 LIFE SKILLS ASSESSMENT AND PATIENT MANAGEMENT

As with any assessment, a life skills assessment raises questions of how to use the information; what effects it might have on the 'therapeutic alliance' (where the latter means the whole range of professionals, family members and friends, and people in the community who provide care for the patient); how it might interact with the clinician's and carer's view of their role; and how it might effect the patient.

Detailed coverage of this area is beyond the scope of this chapter. However, a life skills assessment could contribute significantly to programme planning and placement, especially if we connect the results to both specific likely outcomes and available options for work, housing, etc. In an assessment we will need to prioritize which disabilities to try and reduce, but also which abilities to encourage further and maintain. The advantage of the latter is that by highlighting abilities we can mobilize the strengths of the patient in dealing with the impairments.

12.13.1 INVOLVING THE CLINICIAN

Gaining the co-operation of clinicians involves assuring them that the research/evaluation uses of the instrument are respectful, non-intrusive, and not demeaning or exploitative of the patients or their caregivers. They also need to see how a particular assessment translates into a clinical goal — for example, a low score on self-care implies that a more detailed living skills assessment should be undertaken. Clinicians will also need to accept that associations found in patients as a group actually apply at the individual level. Even if research shows that patients of type 'T' are highly likely to have a particular kind of fate in the community, clinicians are often reluctant to accept that this has anything to say about the likely fate of their type 'T' patient (Meehl, 1973). Finally, low scores must not be seen as an evaluation of the clinician.

12.13.2 INVOLVING THE PATIENT

If the clinician is satisfied, then he can carry out the equally important task of making the patient comfortable with their being assessed by showing that: (a) the patient is not simply being used in a piece of research or for gathering 'government statistics'; (b) the measure is able to convey useful things about the patient to those who have to manage his care; and (c) the staff are able to use the measure to convey useful information back to the patient, by sharing the results with him, and by using them to negotiate a rehabilitation plan or other aspect of management.

A possible further involvement is an assessment by the patients of themselves. While we suggested earlier that self-assessment on the LSP did not provide a very accurate picture compared with other raters, this finding needs to be explored further as we might be able to identify sub-groups who can rate themselves accurately. Nevertheless, provided that the responses are explored in terms of personal validity for the individual with the disorder such an assessment will have its uses. Filling out the assessment can provide an easier way for patients to indicate problem areas and remind themselves — and us — about their strengths. Past assessments can be used as points of comparison, possibly identifying sources of change — 'Last time you were drinking a lot and the neighbours kept calling the police and that's not happening anymore . . . What have you done to stop doing that? . . . Has anything happened to help you do that?' The patient's own assessment can also be contrasted, gently, with a clinician or carer assessment to compare perceptions and provide mutual feedback about the effects of the patient's behaviour.

12.13.3 INVOLVING CARERS AND OTHERS

The case manager also has the task of demonstrating to parents, spouses and similar carers that the assessments have a useful part to play in the care of the patient and are not just statistics. They will need to be assured that they do not reflect upon the quality of their care – they are not tests of family caring for example. With the patient's permission, sharing the results with the caregivers can help them in their difficult role. Similar issues arise with boarding house proprietors, supervisors and people working in hostels.

12.13.4 FEEDBACK OF AN ASSESSMENT

Results from a well-constructed scale can be, and in general should be, discussed with the patient. If the assessment has been made by someone other than the clinician then any issues of confidentiality or the patient's wishes will have to be settled beforehand. Some of the general points that should be considered are: (a) Disability and ability. It is obviously important to give equal weight to both the strengths elicited by an assessment to the weaknesses; (b) Items and sub-scales. It can be overwhelming for a patient to see a large number of items which are causing difficulty for him. It will often be far more helpful to discuss these as part of a sub-scale, that is, as a 'problem area' rather than as an 'host of problems'. This cluster of problems can often be seen as arising from a particular cause — something which will be, and will feel to be, more readily dealt with. A patient who is being violent to others, in turmoil with neighbours and in trouble with the police is faced with a lesser problem if he can see this as a result of 'turbulence' caused by drugs or alcohol. The individual items can of course highlight particular problems that are worth attending to while attempting a fuller solution. (c) Placing the difficulties in context. If a long-term record is available it is often possible to show that the patient has improved over the last twelve months, or that similar difficulties have usually resolved themselves in the past.

12.13.5 IMPLICATIONS FOR THE FAMILY SITUATION

For the person with schizophrenia living in the family, disabilities are likely to be sources of family stress and so will indicate not only areas of change for the patient, but also areas of change for the family. Any family therapy will be able to try and induce adaptation in either the family or the patient. Since members of the family may also have problems with living skills – perhaps showing poor social skills in their contact with patients, intruding on their privacy, or showing violence toward them – an assessment by patients

of key family members is potentially informative.

12.13.6 IMPLICATIONS FOR OTHER SITUATIONS

Just as we might use an assessment to try and restructure the family situation, so we can identify areas where the patient is working or living for change. Take a half-way house as an example. We have some idea of the sort of living skills that do well in that particular accommodation, and so have been directing appropriate patients into it. However we find that there is still an unsatisfactory percentage of patients who do poorly there. We can query our assessment of the patients, but we can also ask the residents with schizophrenia living in the half-way house to assess the key personnel. Hopefully, we will obtain a picture of how the carers appear to the patients, a picture that will help us to understand why some seemingly appropriate patients find it difficult to survive there. Our goal then becomes education of the carers and alterations in the way that the house is run.

ACKNOWLEDGEMENTS

Our thinking on life skills was greatly helped by the people we consulted for a research project funded by the Richmond Implementation Unit of the NSW Department of Health, Sydney, Australia (Rosen *et al*. 1987). Funding for our research has also been provided by the National Health and Medical Research Council of Australia and by the Rebecca Cooper Foundation.

NOTE

1. This example based on case presentation by Dr Kevin Vaughan at Prince of Wales Hospital on 6 April 1990.

REFERENCES

Affleck, J.W. and McGuire, R.J. (1984) The

measurement of psychiatric rehabilitation status: a review of the needs and a new scale. *Br. J. Psychiatry*, **145**, 517–25.

Anderson, R. (1987) The unremitting burden on carers. *Br. Med. J*, **294**, 73.

Andreasen, N. (1982) Negative symptoms in psychiatry: definition and reliability. *Arch. Gen. Psychiatry*, **39**, 784–8.

Andreasen, N. and Olsen, S. (1982) Negative *v.* positive schizophrenia: definition and validation. *Arch. Gen. Psychiatry*, **39**, 789–94.

Andrews, G., Teeson, M., Stewart, G. and Hoult, J. (1990) Follow-up of community placement of the chronic mentally ill in New South Wales. *Hosp. Community Psychiatry*, **41**, 184–8.

Anthony, W.A. and Liberman, R.P. (1986) The practice of psychiatric rehabilitation: historical, conceptual and research base. *Schizophr Bull.*, **12**, 542–59.

Bleuler, M. (1978) *The Schizophrenic Disorders: Long-term Patient and Family Studies*. Yale University Press, New Haven and London.

Chapman, J. (1966) The early symptoms of schizophrenia. *Br. J. Psychiatry*, **112**, 225–51.

Endicott, J., Spitzer, R., Fleiss, J. and Gibbon, J. (1976) The global assessment scale. *Arch. Gen. Psychiatry*, **33**, 766–71.

Falloon, I.R.H., Boyd, J.L. and McGill, C.W. (1984) *Family Care of Schizophrenia: A Problem-Solving Approach to the Treatment of Mental Illness*. Guilford Press, New York.

Glazer, W., Aaronson, H.F., Prusoff, B.A. and Williams, D.H. (1980) Assessment of social adjustment in chronic ambulatory schizophrenics. *J. Nerv. Ment. Dis.*, **168**, 493–7.

Hoult, J., Rosen, A. and Reynolds, I. (1984) Community-orientated treatment compared to psychiatric hospital-orientated treatment. *Soc. Sci. Med.*, **18**, 1005–10.

Katz, M.M. and Lyerly, S.B. (1963) Methods of measuring adjustment and social behaviour in the community: I. Rationale, description, discriminative validity and scale development. *Psychol. Rep.*, **13**, 503–35.

Kuipers, L. and Bebbington, P. (1988) Expressed emotion research in schizophrenia: theoretical and clinical implications. *Psychol. Med*,
18, 893–909.

Meehl, P.E. (1972) Why I do not attend case conferences. In *Psychodiagnosis: Selected Papers*. P.E. Meehl (ed), W.H. Norton, New York, pp. 225–302.

Parker, G., Rosen, A., Emdur, N. and Hadzi-Pavlov, D. (1991) The life skills profile: Psychometric properties of a measure assessing function and disability in schizophrenia. *Acta Psychiatr. Scand.*, **83**, 145–52.

Platt, S. (1985) Measuring the burden of psychiatric illness on the family: an evaluation of some rating scales. *Psychol. Med.*, **15** 383–93.

Platt, S., Weyman, A., Hirsch, S. and Hewitt, S. (1980) The social behaviour assessment schedule (SBAS): rationale, contents, scoring and reliability of a new interview schedule. *Soc. Psychiatry*, **15**, 43–55.

Platt, S.D., Hirsch, S.R. and Knights, A.C. (1981) Effects of brief hospitalization on psychiatric patients' behaviour and social functioning, *Acta. Psychiatr. Scand.*, **63**, 117–28.

Rosen, A., Parker, G., Hadzi-Pavlovic, D. and Hartley, R. (1987) *Developing Evaluation Strategies for Area Mental Health Services in NSW: A Richmond Implementation Research Project*. NSW Department of Health, Sydney.

Rosen, A., Hadzi-Pavlovic, D. and Parker, G. (1989) The life skills profile: a measure assessing function and disability in schizophrenia. *Schizophr. Bull.*, **15**, 325–37.

Schubart, C., Krumm, B., Biehl, H. and Schwarz, R. (1986) Measurement of social disability in a schizophrenic patient group: definition, assessment and outcome over two years in a cohort of schizophrenic patients of recent onset. *Soc. Psychiatry*, **21**, 1–9.

Warner, R. (1988) *Recovering from Schizophrenia: Psychiatry and Political Economy*. Routledge, London.

Weissman, M.M. and Paykel, E.S. (1974) *The Depressed Woman: A Study of Social Relationships*. University of Chicago Press, Chicago.

Weissman, M.M., Sholkomskas, D. and John, K., (1981) The assessment of social adjustment: an update. *Arch. Gen. Psychiatry*, **38**, 1250–8.

Wykes, T. and Sturt, D. (1986) The measurement of social behaviour in psychiatric patients: an assessment of the reliability and validity of the SBS Schedule. *Br. J. Psychiatry*, **148**, 1–11.

Chapter 13

The assessment of severely disabled psychiatric patients for rehabilitation

T. WYKES

13.1 INTRODUCTION

The treatment of schizophrenia must address the biological, social and psychological deficits associated with it. The practice of rehabilitation is a synthesis of all these treatment approaches, and so inevitably this section will overlap with others in this book.

The first issue addressed is the terms that appear in the title. What is meant by rehabilitation and why should this chapter choose to concentrate on the most severely disabled patients?

13.2 A BRIEF HISTORY

The notion that patients should spend as little time in hospital as possible is not a new one. Staff have been energetically discharging patients from large mental hospitals for many decades, although the term 'community care' was not coined until the 1960s. Surveys of patients (e.g. Wing and Brown, 1970) had reported that even those people who had been in hospital for some time could be moved directly to community services. However,

others needed social rehabilitation before being transferred. There was even some optimism that we might be able to dispense with beds in long-term psychiatric care altogether, given the new pharmacological and social treatments for schizophrenia that had become available in that decade.

In the early stages of discharging patients many gains were made merely by providing patients with much needed social stimulation to counter the institutionalization that had developed in a group of patients who now showed little evidence of positive symptomatology (Chapter 1). After some time it became obvious to clinicians that the initial optimism had to be tempered. Many patients were identified who could not be transferred into the community unless other supportive services were provided such as day care and sheltered housing. Surveys of hospitals in the 1970s (Mann and Sproule, 1972; Mann and Cree, 1976) revealed that there was even a group of people who were accumulating in hospitals, despite the advantages of all the new medical and social care. This group of patients became known as the new long-stay. For this group of patients special highly supportive environments known as hospital hostels were suggested, although few have been opened (Wykes, 1982).

It is this 'new' long-stay group and those who require long-term staff input who are considered in this chapter. The group does not consist solely of patients with a diagnosis of schizophrenia but they do form a substantial part. They are currently cared for by a variety of services both in the community and in hospitals. A crude estimate of the numbers of patients with a chronic course of schizophrenia who are in touch with hospital services, living in hostels or group homes or attending day centres can be derived from psychiatric case registers. For Camberwell, a deprived inner urban area of London, the prevalence is about 170 per 100 000 population (Wing, 1983). This figure excludes the group of people 'living rough' which is thought to contain a number who are suffering from schizophrenia.

13.3 WHAT IS REHABILITATION?

Psychiatric rehabilitation is a term that has meant several different things over the past 40 years. It is much easier to say what it will not mean in this chapter. Rehabilitiation is *not* synonymous with resettlement from hospital to the community. Nor is it synonymous with a return to previous levels of functioning, as it might mean in physical rehabilitation. In psychiatry many patients, and especially those who appear in the long-term group, may have been functioning at a poor level prior to the perceived onset of their illness. A return to this level would hardly be a demanding goal. Rather, the approach adopted here is one described by Douglas Bennett. He suggests that we should aim to help patients optimize their social functioning in as normal a social context as possible (Bennett, 1983). For some severely disabled patients this may mean considerable staff effort even to maintain functioning and to prevent deterioration.

Using this definition it is obvious that rehabilitation can be carried out with any patients as long as they are exhibiting a decrement in performance which prevents them from living unsupported. Not only patients with schizophrenia fulfil these criteria: they may have a manic illness or be depressed. They may also exhibit a wide range of disabilities.

The process of rehabilitation has often been narrowly identified with the provision of certain activities, such as low level manual work or supported housing. Whilst not disputing the importance of employment or accommodation there are other significant but less well-developed areas in which rehabilitation needs to take place, such as family roles. In this chapter rehabilitation is viewed in this much wider sense.

In terms of service provision the aim is to provide only the minimum therapeutic dose of support (Birley, 1974). This dose may change over time. Recent studies using computerized life charts have shown that when there is a strict adherence to longitudinal design, it is apparent that there is a broad range of outcomes for chronic patients. Harding *et al.* (1987a, b) have now followed up 269 severely disabled chronic schizophrenic patients over 32 years, and their data have exploded the myth of continuous poor functioning. In their study some patients had windows of good functioning in their lives which sometimes lasted for several years. They explain the illusion of continual poor functioning in several ways. First, clinicians have a great deal more contact with those people who show little improvement or who deteriorate over time. The estimates suggest that clinicians are in contact with the non-recovered group 64 times as often as the intermittently recovered group. Second, clinicians have been taught to expect that chronic severely disabled patients are unlikely to improve very much in the future. Third, the research designs have not been truly longitudinal. Often patients are contacted several times but their functioning is assessed over a very small time period. If life history

Table 13.1 The essential ingredients of a psychiatric rehabilitation programme

Ingredient	Examples of how observed
1. Functional assessment of client skills in relation to environmental demand	1. Client records list client strengths and deficits in relation to environmental demands; strengths and deficits are behaviourally defined and indicate client's present and needed functioning.
2. Client involvement in the rehabilitation assessment and intervention	2. Record forms have places for client sign-off and comments; percentage of clients who sign-off; sample audiotapes of client interviews indicate client's understanding of what programme is doing and why.
3. Systematic individual client rehabilitation plan	3. Written or taped examples of objective, behaviour, step-by-step client plans; a central 'bank' of available rehabilitation curricula; client records specify on which plans client is working.
4. Direct teaching of skills to clients	4. Practitioners can identify the skills they are capable of teaching, describe the teaching process, and demonstrate their teaching techniques. Programme's daily calender reflects blocks of time devoted to skills training.
5. Environmental assessment and modification	5. Practitioners can describe the characteristics of the environment to which client is being rehabilitated and how environment may be modified to support the client's skills level. Functional assessment should have assessed unique environmental demands.
6. Follow-up of clients in their real-life environment	6. Client record indicates a monitoring plan and descriptions of monitoring results; audio-tape of practitioner and client feedback sessions; record keeping forms provide spaces for changes in the intervention plan. Percentage of clients whose plans have changed; number of appointments for 'follow-along' services.
7. A rehabilitation team approach	7. Team members can verbally describe each client's observable goals and the responsibilities of each team member in relation to those goals (may refer to client's records for this information).
8. A rehabilitation referral procedure	8. Client records indicate referral letters requesting specific outcomes by specific dates; telephone referrals demonstrate these same rehabilitation referral ingredients.
9. Evaluation of observable outcomes and utilization of evaluation results	9. Agency records show the pooled outcome data for all clients; agency directors can verbally describe their most significant outcome.
10. Consumer involvement in policy and planning	10. Administrators can list the number of joint meetings with consumers; consumer's ratings of satisfaction with rehabilitation programme.

This table is from Anthony *et al.* (1982)

measures are taken then a different pattern emerges, with functioning in different areas of a patient's life changing at different times and at different rates.

Since the amount of support needed by patients may vary throughout their lives there is a need for the rehabilitation context to be both flexible and well titrated against the needs of individual patients. Table 13.1 shows the components thought by Anthony *et al.* (1982) to make up an ideal rehabilitation programme. It is important that any rehabilitation system defines its aims in this way so that patients can be matched to the appropriate service. Rehabilitation unfortunately has all too often been seen as the provision of a service such as sheltered work. Directing the patient to these services has been seen as equivalent to performing rehabilitation and so few individual plans were made. The emphasis in the table of rehabilitation aims is on individual programmes, observable outcomes and the transfer of skills to other settings.

In order to provide a flexible system of rehabilitation a broad range of supportive service options in both residential and day care must be available. Residential care should stretch from cheap housing (for those who cannot compete financially due to their psychiatric disability) to long-stay hospital hostels (Wykes *et al.*, 1982b; Wykes, 1982i; Garety, 1988). Day care too should cover a wide range, from sheltered work groups in open employment to occupational therapy provided in a hospital ward (e.g. Stein and Test, 1978; Watts, 1983; Holloway, 1988).

In summary, rehabilitation involves equipping patients to function at their optimal level. This is achieved either by intervening directly with the patient or by providing training and support for those who interact with them. It is also important to look at the patient's environment to make sure that it is the most appropriate one for his or her current needs.

13.4 WHY DO YOU NEED ASSESSMENT FOR REHABILITATION?

The definition of psychiatric disorder is broadly based on a subject's description of his or her symptoms. This may not be the only indication of dysfunction. Often there is an inability to perform the common tasks normally required of an adult. These tasks include working, relating to family and friends and looking after one's personal appearance and one's dwelling place. Wing (1978) suggested that these difficulties in social functioning are composed of intrinsic impairments, social disadvantages and adverse self-attitudes. Intrinsic impairments are those which underlie the disorder and are biological or psychosocial. Social disadvantages, such as poverty or homelessness before or after the onset of schizophrenia, can lead to the development of an unnecessary degree of social disablement. An individual's attitude to the impairment of schizophrenia or to the social disadvantage can add a further layer of disablement. This secondary disability can be so severe as to sometimes be indistinguishable from the underlying impairment. For example, some patients become so apathetic within a hospital that they lose all initiative. At its extreme this is known as institutionalism. In its milder forms adverse self-attitudes may mean a loss of confidence in using skills that are unimpaired. Intrinsic impairments, social disadvantages and adverse self-attitudes all contribute to the degree of social impairment.

The process of developing assessments to measure the level of social functioning has also been discussed by John Wing (1990). He categorized the process into three main purposes:

(1) To understand and differentiate between the causes of social disablement.
(2) To devise ways of preventing or reducing the impact of these causes.
(3) To design services that will identify people in need and provide them with effective, acceptable and economic help.

The more we know about the causes of social disablement the better able we should be to plan services and to test methods of prevention and care. The clinician must be willing to participate in this research strategy at all levels. Individual patients must be assessed with a variety of instruments that will provide a baseline of functioning from which to measure change. These assessments should also lead the clinician to plan particular types of intervention. At a higher level, a knowledge of the overall functioning of a group of severely disabled patients will allow the planning of future day and residential provision and its continuing evaluation. Nowhere is the relationship between the researcher and the clinician more crucial than in the development of adequate assessment tools.

The severity of psychiatric illness can be measured by counting up symptoms — e.g. the total PSE score (Wing *et al.*, 1974) — but it is possible for some patients to exhibit symptoms which have little measurable effect on their lives. A more informative scale for rehabilitation purposes is the inability to perform common tasks or social functions. There has been some confusion within this field because social functioning has developed a range of meanings.

13.5 WHAT IS NORMAL SOCIAL FUNCTIONING?

The concept of social functioning embraces all human behaviour so it is difficult to decide which dimensions to include in any particular assessment. Various meanings have been suggested, such as performance in roles, social behaviour and social interaction impairment. Its measurement has been underpinned by a number of different concepts such as social adjustment, fulfilling expected roles, meeting community expectations etc. Defining what is adaptive functioning presupposes a knowledge of what is adaptive and maladaptive.

The establishment of such norms has always

proved problematic. When defining global measures such as family responsibility the coding will inevitably be culturally specific. The cultural bias built into some formal assessments makes it difficult even to consider their use in other societies. Even within one culture expectations will differ with respect to age, social class and sex in a complex manner. For instance, the expectations of child care will be very different for a 30-year-old man and for a 60-year-old. Assessments also have a built-in obsolescence when used in cultures with changing norms. For instance, the role of women has changed considerably since the late 1950s and early 1960s, but this has rarely been reflected in the design and use of social functioning schedules.

There are two main ways of dealing with this problem. One is to specify 'ideal' functioning. But, as was stated earlier this does have its drawbacks. In fact one recently published schedule, The Self-Care Measurement Schedule (Barnes and Benjamin, 1987) includes 'eating a meal in bed', 'not getting up before 10 am' and 'not going shopping' as contributing to a deviant behaviour score. This author and probably some of the readers of this chapter are likely to have scored on all these items in the past month but not to have considered they were deviant. Clare and Cairns (1978) based their level of normal functioning on government statistics such as how people spent their disposable income. Others have used the profile of responses on their instrument when different samples are studied.

The second main approach is to turn the problem on its head and to use a threshold for disability set in such a way that behaviour classified as a problem would be considered abnormal across cultural and subcultural boundaries. This boundary can then be tested on a general population sample. If the number of people scoring on any item is small then the boundary for disability is reinforced.

13.6 DIFFERENT LEVELS OF ASSESSMENT

There are many different layers of social functioning assessment. They are all of use in designing and evaluating individual rehabilitation programmes. For the purposes of this chapter these layers have been divided into social attainments, social roles and instrumental behaviour.

13.6.1 SOCIAL ATTAINMENTS

These are easily identifiable global measures that mark achievements in major role areas such as marital history and employment history. They are generally used to collate historical data. Here as in the other layers of functioning, we come across the problem of what is normal behaviour. For instance, the normality of experiencing several significant heterosexual relationships has been hotly disputed. Social attainment measures are crude and they need to be seen against particular social backgrounds. For example, in weighing the significance of unemployment, community employment figures must be taken into account. Warner (1985) concluded that there was a large negative correlation between the amount of unemployment in the general population and the recovery rates in schizophrenia. Recovery in this context is the return to independent social and financial functioning. In judging the usefulness of social attainment indices the researcher and clinician must take into account both the current and past social expectations. Despite the lack of detail provided by this form of measurement, the fact that a person has been able to persuade an employer to offer a client a job or that he or she has been able to form an attachment to someone else does indicate some socially skilled behaviour in the past. But the absence of these indices does not necessarily indicate disability.

13.6.2 SOCIAL ROLES ARE THE NEXT LAYER DOWN

This type of information provides more detail than the social attainment measures because it measures performance in certain roles. Most researchers have generally agreed on the types of role to be included but the forms of measurement vary significantly. Some questionnaires measure only objective behaviour in a role (e.g. MRC Social Performance Schedule; Hurry and Sturt, 1981; Sturt and Wykes, 1987), others include the subject's feelings about their performance. The inclusion of the client's feelings is likely to confound the measure of performance with symptoms, especially in the severely disabled group where adverse attitudes to impairment are likely to further distort the picture. Another drawback is that the roles studied may be inapplicable for the population being studied. There are numerous preconceptions about the severely disabled group. Many are still involved with their families and some still have an intact marriage. Assessment instruments should therefore not be limited in the sorts of roles they study.

At the lowest level, each role is divided into specific *instrumental behaviours*. For instance, self-care can be divided into ability to look after personal hygiene, cooking, budgeting, and appearance. These more specific items can then be unpacked further (e.g. frequency of washing, need for prompting or actual help in washing). Even these types of behaviours can be further broken down into smaller behavioural units. The level of detail will depend on the need for rehabilitation in each role area.

The wider measures (social attainments and social roles) are useful in first differentiating the problem and providing some background information. The problem areas then need to be described in more detail using the instrumental behaviour-type schedules which assess what the client's behaviour actually is and how it falls short of expected performance. Specific schedules might not be needed for a detailed analysis: carrying out behavioural observations on the individual client may be sufficient. However, there is also a need to use assessments for global behaviours that have some information on comparable populations. These data can be used to set the patient in some sort of context. For example, if he or she is in hospital but has the same level of difficulties as someone in a group home, we might suggest that his current placement is inappropriate and that a transfer to another context would be best. However, there would be some exceptions to this decision rule. For some patients included in this long-term group the overall level of problems may be low, but the particular problems are somewhat intractable or make the client less attractive to community facilities. This is especially true of clients who are sexually disinhibited or who show verbal or physical aggression. These particular problems will initially limit the horizons of any clinician.

In addition to these patient assessments, there are of course many other assessments that may be necessary. Rehabilitation is seen as an interaction between the patient and his or her environment. This environment must be measured in terms of its demand, the level of stress it produces and the opportunities for initiative and choice provided. Relatives' views will also need to be taken into account when making judgments about needs and placement.

13.7 TYPES OF ASSESSMENT

This section provides a few examples of the methods available. It is not a comprehensive list, and the reader who requires more detail on the numerous tools available should refer to reviews in Weissman (1975), Weissman *et al.* (1981), Anthony and Farkas (1982), Beels *et al.* (1984), Kane *et al.* (1985) Wallace (1986), Platt (1986), and other relevant chapters in this book. The reader must be prepared to be somewhat disappointed with the available measures, as the criticisms of most assessments are often quite damning. Hall (1980) in a review

of 29 ward rating scales for the severely disabled population only found two which he thought were acceptable rating instruments. Table 13.2 provides a description of the major criteria to consider when choosing an appropriate assessment schedule.

13.7.1 HIGHER LEVELS OF SOCIAL ATTAINMENTS (e.g. work experience, marital history)

There are several different schedules to collate historical data which are useful because comparison data are available. These schedules are also easy to generate so clinicians should have little difficulty in developing one to meet their needs. A recent NIMH sponsored project on the development of social functioning measures suggested that this area was often neglected in the current literature (Kane *et al.*, 1985). It seems a shame to develop elaborate schedules and omit these very obvious indicators. Examples include the following:

(a) Psychiatric Epidemiology Research Interview (Dohrenwend *et al.*, 1981). This is a self-report schedule covering three areas: job attainment, marital attainment and parental attainment. There are six performance and satisfaction measures. It has been used in a number of studies but few have involved schizophrenic patients. As it is a self-report schedule the data collected may need to be supplemented and verified for the severely disabled group.

(b) Basic Data Schedule (Sturt *et al.*, 1982). This schedule has been used to collect data from the severely disabled group on employment, social relationships and independence (e.g. living arrangements) as well as previous service contacts. The measure is useful in that it codes the best performance as well as the most recent. For example, the last household is coded but so is the maximum level of independence achieved in this category. The data collated on this schedule can be obtained from a variety of sources including the patient, case records, family and key workers.

Table 13.2 Important points to consider when choosing an assessment schedule

1.	Accuracy	Evidence for the accuracy of the information collected would be provided by direct behavioural recordings which can be correlated with informant ratings on an interview schedule. Few assessment instruments provide these data.
2.	Reliability	The information should be reproducible over short periods of time and more importantly two separate raters should code in the same way. If the schedule uses third party informants then the reliability of their information must also be quoted.
3.	Validity	This means that the schedule it is measuring what it says it is measuring. Information is often provided on face validity but concurrent or convergent validity would be preferable (that is, each scale should show how it relates to others and to overt behaviour). Each scale must clearly specify and differentiate between good and poor performance.
4.	Content	It should reflect the concerns of professional groups, e.g. doctors, nurses, social workers, as well as including community and family concerns.
5.	What population?	A schedule designed to measure functioning in the elderly will not be appropriate for young chronic schizophrenics. In this case, the restricted range of some items will give a picture of relatively high functioning in the young chronic patient.
6.	What time frame?	Different time periods may be appropriate for different sorts of behaviours. Low frequency behaviours, e.g. violence, which are important in assessing rehabilitation should be measured over longer time periods in order to maximize the chances of detecting them.
7.	Range of ratings?	This is especially important when choosing an instrument to monitor change over time. Overall behaviour scores show how an individual fits into a population but provide little information on the patterning of disability for rehabilitation. These global measures will also not allow the slower changes in behaviour to be detected. The detection of change is extremely important for supporting staff morale when working with this group.
8.	What settings?	Most behavioural assessments were designed for use in idiosyncratic environments. Institutions often favour particular behavioural styles to cope with the milieu and so care must be taken in transposing schedules across these different environments.

13.7.2 INFORMANT DRIVEN ASSESSMENTS (e.g. role performance, instrumental behaviour

Table 13.3 provides a few examples of the sorts of schedules used in this area. Of the schedules listed here REHAB and SBS are in my opinion the best examples of rating schedules for instrumental behaviours. Both scales have been used with the severely disabled. SBS has more comparative data on community samples and has the virtue of being cheaper but otherwise they are reasonably equivalent. The Life Skills Profile (Rosen *et al.*, 1989 and Chapter 12)

covers many similar areas to REHAB and SBS but it has only recently been developed and it is too early to judge its usefulness in planning and evaluating rehabilitation programmes. SBAS and SPS are the least criticized of the schedules rating social functioning in roles. None of four recommended questionnaires have adopted a concept of 'ideal behaviour'. All of them concentrate on measuring objective performance and where subjective feelings are measured these ratings are separate from the objective score. Both reliability and validity estimates are available for these schedules. All the schedules have been used to rate patients

Table 13.3 Some examples of social role and instrumental behaviour rating scales

Name, source	Areas assessed	Time frame	Data collection method
Katz Adjustment Scale (Katz and Lylerly, 1963)	Symptoms, expected activities	Past few weeks	R — form completed by significant other S — form for patient
Social Adjustment Scale (SAS; Weissman and Paykel, 1974; SAS–SR; Weissman and Rothman, 1976)	Performance and satisfaction in five roles	Past two months SAS and SAS–II past 2 weeks	SAS — rated in interview with patient SAS–SR completed by patient SAS–II for chronic patients
Social Behaviour Assessment Scale (Platt *et al.*, 1983)	Symptoms, role performance subjective and objective burden	Past month	Interview with significant other
Rehabilitation Evaluation of Hall and Baker (REHAB; Hall and Baker, 1983)	Deviant and general behaviours	Past week	Completed by trained direct care staff
Social Performance Schedule (SPS; Hurry and Sturt, 1981)	Eight roles	Past month	Rated in interview with patient
Social Behaviour Schedule (SBS; Wykes and Sturt, 1986)	Instrumental behaviour	Past month	Rated in interview with direct care staff
Community Adaptation Schedule (Burnes and Roen, 1967)	Feelings about about relation-ships and instrumental behaviour	Current	Completed by the patient
Denver Community Mental Health Questionnaire (Ciarlo and Riehman, 1977)	Social inter-action, role functioning and some instru-mental behaviour	Past 24 hrs	Rated during interview with patient
Independent Living Skills Survey (Wallace, 1986)	Social roles and instrumental behaviour	Past month	Rated by relative or member of direct care staff
Morningside Rehabilitation Status Scale (MRSS; Affleck and McGuire, 1984)	Symptoms, social roles, and deviant behaviour	Past month	Rated by trained direct care staff
Life Skills Profile (Rosen *et al.*, 1989)	Social roles and deviant behaviour	Past 6 months	Rated by direct care staff

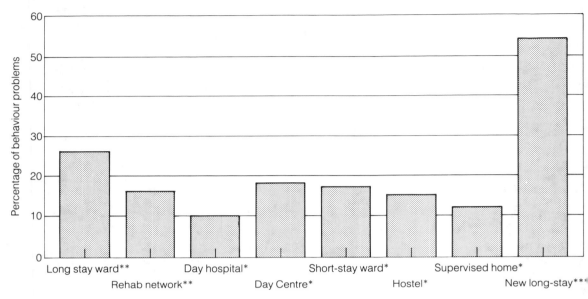

***Wykes, 1982
**Netherne series, Wykes and Sturt (1986)
*Camberwell series, Wykes et al. (1982)

Figure 13.1 Social behaviour problem.

in different service settings (e.g. Hurry and Sturt, 1981; Wykes *et al.*, 1982; Baker and Hall, 1988; Andrews *et al.*, 1990). Figure 13.1 shows the range of ratings on SBS for different community and hospital settings (Wykes and Wing, 1992). This figure shows that patients in services which provide different levels of supervision do show different levels of social functioning problems. In particular, 'new' long-stay patients who are in a hospital-hostel show the highest level of difficulties. These are the patients who despite modern social care still remain in hospital settings.

Although they are expanded versions, it is interesting to note that all four recommended questionnaires are also based on the Wing Ward Behaviour Rating Scale first published in 1961

(Wing, 1961). This schedule was used in the seminal study by Wing and Brown (1970) of three long-stay hospitals, and 29 years since its publication it is still being used in research studies.

The remaining schedules shown in the table are dogged by conceptual difficulties, confusion in the instructions on whether the rater is coding behaviour in the 'sick' or well role and the problem of norms. All of these remaining schedules show reasonable reliability and some even quote data on validity. No schedule is ideal for all areas of functioning and there is a need for continual development. However, there is still a tendency for both researchers and clinicians to 'throw the baby out with the bathwater' and produce idiosyncratic measures that are of little use in assessing patients over time or between settings.

13.7.3 SKILL ASSESSMENT BY ROLE PLAY (see also Chapter 11)

As well as assessing skills by the report of an observer or the patient it is also important to investigate behavioural responses under controlled conditions. In this way the clinician can change some of the environmental or interpersonal contingencies to develop hypotheses about the control of particular behaviours. It may not be possible to assess some interpersonal behaviours in any other way because the opportunities offered to patients have been reduced. For example, we may want to know whether a patient can talk to a stranger and ask for directions. We can encourage him or her to approach in different ways and look to see how the behaviour accomplishes a goal or how far short it is. Role play is often seen as part of a social skills training programme but there are few structured descriptions of how to carry it out or how role play relates to other forms of assessment.

Role play is not an appropriate means of monitoring real changes in the client's behaviour. One of the main problems experienced by rehabilitation consultants is the lack of generalization of skills from one setting to another. This problem has been documented for varying skills training programmes (e.g. Scott *et al.*, 1983; Shepherd, 1983, 1986). It is important to check whether the patient has actually learned a set of skills that can be applied under different conditions or whether he or she has only learned to react appropriately in a simulated situation.

13.7.4 DIRECT BEHAVIOURAL, NATURALISTIC OBSERVATIONS

Observational assessments of behaviour also need to comply with the criteria set out in Table 13.2. Generally, these types of observation are expensive in terms of staff resources. Time samples of behaviour are usually taken as these are less expensive than continuous recordings. One major problem of making these sorts of assessments is to define the time period for observation. When low frequency behaviours are studied then great care must be taken to make sure the most fruitful observation time is chosen. For instance, if the behaviour is improper social contacts, then meal times might be the most efficient observation period.

It is also important to define a meaningful unit of behaviour. For example, instances of delusional speech must be well defined so raters can delineate between utterances. The definition must include when a delusional utterance begins and ends and what content is to be coded as delusional. Delusional speech may otherwise be over-rated because one utterance of several sentences could be coded as two or three, or wishful thinking (e.g. "they're going to let me off my mental health section tomorrow") may also be included in the overall score. A discussion of these and other general problems of behavioural observation is given in Foster *et al.* (1988).

The Time-Sample Behavioural Checklist (TSBC, Paul and Lentz, 1977) is a useful instrument to guide ratings of behaviour. This schedule is based on random, two-second observations made throughout the patients waking hours. The 69 behavioural codes denote not only the actual behaviour but also its context, i.e. the location, presence of others, concurrent activities etc. There is a list of 'crazy' behaviours and a sub-score of inappropriate and appropriate behaviour. The rating is somewhat onerous so only one patient can be rated at a time but the information would be of use in verifying interview and rating scale data as well as providing a way of measuring change over time.

A somewhat less onerous system of ratings is provided in Wykes (1982). In this paper a simple method of time budgeting several patients' behaviour throughout the day was described. The measure was sensitive to changes in environments so that hostel residents were shown to spend less of their time doing nothing than did residents of a traditional hospital ward.

One of the most appropriate ways of monitoring change in a rehabilitation programme is to set behavioural goals which are checked at intervals. These goals can be structured behavioural homework or it can be simple observational records which could be developed for specific individuals' needs.

13.7.5 SELF-ASSESSMENT

The severely disabled patient often has difficulty in reflecting on his or her skills, but this should not preclude the use of structured self-assessments of skills (Table 13.3). Recently MacCarthy et al. (1986) have been successful in having long-term patients appraise their own problems. Unfortunately, there was often little agreement between the patients and their clinicians on the sorts of difficulties that needed to be addressed.

Patiental attitudes need to be assessed not only because clients need to negotiate agreements on rehabilitation plans (Table 13.1), but also to see whether they have any adverse attitudes which might affect the outcome or course of the illness (Wing, 1978). These adverse attitudes might be dealt with explicitly in a rehabilitation treatment plan or they may be monitored to see if increasing success in a programme produces positive effects.

Several studies have used patient attitudes to services as a guide to their usefulness (e.g. Wykes, 1982; Andrews et al., 1990). Patient attitudes have also been used to monitor the progress of patients in transfers between settings (Wykes, 1982). In this last study a number of 'new' long-stay patients were transferred to a hospital-hostel from a traditional hospital ward. Some of the transferred group were opposed to the move and initially were not as satisfied with the new service. Over time the transferred group became more satisfied with their surroundings but were also more vocal about what they would like to see changed about the service. This increasing critical appraisal was seen as an improvement in a group of patients who had appeared quite apathetic in a long stay hospital ward.

13.7.6 SYMPTOMS (see also Chapters 1 and 10)

One scale that may prove useful for symptom assessment is the Krawiecka Scale (Krawiecka et al., 1977). This scale has been used in surveying populations, assessing patients for rehabilitation and in monitoring change (Johnstone et al., 1978; Owens and Johnstone, 1980; Manchandra and Hirsh, 1986). It is relatively easy for untrained raters to use and it can be a substitute for other brief scales such as the Brief Psychiatric Rating Scale (BPRS) (Overall and Gorham, 1962) especially when a limited range of pathology is to be rated. The BPRS covers both florid and deficit symptoms in schizophrenia as well as irritability, depression etc. However, it fails to provide adequate descriptions for rating and several versions have been used with differing scales of severity for each item. The Global Assessment Scale (GAS) (Endicott et al., 1976) uses a patient's symptoms and social functioning to arrive at a measure of overall functioning; therefore it is not recommended if symptom profiles are needed or where particular symptoms are likely to change at different rates.

All of the above types of assessment are useful for the general population of long-term patients irrespective of diagnosis. However, the majority of the group have a diagnosis of schizophrenia and these require some unique assessments of specific disorder. For the design of rehabilitation programmes it is the effect of these symptoms on functioning which is important. For instance, some patients may have delusions which are only apparent under close questioning whereas others appear to talk about their delusions all the time. Although both patients would be rated as exhibiting delusions their functioning is affected in completely different ways.

Symptom assessments such as the PSE (Wing *et al.*, 1974), the BPRS (Overall and Gorham, 1962) and the various negative and positive symptom ratings described in Chapters 2 and 10 may also be useful in designing specific interventions for treating such symptoms. These types of treatments are not now confined to pharmacology. Several psychologists have designed specific interventions for auditory hallucinations, delusions and thought disorder (e.g. Slade, 1972, 1973; Watts *et al.*, 1973).

Monitoring symptoms might also allow a prodromal phase in the patient's illness to be identified. Rehabilitation efforts could then be switched to deal with these symptom exacerbations. For instance, intermittent medication strategies could be allied to psychosocial treatments which reduce the level of environmental stressors.

13.7.7 NEEDS ASSESSMENTS

This type of assessment system was originally devised by Mann and Cree (1976) in a survey of long-stay patients in England and Wales. In their study decisions on a patient's needs for care were taken by various groups of staff. All staff agreed on the need for highly supportive care for the same proportion of patients. Unfortunately, the individuals making up the groups were often different. This model was expanded by Wykes *et al.* (1982, 1985) and further developed by Brewin *et al.* (1987) into the Needs for Care Assessment. Need is said to be present when functioning falls below a specified level. Staff who know the patient make this judgment with the help of a shortened form of SBS. If a need has attracted some intervention that is at least partly effective then it is described as a 'met' need. If no interventions are being carried out at all or the intervention is ineffective then the need is described as

'unmet'. The remaining category is one of 'overmet' need i.e. if the intervention was removed then the patient would not relapse.

The assessment includes guidelines for judging the appropriateness of various interventions and also some information on how to judge when an intervention is ineffective. For instance, Brewin and colleagues provide a list of possible interventions for psychotic symptoms with their effectiveness and acceptability to the patient. This sort of assessment has only recently been developed but it does seem to have some merit in being able to provide a systematic and standardized way in which various treatments can be judged as appropriate and which should be abandoned. Further reliability and validity evaluations should be carried out and further work on the scaling of the effectiveness of treatments has to be developed.

All of the above assessments mainly concentrate on the deficits of a patient's behaviour. Very few schedules stress positive attributes. Although this often leads to more positive views by staff and the behaviours may provide the foundation for any rehabilitative effort.

13.7.8 ENVIRONMENTAL ASSESSMENTS

This category covers not only the actual physical environment but also the emotional environment of the patient. Rehabilitation services are usually assessed in terms of the management practices that they adopt. Raynes *et al.* (1979) developed a series of measures which include client-oriented practices and the extent to which staff felt involved in decision making. Garety and Morris (1984) used modifications of these scales and found higher levels of positive staff interaction in residential settings for the long-term mentally ill in which there were also higher levels of client-oriented management practices.

An alternative approach is to study the restrictiveness and permissiveness of different settings. The Hospital-Hostel Practices Profile (HHPP) has been used to look at hospitals for the long-term mentally ill (Hewitt *et al.* 1975; Ryan, 1979) and a series of hospital- and community-based day and residential services (Wykes *et al.*, 1982). These two approaches are reasonably equivalent and in fact both have been used on a 'new' long-stay hostel and have produced the same results (Wykes, 1982; Garety and Morris, 1984).

Although assessments have been carried out on the restrictiveness of different environments, this has not really been related theoretically to the rehabilitation potential of patients. There is probably a relationship between the level of restrictiveness of an environment and the predictability of that environment. For example, hospital wards are usually (but not necessarily) the most restrictive settings. They provide a predictable rule-governed life which for some patients may be helpful in dealing with their impairment.

This predictability may also help to explain some of the effects of high expressed emotion (EE, Chapter 8) on relapse rate. In a study carried out by MacCarthy *et al.* (1986) families of patients showing high and low EE were asked to make a list of the ways in which they coped with the patient's difficult behaviour, such as staying in bed all day. No particular coping strategy emerged to distinguish the groups, but low EE families tended to be more consistent in their approach. If this result can be replicated it does suggest that predictability, even in the home environment, could be a significant factor in whether patients remain well. Models of the factors involved in environmental demands now need to be developed. These models might then offer a way of differentiating environments for the purposes of rehabilitation. Current classifications deal only with rather broad expectations of functioning such as people having to cook their own evening meal or being expected to make their bed.

13.8 PROBLEMS IN REHABILITATION

It has been noted for many years that some

patients deteriorate when placed in situations requiring more individual choices, for instance in a rehabilitation programme, whereas others improve (Wing and Brown, 1970; Hemsley, 1978). Hemsley (1978) has suggested that the patients who deteriorate have a continuing cognitive abnormality. These patients have adopted certain behavioural strategies, e.g. social withdrawal, to deal with their information overload. Rehabilitative efforts increase the demand for informative processing and therefore patients deteriorate. Other patients, however, have adopted the same strategies but do not now possess the cognitive dysfunction. Rehabilitation programmes are more effective with this latter group because they reduce and replace these maladaptive behaviours. Unfortunately clinicians have not been able to differentiate these groups except on outcome criteria. This has been a great problem for clinicians, as it is often impossible to distinguish these clients from ones who will improve with more social stimulation.

However, recently Wykes and colleagues, in a series of studies on response processing were able to suggest a reaction time measure to distinguish those patients who have a continuing cognitive deficit (Wykes, 1985; Wykes *et al.*, 1992a, 1992b). The group with an underlying cognitive disability could not be distinguished from the rest on the basis of symptoms, social behaviour, service use or social attainments. Both groups showed social withdrawal and poor premorbid functioning, and had been in the longer stay wards for some considerable time. The group without the cognitive disability may be those who in the past were thought to be suffering from institutionalism. Over the following years it was decided to close down the hospital where these patients were based so a rigorous rehabilitation programme was instigated to supplement the existing network. None of the staff had access to the research data, but despite this the follow-up suggests that not one of the patients who showed poor response processing changed their setting to one that would give them more independence. They did move but it was always in the direction of increased care. Many of the other group moved to less dependent settings. These preliminary data suggest that we may be able to supplement our assessment process further and begin to design rehabilitation systems which will allow patients to succeed.

Some experts have suggested that cognitive data will allow the long-stay group to be sifted into those who will benefit from training programmes and those who will not. They have also suggested that this latter group should be excluded from training until a pharmacological control can be found for their impairment. I am more of the opinion that the identification of such a group should drive us to search for other less traditional methods of rehabilitation on the model of special education found in the mental handicap field.

13.9 CONCLUSION

Rehabilitation has developed significantly over the past 50 years and most of the gains that have been made rest on the development, and rigorous testing of assessment procedures. The next challenge is to utilize the detailed analyses from all the theoretical approaches and contributions to the treatment of schizophrenia, combining them into a comprehensive assessment procedure. One attempt at an outline is given in Table 13.4. A generally accepted set of procedures would not only aid service planning but would also enable comparisons of treatments and the extent of the gains made.

After some debate clinicians were able to arrive at a consensus on acceptable forms of symptom assessment. It now falls to those involved in rehabilitation to do the same for social functioning and environmental stress and until a consensus is reached there will be

Table 13.4 A comprehensive rehabilitation package

1. Background information	Social attainment measures (e.g. Basic Data Schedules; (Sturt *et al.*, 1982)
2. Current social functioning	(i) Social role performance (from SBAS; Platt *et al.*, 1983)
	(ii) Instrumental behaviours (SBS; Wykes and Sturt, 1986)
3. Direct observation of problem behaviour	(i) Role play and/or
	(ii) Natural observation
4. Client strengths	Positive features of client's behaviour
5. Environmental assessments	
(a) Services	(i) Setting demands/ opportunities (e.g. HHPP; Wykes *et al.*, 1982)
	(ii) Predictability of setting
(b) Family	(i) Family atmosphere (EE; Vaughan and Leff, 1976)
	(ii) Burden on family (from SBAS; Platt *et al.*, 1983)

problems in communicating both our advances and disappointments.

REFERENCES

Affleck, J. and McGuire, R. (1984) The measurement of psychiatric rehabilitation status. A review of the needs and a new scale. *Br. J. Psychiatry*, **145**, 517–25.

Andrews, G., Teeson, M., Stewart, G. and Hoult, J. (1990) Follow-up of community placement of chronic mentally ill in New South Wales. *Hosp. Community Psychiatry*, **41**, 184–8.

Anthony, W., Cohen, M. and Farkas (1982) A psychiatric rehabilitation treatment program: Can I recognise one if I see one? *Community Ment. Health J.*, **18**, 83–95.

Anthony, W.A. and Farkas, M.A. (1982) A client outcome planning model for assessing psychiatric rehabilitation interventions. *Schizophr. Bull.*, **8**, 13–38.

Baker, R. and Hall, J. (1988) REHAB: A new assessment instrument for chronic psychiatric patients. *Schizophr. Bull.*, **14**, 97–111.

Barnes, D. and Benjamin, S. (1987) The self care assessment schedule SCAS-1. The purpose and construction of a new assessment of self care behaviours. *J. Psychometr. Res.*, **31**, 191–202.

Beels, C.C., Gutworth, L., Berkeley, J. and Struening, E. (1984) Measurements of social support in schizophrenia. *Schizophr. Bull*, **10**, 399–411.

Bennett, D.H. (1983) The historical development of rehabilitation services. In *Theory and Practice in Rehabilitation*, F.N. Watts and D.H. Bennett (eds), John Wiley and Sons, Chichester, pp. 15–42.

Birley, J. (1974) A housing association for psychiatric patients. *Psychiatr. Q.*, **48**, 568–71.

Brewin, C., Wing, J.K., Mangen, S., Brugha, T. and MacCarthy, B. (1987) The principles and practice of measuring needs in the long-term mentally ill: the MRC for care assessment. *Psychol. Med.*, **17**, 971–81.

Burnes, A. and Roen, S. (1967) Social roles and adaptation to the community. *Community Ment. Health J.*, **3**, 153–8.

Ciarlo, J. and Reihman, J. (1977) The Denver Community Mental Health Questionnaire: Development of a multi-dimensional program evaluation instrument. In *Program Evaluation for Mental Health: Methods, Strategies and Participants*. R. Coursey, G. Specter, S. Murrel and B. Hunt (eds), Grune & Stratton, New York.

Clare, A. and Cairns, V. (1978) Design, development and use of a standardized interview to assess social maladjustment and dysfunction in community studies. *Psychol. Med.*, **8**, 589–604.

Dohrenwend, B.S., Cook, D. and Dohrenwend, B.P. (1981) Social functioning in community populations. In *What is a Case?* J.K. Wing, P. Bebbington and L. Robbins (eds), Grant Mcintyre, London, pp. 183–201.

Endicott, J., Spitzer, R., Fleiss, J. and Cohen, J. (1976) The global assessment scale, a procedure for measuring the overall severity of psychiatric disturbance. *Arch. Gen. Psychiatry*, **33**, 766–71.

Foster, S., Bell-Dolan, D. and Burge, D. (1988) Behavioural Observation. In *Behavioural Assessment. A Practical Handbook*. A. Bellack and M. Hersen (eds), Pergamon Press, Oxford, pp. 119–160.

Garety, P. (1988) Housing. In *Community Care in Practice*. A. Lavender and F. Holloway (eds), Wiley and Sons, Chichester, pp. 143–69.

Garety, P. and Morris, I. (1984) A new unit for long stay psychiatric patients: Organisation, attitudes and quality of care. *Psychol. Med.*, **14**, 183–92.

Hall, J. (1980) Ward rating scales for long-stay patients: a review. *Psychol. Med.*, **10**, 277–88.

Hall, J. and Baker, R. (1983) *REHAB, a users manual*, Vine Publishing, Aberdeen.

Harding, C., Zubin, J. and Strauss, J. (1987a) Chronicity in schizophrenia: Fact, partial fact or artifact. *Hosp. Community Psychiatry*, **38**, 477–86.

Harding, C., Brooks, G., Ashkinaga, T. *et al.* (1987b) The Vermont Longitudinal Study of persons with severe mental illness I: Methodology, study sample and overall status 32 years later. *Am. J. Psychiatry*, **144**, 718–36.

Hemsley, D. (1978) Limitations of operant procedures in the modification of schizophrenic functioning: The possible relevance of studies of cognitive disturbance. *Behav. Anal. Mod.*, **2**, 165–73.

Hewett, S., Ryan, P. and Wing, J.K. (1975) Living without mental hospitals. *J. Soc. Policy*, **4**, 391–404.

Holloway, F. (1988) Day Care and Community Support. In *Community Care in Practice*. A. Lavender and F. Holloway (eds), Wiley and Sons, Chichester, pp. 161–86.

Hurry, J. and Sturt, E. (1981) Social performance in a population sample: relation to psychiatric symptoms. In *What is a case?* J.K. Wing, P. Bebbington and L. Robbins (eds). Grant McIntyre, London, pp. 202–13.

Johnstone, E., Crow, T., Frith, C., Carney, M. and Price, J. (1978) Mechanism of the antipsychotic effect in the treatment of acute schizophrenia. *Lancet*, **i**, 848–51.

Kane, R., Kane, R.L. and Arnold, S. (1985) Measuring Social Functioning in Mental Health Studies: Concepts and instruments. *DHSS. Pub. No. (ADM) 85-1384*, US Government Printing Office, Washington.

Katz, M. and Lyerly, S. (1963) Methods for measuring adjustment and social behaviour in the community: I. Rationale, description, discriminative ability and scale development. *Psychol. Rep.*, **13**, 502–35.

Krawiecka, M., Goldberg, D. and Vaughan, M. (1977) A standardized psychiatric scale for rating chronic psychotic patients. *Acta Psychiatr. Scand.*, **55**, 299–308.

MacCarthy, B., Benson, J. and Brewin, C. (1986) Task motivation and problem appraisal in long term psychiatric patients. *Psychol. Med.*, **16**, 431–8.

MacCarthy, B., Hemsley, D., Shrank-Fernandez, C. Kuipers, E. and Katz, R. (1986) Unpredictability as a correlate of expressed emotion in the relatives of schizophrenics. *Br. J. Psychiatry*, **148**, 727–31.

Manchandra, R. and Hirsch, S. (1986) Does propranalol have an antipsychotic effect? A placebo controlled study in acute schizophrenia. *Br. J. Psychiatry*, **148**, 701–7.

Mann, S.A. and Cree, W. (1976) 'New' long stay psychiatric patients: a national sample of fifteen mental hospitals in England and Wales 1972/3. *Psychol. Med.*, **6**, 603–16.

Mann, S.A. and Sproule, J. (1972) Reasons for a six months stay. In *Evaluating a community psychiatric service. The Camberwell Register 1964–1971*, J.K. Wing and A. Hailey (eds), Oxford University Press, London, pp. 233–45.

Overall, J. and Gorham, D. (1962) The Brief Psychiatric rating scale. *Psychol. Rep.*, **10**, 799–812.

Owens, D. and Johnstone, E. (1980) The disabilities of chronic patients – their nature and the factors contributing to their development. *Br. J. Psychiatry*, **136**, 384–95.

Paul, G. and Lentz, R. (1977) *Psychosocial treatment of mental patients*. Harvard University Press, Cambridge MA.

Platt, S. (1986) Evaluating social functioning: A critical review of scales and their underlying concepts. In *The Psychopharmacology and treatment of schizophrenia*. P. Bradley and S. Hirsch (eds), British Association for Psychopharmacology Monograph No. 8, Oxford University Press, London, pp. 263–285.

Platt, S., Weyman, A. and Hirsch, S. (1983) *Social Behaviour Assessment schedule (SBAS)*, Third ed. NFER, Windsor, Berks.

Raynes, N., Pratt, M. and Roses, S. (1979) *Organisational structure and the care of the mentally handicapped*, Croom Helm, London.

Rosen, A., Hadzi-Pavlovic, D. and Parker, G. (1989) The life skills profile: A measure assessing function and disability in schizophrenia. *Schizophr. Bull.*, **15**, 325–44.

Ryan, P. (1979) Residential care for the mentally disabled. In *Community care for the mentally disabled*, J.K. Wing and R. Olsen (eds), Oxford University Press, London, pp. 60–98.

Scott, R., Himadi, W. and Keane, T. (1983) A review of generalisation in social skill training: suggestions for future research. In *Progress in Behaviour Modification*, R. Eisler and P. Miller (eds), Vol. 15, Grune & Stratton, New York, pp. 110–32.

Shepherd, G. (1983) Planning the rehabilitation of the individual. In *Theory and practice of psychiatric rehabilitation*, F.N. Watts and D.H. Bennett (eds), Wiley, Chichester, pp. 329–48.

Shepherd, G. (1986) Social Skills Training and schizophrenia. In *Handbook of Social Skills Training*, Vol 2, C. Hollin and P. Trower (eds), Pergamon, London, pp. 9–37.

Slade, P. (1972) The effects of systematic desensitization on auditory hallucinations. *Behav. Res. Ther.*, **10**, 85–91.

Slade, P. (1973) The psychological investigation and treatment of auditory hallucinations. *Br. J. Med. Psychol.*, **46**, 293–6.

Stein, L. and Test, M. (1978) *Alternatives to mental hospital treatment*. Plenum, New York.

Sturt, E. and Wykes, T. (1987) Assessment schedules for chronic psychiatric patients. *Psychol. Med.*, **17**, 485–93.

Sturt, E., Wykes, T., and Creer, C. (1982) Demographic, social and clinical characteristics of the sample. In *Long term community care in Camberwell, Psychol. Med. Monogr. Suppl. No. 2*. J.K. Wing (ed), Cambridge University Press, Cambridge, pp. 5–14.

Vaughan, C. and Leff, J. (1976) The measurement of expressed emotion in families of psychiatric patients. *Br. J. Soc. Clin. Psychol.*, **129**, 125–37.

Wallace, C.J. (1986) Functional assessment in rehabilitation. *Schizophr. Bull.*, **12**, 604–30.

Warner, R. (1985) *Recovery from Schizophrenia. Psychiatric and Political Economy*. Routledge and Kegan Paul, London.

Watts, F.N., Powell, G. and Austin, S. (1973) The modification of abnormal beliefs. *Br. J. Med. Psychol.*, **46**, 359–63.

Weissman, M. (1975) The assessment of social adjustment by patient self report. *Arch. Gen. Psychiatry*, **32**, 357–65.

Weissman, M. and Bothwell, S. (1976) Assessment of social adjustment by patient self report. *Arch. Gen. Psychiatry*, **33**, 1111–5.

Weissman, M. and Paykel, E. (1974) *The depressed woman: a study of social relationships*. University of Chicago Press, Chicago.

Weissman, M., Sholomkas, D. and John, R. (1981) The assessment of social adjustment: an update. *Arch. Gen. Psychiatry*, **38**, 1250–8.

Wing, J.K., (1978) *Reasoning about Madness*. Oxford University Press, London.

Wing, J.K. (1983) Schizophrenia. In *Theory and Practice of Rehabilitation*. F.N. Watts and D.H. Bennett, (eds), John Wiley and Sons, Chichester, pp. 45–64.

Wing, J.K. (1990) The measurement of 'Social Disablement'. *Soc. Psychiatry*. (in press)

Wing, J.K. and Brown, G. (1970) *Institutionalism and Schizophrenia*. Cambridge University Press, London.

Wing, J.K., Cooper, J. and Sartorius, N. (1974) *The Measurement and classification of psychiatric symptoms: An instruction manual for PSE and Catego systems*. Cambridge University Press, Cambridge.

Wykes, T. (1982) A hostel-ward for 'new' long stay patients: an evaluative study of a 'ward in a house'. In *Long-Term Community Care in Camberwell: Experience in One London Borough, Psychol. Med. Monog. Suppl. No. 2*, J.K. Wing (ed), Cambridge University Press, Cambridge, pp. 59–97.

Wykes, T. (1985) *Cognitive impairment in a psychiatric population – It's relationship to chronic disability and some implications for rehabilitation*. Unpublished M.Phil. Thesis, London University, Institute of Psychiatry.

Wykes, T. and Sturt, E. (1986) The measurement of social behaviour in psychiatric patients: An assessment of the reliability and validity of SBS. *Br. J. Psychiatry*, **148**, 1–11.

Wykes, T. and Wing, J.K. (1992) The size and nature of the problem. In *Residential needs for severely disabled psychiatric patients: the case for Hospital Hostels*. K. Woof (ed), HMSO.

Wykes, T., Creer, C. and Sturt E. (1982a) Needs and the deployment of services. In *Long-Term Community Care in a London Borough, Psychol. Med. Monogr. Supp. No. 2*. J.K. Wing (eds), Cambridge University Press, pp. 41–54.

Wykes, T. Sturt E. and Creer, C. (1982b) Practices of day and residential units in relation to the social behaviour of attenders. In *Long-Term Community Care experience in one London Borough, Psychol. Med. Monograph Supplement No. 2*. J.K. Wing, (ed), Cambridge University Cambridge, Cambridge, pp. 15–28.

Wykes, T., Katz, R. and Sturt, E., (1992a) The prediction of rehabilitative success after three years: the use of social symptomatic and cognitive variables. *Br. J. Psychiatry*, in press.

Wykes, T., Katz, R., Sturt, E. and Hemsley, D. (1992b) *Response processing in a chronic psychiatric group: A possible predictor of rehabilitation failure. Br. J. Psychiatry*, in press.

Chapter 14

Assessment of life events

T.J.K. CRAIG

14.1 INTRODUCTION

There is now a substantive literature attesting to the important role played by recent life events in a number of psychiatric and physical illnesses. For some conditions such as depression, the debate has moved beyond the issue of whether events are aetiological agents to arguments about the strength of the association, and the social and biological vulnerabilities on which they operate. However, for most disorders including schizophrenia, research has not progressed much beyond the first steps towards establishing casual links. The evidence reviewed by Bebbington and Kuipers (Chapter 8) suggests that people who suffer from schizophrenia may be at greater risk of relapse if they are exposed to stressful environments which heighten levels of psychological arousal and that relapse may be prevented by interventions which reduce this exposure. So far, it has only been practicable to attempt such interventions for a narrow subset of chronic stressors (i.e. high 'expressed emotion' family environments). Ideally, it should be possible to develop interventions to reduce the occurrence or impact of other stressful experiences as well, but at present, this seems an unattainable target.

Three factors impede our chances of developing successful interventions. First, the very breadth of circumstances which might produce the sort of arousal which matters and the fact that such circumstances are part and parcel of ordinary life. Second, the apparent impossibility of predicting when such 'events' will occur and third, the short time lag between the event and the relapse, which most studies place at a matter of weeks at most. It stands to reason therefore that any hope of successful interventions will depend on the ability to identify what events matter for which people, to predict periods in a person's biography when these crises are more likely to occur and to develop rapid response strategies (including adjustments to medication) at these times. It has to be admitted that at present these all seem unattainable targets. But developments in the technology of life event assessment are beginning to suggest that this may not be such an impossible task after all. The purpose of this chapter is to review these recent advances in the hope that this may inspire a fresh look at schizophrenia.

14.2 WHAT IS A LIFE EVENT?

The first step in pursuing the aetiological relevance of a particular experience requires a precise definition of the unit of enquiry.

Physical stressors such as extremes of temperature, noise, or the deprivation of nourishment must be clearly distinguished from social experiences. Discrete events which occur abruptly and which are relatively transient need to be distinguished from chronic situational difficulties (such as poor housing conditions) which persist over prolonged periods of time and which may exist without ever producing a discrete event.

Deciding what range of phenomena to study is clearly not enough. Stressors also differ in terms of meaning. Events can only be 'stressful' once they have been appraised and evaluated by the person who experiences them and just what meaning an occurrence will have depends on the extent to which it impinges on a person's plans, goals and concerns (Fridja, 1986). For example, a pregnancy may be desired or wholly unwelcome and a change of job may involve more or less adjustment to new work demands. It might seem therefore, that even if we are able to define events in some arbitrary manner, we will still be unable to assess their likely impact on individuals and the only way to proceed to this level of measurement is to ask people to provide their own classifications as to which of the recent experiences were stressful. However, people may not always be able to give accurate reports of how they felt or responded to an event. Some will deny the impact of events, others will exaggerate claims of distress; people forget how they actually felt at times of crisis; and the full meaning of events may not even be open to conscious awareness or have any rational explanation. Even more problematic from a research point of view is that such an approach does nothing to deal with the possibility that the respondent's account will be influenced by what happened after the event including any subsequent onset of illness.

14.3 MEANINGLESS MEASURES

Small wonder then that first attempts at developing life event rating scales put the issue of meaning firmly to one side. Instead, the emphasis was 'firmly placed on change and disruption from the existing steady state of adjustment and not on psychological meaning, emotional or social desirability' (Rahe, 1969, p. 98). There was some theoretical justification for this. In keeping with Selye's general adaptation theory (1956), events were considered to be important not because they produced emotional reactions, but because they heralded changes in the organism's environment which called for behavioural change and physiological adaptation. The physiological response might be entirely non-specific, but might be enough to precipitate disease in a vulnerable organ which could not 'cope' with the biological strain placed upon it by the process of adaptation.

The Social Readjustment Rating Scale — SRRS (Holmes and Rahe, 1967) was developed as a self-report quantitative assessment of recent change. Accordingly, it concentrated on assessments of events that should produce the greatest demand for 'adaptation' and began with the premise that such events would exert additive effects: each new experience adding to the need for adaptive responses in a linear manner. Since emotional reactions to events were thought to be relatively unimportant (in the sense that these probably reflected the extent of physiological arousal) there was little need to attempt to measure meaning. All that was required was an accurate account of the total number of events over a given time period and a way of scoring the likely adaptive changes that such events would produce. To develop the measure, Holmes and Rahe (1967) combed the medical records of naval personnel for incidents apparently associated with injury or onset of illness, and derived a list of 43 of the more common experiences which seemed to precede illness: all were thought to involve abrupt changes in routine. Since the final measure was the amount of change, scoring initially consisted of asking respondents to indicate which of the list of events they had experienced in the time period under scrutiny and then totalling the number of events. Later amendments attached 'change scores' or weights to each category which could also be added to provide an overall change score. These weights were derived by asking judges to assess the amount of likely disruption to routine caused by each event on the list. The events were then organized in descending order according to the average disruption scores provided by the judges. Finally, to make the scoring even simpler, change values were given to each event reflecting their position in the final hierarchy. For example, death of a spouse is given a weight of 100 and divorce has a weight of 73; a person who is dismissed from work and whose wife gives birth would get a score of 86 (47 + 39).

Set against the haphazard methods of reporting stressors in earlier work, this represented a major advance. At one leap Holmes and Rahe produced a broad list of stressors, a method of data collection using a simple self-report checklist, and a method of quantifying the impact of these stressors based on a simple summation of the individual stress scores. Although subsequently criticized severely, there is no doubt as to the importance of this pioneering work. Unfortunately, the relationships are weak and the result of this effort is rather disappointing.

Respondent-based checklist methods suffer from a number of grave weaknesses. Some of these, although serious, are probably rectifiable and have been tackled by a number of later developments of the method (Tennant and Andrews, 1976).

A more serious weakness concerns the self-report nature of the method of gathering data and this applies equally to all the later derivations of the SRRS. Such checklists are respondent-based measures in the sense that it is left to the respondent to decide which incidents to include and it is he or she who must take on the task of defining the basic unit of experience. So, for example,

in response to a question asking whether a relative has been ill, he or she must decide which relative to include and whether the illness suffered was serious enough to mention. Furthermore, the respondent's choice of relative may well be influenced by some attempt to make sense of the fact that he has developed symptoms of illness himself. The death of an uncle seen once in the last 10 years may only be recorded because the news of the death happened a few weeks before the respondent's own onset of symptoms and the subject is trying to make some sense of why he should have become ill at this particular time. Of course, the influence of such 'effort after meaning' (Bartlett, 1932) can be avoided by carefully instructing the subject as to what type of relatives can be included, how often they ought to have been seen prior to their illness before including them in the response and what illnesses with what level of handicap should be mentioned. These definitions are, however, far too cumbersome to incorporate in a simple checklist. Bias in reporting may also stem from the respondent's personality, attitudes to the questions asked, or even mood on the day the checklist was completed. In short, the SRRS and other checklist instruments have been severely criticized not only in terms of possible sources of measurement bias, but also in terms of inaccuracy in reporting (Brown, 1974, 1981; Jenkins *et al.*, 1979; Wershow and Reinhart, 1974).

A more precise rating technique is an investigator-based interview approach. Here, it is the job of the researcher to judge when sufficient material has been collected to rate an event as present. The technique of such interviewing is critical. A completely standardized interview with no flexibility over the wording of questions and no additional probing has no advantage over self-report checklists, while a completely unstructured interview would run serious risks of bias itself. One study which asked patients to volunteer events found that the likelihood of volunteering an event as 'important' was more likely to occur when the respondent's mood was abnormal and probably reflected the effort after meaning discussed earlier (Lipman *et al.*, 1965). Most modern techniques therefore are based on standard questions supplemented by unstructured probes. Before any interviews are undertaken, the researchers define what classes of experience should be included and draw up detailed rating rules for each. For example, having decided that road traffic accidents should be included as events, the research team goes on to determine whether this category should also include accidents to family members even when the subject is not present at the accident, whether 'family members' include only the immediate household or encompass parents and siblings, how serious the accident must be in order to be included and whether the seriousness of the accident has to be greater when the subject is not involved. This approach has the distinct advantage of getting away from the idiosyncratic reports of respondents while at the same time, through a careful specification of the rules *before* the study begins, providing control over researcher bias (for example, deciding to include an accident might be influenced by the researcher's knowledge that the accident was closely followed by onset of symptoms of the disease that is the subject of the aetiological enquiry).

In recent years, a number of these interview-based measures have been developed. Most popular are the measures of life events developed by Paykel *et al.* (1969), and the Life Events and Difficulties Schedule (Brown *et al.*, 1973; Brown and Harris, 1978). Both demonstrate a number of distinct advantages over the earlier respondent-based approaches. Not least, they permit much higher levels of reliability, and even more important, much higher levels of agreement between respondents and independent sources on the timing and nature of stressors (Brown and Harris, 1978; Paykel, 1983).

The Bedford College Life Events and Difficulties Schedule (LEDS) was developed on the assumption that events productive of general arousal could bring about the onset of schizophrenia in susceptible individuals by means of a simple triggering mechanism (Brown and Birley, 1968). This represented a departure in the conceptualization of what mattered about life events. As already noted, the SRRS assumed that it was behavioural change that was the key factor in explaining the onset of illness. This is not the only possible explanation. Indeed, subsequent research had cast serious doubt on this view and indicated that emotional arousal rather than change *per se* is the key factor responsible for the more common neurohumoral responses to stressors (Mason, 1968a, b) and many of the studies dealing with psychiatric disorder found a greater association with items indicating undesirability than change (Sarason *et al.*, 1978).

For the schizophrenia study, a comprehensive list of incidents was compiled which could be dated to a precise point in time and which were believed to be followed by strong emotion (of either a positive or negative kind). The inclusion criteria for each incident were carefully defined before any data was collected. This resulted in many incidents reported by subjects being excluded from consideration because they did not meet the strict inclusion criteria, but it also provided a common set of standards which allowed comparisons to be made between one individual and another with the certainty that the process of information gathering and rating would correspond closely with that in future studies using the method.

The LEDS also introduced the concept of 'independence' as a means of distinguishing events which might have arisen as a consequence of incipient illness and which therefore should not be included in the most stringent tests of causality. Many disorders impair social role performance and might thus give rise to events. For example, someone might get fired from their job because the incipient onset of schizophrenia had impaired their work capacity or led to unprovoked aggressive outbursts. Clearly such events are the consequence and not the cause of the disorder. One way of getting around this problem is to take particular care over dating event and onset, including only those events which clearly antedate the first signs of illness. Although the LEDS offers meticulous attention to dating, it is still not enough to guard against confounding. Many disorders are presaged by a lengthy and unrecorded prodromal period which may impair functioning at quite a subtle level so that it is not possible to determine the precise date of onset with enough certainty. The LEDS therefore, rates each event on a dimension of 'independence' which records the degree to which it can be said that a crisis would have occurred irrespective of the physical or mental state of the subject at the time. Independent events and difficulties are those which are imposed on subjects and are for all practical purposes outside his or her control (for example, being forced to change residence because of a government redevelopment programme). Of course, independent events exclude many possible stressors and can only give a minimal estimate of the role of event stress. This is useful methodologically though potentially misleading and therefore other events are classified as 'possibly independent' of the disorder in instances when there is no evidence to suggest that they had been related to unusual behaviour of the subject, though this cannot be ruled out on logical grounds. Examples of possibly independent events are marital separations after years of tension or a residence change based on a decision to seek more spacious family accommodation. Finally, these two categories are distinguished from 'illness-related' events such as being dismissed from a job due to carelessness.

By using this measure, it can be argued that if an association emerges between stressors and the onset for events which are logically independent, then any association between the

event and onset cannot be solely due to bias. Furthermore, if such an association holds for the purely independent events, it also makes the existence of a causal link more plausible for those events which can not be said to be entirely independent of the subject's behaviour.

A pilot study in 1960 showed that life events were particularly common in the three weeks prior to onset of florid schizophrenic symptoms. In the main study which followed, these results were confirmed: 60% of the patients had at least one such event compared with an average of only 23% in each of the three preceding 3-week periods, and only 20% of a general population comparison sample (Brown and Birley, 1968).

This study afforded one of the earliest demonstrations of an unambiguous relationship between prior stressful experiences and subsequent illness which could not easily be dismissed on grounds of poor methodology or the inclusion of 'confounded' events. The observed relationship was entirely non-specific. Indeed, Brown and Birley concluded that it seemed any form of emotional arousal including joy and excitement could be enough to precipitate onset. However, the LEDS at that stage of development could not take this any further. The possibility that the nature of the arousal which stressors engender might relate quite specifically to particular disease processes awaited a later development.

14.4 LIFE EVENTS AND MEANING

To recapitulate, by the time that the first LEDS study was under way, evidence was accumulating that it was emotional arousal and not change which was the critical issue and that new measures would have to take meaning into account. Fortunately, there is a way to proceed that can both recognize the fact that an event cannot be stressful until it has been cognitively processed, while at the same time getting away from having to rely on how particular individuals reported that they responded to its occurrence. This approach depends on the fact that human beings have the capacity to empathize with others — to use their own experiences of life to make reasonable guesses about how other people should feel in response to particular crises; and for the most part, to be correct in these guesses of other people's reactions.

First attempts at measuring meaning adopted the most straightforward approach. General meaning was dealt with in the sense that, ignoring how any single individual might react, most events could be broadly classified by the general population as 'desirable' or 'undesirable' or as 'entrances' or 'exits' to the social arena (Paykel *et al.*, 1969, 1971). Although this represented a significant advance over concepts of change and produced many valuable insights, it still did not go far enough. For example, consider the birth of a second child to an affluent, stable family who had made the conscious decision to enlarge their family and contrast this with the unexpected unplanned pregnancy and subsequent birth of a child to an unemployed single mother living in bed-and-breakfast accommodation with no family support. In the general meaning approach, both events are classified as identically desirable entrance experiences. It is 'intuitively' obvious that the two women ought to feel very differently about their pregnancies. If we can make such 'intuitive' judgements for other people once we know the context perhaps we can use this ability to improve the measurement.

Such understanding of other people's hardships is possible where raters and subjects live and have been reared in the same society and provided that they are aware of the circumstances surrounding the event and the subject's goals, choices and plans (Schutz, 1971). This personal context will include information on the person's wider social situation (whether for example, they are married, in a job or striving towards a particular goal), the culture to which they belong and their current sets of hopes and aspirations which are disrupted by the event. Of course, we have no way of knowing that this

is how a particular person *will* respond to a crisis, as even with all the facts at our disposal we can only make an assessment of what the 'average' person in those circumstances ought to feel and what the most likely response will be. The major problem of aetiological study is one of bias and not error. Even if we are wrong in our assumptions some of the time, such errors will only serve to weaken any causal links in our data and must be an improvement over the risks of bias which are inherent in asking people to define stress for themselves. This then is the basis for the *contextual* measure of meaning used by the LEDS. To minimize researcher bias, ratings are made by members of the research team who are ignorant of whether any disorder had developed subsequent to the event and respondent bias is additionally controlled by the fact that for the contextual rating, no attention is paid to what the respondent said he or she felt about the event. This approach allows events to be classified on a number of separate dimensions. For example, the extent to which a particular event would be seen as threatening or unpleasant by people in similar contexts can be rated alongside whether or not most people would have to make life changes or redirect their plans after the event.

For depression, the most crucial dimension has proved to be that of contextual threat. Threat in the LEDS system is measured at two points in time: the immediate impact of the event and the more protracted long-term implications of the event which are still present 10 to 14 days after its occurrence. For ongoing difficulties only the more protracted threat is of course relevant. The Camberwell survey was the first study to utilize the full LEDS (Brown and Harris, 1978). It was designed to investigate the role of stressful experiences in bringing about clinical depression and explored stressors in psychiatric inpatients, outpatients and a general population sample. The only events with causal significance in the onset of depression were those events with severe long-term threat and those with moderate long-term threat that were focused on the subject alone or jointly with another person. Events with only short-term threat, perhaps representing transitory arousal, were of no aetiological importance. In addition, certain markedly threatening long-term difficulties, lasting for two or more years, were more common among the depressed than among the comparison women. Taken together, one or more such events or difficulties had occurred prior to onset in 75% of the depressed patients and 89% of the general population cases but in only 30% of the non-depressed general population comparison women.

The application of the LEDS contextual threat measure to later studies of schizophrenia relapse suggest that the relevant events are at least moderately threatening and that only a small proportion of onsets or relapses seem to be associated with events which have no threat at all (Leff *et al.*, 1973; Leff and Vaughn, 1985). Even at this level of refinement, the association is not strong. For example, the undesirability of life events has been measured in terms of threat (Leff *et al.*, 1973; Leff and Vaughn, 1985), readjustment (Jacobs and Myers, 1976) and objective impact (Day *et al.*, 1987), but none of these studies have produced clear evidence to support the notion of dose-response relationships between the severity of events and onset of illness. One explanation for these observations is that the concept of 'threat' is still too broad to be useful. Onset may be related to some narrower conceptualization of 'threat' or even to an entirely different construct which is not measured by the existing contextual rating scales. This possibility is now taken up.

14.5 SPECIFICITY EFFECTS — ELABORATIONS OF CONTEXTUAL MEASURES

Since this early use of the LEDS, there have been a number of replications of the basic results for depression (e.g. Costello, 1982; Bebbington *et al.*, 1984b; Brown *et al.*, 1986).

For the most part, the stressors involved in bringing about depression involve some degree of loss. Such losses include not only deaths or separations from loved ones, but also the loss of valued roles and cherished ideas such as follows the discovery of a husband's unfaithfulness. Although not systematically explored in the Camberwell survey, there was suggestive evidence to indicate that events not involving loss were more frequently associated with anxiety disorders (Brown and Harris, 1978). This hint that the qualitative aspects of particular experiences might differ for depression and anxiety was explored in a further study of psychiatric disorder. As there is some evidence that only events which involved severe threat were capable of playing a role in the onset of affective disorder, attempts were made to classify all severe events in terms of two qualities. The notion of loss has already been dealt with and with the development of a new scale to rate this was comparatively straightforward. The second quality involved the concept of danger, that is, the degree to which an event suggested or forecast the future occurrence of a specific loss. The rating itself was made in terms of how unpleasant it would be if such a crisis were to occur. It was hypothesized that, as in the Camberwell Study, events characterized by loss would be associated with the onset of depression, while danger events should be associated with anxiety. A new sample was drawn from consecutive female patients of local general practitioners in another London area, and the full LEDS was administered. Ratings of the severity of contextual long-term threat, together with these new dimensions, were made by members of the research team who were unaware of the psychiatric state of the respondent or of her reported reactions to events. Summarizing a somewhat complex analysis, it was shown that loss clearly related to the onset of depression and danger events to the onset of generalized anxiety, with mixed depressive–anxiety disorders relating to the concurrent presence of events with both qualities of loss and danger (Finlay-Jones and Brown, 1981; Finlay-Jones, 1989).

This study was one of the earliest examples of an apparently specific link between one class of experience and one type of illness: since that study similar links have been found for 'goal frustration' events and organic abdominal pain (Craig and Brown, 1984), 'conflict' events and functional dysphonia (House and Andrews, 1988), and 'challenge' events in secondary amenorrhoea (Harris, 1989). Unfortunately, comparable studies have not been undertaken to examine the onset of schizophrenia, although the re-analysis of Brown and Birley's 1968 data raises an interesting possibility. Harris (1987) has recently suggested that a novel contextual measure of meaning — 'intrusiveness' — may be of crucial importance. Her reanalysis of Brown and Birley's (1968) data indicates that events which were characterized by intrusions by outsiders were 20 times as common in the week before the onset of schizophrenia than in the comparison series. These intrusive events included attacks, visits by the police and threatening 'official' communications. There is a suggestive and appealing match between this observation and the well established role of high crtiticism in the home in provoking relapse (Leff and Vaughn 1985; Chapter 8) and between the observations of a higher rate of schizophrenic onset in the early months following first recruitment into the army, an experience which surely exposes subjects to authoritarian and bureaucratic interference (Steinberg and Durrell, 1968). It would be very interesting to know whether the higher incidence of schizophrenia reported in young second generation Afro-Caribbeans (Harrison *et al.*, 1988) might be linked in some way to the sense of alienation and the very real excess of authoritarian intrusiveness to which young black men are exposed in the UK.

14.6 THE CHALLENGE OF BIOGRAPHY

All this amounts to tantalizing evidence for some degree of specificity in the relationship between particular classes of human experience and particular disease entities. However, there is no need to restrict the discussion of specificity to such direct links. There is also the very important issue of how far a particular event is linked to the rest of a person's life when seen in current and biographical terms. It is possible, for example, that a person may be made more vulnerable to a severe loss because of some past loss or because their self-esteem is low following a series of unrelated failures in their life. A central finding of the original Camberwell research was that although most instances of depression in the population are brought about by a severe event, only about a fifth of those who experience such events or difficulties go on to develop depression. In an effort to explain this apparent anomaly, Brown and Harris (1978) developed the notion of vulnerability factors. These were defined in terms of influences which on their own were incapable of producing depression but in conjunction with a provoking agent such as a severe event increased the risk of breakdown. In the original Camberwell study, four such factors were isolated: lack of an intimate confiding relationship, early loss of mother by death or separation, presence of three or more young children at home and lack of employment outside the home. Brown and Harris (1978) suggested that it was possible to see each of these four factors as contributing to low self-esteem. They argued that if self-esteem was low before a major loss, a woman would be less likely to be able to imagine herself emerging successfully from a crisis and would allow her feelings of hopelessness in response to the provoking event to generalize (i.e. to evolve to clinical depression).

Of the many observations arising from this pioneering study, the role of these so-called vulnerability factors has received the greatest critical attention, with some dispute as to whether they constitute only vulnerability or are provoking agents in their own right (e.g. Tennant and Bebbington, 1978; Tennant *et al.*, 1981; Cooke and Hole, 1983; McKee and Vilhjalmsson, 1986). However, the speculations have now received some confirmation in independent replications of the Camberwell study and in a recent prospective investigation in which women classified as scoring highly on a variety of scales measuring negative self-evaluation (i.e. low self-esteem) in the first year of the study were far more vulnerable to breakdown following a major crisis during the two-year follow-up period (Brown *et al.*, 1987).

This prospective investigation also drew attention to yet another type of specific linkage between certain classes of stressors and depression. At the first interview, each woman discussed five areas of her life in considerable detail — her marriage, children, housework, employment and other activities outside the home. She was then rated on a qualitative scale reflecting the strength of her commitment to each of these areas. Women with a severe event that matched this area of commitment in the follow-up year were three times as likely to breakdown than those women with severe events which did not match prior commitment. Matching was judged by whether the severe event was logically part of an area of commitment rated in the first interview (e.g. loss of employment would match prior commitment to employment). Another measure which also demonstrated some specificity in the nature of the causal events concerned conflicts in the role obligations. Here, a rating of 'role conflict' was made during the first interview on the basis of evidence for diverging obligations between two valued roles (e.g. holding down a full time job while rearing a young family). Women rated as having marked or moderate role conflict at first interview were particularly likely to develop depression in the follow up year when an event occurred which underlined her failure in one of the conflicting roles. So for example, the woman whose high role conflict arose from the clash between her

obligations to work and her single-handedly rearing her only child, developed depression when she found out her school-age daughter was pregnant. Role conflict events and commitment events were not related and appeared to be two quite separate routes to depression (Brown *et al.*, 1987).

These results concerning the matching of life events with prior commitments and conflicts indirectly point to something else: that while the context of an event determines whether or not the experience is likely to be viewed as threatening, it may also at times increase the likelihood of the actual occurrence of the event. That this should be the case can be put (somewhat trivially) by the observation that people who stand under trees in thunderstorms are more likely to be struck by lightening than those who remain indoors. The first evidence for this in the LEDS studies came in a study of gastrointestinal disorder (Craig and Brown, 1984), where it was observed that people who developed peptic ulcer disease were more likely to have experienced an event which disrupted intense striving efforts. In the healthy members of the general population, these 'goal frustration' events were much more common among men than among women. Furthermore, interference with work or career ambitions accounted for 70% of the goal frustration events among men whereas for women, three-quarters concerned failure to achieve a desired outcome in personal relationships; a finding which was not unexpected in the light of sociological accounts of how gender roles affect career commitments and aspirations. Amongst the patients, by contrast, there was no sex difference in the rate of goal frustration events and work or career frustration were by far the most common kind of experience reported by both men and women, The patients therefore had a higher than expected proportion of ambitious striving women who were likely to persist in striving until they were met with a goal frustration. There are two non-trivial explanations for this result. First, that it was

247

the nature of their occupational choice that was the most important factor in increasing their exposure to goal frustration events. If so, then the temporal pathway is relatively brief, perhaps reflecting no more than a chance selection into the jobs which carried a high likelihood of frustration. It is also possible that this choice of career was itself driven by even more remote factors involving some personality charateristic of ambition or the outcome of a learning process of prior successes achieved through persistent striving towards difficult targets.

This observation of persistent behaviour leading to an increased risk of exposure to severe events was also observed in later studies of depression. Harris *et al.*, (1987) demonstrated that the quality of care in childhood was related to the likelihood of adult exposure to certain types of severely threatening events which in turn were known to be associated with depression. Additionally, the experience of a premarital pregnancy was associated with experience of a provoking crisis in later life and the risk of a premarital pregnancy was itself associated with earlier lack of care (Brown and Harris, 1989). Brown and Harris (1989) interpret these associations as indicative of a 'conveyor belt' of adversity in which some women passed from one crisis to another, beginning with lack of care in childhood and passing via premarital pregnancies which trapped women in relationships characterized by tension, bitterness and infidelity. These marriages in turn were the source of severe events and major difficulties, both directly (as in the discovery of a spouse's infidelity) and indirectly (e.g. by means of financial problems which arose because the couple had a family to support before they had time to build up any savings). Of course, this is not to say that the pathway is entirely environmentally determined and that the women necessarily had no choice in the matter. It is quite likely that some feature of their personality — for example an attitude

of helplessness or low self-esteem — may have made them less likely to escape from adversity early enough to avoid inevitable future crises or even to have exposed themselves to such crises unnecessarily. Other workers have demonstrated a similar chain of adversity which can at times persist across generations (Quinton and Rutter, 1984) and lead to the startling observation that the risk of exposure to threatening life crises seems to be familiarly determined (McGuffin *et al.*, 1988). At this stage of our understanding, it is not possible to separate the effects of circumstance (being born and reared in socially deprived environments with few chances to escape the treadmill of poverty) from those of personal choice (persistent maladaptive patterns of coping and self-control), but in the case of depression these studies are bringing together causal explanations which integrate the social environment and personality, revealing some of the finer detail of the ways in which objective adversity and personal reactions to this adversity cluster together in specific disorders.

Although no comparable work can be cited in the study of schizophrenia, there is peripheral evidence from a number of studies which suggests that this is an issue worthy of further exploration. For example, the studies carried out in the 1960s which reported on the 30-year outcome of children who had attended child guidance clinics in the 1920s and 1930s and which showed for schizophrenic adults, records of greater maternal dependency, poor parental relationships and overprotection of the child, particularly by the mother (O'Neal and Robins, 1958; Nameche *et al.*, 1964; Waring and Ricks, 1965; Ricks and Nameche, 1966). Might it be possible that these parental behaviours contribute to an individual's later difficulties dealing with stresses of a demanding or intrusive nature?

14.7 THE ADDITIVITY ISSUE

Early life event measures explicitly assumed

that the effects of stress were cumulative (e.g. Holmes and Rahe, 1967). Experience with interview-based measures, however, suggest that if such cumulative effects exist, they do not take any simple linear form (Brown and Harris, 1978). Surtees and his colleagues (Surtees and Ingham, 1980; Surtees and Rennie, 1983; Surtees, 1989) report studies using the LEDS, based on the notion that the threat of life crises decays with the passage of time. The closer events occur to onset the higher the residual adversity and the greater the risk of breakdown. Such causal models, incorporating exponential decay effects and measures of maladaptive coping substantially improve the prediction of depression over that obtained by the use of dichotomized measures based purely on the presence or absence of a severe event.

These results would seem to be in conflict with the model advocated by Brown and Harris (1978, 1989) which places most emphasis on the occurrence of just one severe event (albeit of a rather special type). As these authors point out, the different perspectives may well be the result of technical rather than theoretical importance. Residual adversity scores are determined by the severity of events and their closeness to onset of disorder. Both research groups observe that severe events tend to cluster in the few weeks before onset and so for onset cases, whose adversity score is calculated at the point of onset, there will have been relatively little time for the adversity score to decay. In contrast, residual adversity scores for comparison subjects is calculated at the point of interview and unlike onset cases, severe events in comparison women tend to be evenly distributed over the entire period of scrutiny. It follows that a high residual adversity score is less tied to the presence of a severe event in the comparison women and fewer of the comparison women will be given high adversity scores than are counted as having experienced a severe event, where this is defined as any severe event at any time during the preceding

six months. It follows from this that the decay model will have a more favourable result in terms of indices such as relative risk.

14.8 CRITICISMS OF THE CONTEXTUAL APPROACH

Although the LEDS represents a significant advance over earlier checklist measures of life event stress, it has been suggested that the contextual rating system is liable to confound aspects of biography and prior coping behaviour with aspects that properly belong to the rating of the event alone and that the life events measure is 'more accurately described as a measure of general social stress' (Tennant *et al.*, 1981 p. 381). Such calls for pure measures of events is best set out by Dohrenwend and his colleagues (Dohrenwend *et al.*, 1987). They conceive of life stress as involving three components: events closely preceding the time of interest; ongoing social situations; and personal dispositions (previous psychiatric history, genetic vulnerability and personality factors which influence how people perceive and react to events. They argue that the existing LEDS contextual measure conflates information about the event itself with material on the social context and the individual's biography and that ultimately, it should be possible to produce classifications of events which include all the most important variants of the events for which the unique contributions of social context and biography can be specified.

lthough this would indeed offer an improvement over the LEDS, it is still a good way off. The Psychiatric Epidemiology Research Interview (PERI) contains a list of 102 event categories with weights for each event obtained from averaging the responses of a panel of judges who have been presented with a list of the important variations of these events (Dohrenwend *et al.*, 1978). The list is not exhaustive. For example, as it stands, the central person involved in the event is not specified. The authors themselves have noted the wide variation in judgements of the severity of events according to whether the subject is an acquaintance, a member of the household or a member of the family (and equally wide even within this narrow sub-set). To resolve this difficulty and produce a dictionary of events which covered all the main variants would likely run into tens of thousands of examples. The LEDS manual currently contains just under 5000 vignettes of events in 800 categories and is far from exhaustive (each new study has added further examples). Nor is it clear that in the end, such a list would be substantially different in construction to the rating process used by the LEDS.

14.9 CONCLUSIONS AND FUTURE DIRECTIONS

Advances in our understanding of the aetiological processes involved for conditions such as depression, make clinical interventions aimed at altering or removing these aetiological factors an exciting possibility. In schizophrenia, we are still a good way off being able to formulate such interventions. One way forward is suggested by recent efforts to detect early warning signs of relapse and to abort episodes of illness by adjusting medication at this earliest point (e.g., Birchwood *et al.*, 1989; Chapters 8 and 17). If life events could be recorded prospectively, it might be possible to intervene when they occur, either with adjustments to medication or with specific psychotherapy aimed at reducing arousal. This would, however, require a quite different technology. At present, the LEDS interview takes about 90 minutes to administer with at least as long again in rating and discussing the various qualitative dimensions — clearly an impractical tool if one wished to monitor the occurrence of stressors on a weekly or even monthly basis. One solution might be to develop simpler screening measures and to administer restricted aspects of the full interview only when it seemed likely that an appropriate event had occurred. In one of the few studies which have compared the full LEDS to a checklist measure derived from it, Costello and Devins (1988) had a sample of women fill in a checklist while waiting in their doctor's office and then interviewed these women in their homes within the same week. The checklist had high negative predictive value but its positive predictive value was much less impressive. That is, the majority of women whose full LEDS interview showed they had experienced an event had recorded this event on the checklist. However the determination of which events were 'severe' still relied heavily on the full interview, as it was difficult to estimate long-term threat from the checklist alone. Nevertheless, since the checklist was used in conjunction with the interview, this poor positive predictive value did not threaten the work overall and the instrument appears to be a useful first stage screening device. Costello and Devins attribute the success of the checklist to the fact that it follows the LEDS domains closely and it seems that this particular checklist is more successful at picking up 'severe' events than previous attempts have been (e.g., Katschnig, 1980; Miller and Salter, 1984; Bebbington *et al.*, 1984a).

In conclusion, interview-based measures which rely on 'contextual' assessments of meaning offer the most reliable aetiological importance of stressors even though the measure must remain, at best, an approximation of the true situation. Of these measures, the LEDS currently offers the most flexible approach and holds out the possibility of the exploration of links between specific categories of human experience and specific illness states. The next decade will probably see an increase in the number of qualitative dimensions of events which are assessed and with this, an improvement in our ability to specify the conditions under which disease begins.

REFERENCES

Bartlett, F. (1932) *Remembering: A Study of Experimental and Social Psychology*. Cambridge

University Press, Cambridge, England.

Bebbington, P., Christopher, T., Sturt, E. and Hurry, J. (1984a) The domain of life events; A comparison of two techniques of description. *Psychol. Med.*, **14**, 219–22.

Bebbington, P., Hurry, J., Tennant, C. and Sturt, E. (1984b) Misfortune and resilience: A community study of women. *Psychol. Med.*, **14**, 347–63.

Birchwood, M., Smith, J., Macmillan, F. *et al.* (1989) Predicting relapse in schizophrenia: The development and implementation of an early signs monitoring system using patients and families as observers, a preliminary investigation. *Psychol. Med.*, **19**, 649–56.

Brown, G.W. (1974) Meaning, measurement and stress of life events. In *Stressful Life Events: Their Nature and Effects*. B.S. Dohrenwend and B.P. Dohrenwend (eds), Wiley, New York, pp. 217–43.

Brown, G.W. (1981) Life events, psychiatric disorder and physical illness. *J. Psychosom. Res.*, **25**, 461–73.

Brown, G.W. and Birley, J.L.T. (1968) Crises and life changes and the onset of schizophrenia. *J. Health Soc. Behav.*, **9**, 203–14.

Brown, G.W. and Harris, T.O. (1978) *Social Origins of Depression: A Study of Psychiatric Disorder in Women*. Tavistock, London.

Brown, G.W. and Harris, T.O. (1986) Establishing causal links: The Bedford College studies of depression. In *Life Events and Psychiatric Disorders*. H. Katschnig (ed), Cambridge University Press, Cambridge, England, pp. 107–87.

Brown, G.W. and Harris, T.O. (1989) The LEDS findings in the context of other research: An overview. In *Life Events and Illness*. G.W. Brown and T.O. Harris (eds), Guilford Publications, New York, pp. 385–437.

Brown, G.W., Sklair, F., Harris, T. and Birley, J.L.T. (1973) Life events and psychiatric disorder: some methodological issues. *Psychol. Med.*, **3**, 74–87.

Brown, G.W., Andrews, B., Harris, T.O. *et al.* (1986) Social support, self-esteem and depression. *Psychol. Med.*, **16**, 813–31.

Brown, G.W., Bifulco, A. and Harris, T.O. (1987) Life events, vulnerability and onset of depression: Some refinements. *Br. J. Psychiatry*, **150**, 30–42.

Cooke, D.J. and Hole, D.J. (1983) The aetiological importance of stressful life events. *Br. J. Psychiatry*, **143**, 397–400.

Costello, C.G. (1982) Social factors associated with depression: A retrospective community study. *Psychol. Med.*, **12**, 329–39.

Costello, C.G. and Devins, G.M. (1988) Two-stage screening for stressful life events and chronic difficulties. *Can. J. Behav. Sci.*, **20**, 85–92.

Craig, T.K.J. and Brown, G.W. (1984) Goal frustration and life events in the aetiology of painful gastrointestinal disorder. *J. Psychosom. Res.*, **28**, 411–21.

Day, R., Nielsen, J., Korten, A. *et al.* (1987) Stressful life events preceding the acute onset of schizophrenia: A cross-national study from the World Health Organization. *Cult. Med. Psychiatry*, **11**, 1–123.

Dohrenwend, B.P., Link, B.G., Kern, R., Shrout, P.E. and Markowitz, J. (1987) Measuring life events: The problem of variability within life event categories. In *Psychiatric Epidemiology: Progress and Prospects*. B. Cooper (ed), Croom Helm, London, pp. 103–119.

Finlay-Jones, R. (1989) Anxiety. In *Life Events and Illness*. G.W. Brown and T.O. Harris (eds), Guilford Press, New York, pp. 95–112.

Finlay-Jones, R. and Brown, G.W. (1981) Types of stressful life event and the onset of anxiety and depressive disorders. *Psychol. Med.*, **11**, 803–15.

Frijda, N.G. (1986) *The Emotions*. Cambridge University Press, Cambridge, England.

Harris, T.O. (1987) Recent developments in the study of life events in relation to psychiatric and physical disorders. In *Psychiatric Epidemiology: Progress and Prospects*. B . Cooper (ed), Croom Helm, London, pp. 81–102.

Harris, T.O. (1989) Disorders of menstruation. In *Life Events and Illness*. G.W. Brown and T.O. Harris (eds), Croom Helm, London, pp. 261–94.

Harrison, G., Owens, D., Holton, A. *et al.* (1988), A prospective study of severe mental disorder in Afro-Caribbean patients. *Psychol. Med.*, **18**, 643–57.

Holmes, T.H. and Rahe, R.H. (1967) The Social Readjustment Rating Scale. *J. Psychosom. Res.*, **11**, 213–8.

House, A. and Andrews, H. (1988) Life events and difficulties preceding the onset of functional

251

dysphonia. *J. Psychosom. Res.*, **32**, 331–9.

Jacobs, S. and Myers, J. (1976) Recent life events and acute psychoses: A controlled study. *J. Nerv. Ment. Dis.*, **162**, 75–87.

Jenkins, C.D., Hurst, M.W. and Rose, R.M. (1979) Life changes: Do people really remember? *Arch. Gen. Psychiatry*, **36**, 379–84.

Katschnig, H. (1980) Measuring life stress: A comparison of two methods. In *The Suicide Syndrome*. R. Farmer and S. Hirsch (eds), Croom Helm, London, pp. 116–23.

Leff, J. and Vaughn, C. (1985) *Expressed Emotion in Families*. Guilford Press, New York.

Leff, J.P., Hirsch, S.R., Gaind, R. *et al.* (1973) Life events and maintenance therapy in schizophrenic relapse. *Br. J. Psychiatry*, **123**, 659–60.

Lipman, R.S., Hammer, H.M., Bernardes, J.P. *et al.* (1965) Patient report of significant life situation events. *Dis. Nerv. System*, **26**, 586–9.

McKee, D. and Vilhjalmsson, R. (1986) Life stress, vulnerability and depression: A methodological critique of Brown *et al. Sociology*, **20**, 589–99.

Mason, J.W. (1968a) A review of psychoendocrine research on the pituitary-adrenal cortical system. *Psychosom. Med.*, **30**, 576–607.

Mason, J.W. (1968b) A review of psychoendocrine research on the sympathetic adrenal medullary system. *Psychom. Med*, **30**, 631–5.

McGuffin, P., Katz, R. and Bebbington, P. (1988) The Camberwell Collaborative Depression Study III: Depression and adversity in the relatives of depressed probands. *Br. J. Psychiatry*, **152**, 775–82.

Miller, P. and Salter, D.P. (1984) Is there a short-cut? An investigation into the life event interview. *Acta Psychiatr. Scand.*, **70**, 417–27.

Nameche, G., Waring, M. and Ricks, D. (1964) Early indicators of outcome in schizophrenia. *J. Nerv. Ment. Dis.*, **139**, 232–40.

O'Neal, P. and Robins, L.N. (1958) Childhood patterns predictive of adult schizophrenia: A 30-year follow-up study. *Am. J. Psychiatry*, **115**, 385–91.

Paykel, E.S. (1978) Contribution of life events to causation of psychiatric illness. *Psychol. Med.*, **8**, 245–53.

Paykel, E.S. (1983) Methodological aspects of life events research. *J. Psychosom. Res.*, **27**, 341–52.

Paykel, E.S., Myers, J.K., Dienelt, M.N. *et al.* (1969) Life events and depression: A controlled study. *Arch. Gen. Psychiatry*, **21**, 753–60.

Paykel, E.S., Prusoff, B.A. and Uhlenhuth, E.H. (1971) Scaling of life events. *Arch. Gen. Psychiatry*, **25**, 340–7.

Quinton, D. and Rutter, M. (1984), Parents with children in care. II: Intergeneration Continuities. *J. Child Psychol. Psychiatry*, **25**, 231–50.

Rahe, R.H. (1969) Life crisis and heath change. In *Psychotropic Drug Response: Advances in Prediction*. P.R.A. May, and J.R. Winterborn, (eds), Charles C Thomas, Springfield, Ill., pp. 92–125.

Ricks, D.F. and Nameche, C. (1966) Symbiosis, Sacrifice and Schizophrenia. *Ment. Hygiene*, **50**, 541–51.

Sarason, I., Johnson, J.H. and Siegel, J.M. (1978) Assessing the Impact of Life Changes: Development of the Life Experiences Survey. *J. Consult. Clin. Psychol.*, **46**, 932–46.

Schutz, A. (1971) Concept and theory formation in the social sciences. In *Collected Papers*, Vol. 1. A. Schutz, Nijhoff, The Hague, pp. 48–99.

Selye, H. (1956) *The Stress of Life*. McGraw-Hill, New York.

Steinberg, H. and Durell, J. (1968) A Stressful Social Situation as a Precipitant of Schizophrenic Symptoms: An Epidemiological Study. *Br. J. Psychiatry*, **114**, 1097–1105.

Surtees, P.G. (1989) Adversity and psychiatric disorder: A decay model. In *Life Events and Illness*. G.W. Brown and T.O. Harris (eds), Guilford Publications, New York, pp. 161–95.

Surtees, P.G. and Ingham, J.G. (1980) Life stress and depressive outcome: Application of a dissipation model to life events. *Soc. Psychiatry*, **15**, 25–31.

Surtees, P.G. and Rennie, D. (1983) Adversity and the onset of psychiatric disorder in women. *Soc. Psychiatry*, **18**, 37–44.

Tennant, C. and Andrews, G. (1976) A Scale to Measure the Stress of Life Events. *Aust. N.Z. J. Psychiatry*, **10**, 27–32.

Tennant, C. and Bebbington, P. (1978) The Social Causation of Depression: A Critique to the Work of Brown and his Colleagues. *Psychol. Med.*, **8**, 565–75.

Tennant, C., Bebbington, P. and Hurry, J. (1981) The Role of Life Events in Depressive Illness: Is there a Substantial Causal Relationship? *Psychol. Med.*, **11**, 379–89.

Waring, M. and Ricks, D. (1965) Family Patterns of Children who Become Adult Schizophrenics. *J. Nerv. Ment. Dis.*, **140**, 351–64.

Wershow, H.J. and Reinhart, G. (1974) Life Change and Hospitalization: A Heretical View. *J. Psychosom. Res.*, **18**, 393–401.

Chapter 15

Assessment of family interaction with a schizophrenic member

W.K. HALFORD

I feel empty, a bit of a failure. It's hard to get the energy to do much. I spend a lot of time at home. My folks don't like me hanging out, [they] get on my back to do more, and that makes me feel worse. (A young schizophrenic man in an interview with the author.)

He seems so sad, lonely . . . we try to encourage him to get out, but he just gets so angry. I feel I have lost him, lost contact . . . it's hard to know how to get through. (The young man's mother in a separate interview.)

The feelings reflected in the above quotes capture something of the sense of loss, the confusion, and the problems that often occur when a family member develops schizophrenia. This chapter reviews the assessment of families with a schizophrenic member. The aims in writing the chapter were twofold. First, to provide an analysis of the relationship between family interaction and the functioning and quality of life of each family member. Second, to provide a practical clinical guide to assessment of families.

A central argument developed in this chapter is that good clinical management of schizophrenia usually requires close collaboration with families. The majority of schizophrenic patients reside with their families after hospital discharge (Freeman and Simmons, 1963; Goldman, 1982; Fadden *et al.*, 1987) and family members are important sources of information about the functioning of patients. Furthermore, the interactions between patient and family impact upon the clinical outcome of schizophrenia (Leff and Vaughn, 1985; Koenigsberg and Handley, 1986; Goldstein, 1988). Therapists frequently need to assess, and sometimes to help change, family interaction patterns. In addition, families face a difficult task in supporting their schizophrenic relative, and maintaining a reasonable quality of life for all family members. Many relatives are severely stressed by living with their schizophrenic relatives (Hatfield, 1978; Lefley, 1989), and frequently need assistance in coping with these stresses.

Effective collaboration with families to promote effective coping needs to include education about schizophrenia, as most families have limited understanding of the disorder (Barrowclough *et al.*, 1987; Abramowitz and Coursey, 1989). Providing families with support in the form of discussion which focuses on expression of feeling about the onset of the disorder, and the problems encountered within the family, has been shown to reduce relatives' sense of burden (Leff *et al.*, 1989). Structured training in communication and problem-solving skills has been shown to reduce family conflict, and lead to improved patient functioning (Falloon *et al.*, 1985). Family interventions which incorporate all of these elements have been shown to reduce patient relapse, increase patient functioning, improve family communication, and reduce families' sense of burden (Halford and Hayes, 1991; Chapter 24 of this book).

Assessment is the first step of collaboration with families, as it allows specification of the particular needs of individual families. The review of assessment in this chapter is organized into four sections. The first section is a critical review of the evidence linking family interaction and clinical outcome of schizophrenia. This review provides the empirical and conceptual base for family based assessment and interventions. The second section is a discussion of the model of family interaction relevant to assessment. The final section describes integrating assessment findings, and planning interventions.

15.1 FAMILY INTERACTION AND SCHIZOPHRENIA

There has been a long-standing interest in the association of family interaction and the outcome of schizophrenia (Leff and Vaughn, 1985; Goldstein, 1988). Three related, but somewhat different hypotheses have been forwarded: (1) that disturbed family interaction causes schizophrenia (e.g. Bateson *et al.*, 1956); (2) that certain patterns of family interaction mediate the course of established schizophrenia (e.g. Leff and Vaughn, 1985); and (3) that families are a resource in the rehabilitation of schizophrenia, but that being care-givers to schizophrenic relatives often places considerable burden on families (e.g. Hatfield, 1987). Below research relevant to

each of these hypotheses is reviewed, and then the implications of this evidence for working with families is discussed.

15.1.1 FAMILIES AS THE CAUSE OF SCHIZOPHRENIA

Historically, the first hypothesis advanced about the relationship between families and schizophrenia was that dysfunctional parenting styles caused schizophrenia (e.g. Bateson *et al.*, 1956; Fromm-Reichmann, 1948; Laing, 1965; Wynne and Singer, 1963). The most extensively researched example of this view was the '*double bind hypothesis*', in which it was argued that deviant, internally-inconsistent communication by parents led children to use psychotic behaviour as a coping response. Family therapy was argued to be the appropriate treatment for such dysfunctional communication (Esterton *et al.*, 1965), and was seen as complete treatment for schizophrenia by some writers (e.g. Bowen, 1961).

A large volume of research has accumulated which shows that deviant family interaction is neither necessary or sufficient to produce schizophrenia (Hirsch and Leff, 1975), and family therapy *alone* has not been shown in controlled trials to improve schizophrenic outcome. However, there is a high prevalence of disturbed communication in families in which a member develops schizophrenia, and these communication characteristics antedate the onset of a clear-cut schizophrenia syndrome (Goldstein, 1985). Recent research suggests that a combination of genetic vulnerability and stressful family environment, is associated with high risk for development of schizophrenia (Goldstein, 1985; Tienari *et al.*, 1987; Weintraub, 1987). The causal links between the onset of schizophrenia, genetic vulnerability and family environment are unclear. Premorbid functioning deficits in people who develop schizophrenia may cause communication irregularities within families. Alternatively, deviant communication may interact with biological vulnerability to produce schizophrenia.

At this point in the development of our knowledge it is clear that deviant family interaction alone cannot cause schizophrenia, but it is possible that family communication may interact with other variables to increase the risk of schizophrenia. Further research may lead to family interventions with at-risk individuals to reduce the likelihood of the onset of schizophrenia.

15.1.2 FAMILIES AS MEDIATORS OF THE COURSE OF SCHIZOPHRENIA

Families' responses to the emergence of schizophrenic symptoms have long been argued to mediate the course of the disorder (Brown, 1985). The importance of this hypothesis has increased as more families of schizophrenic patients have taken on the role of primary care givers (Goldman, 1982). Over the last 30 years research testing the hypothesis that family interaction mediates the course of established schizophrenia has been focused primarily on the association of expressed emotion (EE) and relapse in schizophrenic patients (Leff and Vaughn, 1985). The assessment of EE is described in detail later in this chapter. In summary, EE is a composite measure of relatives' reported attitudes and behaviour toward the patient assessed from a semi-structured interview (Goldstein, 1988; Leff and Vaughn, 1985). High EE is operationalized as relatives exhibiting behaviour above certain cut-offs on criticism, emotional over-involvement, or hostility during the interview. High EE is seen as reflecting a psychologically stressful family environment for the patient.

Thirteen studies have been published assessing the relationship between EE and schizophrenic relapse. The results across studies appear inconsistent: nine studies found significantly more patients living with high EE relatives relapsed than patients living with low EE relatives (Brown *et al.*, 1962, 1972; Vaughn and Leff, 1976; Vaughn *et al.*, 1984; Moline

et al., 1985; MacMillan *et al.*, 1986; Neuchterlein *et al.*, 1986; *Karno et al.*, 1987; Leff *et al.*, 1987), but four studies found no significant association between EE and relapse (Köttgen *et al.*, 1984; Hogarty *et al.*, 1988; McCreadie and Phillips, 1988; Parker *et al.*, 1988). The frequency of failures to replicate the EE-relapse association, have led some authors to question if any such association exists (e.g. Parker *et al.*, 1988). However, three of the four studies in which no association between high EE and relapse were found (Hogarty *et al.*, 1988; Köttgen *et al.*, 1984; McCreadie and Phillips, 1988) differed in some important ways from the other studies (see Chapter 8). If the three dissimilar studies are eliminated, nine of the ten studies using similar methodology have found a significant association between high EE and relapse. The mean relapse rate across the ten studies in the high EE families was 58%, and for low EE was 23%. This suggests a strong association.

Even if the results across studies were more consistent, interpretation of the EE-relapse association is contentious. It has variously been suggested that high EE may cause relapse in psychobiologically vulnerable individuals, (Vaughn and Leff, 1976), that EE and patients' symptomatology may be mutually interactive (Leff and Vaughn, 1985), or that EE may be a consequence of patient symptoms rather than a cause (e.g. Hatfield *et al.*, 1987; Kanter *et al.*, 1987).

Available data suggest high EE is probably more than simply the result of patient psychopathology, and it is unlikely that EE is simply a trait of relatives' behaviour independent of patient symptoms. There is evidence that high EE households are stressful for schizophrenic patients. High EE is correlated with negative relative behaviours toward the patient, such as criticism and intrusiveness (Miklowitz *et al.*, 1989). Such behaviours are stressful for patients as they report ongoing subjective tension, and evidence prolonged autonomic arousal when high EE relatives are present (Tarrier *et al.*,

1988). However, high EE also is associated with high levels of criticism by patients of their relatives, poor coping with stress by patients (Strachan *et al.*, 1989), and by greater conditional probabilities of reciprocation of verbal negativity between patient and relatives (Hahlweg *et al.*, 1989). Thus high EE is correlated with a variety of aspects of the interaction between patient and relatives and the precise aspects which may be crucial in determining the course of schizophrenia are unclear.

15.1.3 FAMILIES AS BURDENED CARE GIVERS

Most assessments of families with a schizophrenic member have concentrated on the impact of family interaction on the patient. Many researchers and mental health professionals have failed to recognize the burden that living with a schizophrenic person places on families, and the impact of distressed family interaction on the nonschizophrenic members (Hatfield, 1987; Bernheim and Switaliski, 1988). Relatives often look to therapists for assistance in coping, do not receive the help they want, and express considerable dissatisfaction with the services they receive (Holden and Levine, 1982).

What are the major problems that relatives face? At the time of onset of the disorder relatives often feel a complex range of emotions including shock at the state of their loved one, confusion about the nature of the problem, guilt that they may have caused the disorder, and fear about the future (Hatfield, 1978; McElroy, 1987). Dealing with crisis at the onset, or sudden deterioration of the disorder is often very difficult for families.

Relatives living with chronic schizophrenic patients face numerous other ongoing difficulties such as the economic burden of supporting the patient (as patients are often unemployed), the psychological stress of coping with patients' disturbed behaviour, persistent disruption of household routines by the patient

(e.g. night time wakening and irregular eating habits), and the problems of coping with the social withdrawal and awkward interpersonal behaviour of the patient (Falloon *et al.*, 1984; Hatfield, 1987; Terkelson, 1987). It is not surprising that many families report considerable stress and great dissatisfaction in their relationship with their schizophrenic relative (Hatfield, 1987; Hooley *et al.*, 1987; McElroy, 1987; Bernheim, 1989).

The lack of attention to relatives' needs also is reflected in the reliance on relapse as the primary index of outcome in most family intervention studies. Admittedly, relapse is a major problem in schizophrenia, with 35 to 40% of adequately medicated patients relapsing within 12 months of their last admission (Falloon *et al.*, 1978; Hogarty *et al.*, 1979; Schooler *et al.*, 1980). However, relatives living with patients find the negative symptoms of schizophrenia more distressing than the positive symptoms usually associated with relapse (Leff and Vaughn, 1985; Hooley *et al.*, 1987). Furthermore, it is the negative symptoms of schizophrenia which often are associated with patients having difficulty with independent community living (Liberman *et al.*, 1989). Given that recent research suggests that positive and negative symptoms may reflect relatively independent processes (Lezenweger *et al.*, 1989), it is important that negative symptoms, and their impact on family members, be assessed.

15.1.4 CONCLUSIONS ON FAMILIES AND SCHIZOPHRENIA

The notion of the 'schizophrenogenic family' has been debunked by the research evidence: deviant family interaction does not, by itself, cause schizophrenia. However, disturbed family interaction may be a risk factor which interacts with other variables to increase the likelihood of schizophrenia. An unfortunate side effect of the research on families as the cause of schizophrenia, was for clinicians to blame families for the onset of the disorder. This implication has understandably been resented by some families (Hatfield *et al.*, 1987).

Research on the assessment of families with a schizophrenic member has focused on EE, and the majority of family interventions have emphasized the reduction of EE in the family (Halford and Hayes, 1991. Leff *et al.*, 1982). This emphasis is unfortunate as the high EE concept has been interpreted by some families as another example of professionals blaming families for schizophrenia (Hatfield *et al.*, 1987). Research should seek to define the positive coping responses families make, coping responses which are associated with better patient outcomes, and reduced burden for relatives. Such an emphasis would provide better guidelines for what to teach within family interventions, and reduce the perceptions of families being seen as dysfunctional.

15.2 MODELS OF DYSFUNCTIONAL INTERACTION

Adequate assessment of families with a schizophrenic member has to attend to the needs both of designated patients and their relatives, as optimal family intervention should seek to maximize the quality of life for all family members. Family assessment also needs to focus on the reciprocal nature of interaction between schizophrenic and other family members. In the past there has been a focus either on assessing relatives' behaviours and their influence on patient outcome (e.g. Leff and Vaughn, 1985), or on assessing patient behaviour and its impact on relative's sense of burden (e.g. Platt, 1985; Fadden *et al.*, 1987; Hatfield, 1987). Developments in the conceptualization and assessment of family interaction highlight the importance of the patterns of interaction between family members, which in turn permit targeting and modification of these patterns (Patterson, 1988). Table 15.1 provides a brief overview of some key questions which need to be answered by an assessment of the family.

Table 15.1 Key areas to assess

1. What does each family member know about schizophrenia as a disorder, and the roles of medication and psychological interventions in its management?
2. What does each member perceive as the course and cause of the disorder?
3. Which behaviours within the family are perceived as problematic, and what behaviour changes do members want of each other?
4. How do the patient and other family members cope with the burden of the illness?
5. What are the communication and problem-solving processes within the family, and how effective are these in dealing with existing problems?
6. What accommodation options have the family considered for the schizophrenic member, and how does each member evaluate these options?

What form does dysfunctional family interaction with schizophrenic patients take? Consider the common problems families confront in living with a schizophrenic relative: the withdrawal from activities outside the home, sleeping in during the day, lack of responsiveness to the rest of the family, failing to assist around the home with household chores, the 'crazy talk', and socially embarrassing behaviour. A common reaction of many families to such behaviours is to criticize the person for their behaviour (Leff and Vaughn, 1985).

Patterson's (1982) coercion theory of family processes provides a framework within which the likely impact of family criticism of a schizophrenic member can be analysed. This theory proposes that any family can become trapped into use of aversive methods of controlling each other's behaviour, when these behaviours are negatively reinforced within an escape conditioning paradigm. More specifically, it is argued that negative behaviours such as criticism can lead to escalation in conflict, and that this escalated conflict is aversive for all participants. Such escalation typically is rapidly offset by one or more of the participants terminating the interaction. This offset can be achieved in a variety of ways such as exiting, shouting so loudly or aversively that one person stops, or by abuse. The use of aversive behaviours is negatively reinforced by the offset of the interaction, and this maintains the whole pattern of interaction.

Coercion theory predicts that, if criticism of a schizophrenic relative leads to the temporary termination of the problem behaviour, or offsets arguments about the patient's behaviour, the criticism will be maintained by negative reinforcement. The family may then increase criticism rates. Unfortunately schizophrenic patients seem to be particularly sensitive to criticism. Schizophrenic patients interacting with critical relatives report high levels of subjective stress and have persistent autonomic hyperarousal (Tarrier *et al.*, 1988). Such high arousal is predictive of schizophrenic relapse (Turpin *et al.*, 1988), and indeed patients living with highly critical relatives do relapse more frequently than patients living with less critical relatives (Leff and Vaughn, 1985; Goldstein, 1988). Thus coercive escalation within families might receive immediate reinforcement, but lead to increased risk of relapse in the longer term.

Repeated coercive escalations have a number of deleterious long-term consequences. For example, such patterns often lead marital partners to withdraw and avoid each other (Gottman, in press; Halford *et al.*, 1990), and it is likely that this also occurs in families with a schizophrenic member. Such avoidance probably reduces the psychological stress impinging on patients, and reduces the risk of relapse. It also may lead to relatives being less critical of patients, and being classified as low EE. However, such disengagement also would lower the support available to the patient, and reduce the prompts and reinforcers available for adaptive social behaviour. While reductions in frequency of family contact have been advocated as a desirable outcome for some high EE families (e.g. Leff and Vaughn, 1985), the impact of reduced engagement on patient functioning is untested. The promotion of independent patient functioning through

positive family responding to desired patient behaviours seems preferable to disengagement.

A second possible maladaptive pattern of interaction within families having a schizophrenic member is the 'chronic illness trap' (Fordyce, 1976). A common reaction of many families to a severely disabled member, whatever the specific nature of the disability, is to become overprotective of the person (Burish and Bradley, 1984). This can be maladaptive if such protection inhibits the development of independent coping skills and/or inadvertently reinforces excessive dependence. In schizophrenia the frequency of chronic deficits in self-care, lack of financial independence and social isolation make the chronic illness trap a pattern that is likely to develop and a substantial proportion of relatives become overprotective, self-sacrificing and intrusive in the patients' lives (Leff and Vaughn, 1985). These behaviours are associated with higher risk of schizophrenic relapse for the patient (Goldstein, 1988).

In summary: there is evidence that coercive escalation, avoidance and withdrawal, and the chronic illness trap are common maladaptive interaction patterns within families with a schizophrenic member. Assessment of a family needs to determine if such patterns are of relevance in a particular case. Research on these patterns to date has addressed the impact on patients, but not on relatives. Future research needs to investigate the impact on relatives of various patterns of family interaction.

15.3 METHODS OF FAMILY ASSESSMENT

Table 15.2 identifies in some detail the range of assessment methods available to attempt to answer the questions identified in Table 15.1. It is important to note that some of the measures described in Table 15.2 were not developed specifically for families with a schizophrenic member, but rather are general measures of family functioning which have relevance.

Table 15.2 Key areas for assessment in families with a schizophrenic member

Area of assessment	Methods of assessment	Example instruments
Relative burden	Interview with relative	Social Behaviour Assessment Schedule (SBAS; Platt *et al.* 1978).
	Self-report inventory	Relatives Stress Scale (Greene *et al.* 1982)
Relative responses to patient	Interview with relative	Camberwell Family Interview (Leff and Vaughn, 1985)
	Interview with patient	None published
	Observation	Affective Style Measure (Doane *et al*, 1981)
	Patient report inventory	Perceived Criticism Rating (Hooley, and Teasdale, 1989)
Patient responses to relative	Interview of relative	Social Behaviour Assessment Schedule (Platt *et al.*, 1981)
	Interview of patient	None published
	Observation	Coping Style (Strachan *et al.*, 1989)
Family interaction and problem solving	Interview	None published
	Self-report inventories	Family Environment Scale (Moos and Moos, 1978)
		Areas of Change Questionnaire (Weiss and Perry, 1983; Margolin *et al*, 1983)
	Observation	Interactional Coding System (Hahlweg *et al.*, 1984).
	Self-monitoring	Family Interaction Diary (Halford *et al.* 1990)

15.3.1 RELATIVE BURDEN

Platt (1985) reviewed measures of family burden and noted they varied greatly in method and content of assessment. In method the measures differed in who the informant was, and the procedure of assessment (e.g. self-report questionnaire, standardized interview and unstandardized interview). The content varied in the areas of burden assessed. Some measures focus on a global measure of burden (e.g. Grad and Sainsbury, 1968; Sainsbury, 1975), while others rat e burden derived from

a wide range of sources such as various patient behaviours, financial considerations and so forth (e.g. Spitzer *et al.*, 1971). Finally, the measures differ in the dimensions of burden assessed. Some measures focus on a simple global rating of overall burden (e.g. Sainsbury, 1975), while others rate the effects on specific areas of family functioning. For instance, psychopathology in children, social isolation, and relative anxiety, can be rated as being caused by or exacerbated by the patient's condition. This heterogeneity of measures reveals the lack of consensus about the concept of family burden, which makes it difficult to compare results across different studies.

Some authors distinguish between 'objective burden' and 'subjective burden' (e.g. Hoenig and Hamilton, 1969). The former is seen as a clearly indentifiable stressor on the family (e.g. financial costs of the disorder or an abnormal behaviour of the patient), while the latter is seen as the family's subjective sense of distress in response to the identifiable stressor. In practice this distinction becomes blurred with many measures, as relatives are often the only source of data about the so-called objective burden.

At this point there is no entirely satisfactory measure of family burden. One of the better measures is the Social Behaviour Assessment Schedule (SBAS) which includes a section on relative burden. This scale has high inter-rater reliability (Platt *et al.*, 1978), and is sensitive to clinical change (Platt *et al.*, 1980; Platt and Hirsch, 1981). The SBAS assesses a wide range of effects on family functioning of the patient's disorder, and gives a rating of the relative's overall sense of burden. However, it is time-consuming to administer.

Greene *et al.* (1982) developed a self-report paper and pencil measure of relative burden for care-givers living with elderly demented patients. The measure consists of 34 items assessing relatives' perceptions of the patients' mood and behaviour disturbances, and 15 items assessing relatives' sense of stress in coping. The measure has high internal consistency within its subscales, and high test-retest reliability. The items seem appropriate for assessing family burden in relatives living with schizophrenic relatives, and Abramowitz and Coursey (1989) found the scale sensitive to change produced by an educational support group for relatives of schizophrenic patients. This scale is probably the most cost-effective measure of burden available.

15.3.2 RELATIVES' RESPONSES TO PATIENTS

Camberwell Family Interview. Relatives' responses to patients have been the family variable most often assessed in the relevant literature. Interviews have been the most widely used method for assessing relatives' responses to schizophrenic patients, and the Camberwell Family Interview (CFI) has been the most extensively researched interview method. In the CFI relatives are interviewed individually in a semi-structured format about the patient's most recent episode of their disorder, current symptomatology, the household climate and routine, and the relative's reaction to the patient. The three ratings predictive of relapse derived from this interview are: the number of critical comments made about the patient; a rating on a five-point scale of the relatives' emotional over-involvement (EOI) with the patient; and a dichotomous rating of the presence or absence of hostility toward the patient. A rating of warmth toward the patient, and the number of positive comments made, also are coded (Leff and Vaughn, 1985), but these last two scales have not been found to relate to outcome. In most studies families have been dichotomized into high and low EE on the basis of scores above specified cut-offs on any one of the indices of criticism, EOI or hostility. The most commonly used cut-offs have been six or more criticisms, a rating of 4 or more on the 5 point EOI scale, or a rating of the presence of hostility.

There are considerable difficulties with the assessment of EE using the CFI. Administration takes between 1 and 2 hours, and rating of the resultant audiotape takes a further 3 to 4 hours (Leff and Vaughn, 1985). Training raters to acceptable levels of reliability involves 30 to 40 hours. These time demands are comparable to those required for some other family assessments, such as behavioural coding of family interactional data (Markman and Notarius, 1987), but are prohibitive for routine clinical use. Furthermore behavioural coding yields a complex data set from which the frequency of occurrence of many classes of response, and the sequential relationships between these response classes, can be analysed (Notarius and Markman, 1989). In contrast the CFI provides scores on five scales, only three of which have demonstrated predictive validity, and a dichotomous classification of families.

Besides the time involved in administration of the CFI, the reliability of the assessment method is open to question. High agreement on ratings of each of the CFI scales have been demonstrated on numerous occasions (Leff and Vaughn, 1985). However, in almost all studies raters were trained until they achieved pre-determined agreement levels on a sample of demonstration tapes, but the actual agreement between raters on the tapes in the studies were not assessed (e.g. Vaughan and Leff, 1976; Vaughn *et al.*, 1984; Hogarty *et al.*, 1988; Parker *et al.*, 1988). Furthermore the reliability of rating on individual statements by relatives have not been assessed, only the reliability of overall ratings such as the total number of criticisms. This is not crucial for the use of EE as a predictor of outcome, but it is important if individual statements made by relatives are used to define goals of intervention. In addition, levels of agreement between ratings of interviews of the same relative conducted by different interviewers has not been established. Given the unstructured nature of the CFI, it is questionable if two interviewers independently would elicit similar responses from relatives. Some of the inconsistent findings in the EE research may reflect loss of inter-rater reliability during the lengthy coding process involved in each study, or variable CFI administration across studies.

It is not clear exactly what the CFI measures (Hooley, 1985; Koenigsberg and Handley, 1986). Implicitly it is assumed that relatives' statements made during the CFI correlate with relatives' behaviours when the patient is present. However the CFI is a very indirect measure of the relatives' behaviour toward the patient, and only assessing relatives' responses ignores the possibility that EE reflects an interactional process between patient and relative. Furthermore high EE probably constitutes a heterogeneous grouping of family interaction processes, which may be better understood by being analysed separately. A convention has developed of combining high criticism or high EOI or hostility into a single construct of high EE. In the original development of the CFI the criticism and EOI scales were seen as independent, and subsequent research has shown low to moderate inter-correlation between the scales (Leff and Vaughn, 1985). Furthermore there is some evidence of differential development of high criticism and high EOI, with different patterns of correlations between premorbid adjustment and these different components of EE (Miklowitz *et al.*, 1985).

The CFI is the most widely used method for assessing families with a schizophrenic member. Given this, researchers may need to use the CFI so their results are comparable to the body of related studies. However, the major limitations of the CFI render it of very limited utility for routine clinical assessments. Some authors claim the CFI provides useful additional clinical information (e.g. Vaughn, 1986) but the only empirically validated use is as a marker of high risk for schizophrenic relapse.

Brief measures of expressed emotion. In response to the difficulties associated with use of the CFI, two research teams independently developed quite similar, brief measures of EE. Magãna *et al.* (1986), developed the Five Minute Speech Sample (FMSS) and Schweitzer *et al.* (1988), developed the Videotaped Expressed Emotion measure (VEE). Both the FMSS and the VEE utilize a five minute sample of relative speech about the patient as a means of assessing EE. In both procedures relatives living with a schizophrenic patient are asked to talk for five minutes about 'X as a person, and your relationship with X'. Magāna *et al.* (1986), audiotape the relatives' talk, while Schweitzer *et al.* (1988), videotape the talk. Procedures for coding the recordings vary between the two measures. The VEE uses essentially the same coding system as the CFI, while the FMSS has some variations. (Details of both coding systems can be obtained from the current author on request.)

Both the FMSS and the VEE correlate highly with the CFI in terms of classification of families as high or low EE (Magāna *et al.*, 1986; Schweitzer *et al.*, 1990), though both tend to under-rate (relative to the CFI) the occurrence of high EE. No data has been published on the validity of the FMSS or VEE in predicting relapse in schizophrenia. Both the FMSS and VEE systems have the advantages of being standardized in their administration, and taking relatively little time to administer. Reliable rating of both systems can be achieved with 4 to 5 hours of rater training. In summary the FMSS and the VEE appear to provide similar information to the CFI, but in a much more cost-effective manner. Research is needed on the predictive validity of each system.

Affective Style measure. The Affective Style measure (AS) was developed to measure the dimensions of family interaction assessed by the CFI directly from samples of family interaction (Doane *et al.*, 1981). The AS involves a patient and family engaging in a problem-solving interaction about a topic which is a source of disagreement within the family. The interaction is audiotaped, and then a verbatim transcript is made of the interaction. Transcripts resulting from the AS are coded, with verbal content being classified into a number of categories, the most important of which are the presence of criticisms and intrusive comments.

The AS has good psychometric properties. It can be scored reliably, with kappas greater than 0.8 for agreement between raters on each of the key categories (Doane *et al.*, 1981; Miklowitz *et al.*, 1984). There is evidence of construct validity. Relatives high on criticism during CFI adminstration score high on criticism on the AS, and high EOI relatives during CFI administration score high on intrusive comments (Miklowitz *et al.*, 1984). The AS predicts relapse in discharged schizophrenic patients (Doane *et al.*, 1985) the onset of schizophrenia in vulnerable adolescents (Doane *et al.*, 1981), and changes in the AS following family intervention are correlated with clinical outcome (Doane *et al.*, 1985).

Use of the AS requires extensive training of raters, and the transcription process is very time consuming. The associated costs are prohibitive for routine clinical use, though the AS is useful as a research instrument. The AS does not assess nonverbal behaviour, which is a crucial element of much dysfunctional family interaction (Markman and Notarius, 1987), and this is a significant weakness of the system.

Other methods of assessing relatives' responses to patients. Patient ratings of relative behaviours may be potentially useful in the assessment of families. Parker *et al.* (1979) have developed the Parental Bonding Instrument (PBI), which is a paper and pencil inventory in which respondents report on their perceptions during their first 16 years of life of their relationship with their parents. Scores are derived on two orthogonal scales of parental care and protection. The two scales can be intersected to allow comparison of four broad parenting styles. Schizophrenic patients who rate their parents in the low care, high protection quadrant have a significantly lower average age of onset of schizophrenia than other patients (Parker *et al.*, 1983). Furthermore, they were found to be significantly more likely to be rehospitalized during a 9-month follow-up period after hospital discharge (Parker *et al.*, 1983).

The PBI is retrospective rating of global dimensions of parenting style. If parenting behaviours do influence the course of schizophrenia, the PBI does not provide indications of what behaviours are crucial. However, it is a cost-effective means of detecting patients at high risk of relapse.

Hooley and Teadale (1989) assessed expressed emotion, via the CFI, and perceived criticism by the spouse of hospitalized depressed patients. Perceived criticism was assessed by asking patients to make a rating of how critical their spouse was of them on a 7-point scale. This rating predicted relapse in the patients over the next nine months, and adding EE classification did not significantly improve prediction. The measure has not been applied with schizophrenic patients, and this needs to be done. The cost-effectiveness of the measure suggests it may be useful clinically. More extensive paper and pencil measures of patients' perception of their relatives responses to them are under development by several research groups, but there are no published data available on their utility.

15.3.3 PATIENTS' RESPONSES TO RELATIVES

Social Behaviour Assessment Schedule. Behaviours of the patient within the family have been assessed by interview and observation, and there have been some recent attempts to develop relative-report inventories. The Social Behaviour Assessment Schedule (SBAS) is a structured interview of 329 questions for administration to a relative living with a schizophrenic person (Platt *et al.*, 1980). The interview takes between 1 and 15 hours to administer and yields four summary scores: The severity of the patient's disturbed behaviour; the patient's performance of normally expected social behaviour; the subjective sense of burden the patient's illness imposes on the relative; and a rating of the degree of distress experienced by household members in the process of coping with the disorder. The SBAS has high inter-rater reliabilities on summary scores (Platt *et al.*, 1980), and these scores are sensitive to clinical change following hospital care (Hirsch *et al.*, 1979).

As Wallace (1986) noted, the SBAS is time consuming to administer, and training inter-

viewers to standardize the interview and its coding is a lengthy process. Other instruments are necessary to conduct a functional assessment of patients' living skills or symptomatic behaviour — e.g. Wallace's (1986) Independent Living Skills Survey. However the SBAS is a comprehensive measure of relatives' perception of the patient's behaviour, and the relatives' sense of burden in coping with that behaviour.

Coping Style. The Coping Style measure assesses patients' behaviour during a problem-solving interaction with their relatives (Strachan *et al.*, 1989). Samples of problem solving are audiotaped and transcribed, as for the AS measure of relative behaviours. Patient behaviours are classified into one of seven categories. Patients interacting with high versus low EE relatives have been found to differ on two of these categories: those interacting with low EE relatives use significantly less criticism, and make significantly more autonomous statements. Autonomous statements are defined as a clear statement of intention to achieve a goal, master a task, or engage in an activity that does not involve the relative.

The Coping Style measure can be reliably coded, and covaries with family EE status. However there is no other data available on its validity. Further research is required to assess the relationship of patient coping style to outcome and family functioning.

15.3.4 FAMILY INTERACTION

Areas of Change Questionnaire. The Areas of Change Questionnaire (ACQ) originally was developed to assess requests for behaviour change in maritally distressed couples (Weiss and Perry, 1983), but can be modified to assess the desired behaviour change of family members. In the marital form respondents rate the extent of change they desire from their spouse in particular behaviours. Ratings are made on a 7 point scale from '+3: do much more' to '−3: do much less'. Examples of behaviours rated include 'go out with me', 'start interesting conversations with me', and 'argue with me'.

The sum of the absolute scores of requested change can be used as a measure of dissatisfaction with current behaviour. In the marital form the total score and individual item scores discriminate between distressed and non-distressed couples and the total score correlates negatively with marital satisfaction (Margolin *et al.*, 1983). Individual items provide a very useful clinical guide to behaviours needing to be targeted in interventions. The utility of the ACQ can be further enhanced by the addition of items specifically related to the presence of schizophrenia in the family, such as items on taking medication, staying in bed, and attending clinics.

Family Environment Scale. The Family Environment Scale (FES) consists of 90 true/false items intended to assess the respondents' perception of their family environment on three dimensions: relationships, personal growth, and systems maintenance (Moos and Moos, 1981). These dimensions are measured on 10 subscales. The FES has moderate to high test-retest reliability (Moos and Moos, 1981). Patient ratings of their families as high on conflict and low on emotional expressiveness is associated with higher rates of rehospitalization in schizophrenic patients (Spiegal and Wessler, 1986).

The information gathered by the FES does not provide specific targets for therapeutic change. However, the FES is a cost-effective method of assessing family members' perceptions of family environment. As a research tool this instrument has several advantages over measures of EE, and may become more widely used in the area.

Participant observation measures. In the context of family assessment, participant observation refers to having family members systematically monitor family interactions. Participant observation of family interaction has a number of potential advantages including providing ongoing measurement of behaviour not otherwise accessible, and providing access to family member cognition and affect about day-to-day interactions (Margolin, 1987). Furthermore participant observation overcomes in part some of the problems inherent in global self-report inventories, such as the retrospectivity of assessment. While participant observation methodology has been widely used in marital assessment (e.g. the Spouse Observation Checklist of Weiss *et al.*, 1973), no application of this methodology have been reported with families with a schizophrenic member.

Participant observation can be used to monitor the occurrence of any behaviourally specific target. For example, relatives or patients might monitor the frequency or duration of patient 'crazy talk', time in bed, anger outbursts, silence in the presence of others, self-care behaviours such as hair brushing, or social conversation with family members. The antecedents and consequences of these behaviours also can be tracked, in the standardized behavioural assessment methods described by Liberman *et al.* (1989) and Wallace (1981).

In clinical work I have adapted the Marital Interaction Diary (MID, Halford, *et al.*, in press; Behrens *et al.*, 1990), for use with families with a schizophrenic member. In the MID respondents write down at the end of each day the time spent together, the location and activities involved in time together, and make event records about any stressful interactions. These event records include the antecedents to the stressful interaction, the topic and intensity of the interaction, and how the interaction ended. The MID has acceptable psychometric properties in applications with married couples (Halford *et al.*, in press), but there is no data on its reliability or validity in use with families having a schizophrenic member. Participant observational data gathered from instruments such as the SOC and MID are very useful clinically. The therapist is able to assess where, when and under what circumstance problematic family interaction occurs. Research is needed to assess the utility of

Table 15.3 Brief definitions of the interactional coding system verbal and non-verbal codes

Code	Definition
Verbal	
1. Self disclosure	Direct expression of feelings, wishes or needs.
2. Positive solutions	Specific constructive proposals, or suggested compromise to resolve a problem.
3. Acceptance	Demonstrations of acceptance of the other person by paraphrase, open ended question or positive feedback.
4. Agreement	Agreement by direct agreement, or assent, or acceptance of responsibility.
5. Problem description	Neutral descriptions of problems, or neutral questions seeking problem description.
6. Meta communication	Clarification requests, or comments about the manner in which the topic is being discussed.
7. Listening	This code is used for the listener when double coding of the speaker occurs to ensure an alternating sequence.
8. Criticize	Expressions of dislike or disapproval, or statements likely to demean, the listener.
9. Negative solution	Description of something the speaker wants the listener not to do in order to solve a problem.
10. Justification	Excuses or denial of responsibility for one's behaviour or a problem.
11. Disagreement	Direct disagreement or 'Yes, but' type disagreements.
12. Other	Any response not fitting the above, or which is inaudible.
Nonverbal	
1. Positive	Attending nonverbal behaviour, positive facial expression or voice qualities.
2. Negative	Nonattending, negative facial expression or voice qualities.
3. Neutral	Ambiguous nonverbals, rater unable to judge positive or negative.

such methods in assessing families with a schizophrenic member.

Interactional coding systems. Coding of behaviour based on samples of family interaction has been widely used in assessment of families, particularly in marital asessment (Weiss, 1989), and parent–child interaction (Patterson, 1982). In these applications almost all of the coding systems involve coding the behaviour of all participants in the interaction (Markman and Notarius, 1987). However, in the work on coding interaction of families with a schizophrenic member, most systems used have coded either the behaviour of the patient or the relative. The only coding

system which assesses interaction of participants has been the Interactional Coding System (ICS).

The ICS is an English language adaption of the Katogoriensystem für Partnerschaflichte Interacktion — KPI (developed by Hahlweg *et al.*, 1984). The ICS originally was developed to assess marital interaction. Videotapes are made of the couple or family discussing a specified problem. Responses are defined as any verbalization which is homogeneous with respect to meaning, regardless of length of utterance. Verbal responses of all interactants are classified into one of 12 mutually exclusive content categories. The codes and their

266

definitions are presented in Table 15.3. Each verbal response also is given an accompanying nonverbal rating of affect as positive, negative or neutral.

ICS coding can be done with high levels of inter-rater reliability (Halweg *et al.*, 1984; Halford *et al.*, 1990), though coder training takes 40 to 50 hours. The coding process itself is time consuming, with a 10-minute interaction taking approximately 2 hours to code. The resultant codes can be used to assess the baseline rate of occurrence of response categories, and sequential analysis can be used to assess patterns of interaction (Hahlweg *et al.*, 1989).

Hahlweg *et al.*, (1989) have provided the most detailed account of interaction in high EE families. They found that compared with low EE relatives, relatives classified as high EE on the basis of high criticism in the FMSS exhibited significantly higher levels of negative verbal and nonverbal behaviour, and lower levels of positive verbal and nonverbal behaviours (Hahlweg *et al.*1989). Patients interacting with high EE-criticism relatives made significantly more criticisms, justifications, disagreements, and negative nonverbal behaviour, and there was a trend for less positive solutions. Families classified as high EE-criticism also exhibited high levels of coercive escalation. High EE, over-involved families behaved in a similar manner to low EE families. These findings need replication, but suggest that coercive escalation is relevant to the course of schizophrenia.

The ICS is a very useful research tool but it is too costly for routine clinical use. However, it is possible to use the categories in the ICS and observation of problem-solving interaction to generate clinical hypotheses about the nature of dysfunctional interaction in a particular family.

15.3.5 KNOWLEDGE ABOUT SCHIZOPHRENIA

Knowledge about schizophrenia is presumed to

help families cope effectively with the disorder. However, as Barrowclough *et al.* (1987) noted, it is the functional value of information which is important. That is, the information is valuable to the extent that it allows patient and relatives to respond adaptively to stressors. Consistent with this view, poor knowledge about schizophrenia is associated with greater levels of criticism of the patient by relatives (Barrowclough *et al.*, 1987).

There have been several instruments developed which assess the knowledge of family members about schizophrenia. Some instruments are structured interviews (e.g. Barrowclough *et al.*, 1987), and others are paper and pencil tests (e.g. McGill *et al.*, 1983).The Knowledge About Schizophrenia Interview (KASI) is a semi-structured interview in which relatives are asked about diagnosis, symptomatology, aetiology, medication, course, prognosis, and management of schizophrenia. Interviews are audiotaped and rated. Ratings are intended to assess 'not just the presence of information about schizophrenia, but the effects of that information on the relative's behaviour' (Barrowclough *et al.*, 1987, p. 3). Each knowledge area is assigned a rating from 1 — 'Negative: relative reports knowledge likely to lead to actions detrimental to the patient' to 4 — 'Very positive: relative reports wide knowledge likely to lead to potentially valuable actions in regard to the patient's management'. The KASI has adequate psychometric properties. Interrater reliability of ratings based on audiotapes of KASI interviews are high (greater than 80% agreement in each area). The KASI is sensitive to change from brief educational interventions (Barrowclough *et al.*, 1987).

The Knowledge of Schizophrenia Questionnaire (KSQ) consists of a series of six open-ended questions, followed by 15 multiple choice questions (McGill *et al.*, 1983) which focus on essentially the same content areas as the KASI. The questionnaire is sensitive to changes from educational interventions, and is stable over a

Table 15.4 Family assessment summary form headings

1. Biographical data

2. Assessment instruments used

3. Key problems behaviours from each family member's perspective
   - Behaviours each person believes he or she needs to increase or decrease
   - Behaviours each person believes others need to increase or decrease

4. Behavioural excesses, deficits and assets
   - Based on (3) plus observational, participant observational, and self-report inventory data

5. Antecedents of problem behaviours
   - Where, when and with whom do the behaviours occur?
   - What patterns of family interaction precede the problem behaviours?
   - What events or stressors, both episodic and ambient, may trigger problems?

6. Consequences of problem behaviour
   - What are the intrafamilial and extrafamilial consequences of the problem behaviours, both immediate and delayed?
   - What patterns of family interaction follow problem behaviours?

7. Intrapersonal variables
   - What biological processes (e.g. drug side effects), and psychological processes (cognitive impairments, affect, beliefs) may mediate the patient's target behaviours?
   - What similar processes may mediate relatives' behaviour?

8. Goals of intervention

9. Functional analysis of problem behaviours
   - What hypotheses best fit the assessment data to explain the maintenance of the problem behaviours?
   - What treatment interventions are most likely to modify those mediating variables?

9 month period without intervention. The KASI and KSQ both are suitable instruments for assessing the knowledge of patients and relatives about schizophrenia. The KSQ has the advantage of being quicker to administer, while the KASI yields more information on the functional impact of knowledge.

15.4 INTEGRATION OF ASSESSMENT FINDINGS

The ultimate aims of assessment of family interaction with a schizophrenic member are:

(1) To define the broad goals of intervention.

(2) To specify the behavioural excesses, deficits and assets of each family member.

(3) To generate clinical hypotheses about the functional determinants of problem behaviours within the family.

(4) To develop a collaborative working relationship with the family.

Table 15.4 sets out a summary form for integrating the results of a family assessment and achieving those aims. The assessment would include results from a combination of the measures reviewed in the earlier sections. The form is used to integrate findings, and to document the clinical hypotheses about functional analysis of the problem behaviours.

A brief case example will be used to illustrate the use of the headings in Table 15.4. The presenting family were: Tony H., a 23-year old unemployed male diagnosed as schizophrenic three years ago, who was living with his sister Maureen W. and husband Ben W. The initial presenting concerns were the lack of recovery of premorbid functioning by Tony, his frequent rehospitalizations following relapse (8 episodes in 3 years), and the stress experienced by all family members in coping with the disorder. Each family member completed a modified Areas of Change Questionnaire, was interviewed about the presenting problem, was assessed on their knowledge of schizophrenia, and monitored the occurrence of stressful family interactions for two weeks. In addition the family undertook three problem-solving discussions on areas of conflict between the family members; these discussions were videotaped and coded using the ICS system.

Key problem behaviours from Tony's perspective were the criticism of him by his sister, and the disinterest of his brother-in-law. Maureen saw Tony's failure to seek paid employment, his inactivity outside the family home, failure to do household chores, and excessive sleeping as the key problems. She also reported anxiety and a heavy sense of burden in caring for Tony. Ben reported he resented Tony's lack of financial contribution to the household, was concerned about the stress on Maureen, but felt distant and relatively unaffected by Tony.

Assessment of each family member's knowledge revealed that none of them understood the term 'schizophrenia', Tony and Maureen mistakenly believed neuroleptic medication was only important during acute episodes of schizophrenia, and none of the family knew the effects of psychological stress on schizophrenic relapse. The self-monitoring of stressful interactions revealed frequent (once or twice per day) disagreements between Tony and Maureen on Tony's undertaking of households chores, job seeking and sleeping. Ben rarely was involved in interactions with Tony. The problem-solving interactions revealed high levels of criticism between Tony and other family members, with marked negative escalation. Interviews with the family members revealed that such interactions were typically followed by Tony and the others avoiding each other.

Tony currently was compliant with medica-tion, despite his mistaken belief he did not need to take it, but he had frequently stopped taking it in the past. None of the family members was depressed. Both Maureen and Ben believed Tony's inactivity was due to laziness.

The key goals of intervention were negotiated as: (1) improving the communication and problem-solving processes within the family; (2) learning more about schizophrenia; (3) assisting Tony to become more independent financially and in self-care; and (4) attempting a gradual transition toward Tony living somewhere else with on-going support from Maureen and Ben. It was hypothesized that family members had been trapped into coercive escalation, and that communication and problem-solving training would circumvent this pattern. Lack of knowledge about schizophrenia was thought to have mediated an inappropriate response by each family member, and therefore education was important. Education in this context was not simply information giving, but structured discussion to encourage behaviour change based on new conceptualization of problems. (See Chapter 23 for a discussion of the methods of optimizing the impact of educational interventions.) Finally, it was hypothesized that nonaversive prompting and positive reinforcement of Tony to increase self-care, household chores, and outside activities would increase independent functioning.

15.5 CONCLUSION

Families are the primary care givers for chronic schizophrenic patients. Patients' and relatives' abilities to cope with the numerous burdens of this disorder have profound implications for the quality of life for all family members. Assessment of a particular family's needs must address the patterns of family interaction, help develop goals acceptable to all family members for promoting the patients' independent functioning and identify required knowledge and skills which enable all family members to cope effectively with the burden of schizophrenia.

REFERENCES

Abramowitz, I.A. and Coursey, R.D. (1989) Impact of an educational support group on family participants who take care of their schizophrenic relatives. *J. Consult. Clin. Psychol.*, **57**, 232–6.

Barrowclough, C., Tarrier, N., Watts, S. *et al.* (1987) Assessing the functional value of relatives' knowledge about schizophrenia: A preliminary report. *Br. J. Psychiatry*, **151**, 1–8.

Bateson, G., Jackson, D., Haley, J. and Weakland, J. (1956) Toward a theory of schizophrenia. *Behav. Sci.*, **1**, 252–64.

Behrens, B., Sanders, M.R. and Halford, W.K. (1990) Behavioural marital therapy: An analysis of generalization effects across high and low risk settings. *Behav. Ther.*, **21**, 423–33.

Bernheim, K. (1989) Psychologists and families of the severely mentally ill: The role of family consultation. *Am. Psychol.*, **44**, 561–4.

Bernheim, K.F. and Switalski, T. (1988) Mental health staff and patients' relatives: How they view each other. *Hosp. Community Psychiatry*, **39**, 63–8.

Bowen, M. (1961) The family as the unit of study and treatment. *Amer. J. Orthopsychiatry*, **31**, 40–60.

Brown, G.W. (1985) The discovery of expressed emotion: Induction or deduction. In *Expressed Emotion in Families*. J. Leff and C. Vaughn (eds), Guildford, New York, pp. 1–25.

Brown, G.W., Birley, J.L.T. and Wing, J.K. (1972) Influence of family life on the course of schizophrenic disorders: a replication. *Br. J. Psychiatry*, **121**, 241–8.

Brown, G.W., Monck, E.M., Carstairs, G.M. and Wing, J.K. (1962) The influence of family life on the course of schizophrenic illness *Br. J. Prev. Soc. Med.*, **16**, 55–68.

Burish, T.G. and Bradley, L.A. (eds) (1984) *Coping with Chronic Disease*. Academic Press, New York.

Doane, J.A., Falloon, I.R.H., Goldstein, M.J. and

Mintz, J. (1985) Parental affective style and the treatment of schizophrenia. *Arch. Gen. Psychiatry*, **42**, 34–42.

Doane, J.A., West, K.L., Goldstein, M.J., Rodnick, E.H. and Jones, J.E. (1981) Parent communication deviance and affective style: Predictors of subsequent schizophrenic spectrum disorders in vulnerable adolescents. *Arch. Gen. Psychiatry*, **38**, 679–85.

Esterson, A., Cooper, D.G. and Laing, R.D. (1965) Results of family-oriented therapy with hospitalized schizophrenics. *Br. Med. J.*, **2**, 1462–5.

Fadden, G., Bebbington, P. and Kuipers, L. (1987) The burden of care: The impact of functional psychiatric illness on the patient's family. *Br. J. Psychiatry*, **150**, 285–92.

Falloon, I.R.H., Boyd, J.L. and McGill, C.W. (1984) *Family Care of Schizophrenia: A Problem-solving Approach to the Treatment of Mental Illness*. Guilford, New York.

Falloon, I.R.H., Boyd, J.L., McGill, C.W. *et al.* (1985) Family management in the prevention of morbidity of schizophrenia – clinical outcome of a two-year longitudinal study. *Arch. Gen. Psychiatry*, **42**, 887–96.

Falloon, I., Watt, D.C. and Shepherd, M. (1978) The social outcome of patients in a trial of long-term continuation therapy in schizophrenia: pimozide vs. fluphenazine. *Psychol. Med.*, **8**, 265–74.

Fordyce, W.E. (1976) *Behavioral Methods for Chronic Pain and Illness*. Mosby, St. Louis.

Freeman, H.E. and Simmons, O.G. (1963) *The Mental Patient Comes Home*. Wiley, New York.

Fromm-Reichmann, F. (1948) Notes on the development of treatment of schizophrenics by psycholoanalytic psychotherapy. *Psychiatry*, **11**, 263–73.

Goldman, H.H. (1982) Mental illness and family burden: A public health perspective. *Hosp. Community Psychiatry*, **33**, 560.

Goldstein, M.J. (1985) Family factors that antedate the onset of schizophrenia and related disorders: The results of a fifteen year prospective longitudinal study. *Acta Psychiatr. Scand.*, **71**, 7–18.

Goldstein, M.J. (1988) The family and psychopathology. *Ann. Rev. Psychiatry*, **39**, 283–99.

Gottman, J.M. (in press) How marriages change. In *Depression and Aggression in Family Interaction*. G.R. Patterson (ed). Lawrence Erlbaum, Hillsdale, New Jersey.

Grad, J. and Sainsbury, P. (1968) The effects that patients have on their families in a community care and a control psychiatric service – a two-year follow-up. *Br. J. Psychiatry*, **114**, 265–78.

Greene, J.G., Smith, R., Gardiner, M. and Timbury, G.C. (1982) Measuring behavioural disturbance of elderly demented patients in the community and its effects on relatives: a factor analytic study. *Age and Aging*, **II**, 121–6.

Hahlweg, K., Goldstein, M.J., Nuechterlein, K.H. et al. (1989) Expressed emotion and patient-relative interaction in families of recent onset schizophrenics. *J. Consult. Clin. Psychol.*, **57**, 11–8.

Hahlweg, K., Reisner, L., Kohli, A. et al. (1984) Development and validity of a new system to analyse interpersonal communication: Kategoriensystem für partnerschaftliche interaktion. In *Marital Interaction: Analysis and Modification*. K. Hahlweg and N.S. Jacobson (eds), Guilford, New York, pp. 182–98.

Halford, W.K. (in press) Beyond expressed emotion: Behavioral assessment of family interaction and the course of schizophrenia. *Behav. Assess*.

Halford, W.K., and Hayes, R. (1991) Psychological rehabilitaiton of chronic schizophrenia: recent findings on social skills training and family psychoeducation. *Clin. Psych. Rev.*, **11**, 23–44.

Halford, W.K., Gravestock, F., Lowe, R. and Scheldt, S. (in press) Toward a behavioural ecology of stressful marital interaction. *Behav. Assess*.

Halford, W.K., Hahlweg, K. and Dunne, M. (1990) The cross-cultural consistency of marital communication associated with marital distress. *J. Marr. Fam.*, **52**, 523–32.

Hatfield, A.B. (1978) Psychological costs of schizophrenia to the family. *Social Work*, **23**, 355–9.

Hatfield, A.B. (1987) Coping and adaption: A conceptual framework for understanding families. In *Families of the Mentally Ill: Coping and Adaption*. A.B. Hatfield and H.P. Lefley (eds). Guilford, New York, pp. 60–84.

Hatfield, A.B., Spaniol, L. and Zipple, A.M. (1987) Expressed emotion: a family perspective. *Schizophr. Bull.*, **13**, 221–35.

Hirsch, S.R. and Leff, J.P. (1975) *Abnormalities in Parents of Schizophrenics*. Oxford University Press, London.

Hirsch, S.R., Platt, S.D., Knights, A. and Weyman. A. (1979) Shortening hospital stay for psychiatric care: effect on patients and their families. *Br. Med. J.*, **i**, 442–6.

Hoenig, J. and Hamilton, M.W. (1969) *The Desegregation of the Mentally Ill*. Routledge and Kegan Paul, London.

Hogarty, G.E., McEvoy, J.P., Munetz, M. et al. (1988) Dose of fluphenazine, familial expressed emotion and outcome in schizophrenia. *Arch. Gen. Psychiatry*, **45**, 797–805.

Hogarty, G.E., Schooler, N.R., Ulrich, R. et al. (1979) Fluphenazine and social therapy in the aftercare of schizophrenic patients. *Arch. Gen. Psychiatry*, **36**, 1283–94.

Holden, D.F. and Levine, R.R.J. (1982) How families evaluate mental health professionals, resources, and effects of illness. *Schizophr. Bull.*, **8**, 628–33.

Hooley, J. (1985) Expressed emotion: A review of the critical literature. *Clin. Psychol. Rev.*, **5**, 119–40.

Hooley, J.M. and Teasdale, J.D. (1989) Predictors of relapse in unipolar depressives: Expressed emotion, marital distress, and perceived criticism. *J. Abnorm. Psychol*, **98**, 229–235.

Hooley, J.N., Richters, J.E., Weintraub, S. and Neale, J.M. (1987) Psychopathology and marital distress: the positive side of positive symptoms. *J. Abnorm. Psychol.*, **96**, 27–33.

Kanter, J., Lamb, K.R. and Leoper, C. (1987) Expressed emotion in families: A critical review. *Hosp. Community Psychiatry*, **38**, 374–80.

Karno, M., Jenkins, J.H., de la Selva, A. et al. (1987) Expressed emotion and schizophrenic outcome among Mexican–American families. *J. Nerv. Ment. Dis.*, **175**, 143–51.

Koenigsberg, H.W. and Hanley, R. (1986) Expressed emotion: From predictive index to clinical construct. *Am. J. Psychiatry*, **143**, 1361–73.

Köttgen, C., Sonnichsen, I., Mollenhauer, J. and Jurth, R. (1984) The family relations of young schizophrenic patients: Results of the Hamburg Camberwell Family Interview study I. *Int. J. Fam. Psychiatry*, **5**, 61–70.

Laing, R.D. (1965) Mystification, confusion, and

conflict. In *Intensive Family Therapy*. I. Boszormenyi-Nagy and J.L. Framo (eds), Harper, New York, pp. 112–34.

Leff, J., and Vaughn, C. (1985) *Expressed Emotion in Families*, Guilford, New York.

Leff, J., Berkowitz, N., Shavit, A. *et al*. (1989) A trial of family therapy V. A relatives' group for schizophrenia. *Br. J. Psychiatry*, **154**, 58–66.

Leff, J.P., Kuipers, L., Berkowitz, R. *et al*. (1982) A controlled trial of social intervention in the families of schizophrenic patients. *Br. J. Psychiatry*, **141**, 121–34.

Leff, J., Wig, N.N., Ghosh, A. *et al*. (1987) Influence of relatives' expressed emotion on the course of schizophrenia in Chandigarh. *Br. J. Psychiatry*, **151**, 166–73.

Lefley, H. (1989) Family burden and family stigma in major mental illness. *Am. Psychol.*, **44**, 556–60.

Lezenweger, M.F., Dworkin, R.H. and Wethington, E. (1989) Models of positive and negative symptoms in schizophrenia: an empirical evaluation of latent structures. *J. Abnorm. Psychol.*, **98**, 62–70.

Liberman, R.P., DeRisi, W.J. and Mueser, K.T. (1989) *Social Skills Training for Psychiatric Patients*. Pergamon, New York.

MacMillan, J.F., Gold, A., Crow, T.J., Johnson, A.L. and Johnstone, E.C. (1986) Northwick park study of first episodes of schizophrenia IV: expressed emotion and relapse. *Br. J. Psychiatry*, **148**, 133–43.

Magãna, A.B., Goldstein, M.J., Karno, M. *et al*. (1986) A brief method for assessing expressed emotion in relatives of psychiatric patients. *Psychiatry Res.*, **17**, 203–12.

Margolin, G. (1987) Participant observation procedures in marital and family assessment. In *Family Interaction and Psychopathology*. T. Jacob (ed), Plenum Press, New York, pp. 391–426.

Margolin, G., Talovic, S. and Weinstein, C.D. (1983) Areas of change questionnaire: A practical approach to marital assessment. *J. Consult. Clin. Psychol.*, **51**, 920–31.

Markman, H.J. and Notarius, C.I. (1987) Coding marital and family interactions: current status. In *Family Interaction and Psychopathology*. T. Jacob (ed), Plenum, New York, pp. 329–90.

McCreadie, R.G. and Philips, K. (1988) The Nithsdale Schizophrenia Survey VII. Does relatives' high expressed emotion predict relapse? *Br. J. Psychiatry*, **152**, 477–81.

McElroy, E.M. (1987) The beat of a different drummer. In *Families of the Mentally Ill: Coping and Adaption*. A.B. Hatfield and H.P. Lefley (eds). Guilford, New York, pp. 225–43.

McGill, C.W., Falloon, I.R.H., Boyd, J.L. and Wood-Swerio, C. (1983) Family educational interventions in the treatment of schizophrenia. *Hosp. Community Psychiatry*, **34**, 934–8.

Miklowitz, D.J., Goldstein, M.J., Doane, J.A. *et al*. (1989) Is expressed emotion an index of a transactional process? I. Parents' affective style. *Family Process*, **28**, 153–67.

Miklowitz, D.J., Goldstein, M.J. and Falloon, I.R.H. (1985) Premorbid and symptomatic characteristics of schizophrenics from families with high and low levels of expressed emotion. *J. Abnorm. Psychol.*, **92**, 359–67.

Miklowitz, D.J., Goldstein, M.J., Falloon, I.R.H. and Doane, J.A. (1984) International correlates of expressed emotion in the families of schizophrenics. *Br. J. Psychiatry*, **144**, 482–7.

Mintz, L.I., Nuechterlein, K.H., Goldstein, M.J. *et al*. (1989) The initial onset of schizophrenia and family expressed emotion. Some methodological considerations. *Br. J. Psychiatry*, **154**, 212–17.

Moline, R.A., Singh, S., Morris, A. and Meltzer, H.Y. (1985) Family expressed emotion and relapse in schizophrenia in 24 urban American patients. *Am. J. Psychiatry*, **142**, 1078–81.

Moos, R. and Moos, B.S. (1981) *Family Environment Scale: Manual*. Consulting Psychologists Press, Palo Alto.

Notarius, C.I. and Markman, H.J. (1989) Coding marital interaction: a sampling and discussion of current issues. *Behav. Assess.*, **11**, 1–12.

Nuechterlein, K.H., Snyder, K.S., Dawson, M.E. *et al*. (1986) Expressed emotion, fixed dose fluphenazine decanoate maintenance, and relapse in recent-onset schizophrenia. *Psychopharmacol. Bull.*, **22**, 633–9.

Parker, G., Topling, H. and Brown, L.B. (1979) A parental bonding instrument. *Br. J. Med. Psychol.*, **52**, 1–10.

Parker, G., Fairley, M., Greenwood, J. *et al*. (1983) Parental representations of schizophrenics and their association with onset and course of schizophrenia. *Br. J. Psychiatry*, **141**, 573–81.

Parker, G., Johnston, P. and Hayward, L. (1988) Parental expressed emotion as a predictor of schizophrenic relapse. *Arch. Gen. Psychiatry*, **45**, 806–13.

Patterson, G.R. (1982) *Coercive Family Process*. Castilia, Eugene, Oregon.

Patterson, G.R. (1988) Foreword. In *Handbook of Behavioural Family Therapy*. I.R.H. Falloon (ed), Guilford, New York, pp. vii–x.

Platt, S. (1985) Measuring the burden of psychiatric illness on the family: an evaluation of some rating scales. *Psychol. Med.*, **15**, 383–93.

Platt, S. and Hirsch, S. (1981) The effects of brief hospitalisation upon the psychiatric patient's household. *Acta Psychiatr. Scand.*, **64**, 199–216.

Platt, S., Weyman, A. and Hirsch, S. (1978) *Social Behaviour Assessment Schedule* (2nd ed., revised). Department of Psychiatry, Charing Cross Hospital, London.

Platt, S., Weyman, A. Hirsch, S. and Hewett, S. (1980) The Social Behaviour Assessment Schedule (SBAS): rationale, contents, scoring and reliability of a new interview schedule. *Soc. Psychiatry*, **15**, 43–55.

Sainsbury, P. (1975) Evaluation of community mental health programs. In *Handbook of Evaluation Research*, vol. 2. M. Guttentag and E.L. Struening (eds), Beverly Hills, Sage, pp. 125–59.

Schooler, N.R., Levine, J., Severe, J.B. *et al.* (1980) Prevention of relapse in schizophrenia: evaluation of fluphenazine decanoate. *Arch. Gen. Psychiatry*, **41**, 817–8.

Schweitzer, R., Halford, W.K. and Varghese, F.N. (1988) A brief method of assessing expressed emotion. Paper presented to the Australian Society for Psychiatric Research. Melbourne, Australia.

Schweitzer, R., Halford, W.K., Strachan, A. and Varghese, F.N. (1992) Reliability and validity of a brief measure of expressed emotion. Manuscript submitted for publication.

Hatfield, A., Spaniol, L., Zipple, A.M. *et al.* (1987) Families as a resource in the rehabilitation of the severely psychiatrically disabled. In *Families of the Mentally Ill; Coping and Adaptation* . A. Hatfield and H. Lefley (eds), Guilford, New York, pp. 167–90.

Spiegel, D. and Wessler, T. (1986) Family environment as a predictor of psychiatric rehospitalization. *Am. J. Psychiatry*, **143**, 56–60.

Spitzer, R.L., Gibbon, M. and Endicott, J. (1971) *Family Evaluation Form*. Biometrics Research, New York State Department of Mental Hygiene, New York.

Strachan, A.M., Feingold, A., Goldstein, M.J. *et al.* (1989) Is expressed emotion an index of a transactional process? Patients' coping style. *Fam. Process*, **22**, 169–82.

Tarrier, N., Barrowclough, C., Porceddu, K., and Watts, S. (1988) The assessment of psychophysiological reactivity to the expressed emotion of the relatives of schizophrenic patients. *Br. J. Psychiatry*, **152**, 618–24.

Terkelson, K.G. (1987) The meaning of mental illness to the family. In *Families of the Mentally Ill: Coping and Adaption*. A.B. Hatfield and H.P. Lefley (eds), Guilford, New York, pp. 128–150.

Tienari, P., Sorri, A., Lahti, I. *et al.* (1987) Genetic and psychosocial factors in schizophrenia: The Finnish adoptive family study. *Schizophr. Bull.*, **13**, 477–84.

Turpin, G., Tarrier, N. and Sturgeon, D. (1988) Social psychology and the study of biopsychosocial models of schizophrenia. In *Social Psychophysiology: Theory and Clinical Applications*. H. Wagner (ed), John Wiley and Sons, Chichester, pp. 87–112.

Vaughn, C.E. (1986) Patterns of emotional response in the families of schizophrenic patients. In *Treatment of Schizophrenia: Family Assessment and Intervention*. M.J. Goldstein, I. Hand, and K. Hahlweg (eds), Springer-Verlag, Berlin, pp. 97–108.

Vaughn, C.E. and Leff, J.P. (1976) The influence of family and social factors on the course of psychiatric illness: A comparison of schizophrenic and depressed neurotic patients. *Br. J. Psychiatry*, **129**, 125–37.

Vaughn, C.E., Snyder, K.S., Freeman, W., Jones, S., Falloon, I.R.H. and Liberman, R.P. (1984) Family factors in schizophrenic relapse. *Arch. Gen. Psychiatry*, **47**, 1169–77.

Wallace, C.J., (1981). Assessment of psychotic behavior. In *Behavioral Assessment: A Practical Handbook* (2nd ed). M. Hersen and A.S. Bellack (eds), Pergamon, New York, pp. 328–88.

Wallace, C.J. (1986) Functional assessment in rehabilitation. *Schizophr. Bull.*, **12**, 604–30.

Weintraub, S. (1987) Risk factors in schizophrenia: The Stony Brook High Risk Project. *Schizophr. Bull.*, **13**, 439–47.

Weiss, R.L. (1989) The circle of voyeurs: Observing the observers of marital and family interactions. *Behav. Assess.*, **11**, 135–48.

Weiss, R.L. and Perry, B.A. (1983) The spouse observation checklist: Development and clinical application. In *Marriage and Family Assessment*. E.E. Filsinger (ed), Sage Publications, Beverly Hills, CA, pp. 106–31.

Weiss, R.L., Hops, H. and Patterson, G.R. (1973) A framework for conceptualizing marital conflict, a technology for altering it, some data for evaluating it. In *Behavior Change: Methodology, Concepts, and Practice*. L.A. Hamerlynck, L.C. Handy and E.J. Mash (eds), Research Press, Champaign, Ill, pp. 369–42.

Wynne, L.C. and Singer, M.T. (1963) Thought disorder and family relations of schizophrenics. *Arch. Gen. Psychiatry*, **9**, 191–206.

Chapter 16

Social networks and social support in schizophrenia: correlates and assessment

HENRY J. JACKSON and JANE EDWARDS

This chapter examines the concepts of social networks, their assumed structural parameters and supportive functions. Studies which have investigated social networks of people with schizophrenia are outlined and reviewed and suggestions for future research are made. The topics mentioned previously provide a context for the focus of the chapter, namely reviewing those network tools which might be considered appropriate for schizophrenic patients, bearing in mind that few network measures have been specifically developed for psychotic patients let alone schizophrenic patients. We conclude by making specific suggestions regarding suitable instruments for both clinical and research purposes.

16.1 THE CONCEPTS

A social network is a term used to connote individuals linked by social ties. Implicit is the notion that individuals are in communication with one another (Cohen and Sokolovsky, 1979).

16.1.1 STRUCTURAL CHARACTERISTICS OF NETWORKS

Social networks can be assessed structurally in various ways. For more detail the reader is referred to the excellent article by Morin and Seidman (1986).

- Size refers simply to the number of persons within a network and is negatively correlated with the degree of psychopathology. In general, it would seem the larger the network, the greater the opportunity for alternative sources of support (Sokolove and Trimble, 1986).

- Density refers to the degree of 'interconnectedness, usually defined as the rates of actual links to potential ones' (Morin and Seidman, 1986, p. 263). Dense networks are likely to develop between individuals with common values and goals (Morin and Seidman, 1986).

- Clusters refer to the 'proportion of interconnections between the nuclear family and the friendship network' (Morin and Seidman, 1986). If the clusters are too connected the individual may find it difficult to withdraw from, for example, the family network and seek support from the friendship network.

- Directionality or reciprocity refers to whether a patient receives services or support from a network member (i.e. the relationship is 'dependent') or whether the patient gives and receives services or support to and from the network member (i.e. the relationship is 'reciprocal').

• Multiplexity refers to the different functions a relationship may perform. For example, an individual might provide information about certain types of community services, lend money and provide opportunities for a patient to discuss issues and concerns. It has been suggested that multiplex relationships are superior to uniplex ones, since some functions of a multiplex relationship may be available at a particular time even if others are not (Morin and Seidman, 1986; Sokolove and Trimble, 1986). For example, a network member may not have any spare time on a particular day to listen to the patient describe his problems with his landlord, although he may be prepared to lend the patient money to pay for a ticket to gain admission to the movies.

• Stability refers to the duration of the relationship.

• Flexibility refers to the sum of the number of network members, the number of clusters, the degree of multiplexity, and the level of acceptance. Flexibility reduces dependency on any one network member and allows the patient to rely on other network members for different requirements. However, Morin and Seidman (1986) admitted that further research was required to arrive at the weightings to be given to these components and so allow the formulation of an appropriate algorithm for obtaining an index of flexibility.

16.1.2 THE SOCIAL SUPPORT FUNCTION OF NETWORKS

In an omnibus review, Cohen and Wills (1985) observed that measures of structural characteristics such as size or density of networks, do not provide sufficiently fine-grained measures of the functions provided by those social structures. Correlations between number of social connections and functional support typically vary between 0.20 and 0.30 (Cohen and Wills, 1985). A great deal of functional support may be obtained from one significant relationship, as opposed to multiple superficial relationships.

Social support could help one avoid or prevent certain potentially stressful problems (e.g. money difficulties), or attenuate the individual experiencing a severe stress reaction to a significant life event (e.g. break-up of a relationship; Lin *et al.*, 1981; Cohen and Wills, 1985). Presumably this buffering effect would occur by the supportive person providing information or solutions to the problem, reducing the perceived importance of the problem, distracting the individual, or providing instrumental help (e.g. money or materials). For the individual such support may restore feelings of helplessness, create a better mood, and improve self-esteem (Cohen and Wills, 1985; Schradle and Dougher, 1985).

Although cognizant that social support is but one function of a social network, it remains the essential focus of our current interest. Whilst our emphasis will be on the ameliorative effects of social intercourse, interpersonal exchanges can also be toxic, depending both on endogenous factors such as the individual's premorbid personality and current mental state (Hammer, 1981; Henderson, 1984), as well as exogenous influences such as the stress produced by demanding or intrusive individuals (Hamilton *et al.*, 1989).

16.2 SOCIAL NETWORKS OF PEOPLE WITH SCHIZOPHRENIA

Studies published over the last decade which investigated social networks of schizophrenic patients are displayed in Table 16.1. Studies which investigated the social networks of relatives of schizophrenic patients (e.g. Anderson *et al.* (1984) are not reviewed. Studies are grouped according to design and notes are made regarding patient status, composition and age of the sample, and type of assessment techniques

Table 16.1 Correlates of network or support variables in schizophrenia

Study	Status	Sample	Age	Social network or support measures
Single sample, Cross-sectional				
Mitchell (1982)	o/p	35 outpatients 'majority schizophrenic' (22 men, 13 women) 35 of their family members	M = 37.9 years	Own scale
Mitchell and Birley (1983)	o/p	'chronic' (25 men, 16 women) 22 schizophrenia 7 bipolar 12 neurosis/personality disorder	Middle-aged	Unspecified interview
Dozier et al. (1987)	o/p	'chronic' 18 schizophrenia 5 bipolar 7 borderline personality disorder	Range 21–40 M = 31 years	Own semi-structured interview
Earls and Nelson (1988)	o/p	89 'long term' schizophrenia depressive bipolar	Range 18–65 M = 38 years	Modified Arizona Social Support Interview Schedule
Hamilton et al. (1989)	o/p	39 males with DSM-III schizophrenia	M = 33 years	Pattison Psychosocial Kinship Inventory
Sullivan and Poertner (1989)	o/p	213 'long term mental patients'	...	Own seven-item scale,
Single sample, 'Longitudinal'				
Breier and Strauss (1984)	o/p	3 schizophrenia 8 bipolar 5 schizo-affective 4 major depression	Range 20–41	Own semi-structured interview
Comparison groups				
Tolsdorf (1976)	i/p	10 first admission schizophrenia 10 medical patients	...	Own instrument, unspecified format
Cohen and Sokolovsky (1978)	o/p	11 schizophrenia with chronic residual symptoms 21 schizophrenia with minimal residual symptoms 12 controls with no known psychotic history	Range 24–66 M = 43 years	Own scale
Froland et al. (1979)	i/p/o/p	30 state hospital patients 20 day hospital patients 27 outpatients (clinic) 30 general population sample	Ms varied for each group = 31–36 years	Own scale
Lipton et al. (1981)	i/p	15 first admission schizophrenia 15 multiple admission schizophrenia	Range = 18–34 M = 25.7 years Range = 19–38 M = 27.6 years	Instrument in Cohen and Sokolovsky (1979)
Isele et al. (1985)	i/p	First admission 69 schizophrenia 60 normal controls	Range 16–40 years M = 24.7 years Range 15–40 years M = 26.2 years	Own instrument
Erickson et al. (1989)	...	First admission 72 schizophrenia 74 major depression/bipolar 122 'normals'	Range 15–50 M = 25.2 years	Interview Schedule for Social Interaction

... = Not reported; o/p = Outpatient; i/p = Inpatient

used. The assumption is that studies employing between-group designs yield stronger data than single-sample designs.

16.2.1 SINGLE SAMPLE, CROSS-SECTIONAL

Studies included under this rubric are defined as describing and reporting data for one group, these data being obtained at a solitary point in time. Many of the single-sample, cross-sectional studies used mixed psychiatric samples which included schizophrenic patients. Separate results from specific diagnostic groups went unreported.

The cross-sectional study by Mitchell (1982) is not concerned with social network size or degree of social support *per se*, but rather with those factors which affect network size and degree of support. Patient psychopathology was assessed on the Psychoticism factor of the Katz Adjustment Scale (Katz and Lyerly, 1963). The patient's problem-solving skills, the family environment, and the family's social resources were also assessed. Demographic indices were not significantly related to social network variables. Better problem-solving skills were associated with having more intimates and greater support from the family, and less psychopathology was associated with having a greater number of intimates and greater support from peers. However, the more contact the family had with their own friends, the less support the patient received from their own family. One possible explanation proposed by Mitchell is that the patient's psychopathology not only alienates support from non-kin, but also prompts family members to seek high levels of contact with friends.

Mitchell and Birley (1983) described their sample as chronic with an average of six admissions. More detailed illness and hospitalization data were not provided. Information on the network included the people with whom subjects had some contact over the past year, their primary group (all relatives and friends with whom they had regular contact) and their confidant (the person in the primary group whom they regarded as most important). The mean primary group size was 7.0, being less for men than women. Twenty of the 41 subjects could name a frequent confidant. Fewer men (41%) than women (63%) were satisfied with their social contacts. Although results were not reported for different diagnostic groups, the findings indicate that patients with later onset of illness were more likely to possess a larger network and a confidant.

Dozier *et al.* (1987) interviewed 30 patients under the age of 40 who had been hospitalized at least six times in the previous four years. The subjects were asked to identify all persons important to them (persons with whom they had had contact in the past two weeks), and further, nominate which members of their networks knew other network members (i.e. had a conversation with one another in the past two weeks). Network size averaged 16 persons, and the average density was 0.51. Time spent in hospital was not related to network size but patients with networks of very low or high density obtained higher numbers of days in hospital than those with moderately dense networks. Dozier *et al.* suggested that a moderately dense network was optimal for psychologically vulnerable individuals because it could be maintained under stress. Problems with this study included the small sample size, the lack of symptom measures and limited sample descriptions.

Earls and Nelson (1988) examined 89 psychiatric clients between the ages of 18–65 who had been hospitalized for psychiatric problems at least twice. Network size was determined by averaging the total number of people who provided support. Total support satisfaction was assessed with the use of a three-point scale. Results indicated that network size was not significantly correlated with the clients' satisfaction over the support they received. However, the more frequent contact patients enjoyed with network members, the larger their network and the more satisfied they were with network support. Earls and Nelson commented on the need for a larger sample and queried the representativeness of the study sample.

Hamilton *et al.* (1989) undertook a significant cross-sectional study which examined the relationship of symptomatology to social networks. Positive and negative symptoms of 39 males with DSM–III (American Psychiatric Association, 1980) diagnoses of chronic schizophrenia (11 years since diagnosis) were assessed. Symptoms were rated on the Schedules for the Assessment of Positive and Negative Symptoms — SAPS and SANS — (Andreasen, 1983, 1984), and the Negative Symptom Rating Scale — NSRS (Iager *et al.*, 1985). Patients' networks were examined using a modified version of the Pattison Psychosocial Kinship Inventory — PPKI (Pattison and Pattison, 1981). Size of network (number of kin and non-kin), frequency of contacts, multiplexity and instrumentality (how frequently each member provided support) were measured. Since the NSRS and SANS correlated very highly, only data for the NSRS were reported.

The SAPS did not correlate with any network variable, level of negative symptoms or duration of illness. The patients reported about 13 people in their total network, about six multiplex individuals and seven reciprocal individuals. Essentially, the NSRS did not correlate with medication dose or the PPKI. However, there were significant correlations between negative symptom (NSRS) scores and reduced network size, multiplexity, reciprocity, and instrumentality for 'non-kin' relationships. The results suggested that kin remained important, regardless of whether the patients were able to maintain multiplex, reciprocal and instrumental relationships. Hamilton *et al.* (1989) concluded that 'once the course of illness is chronic, the negative symptoms of schizophrenia, not the positive symptoms, are associated with network distruption' (p. 628).

That remains one of the more sophisticated studies in the area, as it controlled for the degree of schizophrenic symptomatology, medication dose, duration of illness, and utilized an acknowledged social network instrument. Unfortunately, phenomena which can mask negative symptoms were not indexed (e.g. side effects and depression), inter-rater reliability data for the symptom measures went unreported, data pertaining to length and duration of inpatient hospitalization were not collected, and structured interviews were not employed to confirm DSM–III diagnoses.

Sullivan and Poertner (1989) included 213 long-term mentally ill individuals from a variety of settings. The study provided no details of diagnoses, illness severity and duration, drug dose information, nor number of admissions. The seven-item scale examined network size, reciprocity, instrumental and emotional aid. The essential finding was that the individuals had very small social networks dominated by family members.

Cross-sectional studies imply an immutability in a patient's network, rather than viewing it as a changing dynamic process. Individuals may temporarily or permanently drop out of a patient's network due to a change in the patient's mental state or behaviours or because of the support person's reactions to the mental illness. Support individuals may also withdraw because of their own mental state problems, changes in their own employment and environment, and changes in other relationships (e.g. marriage).

16.2.2 SINGLE SAMPLE, LONGITUDINAL

An important study by Breier and Strauss (1984) employed bi-monthly interviews to document the change in social needs of 20 patients during a one-year period following hospital discharge. Using semi-structured interviews, they attempted to identify the specific qualitative factors within a social relationship that might prove useful for patients recovering from psychosis. Twelve useful functions were identified: ventilation; reality-testing; material support; social approval and integration; constancy; motivation; modelling; symptom-monitoring; problem-solving; empathic understanding; reciprocal-relating; and insight.

Breier and Strauss identified two phases in the year following hospital discharge, namely convalescence and rebuilding. The first phase involved recovery from the illness and leaving hospital. Ventilation and reassurance were described by patients as the most beneficial functions of the social network during this phase. Social relationships were one-sided with the patient being dependent. In the second phase patients were somewhat more reintegrated, and motivation, reciprocal-relating and symptom-monitoring were described by patients as being the most important functions of their social relationships. Breier and Strauss (1984) agree that a large social network is likely to buffer against stress. However, major problems with the study, acknowledged by the authors, are that they may have preselected a high functioning group and that a one-year follow-up period may have been too short to detect differences among the diagnostic groups. Only patients who had held a job at some time during the year before entrance into the project were selected.

16.2.3 COMPARISON GROUPS

Tolsdorf (1976) compared 10 recently hospitalized first admission schizophrenics, with 10 recently hospitalized medical patients matched for age, marital status, education, and socio-economic status. Essentially no differences were found between the two groups in terms of size and density of network. Nonetheless, in the schizophrenic group, there were fewer numbers of multiplex persons, a smaller proportion of multiplex relationships, a greater proportion of kin and a greater proportion of nonreciprocal relationships. Formal diagnostic and symptom measures were not employed in this study.

Cohen and Sokolovsky (1978) examined networks in three groups of people living in the same Manhattan hostel. One group was assessed as suffering from schizophrenia with moderate or severe residual symptoms (SR). The second group suffered from schizophrenia with minimal or no chronic residual symptoms (S), whilst a third group had no known psychotic history (NP) but may have experienced other psychopathology. There were no differences between the groups in sex or ethnic composition. A consensus diagnostic approach was utilized, although no formal structured instruments were employed to arrive at diagnoses. The more chronic SR group had fewer kin and non-kin relations ($M = 10.3$) and multiplex individuals ($M = 4.3$) when compared to the S group (total contacts $M = 14.8$, multiplex individuals $M = 6.7$) and the NP group (total contacts $M = 22.5$, multiplex individuals $M = 12.1$). The SR group engaged in the least amount of reciprocity. Shortcomings of this study include the non-use of formal diagnoses or formal measures of symptom-atology and the apparent omission of demographic and illness-related variables.

Froland *et al.* (1979) studied the social networks of a sample comprising three groups of patients and one group drawn from the general population. Results revealed that the networks of the three treatment groups were smaller in size, that patients had fewer long-term friends and their relationships were more unstable compared with those of the general population group. The state hospital group, which had the greatest number of prior hospitalizations and presumably had a high proportion of schizophrenia sufferers, had the smallest network size, few reciprocal exchanges, lower stability of support and less contact with family and friends. Froland and his colleagues asserted that a poorly functioning social network was a strong predictor of poor social adjustment, although the study did not clarify the direction of any causal influence. Diagnostic and symptom data were omitted and no indication of illness-related parameters was given.

The investigation of Lipton *et al.* (1981) compared the social networks of first-admission with multiple-admission schizophrenic persons. Size, density, directionality, frequency of social contact and multiplexity were among those parameters investigated. The first-admission patients reported significantly larger and higher density networks, and more multiplex relationships than the multiple-admission patients, who possessed more than a two-year history of psychiatric illness. Although not significant, the multiple-admission group tended to have high levels of dependency and lower levels of reciprocal relations than the comparison group. Between the two groups, no significant differences were found in terms of the number of kin within networks, suggesting kin still remained tied to the patient, at least at this conjectured intermediate stage of illness. The prime weaknesses of this study reside in the non-use of symptom measures and accurate indices of the illness or hospitalizations.

Isele *et al.* (1985) presented results from a prospective study of first-onset schizophrenic patients' premorbid social situation and adjustment compared with normal controls, using an unpublished tool (the Social Adjustment Scale). The schizophrenic sample consisted of 69 persons hospitalized for the first time in their life. The control sample comprised 60 people selected at random from a rural community, none of whom had ever received psychiatric treatment. It was decided *a priori* that the interview should refer to a period of two months prior to the onset of symptoms and for the controls the two months preceding the interview. Comparison between these two samples showed significant differences for nearly all areas assessed, suggesting premorbid disablement of the schizophrenic group for both the quantitative and qualitative aspects of social functioning. Compared with healthy people, the size of the schizophrenics' social network was markedly reduced and often characterized by

a strong link to their family of origin. In general, the schizophrenic patients failed to establish close relationships or engage in social contact. Moreover, they tended to withdraw from existing relationships, especially heterosexual relationships. Even when the schizophrenic patient appeared to be functioning well according to formal criteria such as partnership or employment, further analyses often revealed problems such as conflicts at work or reticence with partners. Unfortunately Isele *et al.* did not control for hospitalization or the degree of symptomatology. Further, examination of the period two months prior to hospitalization may be insufficient as the onset of the psychotic episode may have been an insidious process, extending over a long period of time.

In an intriguing investigation, Erickson *et al.* (1989) examined the social relationships of patients with a first psychotic episode and compared them with volunteers who were obtained from the community via quota sampling and matched on sex and age. At intake and 18-month follow-up, the Present State Examination (Wing *et al.*, 1974) was administered to each member of the psychotic group. Case conferences produced 'best estimate' consensus psychiatric diagnoses. The ISSI (Henderson *et al.*, 1981) was used to identify all 'family and friends with whom the individual is close to, fond of, or attached to', the availability of social resources and the adequacy of their social relationships. The DSM–III Axis V (APA, 1980) indexed the highest level of adaptive functioning at baseline and 18-month follow-up.

DSM–III schizophrenic and bipolar/major depressive (psychotic) patients were contrasted with the community volunteers at the initial assessment. The schizophrenic patients had the least number of friends (3.6 ± 3.1) followed by the affective disorder patients (5.0 ± 4.7) with the community volunteers having the largest number of friends (6.3 ± 4.6). The schizophrenic patients identified fewer family members (3.7 ± 2.7) than the affective (4.4 ± 3.2) and community groups (4.6 ± 2.9). Schizophrenic patients had fewer close and confiding relationships than the other two groups, but there were no significant group differences among the three groups regarding the adequacy of perceived social support derived from acquaintances, but there was a trend favouring the community group.

At the 18-month follow-up, 127 psychotic patients and 87 normals were still retained for study. Results demonstrated that schizophrenics functioned worse than affective psychotic individuals at 18-month follow-up. Initial assessment Axis V ratings were highly correlated with the same ratings completed at 18-month follow-up. Multiple regression analyses with the 18-month follow-up as the criterion variable indicated that the initial assessment Axis V rating, age, sex, number of non-kin in the network, and interactions between diagnoses and ISSI variables, all contributed significantly to the variance. Having a greater number of non-kin was positive for both psychotic groups. Greater availability of acquaintances was better for the schizophrenic group but not for the affective group. In contrast, possessing larger numbers of kin was toxic for schizophrenic patients but ameliorative for affective disorder patients. The negative association between kin and schizophrenia might imply that expressed emotion is high within the family, or that in contrast to friends, the family demands too much intimacy and closeness of contact.

Although impressive in terms of the scale of the investigation it is unfortunate that the network measures taken at baseline were not repeated at 18-month follow-up. Measures of individual symptoms were not reported, so that it was not possible to assess whether they made differential contributions to level of functioning. The percentages of patients in each group who had recovered or relapsed were omitted. Mean levels in Axis V ratings went unreported and the rating itself appears a relatively flimsy, composite and global measure which

confounds level of symptoms with degree of social functioning. The use of two assessors would have increased confidence in the Axis V rating as the sole dependent measure. Erickson *et al.* (1989) acknowledge that they may have failed to account for the influence of non-included independent variables and moreover that the small social network reported by the schizophrenic patients at entry may be due to social ineptness, poor premorbid personality, or an insidious psychotic process.

16.2.4 SUMMARY OF THE LITERATURE ON SCHIZOPHRENIA AND SOCIAL NETWORKS

The literature is summarized with respect to four important questions raised by Henderson in 1980 which are still pertinent today.

Is the network reduced and impaired in quality in patients with recent-onset schizophrenia? The current literature affirms that this is the case. Even at first admission, schizophrenic individuals possess smaller networks than comparison groups comprising normals, hospitalized patients with medical illness, and patients with affective disorders. Networks are dominated by family members and are less reciprocal and multiplex. With continued development of the illness individuals' social networks shrink further. This may be due to withdrawal initiated by the patient or the result of the stigmatizing process. Patients with more psychopathology or severe residual or negative symptoms possess the lowest levels of social support, network size, instrumentality, reciprocity and multiplexity. Family members assume increasing importance as friendship networks diminish. Family climate and its potential for triggering subsequent psychotic illness then takes on increasing significance (see Chapters 8, 15 and 24).

Although the Froland *et al.* (1979) study has some important limitations it does suggest that stability and reciprocity are very important parameters of social adjustment, especially for chronic patients. Family and friends may only continue to support chronic persons as long as there is reasonable reciprocity in the relationships. If this does not occur, family and friends may, due to the burden, become less involved with the patient who may turn increasingly to professionals for aid and support. The earlier the onset of illness the smaller the network: the data also indicate that those patients with an early onset of illness are less likely to have a confidant (Mitchell and Birley, 1983). In one study (Dozier *et al.*, 1987) network density, not network size, was predictive of hospital duration. Finally, the more frequent the patient's social contact, the more likely the patient is to have a larger social network (Earls and Nelson, 1988).

Is the reduced network primary or secondary to the psychoses? Whilst the evidence indicates that the networks of psychiatric patients are impoverished, it does not demonstrate whether this is a function of illness chronicity, severity of symptomatology, or prodromal deterioration. Moreover, other variables (e.g. social competence, personality) may be involved in modulating both levels of support and symptomatology (Cohen and Wills, 1985). Networks and support should be assessed prior to the first admission of a schizophrenic individual, perhaps in 'high-risk populations', such as the close biological relatives of a clearly diagnosed schizophrenic proband (Weintraub, 1987).

What is the effect of premorbid personality on one's network? Clearly individuals differ in their need for social affiliation. This question demands that researchers assess premorbid personality, but this was not undertaken by any of the reviewed studies. Instruments such as the Structured Interview of DSM–III-R Personality Disorder (Pfohl *et al.*, 1990) or the Personality Disorder Examination (Loranger, 1988) would be eminently suitable for this purpose.

If the network is impaired qualitatively or quantitatively what does this mean for prognosis? A patient's impaired network

appears to be correlated with a poor prognosis (e.g. Erickson *et al.*, 1989; Froland *et al.*, 1979). The cause of that poor prognosis is as yet unknown, at least partly because of the inadequate methodologies adopted by the various researchers.

16.2.5 CRITIQUE

It is apparent that there have been relatively few published studies regarding applications to schizophrenia over the last decade. Programmatic research is totally lacking in this area. Rather, the literature consists of widely disparate studies, each using different measurement strategies. It should be noted that network size is assessed in contrasting ways by these techniques and that these differences may be contributing to discrepant results across the studies.

Sample descriptions were frequently missing or inadequate. For instance, patients were not normally diagnosed using semi-structured interviews such as the Structured Clinical interview for DSM–III-R (Spitzer *et al.*, 1986) and the diagnostic groups were typically heterogeneous. Details of length of illness, numbers and lengths of hospitalizations, medication doses and demographic factors were frequently unreported. Little cognizance was given to factors impacting significantly on the social networks of patients. Similarly, little distinction was made between chronic and recent-onset schizophrenic patients or between schizophrenic sub-groups. There was also little recognition of discontinuities between various 'disorders' such as depression versus schizophrenia. Severity and type of symptomatology was measured in only one of the reviewed investigations (Hamilton *et al.*, 1989). Other biological influences such as medication side effects went unexamined.

Hamilton *et al.* (1989) queried whether the lack of a relationship between social support and positive symptoms would hold for unmedicated patients. In the absence of research data, we expect that positive symptoms may be related to social network deficits for patients who default on medication or whose florid, positive symptoms are not substantially ameliorated by medication.

Notwithstanding methodological criticisms of the extant literature, there are more substantial issues which can be raised which extend in some cases beyond the research strictly pertaining to schizophrenic patients.

First, as underscored by Schradle and Dougher (1985) and Veiel (1985), we still are no closer to pinpointing the major active ingredients of social support and their comparative values (e.g. practical help, problem-solving). Further, we need to explore whether the degree of obtained support depends on the individual's level of pathology, and/or the interaction of pre-existing pathology and specific life events. The mechanisms through which social support may function to mediate stress also need to be determined.

Second, social support and network size are always in a state of flux. With a frequently fluctuating disorder such as schizophrenia, this may be even more the case. Networks and support may interact with symptoms, causing variability over time. This necessitates the utilization of designs where symptoms and network/support parameters are repeatedly sampled over time.

Third, symptoms may alter a personal network, but they also threaten the validity of the patients' reports about social networks and the social support benefits derived from the same (Henderson, 1980). Even if recovered from florid symptomatology, patients may still possess residual symptoms. Hamilton *et al.* (1989) investigated this issue, by comparing the PPKIs completed by patients, with those completed by a family member or significant friend. Good correlations were generally obtained between patient and family members' reports, particularly with regard to patient–family contact. Hamilton *et al.* (1989) maintained that the poorer correlations between

patient and family/friends' reports concerning acquaintances and non-kin were not surprising, as family members may simply have been unaware of all the patient's social contacts made through work or recreation.

Fourth, perhaps as a sequela of psychopathology, demographic variables which may affect social networks in schizophrenia include lower class and status, ethnic marginality, migration and mobility across geographic regions (Hammer *et al.*, 1978; Henderson, 1980). Such factors were generally not considered in the literature we reviewed.

Fifth, a social desirability factor may be operative when assessing social networks and/or social support (Henderson, 1984): individuals may be loath to admit to the limited number of individuals comprising their networks. Therefore, they may exaggerate the numbers of social ties and overestimate the amounts of support they acquire (Beels *et al.*, 1984). Only McFarlane *et al.* (1981) examined this issue.

Finally, in the general social network/support literature, there is a confounding of life events with social support (Cohen and Wills, 1985). For example, consider a parent's death. This is clearly a major life event which simultaneously results in a reduction in one's social network/support. One possible way to obviate such a confound is to remove such exit events from either the life events instrument or the social support scale. Not one of the studies reviewed endeavoured to measure life events.

16.2.6 SOME FUTURE DIRECTIONS FOR RESEARCHING NETWORKS IN SCHIZOPHRENIA

We argue that the most exacting attempts should be made to employ only first-admission patients with schizophrenia. Such patients should be diagnosed with semi-structured diagnostic instruments such as the SCID–II (Spitzer *et al.*, 1986) and the complete range of demographic and illness-related variables should be reported and subjected to statistical analysis. Patients should only be assessed on social network/ social support instruments when recovered from their acute illness. A patient's description of their social network may be distorted by florid psychotic illness, e.g. due to paranoid ideation concerning family members. Likewise, attempts should be made to accurately assess premorbid personality/disorders in first-admission schizophrenic patients. Such patients are likely to have family members available as informants to aid in the differentiation between the prodromal phase of a schizophrenic illness and relevant personality disorders. Biases attendant in retrospective reporting may be attentuated when family informants have a shorter time period to review their own accuracy of recall. The presence of a pre-existing personality disorder, particularly of the type where there is minimal desire for social interaction, may arguably mean that on recovery from the initial florid episode, social network analysis reveals only a small group of family members providing limited support. This may reflect the patient's lifelong lack of desire for social affiliation, rather than a deterioration in social competence or social contacts subsequent to a psychotic episode.

Cross-sectional comparisons may elucidate whether the social networks of first-admission schizophrenics are diminished compared with 'normal'. Perhaps more helpful comparisons might involve other psychiatric patients with bipolar illness or recurrent major depressive disorder. Equally valuable would be the inclusion of a chronically medically disordered group, e.g. those patients with diabetes or epilepsy. In short, this could allow one to determine whether a reduction of social networks and support is specific to schizophrenia. Research which matches those groups of patients in terms of age, age of onset, IQ, education, and length of illness would be particularly welcome.

The adoption of a longitudinal repeated-measures design which incorporates a between-groups comparison would of course constitute the superior design. Such a design would permit the determination of whether change over time occurs in response to symptoms, life-events or daily hassles. One could, for instance, determine whether social networks and degree of social support inevitably deteriorated over time compared to other diagnostic groups, and whether deterioration was related to illness-related factors or whether a more complex reciprocal relationship exists. Whether large and/or moderately dense relationships have a stress-buffering function could also be investigated, with illness-related and symptom measures functioning as dependent variables.

Certainly the interaction between personality, life events, symptoms and also social competence, needs to be assessed longitudinally. In fact, the assumed relationship between social competency and social networks has not ben researched (Cohen and Wills, 1985). It may be that socially competent individuals are more capable of forming strong networks and of coping more effectively with stressful life events or daily hassles. On the other hand, it seems theoretically possible that a patient might be deficient in social competency and yet possess a 'sound' social network: the family's financial resources might allow them to purchase an extensive professional support network for an individual. The issue begs closer scrutiny as social skills training may help a patient improve their social competency and in turn, aid in extending their social networks/social supports.

16.3 ASSESSMENT

An historical examination of measurements of social support in schizophrenia is to be found in the excellent review by Beels *et al.* (1984). To aid the reader we have presented social network assessment tools in Table 16.2.

Table 16.2 Network assessment instruments

Authors	Name of instrument	Focus of assessment	Samples studied
Semistructured interviews			
Garrison and Podell (1981)	Community Support System Assessment	Informal and formal social support networks,	...
Sokolove and Trimble (1986)	...	Stress and support in social networks of chronically mentally ill	...
Cheers (1987)	Social Support Network Map	Educational purposes. Obtains and structures information on social support	...
Structured interviews			
Henderson *et al.* (1981)	Interview Schedule for Social Interaction	Availability and adequacy of social relationships	Pilots: 130 subjects from two psychiatric clinics; 150 people randomly selected from two Canberra suburbs. Main study: 756 householders
Pattison and Pattison (1981)	Pattison Psychosocial Kinship Inventory	Structure of social networks	...
Phillips (1981)	... (Questions listed)	Social networks and social participation	1050 non-psychiatric persons living in Northern California
Brugha *et al.* (1987)	Interview Method of Social Relationships	Personal social resources and support	90 and 116 depressed patients
Self-report inventories			
McFarlane *et al.* (1981)	Social Relationship Scale	Quantitative and qualitative aspects of the network	15 referred married couples; 18 parent-therapist couples; 78 college students; 19 post-graduate students; 518 general population
Marziali (1987)	People in Your Life Scale	Social network and social support	511 psychiatric and non-psychiatric patients; 42 patients treated in psychodynamic therapy
Power *et al.* (1988)	Significant Other Scale	Perceived social support: emotional and practical	135 female psychology students

... = not specified in article

16.3.1 SEMI-STRUCTURED INTERVIEWS

Garrison and Podell (1981) advocated the integration of an open-ended clinical interview into the standard clinical intake and psychiatric assessment interview. Two versions of the Community Support System Assessment (CSSA) were outlined. The first version comprises six interview items, contained in the appendix, which can be collected at intake with minimal instructions. The second version of the CSSA includes an expanded genogram, a reconstructed week, and an open-ended history of help-seeking. The latter interview takes at least one hour to complete. The psycho-metric properties of both instruments are not discussed.

Sokolove and Trimble (1986) developed a list of 14 questions to assess the characteristics of a patient's social network, including the number of people in the network, the types of roles assumed in each relationship, multiplexity, directionality, and the nature of behavioural exchanges in each relationship. Quantitative data supporting the psychometric properties of the instrument were not provided.

Cheers (1987) outlined a Social Support Network Map which could be useful as an educational tool in the training of clinicians. Measures of support size, density, directionality and intimacy could be obtained from the map. The map may be useful in generating hypotheses in order to conduct more controlled research. Psychometric indices were not reported.

16.3.2 STRUCTURED INTERVIEWS

Items in Henderson *et al.*'s (1981) Interview Schedule for Social Interaction (ISSI) refer to acquaintances and work associates, friends, close attachment figures, and other individuals with whom the individual enjoys social interaction. Questions are asked about the availability of a given type of social relationship, followed by an item on the adequacy of this relationship for the respondent. At the end of the section on relationships, questions are asked about the amount of change over the previous 12 months. The ISSI, which is clearly set out and easily entered into a computer for scoring, takes approximately 60–90 minutes to complete.

Henderson *et al.* provide reliability indices of internal consistency and test-retest. Most coefficients reached a satisfactory level (i.e. about 0.70). Validity of the instrument has been examined by comparing ISSI scores in several sociodemographic groups, questioning informants, and examining the relationship between the ISSI and measures of response style. Henderson *et al.*'s comprehensive book provides detailed information on the psychometric characteristics of the ISSI, together with the interview and instructions.

Pattison and Pattison (1981) developed the Pattison Psychosocial Kinship Inventory (PPKI) to determine the number of people, relationships, and interactions in the social networks of both normals and individuals with various states of psychopathology. Five zones of relationships were considered: personal; intimate; effective; nominal; and extended. Data were obtained on the number of people in the network, the relationship between network members, and the nature of the interactions between them. Psychometric properties of the inventory are not described.

Phillips (1981) interviewed people living in Northern California communities with the aim of gathering information on the individuals who were significant in respondents' lives. The eight network variables Phillips examined were size, density, number of instrumental supports, number of confidants, number of kin, number of dependent others, number of social contexts, and range of socializing. The duration of the interview was not reported. Phillips suggested that the interview, which is outlined in the article, may not be suitable for persons living in residential care environments or for persons with severely restricted social contacts.

The interview has not, to our knowledge, been employed with psychiatric patients.

Brugha *et al.* (1987) developed the Interview Method of Social Relationships (IMSR) which is a modified and shortened (15–20 minutes) version of Henderson *et al.*'s (1981) ISSI. The information obtained from the IMSR can be stored in a hierarchical data base management system, allowing flexible access to the data. Measures of network size, density, clusters, the number of non-primary group contacts, qualitative information about personal relationships and support in relation to adversity (life events and difficulties), can be obtained. Inter-rater agreement, test-retest reliability and internal consistency figures were reported for depressed patients by Brugha *et al.* (1987).

With one exception inter-rater agreements for categorical variables were 0.85 or better for ordinal data. Only four of the 13 measures obtained weighted kappa figures which were less than 0.90. Internal consistency was also good. The number of contacts within the subjects' primary group was highly positively correlated with its size ($r = 0.82$), and overall dissatisfaction with social support was positively correlated with dissatisfaction with the amount of interaction. Test-retest reliability, where the interval between the two assessments was on average four months, was moderate to excellent (r's $= 0.42$ to 0.73) for structural aspects of the network (e.g. size, density). However, adequacy of social interaction ($r = 0.14$) and satisfaction with social support ($r = 0.39$) demonstrated less stability over time.

16.3.3 SELF-REPORT INVENTORIES

McFarlane *et al.* (1981) developed the Social Relationship Scale (SRS) which focuses on both the quantitative and qualitative aspects of social relationships. The SRS examines categories of potential areas of stress: work; money and finances; home and family; personal and social; personal and health; and issues that relate to society in general. Subjects are asked to list individuals and type of relationship (e.g. friends, co-workers, close relatives) with whom they have had discussions about each of the above problem areas. Subjects rate on a seven-point scale the helpfulness of discussions they had with each person. They are also asked to indicate those individuals listed who come to the subject for similar kinds of discussion (reciprocity or directionality). Measures of size, directionality and multiplexity can be obtained.

The work undertaken on the instrument is most impressive compared with other social network measures. Content validity was investigated with four senior clinicians describing information they believed was missing in a preliminary version of the SRS. Criterion validity was examined by comparing 'stable' married couples with married couples who came into treatment regarding family difficulties. The 'stable' group rated their spouses as significantly more 'helpful' overall and more helpful in the 'home and family' category. Test-retest reliability data were obtained by administering the SRS to 78 community college students on two occasions separated by a one-week interval. Correlations for the extent of network ranged from 0.62 to 0.99 (median = 0.91) depending on the relationship category (e.g. parents, friends, physician). Correlations for the average helpfulness score were also acceptable and ranged from 0.54 to 0.94 (median = 0.78), again depending on the category (e.g. work, money, home). Response bias was explored with 19 postgraduate students. It was calculated that the SRS instructions did not appear 'to elicit a socially desirable response regarding the average helpfulness of people in the social network' (p. 93). McFarlane *et al.* (1981) provided extensive data based on 518 'normal' individuals. The present authors have found the SRS to be a useful tool with schizophrenic patients, although they may require active guidance to complete the instrument. The completion time is only about 30 minutes.

The major problem with the SRS is the number of variables indexing network size, support, multiplexity, reciprocity (directionality) and the complexity of the scoring procedure. For research and where large samples are examined, computer scoring is a necessity. If the practitioner uses the SRS only occasionally, manual scoring, although time-consuming, is viable.

Marziali (1987) aimed to develop a measure of social support that would function as a measure of psychotherapy outcome. The 23-item People in Your Life (PIYL) measure obtains through self-report, the number of friends and close attachment figures available to an individual, as well as an estimate of the degree of satisfaction with those people, using four-point scales. The instrument was derived from Henderson *et al.*'s (1981) ISSI which was converted into a self-administered questionnaire. The psychometric properties of the PIYL are well-documented (Marziali, 1987). The development study used 251 psychiatric outpatients whose diagnoses were not given and 260 non-patients who were solicited through posters displayed in a public utility office building. Marziali determined weighting for the various levels of satisfaction by utilizing Guttman's (1941) optimal scaling procedure. A principal component factor analysis was undertaken on the satisfaction items and this yielded two factors: 'intimate satisfaction' and 'friendship'. Alpha coefficients were 0.88 or better for the two satisfaction sub-scales that were derived from these factors and for their two structural counterparts (the number of people with whom the individual was intimate and the number of friends). Test-retest reliabilities with an intertest interval of two-three weeks, were between 0.71 and 0.83 for the overall combined sample but lower for the patient sample ($r = 0.46$ to 0.78).

Analyses were also undertaken on the relationship of the PIYL with demographic variables and symptom scores (using the Behaviour Symptom Index of Derogatis, 1983). These showed that for the patient group, socio-economic status, age and sex influenced the number of available friends and intimates. Patients had fewer intimate relationships and were less satisfied with their friends and intimates than were non-patients. Psychopathology as indexed by the Behaviour Symptom Index had a strong association with fewer friends and less satisfaction with friends and intimates for patients and non-patients alike.

In a second study reported by Marziali (1987), the effects of brief psychotherapy on 42 psychiatric outpatients with unspecified diagnoses were examined. The intervention led to positive changes in the patients' perceptions of both the quantity and quality of social support. Measures of predictive and concurrent validity were obtained and were supportive of the validity of the PIYL.

The PIYL can be employed in an interview format, provided that the subjects' responses are coded on the four-level satisfaction scale (Marziali, personal communication, November, 1988). We have used the PIYL in an informal trial basis with recent-onset psychotic patients when they were nearing discharge. We found that the PIYL was too complex for those patients when used as a self-report measure, and they required assistance in responding to the various items. Other problems with the PIYL include the somewhat repetitious items and the fact that some of the items pertaining to neighbourhood and work did not appear pertinent to out patient population.

Power *et al.* (1988) perceived current measures as inadequate and designed the Significant Other Scale (SOS). The SOS is comprised of a grid with ten items assessing emotional and practical support and 12 categories of potential role relationships. Test-retest reliability is reported to range from 0.73 to 0.83. It is estimated to take 30 minutes to complete. The explication of the instrument renders it difficult for us to comment on its utility.

16.3.4 CRITIQUE OF ASSESSMENT INSTRUMENTS

Muriel Hammer (cited in Beels *et al.*, 1984) aptly summarized the situation regarding social network assessment as follows: 'Most instruments . . . have no published results to date of reliability testing, and different instruments have not been tested against each other. Moreover, no systematic approach has been presented for establishing criteria of adequacy, for different purposes, for the levels of reliability obtained' (p. 405). Indeed, the interview methods of social network assessment, both semi-structured and structured, appear to largely ignore the issues of reliability and validity (with the exceptions of the SMIR and ISSI). To that extent, the self-report inventories, the SRS and PIYL in particular, seem to fare considerably better.

Few of the instruments have been specifically designed for psychiatric patients. Instruments that are too lengthy or complex are inappropriate for schizophrenic patients. Often the repetitiveness of an instrument is demoralizing for a client who obviously has few social contacts. Those instruments which have been specifically designed for psychiatric patients (e.g. Sokolove and Trimble, 1986) appear suitable only for chronic schizophrenics and fail to consider the heterogeneity of schizophrenia. There also seems to be a dilemma implicit in the literature regarding research versus clinical needs (e.g. Cheers, 1987; Sokolove and Trimble, 1986). This is a false dichotomy: instruments can be designed which suit both research and clinical needs. Sokolovsky and Cohen (1981) noted that social network instruments should examine the qualitative and quantitative aspects of networks, and the subjective and objective factors, for which behavioural indices are necessary; and adopt a broader time frame. Questions need to be asked regarding fluctuations in a network on a daily, monthly, or yearly basis, recognizing that the size and type of network and support can vary across time (Cohen and Wills, 1985).

From our reading of the literature, we believe it sensible to focus attention on further investigating the psychometric properties of those instruments which have already undergone some degree of development. The SMIR, ISSI, SRS and PIYL meet this criterion, and could be further refined by researchers working independently of the authors of those tools. Although both the SRS and PIYL were originally designed as self-report instruments, interviewer-conducted, informant-report and self-report formats could be tested against each other with various groups of schizophrenic patients and other specific diagnostic samples. Assuming a vigorous methodology was utilized, incorporating multiple instruments would permit examination of the contribution of instrument variance to results concerning network size.

16.4 CONCLUSION

To date, research on the social networks of persons with schizophrenia suffers from many shortcomings and leaves many questions unanswered. However, at the very least, the material reviewed in this chapter should provide clinicians with a critical evaluation of relevant studies and also alert them to issues concerning correlates of networks. Similarly, there are many inadequacies in the instruments used to assess social networks and the manner in which such tools have been evaluated. From our review we conclude that the most promising social network instruments available for use with this population suitable for both clinical and research purposes, are the SRS and the PIYL. Clinicians are encouraged to routinely incorporate a social network instrument into their psychiatric assessment battery. That battery should, of course, include standardized instruments designed to aid in diagnosis and measure mental state, life events and personality.

ACKNOWLEDGEMENT

We express our gratitude to Pam Lambert for typing the manuscript.

REFERENCES

American Psychiatric Association (APA) (1980) *Diagnostic and Statistical Manual and Mental Disorders, 3rd ed. (DSM–III).* Washington, DC,

Anderson, C.M., Hogarty, G., Bayer, T. and Needleman, R. (1984) Expressed emotion and social networks of parents of schizophrenic patients. *Br. J. Psychiatry*, **144**, 247–55.

Andreasen, N.S. (1983) *The Scale for the Assessment of Negative Symptoms (SANS).* The University of Iowa, Iowa City.

Andreasen, N.C. (1984) *The Scale for the Assessment of Positive Symptoms (SAPS).* The University of Iowa, Iowa City.

Beels, C.C., Gutwirth, L., Berkeley, J. and Struening, E. (1984) Measurements of social support in schizophrenia. *Schizophr. Bull..*, **10**, 399–411.

Breier, A. and Strauss, J. (1984) The role of social relationships in recovery from psychotic disorders. *Am. J. Psychiatry*, **141**, 949–55.

Brugha, T.S., Sturt, E., MacCarthy, B. *et al.* (1987) The interview measure of social relationships: The description and evaluation of a survey instrument for assessing personal social resources. *Soc. Psychiatry*, **22**, 123–8.

Cheers, B. (1987) The social support network map as an educational tool. *Aust. Soc. Work*, **40**, 18–23.

Cohen, C.I. and Sokolovsky, J. (1978) Schizophrenia and social networks: Ex-patients in the inner city. *Schizophr. Bull.*, **4**, 546–60.

Cohen, C.I. and Sokolovsky, J. (1979) Clinical use of network analysis for psychiatric and aged populations. *Community Ment. Health J.*, **15**, 203–13.

Cohen, S. and Wills, T.A. (1985) Stress, social support, and the buffering hypothesis. *Psychol. Bull.*, **98**, 310–57.

Derogatis, L.R. (1983) *Administration and Procedures: BSI Manual I.* Clinical Psychometric Research, Towson, Maryland.

Dozier, M., Harris, M. and Bergman, H. (1987) Social network density and rehospitalization among young adult patients. *Hosp. Community Psychiatry*, **38**, 61–5.

Earls, M. and Nelson, G. (1988) The relationship between long-term psychiatric clients' psychological well-being and their perceptions of housing and social support. *Am. J. Community Psychol.*, **16**, 279–93.

Erickson, D.H., Beiser, M., Iacono, W.G. *et al.* (1989) The role of social relationships in the course of first-episode schizophrenia and affective psychosis. *Am. J. Psychiatry*, **146**, 1456–61.

Froland, C., Brodsky, G., Olson, M. and Stewart, L. (1979) Social support and social adjustment: implications for mental health professionals. *Community Ment. Health J.*, **15**, 82–93.

Garrison, V. and Podell, J. (1981) 'Community support systems assessment' for use in clinical interviews. *Schizophr. Bull.*, **7**, 101–8.

Guttman, L. (1941) The quantification of a class of attitudes: a theory and method of scale construction. In *The Prediction of Personal Adjustment.* Committee on Social Adjustment (eds), Social Science Research, New York, pp. 319–48.

Hamilton, N.G., Ponzoha, C.A., Cutler, D.L. and Weigel, R. M. (1989) Social networks and negative versus positive symptoms of schizophrenia. *Schizophr. Bull.*, **15**, 625–33.

Hammer, M. (1981) Social supports, social networks and schizophrenia. *Schizophr. Bull.*, **7**, 45–57.

Hammer, M., Makiesky-Barrow, S. and Gutwirth, L. (1978) Social networks and schizophrenia. *Schizophr. Bull.*, **4**, 522–45.

Henderson, A.S. (1984) Interpreting the evidence on social support. *Soc. Psychiatry*, **19**, 49–52.

Henderson, S. (1980) Personal networks and the schizophrenias. *Aust. N.Z.J. Psychiatry*, **14**, 255–9.

Henderson, S., Byrne, D.G. and Duncan-Jones, P. (1981) *Neurosis and the Social Environment.* Academic Press, Sydney.

Iager, A.C., Kirch, D.G. and Wyatt, R.J. (1985) A negative symptom rating scale. *Psychiatry Res.*, **16**, 27–36.

Isele, R., Merz, J., Malzacher, M. and Angst, J. (1985) Social disability in schizophrenia: the controlled prospective burgholzi study. *Eur. Arch. Psychiatry Neurol. Sci.*, **234**, 348–56.

Katz, K.M. and Lyerly, S.B. (1963) Methods of measuring adjustment and social behaviour in the community: I. Rationale, description, discriminative validity and scale development. *Psychol. Rep.*, **13**, 503–35.

Lin, N., Dean, A. and Ensel, W.M. (1981) Social support scales: a methodological note. *Schizophr. Bull.*, **7**, 73–89.

Lipton, F.R., Cohen, C.I., Fischer, E. and Katz, S.E. (1981) Schizophrenia: A network crisis. *Schizophr. Bull.*, **7**, 144–51.

Loranger, A.W. (1988) *Personality Disorder Examination (PDE) Manual*. D.V. Communications, Yonkers, New York.

McFarlane, A.H., Neale, K.A., Norman, G.R., Roy, R.G. and Streiner, D.L. (1981) Methodological issues in developing a scale to measure social support. *Schizophr. Bull.*, **7**, 90–100.

Marziali, E.A. (1987) People in your life: development of a social support measure for predicting psychotherapy outcome. *J. Nerv. Ment. Dis.* **175**, 327–38.

Marziali, E.A. (1988) Personal communication, Clarke Institute of Psychiatry.

Mitchell, R.E. (1982) Social networks and psychiatric clients: The personal and environmental context. *Am. J. Community Psychol.*, **10**, 387–401.

Mitchell, S.F. and Birley, J.L.T. (1983) The use of ward support by psychiatric patients in the community. *Br. J. Psychiatry*, **142**, 9–15.

Morin, R.C. and Seidman, E. (1986) A social network approach and the revolving door patient. *Schizophr. Bull.*, **12**, 262–73.

Pattison, E.M. and Pattison, M.L. (1981) Analysis of a schizophrenic psychosocial network. *Schizophr. Bull.*, **7**, 135–43.

Pfohl, B., Stangl, D. and Zimmerman, M. (1990) *Structured Interview for DSM–III–R Personality Disorder (SIDP–R)* (9-1-89). Department of Psychiatry, University of Iowa, Iowa City.

Phillips, S.L. (1981) Network characteristics related to the well-being of normals: a comparative base. *Schizophr. Bull.*, **7**, 117–24.

Power, M.J., Champion, L.A. and Aris, S.J. (1988) The development of a measure of social support: The significant others (SOS) scale. *Br. J. Clin. Psychol.*, **27**, 349–58.

Schradle, S.B. and Dougher, M.J. (1985) Social support as a mediator of stress: Theoretical and empirical issues. *Clin. Psychol. Rev.*, **5**, 641–61.

Sokolove, R.L. and Trimble, D. (1986) Assessing support and stress in the social networks of chronic patients. *Hosp. Community Psychiatry*, **37**, 370–2.

Sokolovsky, J. and Cohen, C.T. (1981) Toward a resolution of methodological dilemmas in network mapping. *Schizophr. Bull.*, **7**, 109–116.

Spitzer, R.L., Williams, J.B.W. and Gibbon, M. (1986) *Structured Clinical Interview for DSM–III–R — Disorders (SCID–II)*. Biometrics research Department, New York State Psychiatric Institute, New York.

Sullivan, W.P. and Poertner, J. (1989) Social support and life-stress: a mental health consumer's perspective. *Community Ment. Health J.*, **25**, 21–32.

Tolsdorf, C.C. (1976) Social networks, support, and coping: An exploratory study. *Family Process*, **15**, 407–17.

Veiel, H.O.F. (1985) Dimensions of social support: A conceptual framework for research. *Soc. Psychiatry*, **20**, 156–62.

Weintraub, S. (1987) Risk factors in schizophrenia: The Stony Brook high-risk project. *Schizophr. Bull.*, **13**, 439–50.

Wing, J.K., Cooper, J.E. and Sartorius, N. (1974) *The Measurement and Classification of Psychiatric Symptoms*. Cambridge University Press, London.

Chapter 17

Predicting and controlling relapse in schizophrenia: early signs monitoring

FIONA MACMILLAN, MAX BIRCHWOOD and JO SMITH

A consultant psychiatrist working in The Mental Health services in the UK may expect to see perhaps eight to twelve new cases of schizophrenia in a year: however the known individuals suffering from schizophrenia may number 100 to 120 for a catchment area of 45 000. In some settings, characteristically that of a deprived inner city area, this number may be greatly exceeded. The service provision for this group may have to be flexible to accommodate a broad range of age, disability, and social settings. Although there is a marked tendency for the deficits associated with schizophrenia to increase with duration of illness (Owens and Johnstone, 1980) there will be individuals for whom youth is no protection from severe disability, and some aging individuals whose disabilities may be less than expected.

Relapse is a constant preoccupation of the services and patients and carers. Estimates vary, but one might expect approximately 30% of individuals to relapse within one year of an acute episode. The use of long-term neuroleptic prophylaxis may halve the relapse rate from 60 to 30% over two years (Davis, 1975). Even the most enthusiastic advocate of drug management would not suggest that such therapy ablates relapse. Individuals who remain relapse/readmission free for many years, in receipt of maintenance therapy, may return to their past pattern of recurrent relapse upon cessation of maintenance therapy (Johnson et al., 1983). So powerful was this finding that Johnson discontinued his study of this aspect of maintenance therapy before completion. Similarly, the addition of psychosocial interventions to medication may reduce relapse rates further (Tarrier et al., 1988), but few would argue that even the most ideal environment would eliminate the potential for relapse (Hogarty et al., 1986; Chapter 24).

Clinicians may have modest ability to anticipate individuals' potential for relapse even when the individual is well known. In a small study of 14 patients, Pyke and Seeman (1981) demonstrated the practical difficulty in predicting the potential for relapse when they exposed patients on maintenance therapy to a six-week period free of drug treatment, repeated at six-monthly intervals, aimed to reduce or discontinue the maintenance therapy. The cohort was drawn from ordinary clinical practice, including some individuals with tardive dyskinesia, some who were well and

and symptom free, and a small group with residual symptoms who insisted on participation against the judgement of the clinicians. Eight patients suffered recurrences, four of whom required inpatient treatment. A patient who had been symptom free and well for 11 years on small doses of oral neuroleptic suffered an acute relapse three months after discontinuation, another who participated against the advice of clinicians, remained well and symptom free for two-and-a-half years following discontinuation.

Studies of very large groups exposed to dose manipulations of neuroleptic therapy (Kane, 1986) suggest that the response of individuals is difficult to predict. Kane suggests that elucidation of sub-groups is necessary to determine those individuals who may remain well on minimal doses. This is extremely difficult in clinical practice and may confound routine use of low-dose strategies.

Although clinicians may be only modest predictors of relapse potential in individuals, this does not prevent early recognition of loss of well-being, nor preclude early intervention. For example, many clinicians will recognize the repeated appearance of individuals at clinics and services with some minor request that raises the question of impending relapse in the minds of staff. McCandless-Glincher *et al.* (1986) studied 62 individuals attending maintenance therapy and enquired about their recognition of and response to reduced well-being. The patients were drawn from those routinely attending two medical centres, and the age (20–75 years) and mean illness duration (28 years) suggest that such a group would be well represented in ordinary clinical practice. Sixty-one said they could recognize reduced well-being; of these 13 relied upon others to identify symptoms for them. Nine were assisted by others and 36 identified the problem themselves. The majority of patients (50 out of 61) initiated some change in their behaviour when they recognized reduced well-being. This change included engaging in diversionary activities, seeking professional help, and resuming or increasing their neuroleptic medication. Only three of this group had ever been encouraged to self-monitor by mental health professionals, and a further seven had received encouragement from relatives. Thus these schizophrenic patients had initiated symptom monitoring and a range of responses almost entirely at their own initiative.

The authors draw attention to the emphasis generally placed on compliance rather than monitoring in routine clinical settings. The role of compliance in the prevention of relapse has perhaps been over-emphasized (Schooler, 1986), and the structure of many clinics does not facilitate close monitoring with a view to early intervention. Routine medical assessment often relies upon changing junior staff and rarely occurs at frequent intervals, resulting in a slow change of therapy rather than a responsive system.

In essence, there may be a relatively untapped pool of information which is not being accessed adequately enough to initiate early intervention, except perhaps by patients themselves. If individuals can recognize and act on symptoms suggestive of reduced well-being, then it is possible that patterns of prodromal episodes heralding relapse may be apparent and identifiable. Studies of relapse prodromes in research centres support this possibility, but these studies have only recently begun to influence routine clinical practice.

17.1 STUDIES OF PRODROMES

17.1.1 CLINICAL STUDIES

While reports of clinical studies lack observational rigour and objectivity they have provided important insights into the phenomenology of decompensation. The most common approach is the detailed case study that retrospectively gathers information from the patient and family members after a relapse (e.g. Chapman, 1966). Past reviewers of the early literature (Donlon and Blacker, 1975; Docherty *et al.*, 1978) distinguished four sequential stages of relapse. Although the clinical literature is not sufficiently powerful to clearly support the validity of these stages and their suggested sequential relationship, they provide a useful framework for descriptive purposes.

The first stage, described by many authors, is a feeling of loss of control over cognitive and perceptual processes. McGhie and Chapman (1961) and Bower (1968), and Freedman and Chapman (1973) describe cases where the individual is initially aware of *heightened* mental efficiency, creativity and general well-being. Birchwood *et al.* (1989) described a patient who abruptly discontinued medication due to a sensation of well-being, only to relapse; and a further two cases who experienced a similar feeling of well-being prior to the onset of decompensation. However, this 'euphoria' quickly subsides as the individual begins to experience a diminution of control over cognitive-perceptual processes. This is described in most of the clinical reports as a feeling of over-stimulation, involving a difficulty in preventing internal or external events invading consciousness (e.g. Chapman, 1966). 'Visual, proprioception and time distortions are common resulting in visual illusions and feelings of derealisation and depersonalisation . . . irrelevant thoughts and feelings appear from nowhere and cannot be separated from more meaningful ones . . . the patient becomes a passive recipient . . . past memories and present occurrences, varying in length, relevance and emotional tone that run through his mind, leaving him fearful and perplexed' (Donlon and Blacker 1975, p. 324). Perhaps not surprisingly it has been reported that patients will consult their physicians with vague, diffuse symptoms which are suggested to be the result of activated biological systems (Offenkrantz, 1962).

The onset of depressive-like symptoms is widely reported in the second stage and is regarded by some as a psychological reaction to deteriorating mental processes. These include low mood, lowered self-esteem, vegetative signs and social withdrawal (Cameron, 1938; Stein, 1967; Donlon and Blacker, 1975). Chapman's (1966) classic study notes an absorbing self-concern and preoccupation with aberrant mental functions and experiences. The uncertainty this creates may be responsible for obsessional rituals which Chapman notes as characteristic of the prodrome in some of his patients. Those with prior experience of relapse may feel a sense of foreboding; this, in the context of intact insight, may be the trigger for self-administration of medication observed by Brier and Strauss (1983) and McCandless-Glincher *et al.* (1986). Needless to say, these changes are clearly associated with impairment of role performance.

Some authors describe a further third stage characterized by impulsivity, exaggeration of normal emotions and an inability to exercise control over the expression of personal thoughts. 'She began atypically to lose her temper and spend money freely . . . she bought an automobile and drove it impulsively without a licence . . . (she acted) in a rebellious urge to obtain what she wanted for her life' (Docherty *et al.*, 1978, p. 424. The disinhibition tends to be progressively more primitive, including sexuality, rage, demands for attention and concerns about death — e.g. 'I'm not afraid of anyone anymore, I hate everyone, hate good, I'm going to burn the world' (Docherty *et al.*, 1978, p. 424.

Many of the cases described in the clinical studies suggest a fourth stage which includes experiences of 'pre-psychotic' thinking: these include delusional mood, ideas of reference, a sense that one's thoughts have an alien quality, and losing trust in people. Perceptual misinterpretations are frequently reported and delusion-like explanations may be entertained to make sense of these experiences.

The clinical studies do not reveal a homogeneous picture of prodromes of schizophrenia, partly because they are a based on observations of over 30 patients taken in different epochs by clinicians schooled in different psychiatric traditions. There is some consensus in observation of pre-psychotic changes (anxiety/agitation and dysphoria) but less agreement in respect of other 'borderline' symptoms (disinhibition and 'pre-psychotic' thinking). However, it is possible that the transition to full relapse may be as variable *between* subjects as the characteristics of an episode itself. The strong emphasis on phenomenology in these studies have shown that early signs of relapse are inappropriately caricatured as 'neurotic' symptoms' i.e. in terms of Foulds' (1976) notion of a hierarchy of psychiatric illness, according to which schizophrenia, at the top of the hierarchy, will concurrently incorporate dysphoria, anxiety and other neurotic symptoms. The loss of control over normal mental processes is widely observed and probably plays a significant role in the genesis of 'neurotic' symptoms giving them a unique character. In fact, in the retrospective study by Hirsch and Jolley (1989), 'fear of going crazy' was the most prevalent early symptom reported by 70% of their relapsing patients.

The clinical studies have at best offered a set of hypotheses for further examination. They have not provided information about the duration of prodromes, the validity of the 'stages', their sequential relationship, nor the survival of insight. All of these aspects are prerequisites for clinical application.

17.1.2 RETROSPECTIVE STUDIES

The interview study by Herz and Melville (1980) in the USA attempted systematically to collect data from patients and relatives about early signs of relapse. It is widely regarded as definitive since they interviewed 145 schizophrenic sufferers (46 following a recent episode) as well as 80 of their family members. The main question, 'could you tell that there were any changes in your thought, feelings or behaviours that might have led you to believe you were becoming sick and might have to go into hospital?', was answered affirmatively by 70% of patients and 93% of families. The overall agreement between patients and families was 66%. The study did not however determine the reasons for the discrepancy between patients and family members.

Generally the symptoms most frequently mentioned by patients and family members were dysphoric: eating less (53%), trouble concentrating (70%), troubled sleep (69%), depression (76%) and seeing friends less (50%). The most common 'early psychotic' symptoms were hearing voices (60%), talking in a nonsensical way (76%), increased religious thinking (48%) and thinking someone else was controlling them (39%).

A similar British study (Birchwood *et al.*, 1989) interviewed relatives of 42 CATEGO 'S' schizophrenic patients recently admitted or discharged from inpatient care. All relatives recalled 'early signs' but 19% could not specify when they occurred. Table 17.1 summarizes results of this study together with parallel data from Herz and Melville (1980). There is considerable agreement in the content of the early signs although somewhat less in their relative frequency. Both studies concur in finding 'dysphoric' symptoms the most commonly prevalent. In the Herz and Melville study, although more families than patients reported the presence of early signs, there was considerable concordance between patients and families in the content and relative significance of early symptoms. There was substantial agreement between patients that non-psychotic symptoms such as anxiety, tension and insomnia were part of the prodrome but less agreement as to the characteristics of the earliest changes. Fifty-percent of the patients felt that the characteristic symptoms of the prodrome were repeated at each relapse. A number of these patients also reported that many of the non-psychotic symptoms persisted between episodes of illness, an issue to which we shall return.

Table 17.1 Percentage of relatives reporting early signs

Symptom category	Birchwood et al. (1989) (n = 42)		Herz and Melville (1980) (n = 80)	
	(%)	Rank*	(%)	Rank*
Anxiety/agitation				
Irritable/quick tempered	62	2(eq.)	—	—
Sleep problems	67	1	69	7
Tense, afraid, anxious	62	2(eq.)	83	1
Depression/withdrawal				
Quiet, withdrawn	60	4	50	18
Depressed, low	57	5	76	3
Poor appetite	48	9	53	17
Disinhibition				
Aggression	50	7(eq.)	79	2
Restless	55	6	40	20
Stubborn	36	10(eq.)	—	—
Incipient psychosis				
Behaves as if hallucinated	50	7(eq.)	60	10
Being laughed at or talked about	36	10(eq.)	54	14
'Odd behaviour'	36	10(eq.)	—	—

*There were many other symptoms assessed. Percentages are only shown for parallel data.

Both studies carefully questioned respondents about the timing of the onset of the prodrome. Most of the patients (52%) and their families (68%) in the Herz and Melville study felt that it took more than a week between the onset of the prodrome and a full relapse. Only 10% of patients and families believed that the time period was less than a day. Similarly, Birchwood *et al.* (1989) found that 59% observed the onset of the prodrome one month or more prior to relapse, and 75% two weeks or more. Nineteen percent were unable to specify a time scale.

These studies systematize relatives' and patients' experiences of the prodromal period, finding the characteristic symptoms to be predominantly non-psychotic, and of sufficient duration to enable the implementation of an early intervention strategy. Such a strategy would require the compliance of the patient, which might not always be forthcoming without sustained insight. Heinrichs *et al.* (1985) examined the survival of insight retrospectively

in a group of 38 DSM–III schizophrenics who had relapsed. A systematic retrospective case note analysis indicated that insight was present in 63% of relapses, a figure confirmed by an independent interview with the responsible clinicians. They also found that early insight predicted a much better response to early intervention, aborting relapse through raised medication. In those with early insight, 92% responded well to rapid intervention as opposed to 50% without early insight.

17.1.3 PROSPECTIVE STUDIES

The true predictive significance of prodromal signs can only be clearly established with prospective investigations. Such studies need to examine three issues: (a) whether prodromes of psychotic relapse exist; (b) to what extent there are similarities and differences to those identified in the clinical and retrospective studies, and (c) how often the 'prodromes' fail as well as succeed to predict relapse (i.e.

'sensitivity' and 'specificity'). The clinical implications of this research will largely depend on the degree of specificity which early signs information affords. In particular a high false positive rate will tend to undermine the use of an early intervention strategy that uses raised doses of neuroleptic medication since in such cases, patients will have been exposed to additional medication needlessly.

The first prospective study of prodromal signs was reported by Marder *et al.* (1984). In the course of a study comparing low and standard dose maintenance medication, patients were assessed on a range of psychiatric symptoms at baseline, two weeks later, monthly for three months and then every three months. Relapse was defined as the failure of an increase in medication to manage symptoms following a minor exacerbation of psychosis/paranoia ratings. Thus under this definition it is not known how many genuine prodromes were *aborted* with medication and whether those that responded to medication were similar to those that did not. Of the 41 DSM–III chronic schizophrenic men who took part in the study, 14 relapsed. Patients were assessed using the Brief Psychiatric Rating Scale (BPRS), a standard psychiatric interview scale (Overall and Gorham), 1962), and a self-report measurement of psychiatric symptoms, the SCL–90, which is a 90-item symptom checklist (Derogatis *et al.* 1973). Changes in scores 'just prior to relapse' were compared with the average ('spontaneous') change for a given scale during the course of the follow-up period. Marder *et al.* (1984) found increases in BPRS depression, thought disturbance and paranoia and SCL-90 scores for interpersonal sensitivity, anxiety, depression and paranoid ideation prior to relapse. Marder *et al.* (1984) note that the changes they observed were very small (equalling 2 points on a 21-point range) and probably not recognizable by most clinicians. A discriminant function analysis found the most discriminating ratings were paranoia and depression (BPRS) and psychotism (SCL–

90). They suggest 'such a formula if used in a clinic could probably predict most relapses although there would be a considerable number of . . . false positives' (p. 46). While this study strongly supports the presence of the relapse prodrome, and some of the characteristics described by Herz and Melville (1980), the study was unable to control for timing. The last assessment before relapse varied from between 1 and 12 weeks, weakening the observed effects. One would anticipate the prodrome to be at its maximum in the week or two prior to relapse; assessments carried out prior to this would measure an earlier and weaker stage of the prodrome.

Subotnik and Nuechterlein (1988) considerably improved upon the Marder study by administering the BPRS bi-weekly to 50 young recent-onset schizophrenic patients diagnosed by RDC criteria. Twenty three patients relapsed and their BPRS scores 2, 4 and 6 weeks prior to the relapse were compared with their scores in another six-week period not associated with relapse and with scores of a non-relapse group ($N=27$) over a similar period. This research found that BPRS Anxiety-Depression (which includes depression, guilt and somatic concern) and Thought Disturbance (hallucinations and delusions) were raised prior to relapse. Increases in 'odd thought content' were more prominent as relapse approached (2–4 weeks prior to relapse). The contrast with the non-relapsed patients revealed a rise in low-level 'psychotic' symptoms as part of the prodrome, but not of the non-psychotic items (depression, somatic concern, guilt etc.). This suggests that the non-psychotic symptoms are sensitive to relapse but not specific to it. If however, they were followed by low-level psychotic symptoms, then this study suggests that relapse is more probable. It is also possible that elevations in anxiety-depression may be predictive in certain individuals. Subotnik and Nuechterlein note: '. . . mean elevations in prodromal symptoms were small . . . 0.50–1.00 on a 7-point scale . . . but in three patients no prodomal symptoms were present . . . in several others they did not begin to show any symptomatic change until 2–4 weeks prior to relapse . . . thus lowering the magnitude of the means' (p. 411). These results support clinical observation, that the nature and timing of prodomal signs are like relapse itself — not universal, but including considerable between-subject variability. Nevertheless Subotnik and Nuechterlein reported that a discriminant function using two BPRS 'psychotic' scales correctly classified 59% of relapses and 74% of non-relapse periods, suggesting a false positive rate of 26%.

Hirsch and Jolley (1989) in the course of an early intervention study measured putative prodromes ('neurotic or dysphoric episodes') in a group of 54 DSM–III schizophrenics using the SCL–90 and Herz's ESQ, the Early Signs Questionnaire (Herz *et al.*, 1982). Patients and their key workers received a one-hour teaching session about schizophrenia, particularly concerning the significance of the 'dysphoric' syndrome as a prodrome for relapse. This enabled them to recognize 'dysphoric episodes', a task made easier since all subjects were symptom-free at the onset of the trial. The SCL–90 and the ESQ were administered at each dysphoric episode, and then weekly for two further weeks; otherwise each was rated monthly. Relapse was defined as the re-emergence of florid symptoms including delusions and hallucinations. Fifty-three percent of the relapses were preceded by a prodomal period of dysphoric and neurotic symptoms within a month of relapse. These prodromes were defined clinically but confirmed by SCL–90 scores which were similar to those reported by the other two prospective studies and included depression, anxiety, interpersonal sensitivity and paranoid symptoms. Interpretation of this study is complicated by the design in which half the subjects received active and half placebo maintenance medication and all patients showing signs of dysphoric (prodomal) episodes were given additional

Table 17.2 Frequency of emergent symptoms during prodromal episodes, using the Herz early signs questionnaire.

Emergent symptom	Prodromal episodes % (n=44)
Fear of going crazy	70
Loss of interest Discouragement about future	60–70
Labile mood Reduced attention and concentration Preoccupation with 1 or 2 things	50–60
Feelings of not fitting in Fear of future adversity Overwhelmed by demands Loss of interest in dress/ appearance Reduced energy Puzzled/confused about experience Loss of control Boredom Thoughts racing Indecisiveness	40–50
Distanced from friends/family Feeling that others don't understand Disturbing dreams Loneliness	30–40
Reduced sex drive Fear of being alone Increased energy	20–30
Increased perceptual intensity Increased sex drive Depersonalization Religious preoccupation	10–20
Ideas of reference Elevated mood Risk taking	0–10

Data are from Hirsh and Jolley (1989).

active medication (haloperidol, 10 mg per day). Dysphoric episodes were much more common in the placebo (76%) than in the active group (27%), but the prompt pharmacological intervention does not allow us to ascertain whether these dysphoric episodes were part of a reactivation of psychosis (i.e. true prodromes) aborted by medication and to what extent these included 'false positives' related, perhaps, to the use of placebo.

This study confirms the existence of a prodromal period of approximately four weeks' duration characterized by non-psychotic symptoms including (a) mild depression or dysphoria, anxiety and interpersonal sensitivity, and (b) low-level psychotic symptoms including suspiciousness, ideas of reference and a feeling that the individual does not 'fit in' with others around him. One of the most interesting aspects of the study was the result of administering the ESQ interview questionnaire designed by Herz and Melville, reproduced in Table 17.2. This shows the importance of symptoms of dysphoria/depression and general blunting of drives and interests and highlights the phenomenological experience of psychotic decompensation, which are not generally part of the psychopathology examined by BPRS and SCL–90. Experiences such as 'increased perceptual intensity', 'puzzlement about objective experience', 'racing thoughts' 'loss of control' and 'fear of being alone' capture the phenomenological schemas which were described so lucidly in the clinical studies.

The most recent prospective study was conducted by Birchwood *et al.* (1989) who attempted to develop a scale designed to tap the specific characteristics of the prodrome rather than that of general psychopathology. Construction of the scale was informed by the previous retrospective study reported and underwent extensive psychometric validation. Birchwood *et al.* (1989) went one stage further than previous studies and developed scales to be completed by both the patient *and* an observer (e.g. relative, carer, hostel worker). There were four concerns (relating to the clinical application of early signs monitoring) that influenced this development:

(1) Identification of 'early signs' by a clinician requires intensive, regular monitoring of mental state at least bi-weekly which is rarely possible in clinical practice.

(2) Some patients choose to conceal their symptoms as relapse approaches and insight declines (Heinrichs *et al.*, 1985).

(3) Many patients experience persisting symptoms, deficits or drug side effects. These symptoms will obscure the visibility of the prodromes. Indeed the nature of a prodrome in patients with residual symptoms (*vs.* those who are symptom-free) has not been studied and is important since in clinical practice the presence of residual symptoms is the norm.

(4) The possibility is raised that the characteristics of prodromes might vary from individual to individual and that this information may be lost in scales of general psychopathology.

The authors developed an ongoing system of measurement, where patients and observers completed the scale bi-weekly; at out-patient clinic attendance, with a community psychiatric nurse or through the mail. These data were then plotted in an ongoing fashion (Figure 17.1). The behavioural observations by the observers might provide additional information if the individual under-reported or lost insight. Changes in baseline levels were readily apparent, which is particularly important if the individual experiences persisting symptoms.

The authors report an intensive investigation of 19 young schizophrenic patients diagnosed according to the broad CATEGO 'S' class. All except one were on maintenance medication and monitored in the context of a routine clinical service and were not involved in a drug trial. Eight of the 19 relapsed in the course of 9 months and of these, 50% showed elevations on the scales between two and four weeks prior to relapse. A *post hoc* defined threshold on their scale (> or < 30) led to a sensitivity of 63%, specifity of 82% and an 11% rate of false positives.

This study was a clinical investigation to see how prodrome monitoring might be applied in

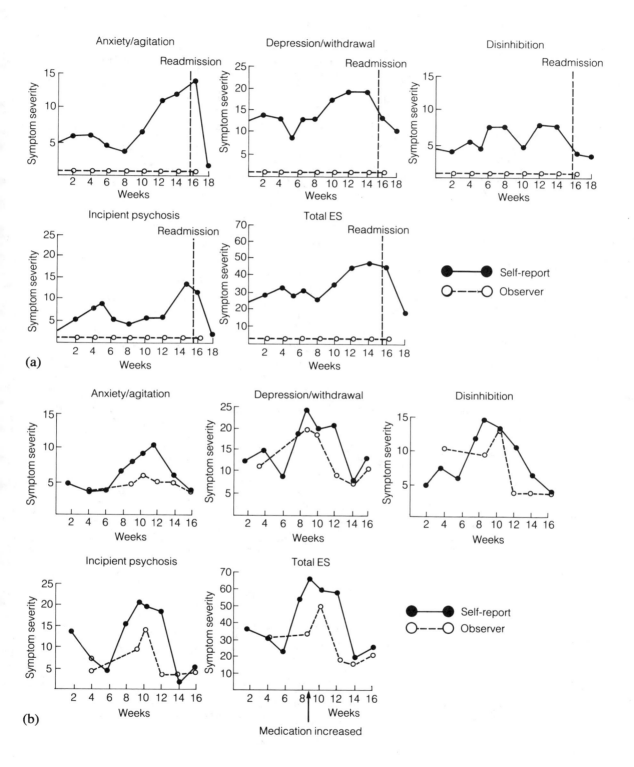

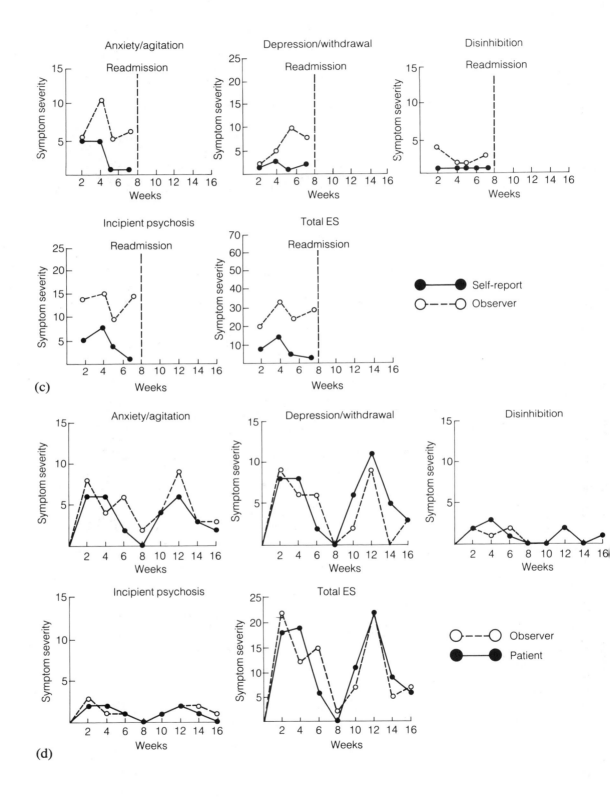

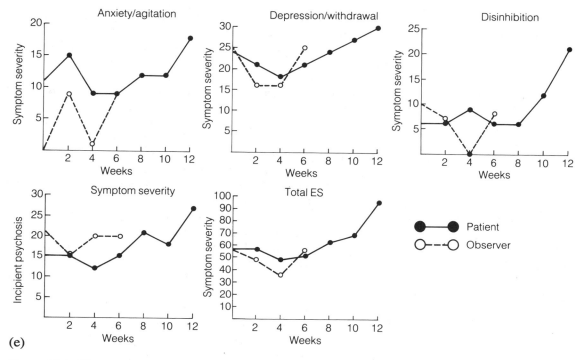

Figure 17.1 Five prodromes detected using the ESS scales.

the clinical setting and to examine in more detail idiopathic aspects of the prodromes. Figure 17.1 shows some of the results of individual prodromes. Figure 17.1a is that of a young male who relapsed 16 weeks following discharge. In this case the first change was that of dysphoria/withdrawal which was apparent five weeks prior to relapse. One to two weeks later he became steadily more agitated and within two weeks of relapse, low level (incipient) psychotic symptoms appeared. Disinhibition was unaffected. In contrast the individual shown in Figure 17.1b had dysphoria/withdrawal and incipient psychotic symptoms simultaneously together with signs of disinhibition; anxiety/ agitation did not peak until somewhat later. It is interesting to note that the observer's behavioural observations showed striking concordance with self-report in respect of dysphoria but lagged behind by one to two weeks in respect of the behavioural concomitants of incipient psychosis. These two examples also reveal an apparent *improvement* in well-being just prior to the onset of the prodromes. The third case (Figure 17.1c) is a young male where the rise in anxiety/agitation, dysphoria and incipient psychosis were noted by the observer, but the individual reported a slight rise in symptoms followed immediately by a sharp fall, presumably due to loss of insight. Case four (Figure 17.1d) demonstrates a definite rise in the scales which returned to baseline four weeks later and was not followed by a relapse. While the scores did not rise above the 30-point threshold, the apparent rise might be regarded as a 'false alarm'. The patient had learnt he had secured employment which seemed to be associated with a feeling of well-being noted by the individual and his mother; as the start of his job approached, his symptoms increased then returned to baseline a few weeks after the start of his job. What was witnessed here was probably the impact of a stressful life event that on this occasion did not culminate in relapse.

The patients in this study were drawn from an outpatient clinic. Many had residual symptoms which were reflected in their baseline scores: Case 1 had moderate negative symptoms and partial delusions; case 2 also had moderate negative symptoms and heard a 'voice' that she knew was part of her illness; case 3 was asymptomatic. Clinically the detection of a prodrome in those with residual symptoms is not easily done by reference to absolute scores: comparisons with a baseline are clearly important here. The issue is raised as how *severe* residual symptoms need to be before the concept of 'relapse' and therefore of a 'prodrome' becomes meaningless. In the cases we have monitored, prodromes have been apparent in those with 'mild to moderate' residual positive or negative symptoms as long as some insight is available. In case 5 (Figure 17.1e) a young female continued to hear voices which caused her considerable distress. She had retained some insight but steadily lost it as she found the voice content increasingly plausible. Two weeks prior to this she became more withdrawn and self-absorbed and her psychotic symptoms became more generalized. In this case, as in others with severe residual symptoms, early intervention by way of raising medication is questionable as such patients are often already on high doses and limited improvement is likely from an increased dose. Other forms of intervention such as stress management in conjunction with other forms of intensive support (e.g. increased day care attendance) may need to be explored with such cases.

17.2 CONTINUING QUESTIONS

The results of the four prospective studies are consistent with the clinical and retrospective studies, particularly supporting Herz and Melville's (1980) seminal investigation. The studies all found that psychotic relapse was preceded by the now familiar set of non-psychotic, 'dysphoric' symptoms including anxiety, dysphoria, interpersonal sensitivity/withdrawal and low-level psychotic thinking including ideas of reference and paranoid thoughts. In two of these studies (Marder *et al.*, 1984; Hirsch and Jolley, 1989) the observations were confounded with a targeted medication strategy, so it was not clear how many of their putative prodromes were actually false positives. It is also possible that the use of an early intervention strategy exaggerated the magnitude of the recorded prodromes. Under normal conditions the baseline levels of psychopathology would be increased in the non-relapsed patients by transient fluctuations in dysphoric symptoms which were not part of a relapse (i.e. the false positives) which might respond to medication, thus reducing the contrast between relapsed and non-relapsed groups.

The possibility of between-subject variability in the nature and timing of prodromes will however act to reduce their apparent amplitude in group studies. Subotnik and Nuechterlein (1988) reported that some patients showed no prodromal symptoms. Among the patients that did show prodromal signs, some were elevated six weeks prior to relapse while in others this occurred a full month later, thus lowering the mean value for the whole group within the time frames (six, four or two weeks prior to relapse). The study by Birchwood *et al.* (1989) raises further potential complications as not only does it reveal differences in the amplitude and timing of symptoms, but also indicates that the pattern of prodromal symptoms shows subject variability: some may 'peak' on anxiety symptoms, others on disinhibition, and so forth.

The prospective studies have thus raised a number of questions. They have confirmed the existence of prodromes of psychotic relapse, but their limitations have not enabled a clear picture to emerge of the true predictive significance of apparent early warning signs. If the work of Birchwood *et al.* (1989) is borne out, then group studies in the mould of Subotnik and Nuechterlein (1988) would be inherently limited as they could not capture the apparent qualitative and quantitative differences between patients in their early signs symptoms. This is supported by Subotnik and Nuechterlein's finding that greater prediction came when patients were compared against their own baseline rather than that of other patients. It may be more appropriate to think of each patient's prodrome as a personalized 'relapse signature' which includes core or common symptoms together with features unique to each patient. If an individual's relapse signature can be identified, then it might be expected that the overall predictive power of 'prodromal' symptoms will be increased. Identifying the unique characteristics of a relapse signature can only be achieved once a relapse has taken place; with each successive relapse further information becomes available to build a more accurate image of the signature. This kind of learning process has been acknowledged by patients (Brier and Strauss, 1983) and could be adapted and developed by professionals and carers as well.

An issue not directly examined in the prospective studies concerns the existence of a prodrome of relapse where the individual continues to experience significant residual symptoms. Where the patient experiences continued negative symptoms such as anergia, alogia and withdrawal, a prodrome presumably will involve an apparent *exacerbation* of these symptoms as shown in some of the cases in Figure 17.1. Where individuals continue to suffer from symptoms such as delusions and hallucinations, a 'relapse' will involve an exacerbation of these symptoms; whether these relapses will also be preceded by prodromes of a similar character

is unknown. Patients in the Hirsch and Jolley and Subotnik and Nuechterlein studies were generally symptom-free; there was somewhat more variability in residual symptoms than in the Birchwood and Marder studies. In view of the large numbers of patients with even moderate residual symptoms, this issue deserves serious and careful examination.

Patients participating in the prospective studies generally were young (18–35 years) with a relatively brief psychiatric history. Such individuals are more prone to relapse and tend to be recruited at acute admission or because they were thought to be appropriate for low dose or intermittent drug strategies (Hirsch and Jolley, 1989). The application of this methodology to older, more stable individuals is another important area for further investigation.

In summary, a great deal more careful research is required to expand the knowledge base of this developing area to facilitate more widespread and realistic clinical application.

17.3 IMPLICATIONS AND CLINICAL APPLICATIONS

The clinical application of early signs monitoring offers considerable opportunity for improving care. However, if the encouraging results of the early intervention studies employing targeted medication are to be realized in clinical practice, careful thought must be given to the identification of individual 'relapse signatures', the design of monitoring methodology and the nature of the service response to secure these advances for the well-being of patients.

17.3.1 IDENTIFICATION OF INDIVIDUAL RELAPSE SIGNATURES

The relationship between early signs of decompensation and actual psychotic relapse remains unclear. There is unlikely to be a simplistic relationship and evidence suggests that false positives and negatives will occur. One means to improve the specificity of early signs may be to harness additional information relating to idiosyncratic signs for a given individual.

This information can be obtained by interviewing the individual and his or her nearest relative concerning the nature and timing of early signs preceding the last relapse episode. Experienced clinic staff, who often have years of regular contact with a client, can also provide useful information concerning certain key changes which in themselves might go unnoticed but for a given individual is highly predictive of relapse. The fuller 'relapse signature' that is so obtained can be harnessed into the early signs monitoring procedure and used as a hypothesis predicting specific idiosyncratic signs which will occur at subsequent relapse of a given individual. This can be tested out prospectively to assess how well this signature bears out with respect to the next episode. Any additional early signs observed at the next relapse can be added to the signature thereby increasing the accuracy of prediction with each relapse.

17.3.2 MONITORING METHODOLOGY

The strategy of close monitoring by highly trained personnel is impractical in routine care. On the other hand, the use of close monitoring by staff for particular target groups who have a high relapse risk is limited by the ability to reliably select high potential relapsers. The methodology adopted by Birchwood *et al.*, (1989), harnessing the experiences of patients and their carers in a routine in-service setting, may be most easily applied clinically. This offers the potential for documenting information relating to early signs of relapse for a substantial group of patients, with relatively limited input of professional time. However it is still probable that a substantial group of patients, who retain very little insight or where loss of insight occurs very early in decompensation, may be unable or unwilling to entertain self-monitoring and are also least likely to consent to observation by another. There are no easy solutions to these problems, although education about the illness

may, in some cases, improve insight and key personnel in the individual's life can be trained to monitor and recognize specific early warning signs and to initiate preventative strategies such as increasing medication or seeking professional help easily if relapse is predicted.

Nothwithstanding its potential therapeutic value, the notion of self-monitoring does raise a number of concerns about sensitizing patients and carers to disability, promoting the observations as critical responses, burdening individuals and carers further with requests for repetitive information at frequent intervals, or increasing the risk of self-harm in an individual who becomes demoralized by an impending relapse. There is no real evidence that self-monitoring is likely to increase the risk of self-harm. Indeed, florid and uncontrolled relapse may be more dangerous and more damaging. Engaging patients and carers more actively in the management of the illness may also promote a sense of purposeful activity and have therapeutic benefits *per se*. The repetitive nature of the procedure may be self-defeating in the long term and indeed wasteful in well established patients. Instituting monitoring at times of stress may be a reasonable alternative to continuous monitoring in some individuals. Despite these limitations, if early signs monitoring fulfils even part of its promise, it may for many patients with recurrent episodes, promote learning and lead to increased opportunity for combined efforts to control exacerbations due to stress.

17.3.3 THE SERVICE RESPONSE

For the group of patients who routinely attend clinical appointments, information from monitoring by patients and carers has an identified route of access. If this route were formalized it might be possible to ensure clear responses from the service. However, not all patients attend services and the move away from an institutional model is likely to further devolve care away from current services. The difficulty in accessing traditional psychiatric services has been well documented. Creer and Wing (1974) and Johnstone *et al.* (1984) describe patchy access to care with particular problems for relocated patients and families. The implementation of case management for the long-term mentally ill may ensure constant service links at a distance, and the utilization of psychiatric services during critical periods, but will necessarily require information concerning early signs of relapse to be adequately assessed and harnessed. The nature of the service response to information concerning early signs of decompensation is still an open question. Most clinical trials have employed pharmacological interventions upon recognition of early signs of decompensation (Jolley and Hirsch, 1989). Within defined cohorts (as in clinical trials) the use of targeted medication has not been sufficient to cope with individual variation. In the clinical setting where there is a very wide range of maintenance therapy and where the dose and duration is likely to be vary considerably between individuals, targeted medication would require to be individually tailored. However the implementation of strategies that are already recognized by patients and carers as useful would often be entirely appropriate. Indeed the work by McCandless-Glincher *et al.* (1986) is particularly encouraging since it suggests that very nearly all patients recognize loss of well-being and the majority institute some change in behaviour at their own initiative in response to this, including engaging in diversionary activities, seeking professional help or resuming and increasing neuroleptic medication. In the face of this information, individuals might be encouraged to employ self-management strategies such as stress management procedures or symptom control strategies (Brier and Strauss, 1983) to initiate preventative actions. Examples may include increasing the frequency of day centre attendance, requesting brief admission, or enlisting professional support to assist in symptom management. To achieve these ends may require radical service change in the direction of the development of a more responsive and flexible service than currently exists. The resultant service would need to be proactive rather than reactive and responsive to the needs and concerns of individuals and their carers if these alternative preventative strategies are to be viable.

In summary, routinely monitoring early signs to identify individual relapse signatures opens the possibility for individuals to recognize and act on symptoms suggestive of reduced well-being and to initiate early intervention strategies to prevent relapse. However, if the promising results of the research studies are to be systematically applied and incorporated into routine clinical practice a viable system of monitoring needs to be established in order to access information routinely and accurately. The service structure also needs to be adapted in order to facilitate this and to be able to respond flexibly and promptly when relapse is predicted. It is to this end that the authors' research efforts are devoted.

REFERENCES

Birchwood, M., Smith, J., Macmillan, F. *et al.* (1989) Predicting relapse in schizophrenia: the development and implementation of an early signs monitoring system using patients and families as observers. *Psychol. Med.*, **19**, 649–56.

Bower, M.B. Jr. (1968) Pathogenesis of acute schizophrenic psychosis — an experimental approach. *Arch. Gen. Psychiatry*, **19**, 348–55.

Brier, A. and Strauss, J.S. (1983) Self-control in Psychiatric Disorders. *Arch. Gen. Psychiatry*, **40**, 1141–5.

Cameron, D.E. (1938) Early schizophrenia. *Am. J. Psychiatry*, **95**, 567–8.

Chapman, J. (1966) The early symptoms of schizophrenia. *Br. J. Psychiatry*, **112**, 225–51.

Creer, C. and Wing, J. (1974) *Schizophrenics at home*. National Schizophrenia Fellowship, Surbiton, Surrey.

Davis, J.M. (1975) Overview: Maintenance therapy in psychiatry: I. Schizophrenia. *Am. J. Psychiatry*, **132**, 1237–45.

Derogatis, L., Lipman, R. and Covi, L. (1973) SCL – 90: An outpatient psychiatric rating scale — preliminary report. *Psychopharm. Bull.* **9**, 13–17.

Docherty, J.P., Van Kammen, D.P., Siris, S.G., and Marder, S.R. (1978) Stages of onset of schizophrenic psychosis. *Am. J. Psychiatry*, **135**, 420–6.

Donlon, P.T. and Blacker, K.H. (1975) Clinical Recognition of Early schizophrenic decompensation. *Disord. Nerv. Sys.*, **36**, 323–30.

Foulds, G.W. (1976) *The Hierarchical Nature of Personal Illness*. Academic Press, London.

Freedman, B. and Chapman, L.J. (1973) Early subjective experience in schizophrenic episodes. *J. Abnorm. Psychol.*, **82**, 45–54.

Heinrichs, D., Cohen, B.P. and Carpenter, W.T. (1985), Early insight and the management of schizophrenic decompensation *J. Nerv. Ment. Dis.*, **173**, 133.

Heinrichs, D.W. and Carpenter, W.T. (1985) Prospective study of prodromal symptoms in schizophrenic relapse. *Am. J. Psychiatry*, **143**, 371–3.

Herz, M. and Melville, C. (1980) Relapse in schizophrenia. *Am. J. Psychiatry*, **137**, 801–12.

Herz, M.I. Syzmonski, H.V. and Simon, J. (1982) Intermittent medication for stable schizophrenic outpatients. *Am. J. Psychiatry*, **139**, 918–22.

Hirsch, S.R. and Jolley, A.G. (1989) The Dysphoric Syndrome in schizophrenia and its implications for relapse *Br. J. Psychiatry*, **155**, 46–50.

Hogarty, G.E., Anderson, C.M., Reiss, D.J. *et al.* (1986) Family psychoeducation, social skills training and maintenance chemotherapy in the after care treatment of schizophrenia: I. One year effects of a controlled study on relapse and expressed emotion. *Arch. Gen. Psychiatry*, **43**, 633–42.

Johnson, D.A.W., Pasteski, G., Ludlow, J.H. *et al.* (1983) The discontinuance of maintenance neuroleptic therapy in chronic schizophrenic patients. *Acta Psychiatr. Scand.*, **67**, 339–52.

Johnstone, E.C., Owens, D.G.C., Gold, A., *et al.* (1984) Schizophrenic patients discharged from hospital: A follow-up study. *Br. J. Psychiatry*, **145**, 586–90.

Kane, J.M., Woerner, M. and Sarantakos, S. (1986) Depot neuroleptics: A comparative review of standard intermediate and low dose regimes *J. Clin. Psychiatry*, **47**, May Supplement, 30–3.

Marder, S., Van Putten, T., Muntz, J. *et al.* (1984) Maintenance therapy in schizophrenia: new findings. In J. Kane (ed), *Drug Maintenance Strategies in Schizophrenia*. American Psychiatric Press, Washington D.C. pp. 31–49.

McCandless-Glincher, L., McKnight, S., Hamera, E. *et al.* (1986) Use of symptoms by schizophrenics to monitor and regulate their illness. *Hosp. Community Psychiatry*, **37**, 929–33.

McGhie, A. and Chapman, J. (1961) Disorders of attention and perception in early schizophrenia. *Br. J. Med. Psychol.*, **34**, 103–16.

Offenkrantz, W.C. (1962) Multiple somatic complaints as a precursor of schizophrenia *Am. J. Psychiatry*, 119, 258–9.

Overall, J.E. and Gorham, D.R. (1962) The brief psychiatric rating scale. *Psychol. Rep.*, **10**, 799–812.

Owens, D.G.C. and Johnstone, E.C. (1980) The disabilities of chronic schizophrenia. Their nature and factors contributing to their development. *Br. J. Psychiatry*, **136**, 384–95.

Pyke, J. and Seeman, M.D. (1981) 'Neuroleptic free' intervals in the treatment of schizophrenia. *Am. J. Psychiatry*, **138**, 1620–1.

Schooler, N.R. (1986) The efficacy of antipsychotic drugs, and family therapies and the maintenance treatment of schizophrenia *J. Clin. Psychopharmacol.*, **6**, 115–95.

Stein, W., (1967) The sense of becoming psychotic. *Br. J. Psychiatry*, **30**, 262–75.

Subotnik, K.L. and Nuechterlein, K.H. (1988) Prodromal signs and symptoms of schizophrenic relapse. *J. Abnorm. Psychol.*, **97**, 405–12.

Tarrier, N., Barrowclough, C., Vaughn, C. *et al.* (1988) The community management of schizophrenia: a controlled trial of behavioural intervention with families to reduce relapse. *Br. J. Psychiatry*, **153**, 532–42.

Chapter 18

The clinical prediction of dangerousness

PAUL E. MULLEN

18.1 INTRODUCTION

This chapter will examine the problems inherent in the clinical prediction of dangerousness. The focus will be on those with schizophrenic disorders but inevitably the review will have to cover a range of factors potentially relevant to the issue of prediction. Monahan (1984) highlighted the changing attitudes towards the prediction of violent behaviour. Twenty years ago the capacity of psychologists and psychiatrists to predict future dangerousness was accepted with little reservation. Such predictions were increasingly built into processes governing both civil commitment and the continued containment of convicted felons. The situation changed in the 1970s in response to research which cast doubts on the reliability of prognostications about dangerousness. The point was reached where psychologists and psychiatrists were regarded as having no knowledge or skills at all in predicting dangerousness (Steadman, 1980). In recent years a second generation of research is producing another shift in attitude to a middle ground characterized by Monahan (1984) in the phrase 'little is known about how accurately violent behaviour can be predicted in many circumstances but it may be possible to predict it accurately enough to be useful in some policy decisions'.

Dangerousness conjures up in our minds a thing hurtful and injurious. The dangerous offender is equated with the violent offender. One definition of dangerousness is 'a propensity to cause serious physical injury or lasting psychological harm to others' (Butler, 1975). This is open to objection as it both omits the element of fear and incorporates psychological harm. The latter element, though often all too real, is intangible, easy to claim and impossible to exclude (Scott, 1977). Fear, as Gunn (1982) has argued, is at least as important in the apprehension of danger as any statistical calculation of actual risk. A large proportion of the female population of Leeds, during the years when Peter Sutcliffe, the Yorkshire Ripper, stalked their streets, perceived their city as having become threatening and dangerous. The city dwellers of America increasingly see vast areas of their urban environment as dangerous because of their fear of violent street crime. A dispassionate account of the actual risk to a Yorkshire lass or a Manhattan worthy of falling victim to violence and its relative insignificance next, say, to the perils of driving home, would be unlikely to assuage the anxiety or decrease the belief that their world was dangerous. How an individual or group is perceived contributes to whether they are considered dangerous. Large males, particularly if they are from minority groups, when admitted as patients on psychiatric wards are likely to be regarded by staff as potentially dangerous irrespective of their previous behaviour and present state. Fear, unless controlled or allowed for, contaminates attempts to systematically assess dangerousness.

Fear may be more damaging, in all senses, than what is feared. American families who keep guns in their homes, often on the pretext of protecting themselves against violent criminals, are far more likely to fall victim to their own weapons than are the fantasized intruders. In King County, Washington State, of 398 firearm-related deaths within the home, only nine involved intruders or would-be assailants; the rest arose from accidents, suicides and domestic disputes (Kellermann and Reay, 1986).

Dangerousness is a quality of actions or events. A person cannot be dangerous. It is actions, and in only rare instances attributes, such as being a carrier for an infection, which renders an individual dangerous. It is what we do, not what we are, which is violent and therefore dangerous. The platitude is important for it is tempting to reify dangerousness and make it a quality of an individual or group of individuals. Those diagnosed as having a schizophrenic illness are more likely to find themselves charged with violent crimes (Chapter 9). This correlation is best understood by viewing a schizophrenic disorder as a risk factor which, in combination with other factors may release violent actions. Those with a schizophrenic illness are not predestined to violence. What they may be, is peculiarly vulnerable to particular situations and provocations. To label those with schizophrenia as dangerous is both inaccurate and unhelpful. To recognize that some with this disorder can be identified as being at risk, is to begin to question what will ameliorate and what exacerbate that risk.

18.2 DESCRIBING AN INDIVIDUAL'S VIOLENCE

A simple model for an act of individual violence is useful for the practitioner. Violence often occurs in a context which is provocative to the attacker. It matters not how reasonable others, or even the individual themselves, with the benefit of hindsight, consider the response. The exceptions are instrumental violence where it is used as a means to an end, such as chasing the security guard to reach the money, and acts of revenge where the provocation predates the act by sufficient time for the passion to settle and plans to be laid. The attacker has predispositions such as beliefs, knowledge and desires which, though they manifest intermittently, may be long standing. They may have a tendency to cope with stressful situations by becoming belligerent and hostile. The mental state at the time of the violence can be important: for example, consciousness may be impaired by intoxication, perception disordered by hallucination or they may be in the grip of an overwhelming affective state characterized by fear or rage. From the context, the predispositions and the mental state arise intentions which may or may not culminate in action. The factors which may increase the likelihood of a violent outcome and those which inhibit such actions are complex. Some are situation-specific, such as the availability of weapons, the proximity to the potential victim and the presence or absence of other people; whilst others, such as skills in the exercise of violence, are continuing attributes of the individual. Violence initiated and carried through by a single perpetrator is clearly different from group violence. Violence which begins as a defensive or retaliatory response has to be understood differently from that of the first strike variety, though the first blow may be the pre-emptive attack of an individual in fear of imminent assault. Finally, acts have outcomes and the outcome may reflect the violence of the attack or be more a product of chance. One of our patients tried on a number of occasions to poison her husband, but he was peculiarly resistant to the effects of the rat poison and the worst result was a bout of vomiting, whereas another man found himself facing a manslaughter charge after irritably pushing someone who annoyed him. Thus a description of the individual's act of violence should include the context of the conflict, the individual's predispositions, state of mind and intentions at the time together with the factors influencing self control in the perpetrator. Finally, the actions of the victim at the time which may have contributed to the violence or have avoided a worse outcome need to be addressed.

An example is provided by a recent case of ours in which a young man was charged with murder. He had developed a propensity to be possessive following being deserted by his first wife. He had grown up in a disorganized and frequently violent family and what positive regard he had received in youth had come from an adolescent peer group of delinquent habits. The killing occurred in the context of a dance at which his girlfriend had become somewhat intoxicated and flirtatious. He had objected to her dancing with another man and she had told him exactly where he could put his objections. His mental state was clouded by alcohol, he was preoccupied by suspicion and jealously and enraged by her insults. He had grabbed a bottle from a table and threatened her with it. She had said he wouldn't dare use it. This was a fatal miscalculation. The concatenation of predispositions, mental state, reduced self-control and provocation which activated pre-existing vulnerabilities, conspired to produce the killing. It is possible that the absence of even one of these factors would have been sufficient to tip the balance against an actual assault.

18.3 PREDICTION

The prediction of dangerousness is an exercise in estimating the probability that the events necesssary to precipitate a particular individual into violent action will recur (Mullen, 1984). Recur is used, in preference to occur, as attempts to predict dangerousness in those who have never acted violently is so fraught with problems as to be best avoided.

Health professionals are no strangers to the prediction of probabilities. The everyday decisions about the assessment and management of clinical problems are judgements of probability. Decision analysis has made practitioners more aware of their reliance on probabilities, and in many cases their woeful lack of empirical data on those very factors on which decisions are based. The lack of hard data is nowhere more obvious than in the area of predicting dangerousness.

Critics of psychiatric practice point to the frequency with which false positives occur in predicting dangerousness. The assumption underlying this criticism is that dangerousness is an all-or-nothing judgement and that if violence does not eventuate, then the attribution of dangerousness was false. To be fair to these critics, many psychiatrists talk and act as if they shared this conception of dangerousness as an absolute quality of a person. As already noted, dangerousness is a quality of actions and actions arise from a complex interaction of psychological, social and occasionally biological factors. Predictions in this field are estimates of probability and should ideally be stated as such. To put a figure on such predictions, such as 70% or 32% is rarely possible, and would suggest spurious certainty. To be clear about the general probability is, however, essential.

The problem is that probability judgements are converted into all-or-nothing decisions. The courts either release or confine, you cannot be 70% to 80% imprisoned. In medicine, probabilities are frequently converted into concrete actions; the probability of the patient having an inflamed appendix is in the region of 60%, but the patient goes to theatre 100%. The two situations differ, however, in important regards. An appendicectomy is decided on in the interests of the sufferer with abdominal pain, whereas the confinement may be largely or solely in the interests of others and against those of the supposedly dangerous individual.

Predicting is difficult in situations where there is a low base rate for the event. If, for example, the annual rate of serious violence in a community is 20 per 10 000, then a predictor with a sensitivity and specificity of 95% would correctly identify 19 potential assailants, but incorrectly stigmatize 500 innocents. If, as a matter of social justice, you required that not more than one innocent should be confined for every three who were truly dangerous, then you would require a predictor which was 99.9993% accurate.

These difficulties have led some to argue that mental health professionals should only attempt predictions of dangerousness in populations which have already engaged in repeated violence and will therefore present a high base rate for future offending (Megargee, 1976). This, unfortunately, ignores the different but equally problematic factors influencing attempts to use a weak predictor in situations where strong predictors are operative. In offences involving violence, a study from the UK reported that the reconviction rate reached 40% after two prior convictions (Walker *et al.*, 1976). If the presence of a particular mental abnormality is associated with a rate of violent reoffending of 10%, then in a group of offenders with a base rate of 40%, those who are also mentally abnormal will have a 46% risk of further violence. This assumes that your diagnostic acumen enables you to correctly identify all subjects. In practice a relatively weak predictor will not operate effectively against a high base rate.

Those clinicians who would justify a patrician disdain for the attempt to predict dangerousness have ample arguments to bolster their position. This posture is however, difficult to sustain for those whose work brings them in contact with the mentally abnormal offender

or the objecting and objectionable among the seriously mentally disturbed. Civil commitments and criminal proceedings raise questions of dangerousness and if the clinicians decline to address the question, their parents may be disadvantaged or their professions by-passed. Those who confront the necessity of providing opinion and guidance on the risks of future violence need to know what factors may have some relevance to the question and which can be discounted. Predictions should be advanced with modesty for they are always fallible and often erroneous. The opinions expressed are best accompanied by a clear outline of the factors on which they are based to allow scrutiny and critical appraisal. The statement of the relevant issues, without a definite opinion, will often suffice in a criminal court but in many civil procedures committal decisions will reflect overtly or covertly the practitioner's estimate of the risks of future violence. Predictions of dangerousness are estimates and opinions, not facts, they are open quite properly to argument and rejection by others. When courts or other bodies decline to endorse our opinions, this is not a matter for righteous anger, hurt pride, or even irritation.

18.4 FACTORS IN PREDICTING DANGEROUSNESS

A number of factors have been claimed at one time or another to assist in predicting future dangerousness. Studies which assess the accuracy of such predictions, both by mental health and other professionals, suggest limited efficacy. Criminological prediction studies, including those attempting to predict reoffence, both violent and otherwise among juveniles, ex-prisoners and probationers, rarely achieve a correlation between prediction and future conviction of better than 0.4 (Simon, 1971).

18.4.1 GENDER AND AGE

Violent offending is not a form of behaviour

which is distributed evenly through the population. The first and most obvious characteristic of violent offenders is that they are predominantly male. Even in serious domestic violence men are usually the perpetrators and women the victims. The second most obvious feature is that they are young. The median age of arrest for aggravated assault in the USA is about 25 years, and for murder, 26 years (Glaser, 1975). In the mentally disordered however, the preponderance of the young and the male is less marked. In schizophrenia advancing age and female gender do not bring the same guarantees of non-violent behaviour.

18.4.2 SOCIAL CLASS

The offenders who appear before our courts and populate our penal institutions are drawn disproportionately from the lower socioeconomic classes (Pritchard, 1977; Silberman, 1978). Criteria for poverty, in this context, are relative rather than absolute, for clearly the most socially deprived of Western nations compare favourably in terms of actual income with the comfortably off in other parts of the world. Anomie, the lawlessness generated by a sense of exclusion from the rewards and regard of one's own society, is a time-honoured explanation for criminality. Low status is a risk factor for offending and a poor prognostic indicator for reoffence. Those disabled by schizophrenia are all too often drawn into the impoverished and drifting populations of the excluded and rejected. With their recruitment into such groups comes increased risks of offending, arrest and reoffence.

Those who are both economically deprived and members of a definable minority group within a society are at particular risk for offending and arrest. Figures from the USA suggest black Americans are seven times more likely to be arrested for both poverty and violent offences (Blumstein and Cohen, 1987). In New Zealand nearly half of prison inmates are recorded as of Maori origin though they form only about 10% of the general population (Braybrook and O'Neill, 1988). Care in interpreting such data has to be emphasized for there are significant confounding variables such as differential arrest rates between ethnic groups and deficits in the data consequent on poor ascertainment of ethnic origin. The significant variable is almost certainly the social and economic deprivation to which such ethnic minorities are subject and has nothing to do with ethnicity *per se*. That being so, ethnicity should not be employed as a predictive variable.

18.4.3 PAST BEHAVIOUR

That past behaviour predicts future behaviour is the pre-eminent truism of this area of discourse. The probability of reconviction increases with the number of previous offences (Monahan, 1981). Those who have an established pattern of offending, particularly when it is committed in adolescence, are likely to continue to behave in a similar manner through their youth and early adult life. This is particularly so for those whose criminality ranges widely over offences against both property and the person. Given that an individual has an established record of antisocial and violent conduct, given that the social, economic, interpersonal, biological and psychological contingencies are likely to remain much the same, then the future may well be consistent with the past. In practice such convenient stability does not occur and clinicians are called upon to prognosticate in situations where some, or all, of these contingencies are in flux. Further, many of those we see do not have a long history of consistently antisocial conduct, but a past history of isolated or episodic disturbance in the context of specific mental or social disorder. The fact that past behaviour predicts future behaviour should not be confused with the assumption that any act committed in the past is likely to be repeated. It is clear that isolated acts which deviate in considerable degree from the individual's normal patterns of conduct are far less likely to recur than are the mundane regularities which characterize the rest of their past behaviour. The most serious crimes such as murder and potentially lethal assaults, have the least likelihood of repetition, whereas petty theft has one of the highest recidivism rates (Neithercutt, 1972). Naïve assumptions about the repetition of offending are themselves dangerous in clinical practice.

18.4.4 TYPE OF OFFENCE

The category of offence is of little assistance in predicting recurrence. Sexual offences, for example, have a low rate of reconviction and recurrence overall, yet some sexual offenders are among the most dedicatedly recalcitrant of villains. Scott (1977) commented that offence entities all comprise a majority of cases where there has been a single and temporary infringement and a malignant minority who go on to offend repeatedly. To separate the groups after a first offence is rarely possible.

The details of the offence are more informative than the legal category. The context, the relevant predispositions, the mental state and the balance between self control and provocation all give information about how likely the individual is to be exposed to a similar or related situation. The presence of an essential, but unique, constituent in the pattern can be reassuring. An example would be a confused state following inadvertent poisoning or injury. The identical state of mental confusion induced by excess alcohol in an habitual drunkard would be far less reassuring, given the likelihood of it recurring. An opinion occasionally advanced is that the offence is unlikely to be repeated if for example the offender has killed the only mother he had. In practice, most of us have the capacity to reproduce our relationships, filial, fraternal or whatever, particularly when the original models have been conflicted and intense.

In reconstructing the crime, all available evidence should be consulted. Relying solely on the offender's account is an error, however honest and open it may appear. The temptation to play detective by demanding from the offender a detailed, blow-by-blow account, is usually a self-indulgence rather than a contribution to assessment. In practice, we often find ourselves asked to give opinions on those whose offences are in the distant past. This increases the need to consult contemporary court and psychiatric records rather than excusing us the trouble of searching them out. Self-justification and editing the memory begins in most of us almost immediately following a criminal act and many an offender has usually managed a complete rewrite of events after a few years. Previous interviews which have included leading questions and suggestions go a long way to shaping the offenders subsequent accounts. The statements, depositions, pathologist's or other medical records of victim and perpetrator form the most reliable and acceptable basis on which to reconstruct the offence.

18.4.5 THE EXTENT OF VIOLENCE EMPLOYED

In homicide cases a great deal of importance is often attributed to the extent of the violence employed. It is sometimes asserted that multiplicity of stabs, shots or blows indicates insanity or viciousness and as a result predicts future dangerousness. Scott (1977), on the basis of his own material, suggested that excessive violence does not warrant the importance assigned to it. He suggested that it often arises from inexperience, panic and the difficulty of actually killing a healthy victim. He noted that the defencelessness of the victim seemed paradoxically to unleash unbridalled savagery.

18.4.6 REMORSE AND ACKNOWLEDGEMENT OF GUILT

The expression of appropriate remorse and

acceptance of guilt is still often employed as a criterion for assessing dangerousness and a prerequisite for release. This simple faith in the power of contrition would be more impressive if we were better able to identify this elusive quality. Calculating criminals are usually able to provide the cry of *mea culpa* in a form impressive to most interrogators. Those who decline to satisfy the moral qualms of those in power over them are at risk of extending their incarceration. Those with schizophrenic illnesses may be singularly disadvantaged by such a criterion as either from emotional blunting, apathy or negativism they may be unable to express an emotionally convincing contrition. In my experience, some offenders are genuinely puzzled about how they came to commit their crimes, particularly if deluded or otherwise mentally disordered at the time, and the more thoughtful amongst this group have difficulty asserting wholeheartedly both remorse and the conviction it could not happen again. Those whose acts have been committed when mentally disordered may reasonably argue that they, like the courts, hold themselves to be not guilty by reason of insanity. One patient of mine who had killed his brother in a state of manic excitement continued to assert that he could not accept responsibility for his actions, nor could he feel confident that he might not repeat such an offence were a manic state to recur. This sober and intelligent self-appraisal led a number of experts to judge him unsafe for release, whereas it might more plausibly have encouraged their confidence in the man's willingness to submit to ongoing supervision.

18.4.7 PERSONALITY FACTORS

The offender's personality is central to attempts to predict future behaviour. Given that personality includes such factors as motivation, habit, strength and impulsivity, if accurate measures were possible then the assessment of future dangerousness would be improved. In practice, the use of standardized instruments for assessing personality traits have made little contribution to the prediction of dangerous behaviour (Megargeee, 1982). There are considerable problems attendant on attempts to predict factors such as future academic performance, even with well standardized instruments that are presented in controlled circumstances and with objectives that are shared by tester and tested. In dangerousness the variables are so much greater and little community of interest exists between the tested and tester. Megargee (1976) concluded that though personality assessment devices can distinguish normals from people who have engaged in dangerous behaviour in the past, such tests fail to adequately distinguish between violent and non-violent criminals and their validity for any long-term prediction is dubious.

The attractions of an objective measure of dangerousness that is based on empirical data are immense. Responsibility could be shifted from the individual to science itself. To date, however, psychological tests in this area offer little more than spurious certainties and scientism.

There have been numerous attempts to categorize the personality characteristics of violent offenders. The literature on psychopathic disorder relies extensively on past offending and socioeconomic instability in the individual and his environment. Circularity is endemic in this literature. One of the attempts to provide a personality profile of the potentially dangerous individual was that of Kozol *et al.* (1972). He highlighted hostility, lack of compassion, a sense of resentment, rejection of authority, self-interest, poor impulse control, immaturity, a distorted view of reality, an enjoyment of witnessing and inflicting suffering and a history of violence. Few could argue with the proposition that those with such characteristics are potentially dangerous. Studies of violent and socially deviant populations consistently find high rates of personality disorder (West, 1982; McManus *et al.*, 1884; Blackburn *et al.*, 1990) but to date this has not allowed any systematic assessment of personality which could be used predictively.

18.4.8 CONDUCT DISORDERS OF CHILDHOOD

The conduct disorders which occur in childhood are, to some extent, predictors of later adolescent and adult aggression (Robins, 1966). Conduct disorder is defined by a persistent pattern of seriously disruptive behaviour, which involves a violation of age-appropriate norms and usually inflicts damage on property, other persons or themselves. In pre-adolescent children the frequency of such disorders is estimated at between 4% and 8%. Most conduct disordered children do not, however, grow up to be criminals in adolescence and adulthood. Conduct disorder in childhood is a warning and a risk factor, not the harbinger of an immutable progress to violence.

The earlier the onset of an established pattern of conduct disorder, the more likely seems a progress to later criminality. Lying and stealing outside the home from an early age has been found to predict progress to adolescent delinquency. In one study it was found that by ten years of age teachers and peers had identified a group of impulsive, aggressive and inconsiderate children who subsequently progressed to criminal delinquency (West and Farrington, 1977). In general, poor relationships in children and early adolescents, which usually reflect an inadequately socialized personality, predict future delinquency.

Conduct disorder is associated with a number of deleterious social influences, including low income, broken homes, criminality in parents, and harsh and inconsistent parental discipline, with low income being the strongest association (Offord, 1990). The conduct disorder of younger children often arises from the experience of disadvantage. Conduct disorder would appear to be in large part, a preventable social disorder.

In clinical practice a history of conduct disorder from an early age in an adult criminal suggests ingrained and persistent behavioural difficulties. In combination with a schizophrenic illness such a history is worrying.

18.4.9 BRAIN DAMAGE AND DISORDER

Offenders in general, and violent offenders in particular, are more likely to show unusual cerebral structure and function than their non-criminal peers, but the nature of this relationship remains unclear (Taylor, 1985). Though there are higher rates of epilepsy among institutionalized male offenders, a direct link between an epileptic fit and an offence is rare (Gunn, 1977). Social rather than biological factors probably explain the excess of epileptics among prisoners. The assumption of a link between apparently inexplicable crimes and epilepsy, which dates at least back to Henry Maudsley (1900), continues to appeal to the judicial mind, but is given little support from systematic studies (Fenton *et al.*, 1974). Brain damage, particularly frontal lobe damage, may produce personality change and anecdotal accounts of links to serious violence abound. Hafner and Boker (1982) found a small group of offenders with acquired brain damage who were disposed to act violently, but concluded that the cause could hardly be the brain damage alone. They claimed that a multiplicity of social factors and pre-existing personality traits interacted with the organic impairment to produce the violent outcome.

In practice, violent offending emerging in the context of brain disease or obvious cerebral pathology, gives rise to real anxieties about recurrence if the brain disorder is not open to modification. Whatever the results of surveys, such as those of Hafner and Boker (1982), clinicians have usually learnt to be wary of offenders where the sudden emergence of criminal deviance has followed serious head injury or other cerebral insult.

18.4.10 CHROMOSOMAL ANOMALIES

The possible association of sex chromosome anomalies with violent offending has created considerable interest and debate. The report that a number of men with 47,XYY and 48,XXYY chromosomal patterns had been identified among violent, mentally abnormal offenders, led to speculation on a casual link. Systematic studies cast doubt on whether there is any real increased propensity to criminal, let alone violent, behaviour when there are such chromosomal abnormalities (Pitcher, 1982). Whatever tenuous link might exist, such chromosomal abnormalities have no known predictive value.

18.4.11 THREATS OF VIOLENCE

Threats to kill often precede violent assaults. Equally, such threats are commonplace particularly among the disturbed and deluded individuals with schizophrenia. Macdonald (1960) studied a group of 100 subjects who had made threats on the lives of others. Two of these subjects killed during the initial follow-up period. This was a highly selected group, but nevertheless it highlights the importance of treating such threats seriously. Those who threaten violence are often at even greater risk themselves, both from their aggression turning inward to suicidal behaviour and from provoking pre-emptive attacks.

Macdonald (1961) considered that parental brutality and the triad of childhood fire-setting, cruelty to animals and enuresis were indicators of a propensity to violence. Childhood cruelty to animals has been linked to late aggression towards people (Felthous and Kellert, 1987). Sadistic and violent fantasies which lead on to acts of brutality towards animals appear in the biographies of some sadistic murderers. The association, though far from common, is sufficiently chilling to impress those who encounter such cases with the dangerousness of those who begin to practice their violent fantasies on animals.

18.4.12 PSYCHIATRIC SYMPTOMS

The general relationship between schizophrenia and a propensity to behave violently is discussed in Chapter 9. There does appear to be an increased risk that those with established schizophrenic illnesses, particularly with predominantly persecutory delusions, are at greater risk for acts of violence.

Morbid jealousy deserves its sinister reputation (Mullen and Maack, 1985) and threats of violence in paranoid patients, particularly when directed at those in a close relationship, should always be taken seriously. The available evidence suggests that those at highest risk for acts of violence have established illnesses for which they have received care in the past, but have drifted away from treatment services.

18.4.13 SUBSTANCE ABUSE

The role of alcohol and drug abuse in dangerous behaviour remains controversial (Brain, 1986). In practical terms however patients already disabled by schizophrenia are often rendered more difficult and impulsive when intoxicated. This is particularly so in my experience when they make regular use of cannabis which can intensify suspiciousness and persecutory delusions. The coexistence of substance abuse and schizophrenia leads to difficulties in providing adequate supervision, accelerates social and economic decline, impairs compliance and increases the risk of conflict with those who come into contact with the patients.

18.5 THE ASSESSMENT PROCESS

The clinical approach to the prediction of dangerousness should, it has been argued be augmented or even replaced by an actuarial approach (Monahan, 1984). The problem is not with the theoretical advantages of a systematic assessment instructed by actuarial information: the problem is the current lack of the actuarial data required. In the absence of information which would provide for actuarially based prediction we have to rely on systematic assessments which are open to scrutiny and discussion and we would be well advised to involve multidisciplinary teams in all such assessments (Travin and Bluestone, 1987; Marra *et al.*, 1987).

The factors which need to be taken into account in assessing dangerousness can be summarized as follows:

1. Being a male
2. Being young.
3. Coming from an economically deprived sub-group.
4. Substance abuse.
5. Lacking social supports.
6. Having an established pattern of violent behaviour.
7. Having a personality structure given to conflict, lacking impulse control and marked by a paucity of feelings for others.
8. Having shown conduct disorder as a child and delinquent behaviour as an adolescent.
9. The previous offence or offences, taking particular note of:
   (a) The context.
   (b) The predispositions revealed.
   (c) The state of mind at the time.
   (d) The behaviour of the victim.
   (e) The intentions of the perpetrator.
   (f) The outcome for the victim and the subsequent behaviour of the attacker.
10. Mental disorder, having regard to:
    (a) Its type and likely natural history.
    (b) The associated disturbances of mental state.
    (c) Its relationship, if any, to previous offences.
    (d) Its likely effect on social and economic supports.
    (e) Its manageability.

The prediction of dangerousness is dubious business, but on occasion it is our business. In situations of uncertainty and doubt, the only help is clinical method, applied with meticulous attention to detail and a knowledge of which factors do and which do not relate to violent behaviour.

REFERENCES

Blackburn, R., Crellin, C., Morgan, E. and Tulloch, R. (1990) Prevalence of personality disorders in a special hospital population. *J. Forensic Psychiatry*, **1**, 41–52.

Blumstein, A. and Cohen, B. (1987) Characterizing criminal careers. *Science*, **237**, 985–91.

Brain, P.F. (1986) *Alcohol and Aggression*. Croom Helm, London.

Braybrook, B. and O'Neill, R. (1988) *A Census of Prison Inmates*. Crown Printers, Wellington.

Butler, R.A. (1975) *Report of the committee on mentally abnormal offenders*. HMSO London.

Felthous, A.R. and Kellerent, S.R. (1987) Childhood cruelty to animals and later aggression against people: a review. *Am. J. Psychiatry*, **144**, 710–17.

Fenton, G.W., Tennent, T.G., Fenwick, P.B.C. and Rattray, N. (1974) The EEG in antisocial behaviour. *Psychol. Med.*, **4**, 181–6.

Glaser, D. (1975) *Strategic Criminal Justice Planning*. US Govt Printing Office, Washington.

Gunn, J. (1977) *Epileptics in Prison*. Academic Press, London.

Gunn, J. (1982) An English psychiatrist looks at dangerousness, *Bull. A.A.P.L.*, **10**, 143–53.

Hafner, H. and Boker, W. (1982) *Crimes of Violence by Mentally Abnormal Offenders*, (trans. by H. Marshall), Cambridge University Press, Cambridge.

Kellerman, A.L. and Reay, D.T. (1986) Protection or peril: An analysis of firearm related deaths in the home. *N. Engl. J. Med.*, **314**, 1557–60.

Kozol, H.L., Boucher, R.J. and Garofalo, R.F. (1972) The diagnosis and treatment of dangerousness. *Crime Delinquency*, **18**, 371–92.

Macdonald, J.M. (1960), The threat to kill. *Am. J. Psychiatry*, **120**, 125–30.

Macdonald, J.M. (1961) *The Murderer and his Victim*. C.C. Thomas, Springfield.

Marra, H.A., Konzelman, G.E. and Giles, P.G. (1987) A clinical strategy to the assessment of dangerousness. *Int. J. Offender Ther. Criminol.*, **31**, 291–9.

Maudsley, H. (1900) *Responsibility in Mental Disease*. Appleton, New York.

McManus, M., Alessi, N.E., Grapentine, W.L. and Brickman, A. (1984) Psychiatric disturbances in serious delinquents. *J. Am. Acad. Child Psychiatry*, **3**, 602–15.

Megargee, E.I. (1976) The prediction of dangerous behaviour, *Crim. Justice Behav.*, **3**, 3–21.

Megargee, E.I. (1982) Psychological determinants and correlates of criminal violence. In *Criminal Violence*. M.E. Wolfgang and N.A. Weiner (eds), Sage, California, pp. 81–170.

Monahan, J. (1981) *The Clinical Prediction of Violent Behaviour*. United States Department of Health and Human Service, Maryland.

Monahan, J. (1984) The prediction of violent behaviour: toward a second generation of theory and policy. *Am. J. Psychiatry*, **141**, 10–5.

Mullen, P.E. (1984) Mental disorder and dangerousness. *Aust. N.Z. J. Psychiatry*, **18**, 8–19.

Mullen, P.E. and Maack, L.J. (1985) Jealousy, Pathological Jealousy and Aggression. In *Aggression and Dangerousness*. D.P. Farrington and J. Gunn (eds), Wiley, London, pp. 103–26.

Neithercutt, M.G. (1972) Parole violation patterns and commitment of offence. *J. Res. Crime Delinquency*, **9**, 87–98.

Offord, D.R. (1990) 27 Social factors in the aetiology of childhood psychiatric disorders. In *Handbook of Studies on Child Psychiatry*. B. Tony, J. Werry and G. Burrows (eds),

Elsevier Press, Amsterdam, pp. 55–68.

Pitcher, D.R. (1982) Chromosomes and violence. *Practitioner*, **226**, 497–501.

Pritchard, D. (1977) Stable Predictors of Recidivism. *J. Suppl. Abstract Serv.*, **7**, 72.

Robins, L.N. (1966), *Deviant Children Grown Up: A Sociological and Psychiatric Study of Sociopathic Personality*. Williams and Wilkins, Baltimore.

Scott, P.D. (1977) Assessing dangerousness in criminals. *Br. J. Psychiatry*, **131**, 127–42.

Silberman, C.E. (1978) *Criminal Violence, Criminal Justice*. Random House, New York.

Simon, F.H. (1971) *Prediction Methods in Criminology*. HMSO, London.

Steadman, H.J. (1980) The right not to be a false positive: Problems in the application of the dangerousness standard. *Psychiatr. Q.*, **52**, 84–9.

Taylor, P.J. (1985), Forensic Psychiatry. In *Essentials of Postgraduate Psychiatry*. P. Hill, R. Murray and A. Thorley (eds), Grune and Stratton, London, pp. 571–97.

Taylor, P.J. and Gunn, J. (1984) Violence and psychosis. *Br. Med. J.*, **289**, 9–12.

Travin, S. and Bluestone, H. (1987) Discharging the violent psychiatric inpatient. *J. Forensic Sci.*, **32**, 999–1008.

Walker, N., Hammond, W. and Steer, D. (1976) Repeated violence. *Crim. Law Rev.*, 463–72.

West, D.J. (1982) *Delinquency: Its Roots, Careers and Prospects*. Heinemann, London.

West, D.J. and Farrington, D.P. (1977) *The Delinquent Way of Life*. Heinemann, London.

Part Three
Treatment of Schizophrenia

Introduction

This section attempts to cover a range of pharmacological and psychological interventions that apply to schizophrenia. The emphasis is on interventions that have established their utility in controlled trials, or when these are not yet available, they are consistent with studies on predictive factors. With regard to psychological treatments, these criteria result in a bias toward cognitive–behavioural approaches, since they currently have the most substantial empirical support.

Chapter 19 begins this section with a review of pharmacological treatments for schizophrenia, examining their effects on the treatment of episodes and their role in long-term maintenance. The author highlights strategies to reduce the risks of side effects and improve compliance. He also discusses the relationships between neuroleptic treatment and psychosocial interventions.

Chapter 20 takes up the issue of adherence to treatment, and outlines the evidence on associated factors. From this analysis the authors derive a set of practical guidelines for clinicians that are likely to improve adherence and maximize self-regulation. The chapter concludes with a brief case example.

In recent years, a number of studies have suggested that schizophrenia sufferers also use a variety of psychological strategies to control their symptoms. Chapter 21 reviews these data and examines the evidence on psychological interventions to improve symptom control. It describes a new approach called Coping Strategy Enhancement (CSE), developed by the author and his colleagues, and details its application to a single case. The chapter concludes with a report of preliminary results from a controlled trial of CSE versus training in problem solving.

Of the functional deficits associated with schizophrenia, perhaps the problems in social skills have the most widespread impact. Chapter 22 summarizes the content of behavioural social skills training, and provides sample outlines of sessions from a therapist manual. A critical review of the literature is presented, and the authors discuss potential directions for further research and development.

Chapter 23 focuses on training sufferers in other life skills. It reviews the contributions of token economies and community support programmes, and outlines the module approach of Liberman and his colleagues. The scope of the modules is summarized and the structure of the skills training procedure is described.

Earlier chapters on social factors suggested that intrusive or critical interactions within the household may have a powerful impact on the course of schizophrenia (Chapters 8 and 11). Chapter 24 reviews the literature on psychosocial interventions for families. It outlines an an interactive model of family influences and uses the model to construct an intervention strategy that is currently being evaluated in the author's research.

The final two chapters examine treatment and prevention in the community, taking up some of the issues that are raised in earlier contributions and discussing their implications for health service provision. Chapter 25 examines the relative utility of brief versus extended hospital admissions, and also compares admissions with community care. It stresses the importance of continuity of care and supports the case management concept.

Chapter 26 extends the community intervention model to include preventative strategies. It draws on concepts and methods that appear in previous chapters to outline a comprehensive approach to primary, secondary and tertiary prevention of schizophrenia. A project is described which applies the authors' approach in a rural community.

Part Three exemplifies the two main messages in the book. One is that schizophrenia requires an integration of pure and applied research, and readers who are interested in particular topics are encouraged to look at relevant chapters from all three units. The second message is that integration is needed across specialist areas, and the contributions to this section emphasize a coalition between disciplines and between professionals, families and sufferers. Only with such a coalition can we adequately address the problems that are posed by this complex and serious disorder.

David J. Kavanagh

Chapter 19

Pharmacological treatment of schizophrenia

STEPHEN R. MARDER

Neuroleptic medications (also referred to as antipsychotics) are a group of compounds that have been found to be effective for treating the symptoms associated with acute schizophrenia and for the prevention of relapse in schizophrenic patients who have recovered from psychosis. As the result of a large body of research, these drugs have become standard treatments for nearly all patients who suffer from schizophrenia. However, these drugs have a number of important limitations: they are not effective for all patients, they have a number of serious adverse effects, and they are limited in what they can do.

19.1 EFFECTIVENESS OF NEUROLEPTICS

Numerous well-controlled studies have established that this group of drugs has antipsychotic effects in schizophrenia. A few studies that used very low doses — less than 400 mg of chlorpromazine daily — were equivocal; higher dosages, almost without exception, led to clear-cut improvement. Cole and Davis (1969) also compared the results of studies that were characterized according to their overall quality. Those studies with significant methodological problems were more

likely to find drugs ineffective. On the other hand, the most carefully designed studies (double-blind, placebo-controlled studies with random allocation to treatment) were unequivocal in demonstrating that neuroleptics had substantial beneficial effects.

All of the symptoms associated with schizophrenia are affected to some degree by neuroleptics. The so-called positive symptoms which include hallucinations, delusions, and disorganized thoughts are more responsive to drug treatment than are negative symptoms such as blunted affect, emotional withdrawal, and lack of social interest. Frequently, positive symptoms will be eliminated by drug treatment, while negative symptoms are only modestly improved and continue to impair the patient's social recovery. A substantial proportion of schizophrenic patients — about 10 to 20% — fail to demonstrate substantial improvement when they are treated with neuroleptics. This sub-group of treatment refractory schizophrenic patients often requires long-term care (Kane, 1989).

The time course of improvement from neuroleptics differ among patients. Patients who are agitated or excited will usually experience a calming effect that begins within hours of the start of drug treatment. However, symptoms such as hallucinations, delusions, and disturbed behaviours may not begin to improve for several days and sometimes not for several weeks. Once patients begin to improve, it may take months before they achieve maximum benefit. This slow time course can become a problem if the clinician believes after a week or two that a patient is not responding because the wrong drug or dose was prescribed. This may result in a change in drug or an increase in dose that is unnecessary. If the dose is increased and the patient improves a few days later, the prescriber may wrongly conclude that the higher dose was needed, despite the fact that the individual may have done just as well on the lower dose.

Although neuroleptics seem to act on the process that leads to psychotic thinking in schizophrenics, they are not exclusively 'anti-schizophrenic'. Other illnesses such as depression, mania, and organic brain syndromes such as Huntington's disease or Alzheimer's disease can lead to psychotic thought processes. In all of these the psychosis may respond to neuroleptics.

19.2 COMPARING NEUROLEPTICS

Table 19.1 lists the different classes of neuroleptics that are currently prescribed in the US. Although many neuroleptics are available, none has been shown to be more effective than any other. (A possible exception is clozapine which appears to be superior in treating severely ill patients who are poor responders to other drugs.) In the past it was believed that different types of schizophrenia responded better to certain types of drugs. For example, it was believed that chlorpromazine, a drug with considerable sedative side effects, was better for agitated or excited patients whereas haloperidol, a drug that is only minimally sedating, was better for more withdrawn patients. This has not been supported by empirical research and it is currently believed that all of the classes of neuroleptics are equally efficacious for

all of the different manifestations of the illness (Kane, 1989). These observations are based on the average responses of groups of patients and cannot be strictly applied to individual cases. It is possible that a particular patient may do well to one drug and be unimproved or even worsened by another. Thus, a record of a good or poor response to a particular drug should be an important factor in selecting that drug.

The most important differences among neuroleptics are in their side effects. For simplicity, these drugs are usually divided into two groups: high-potency drugs including fluphenazine, haloperidol, thiothixene, and trifluoperazine, and low-potency drugs including chlorpromazine and thioridazine. High-potency neuroleptics are prescribed in much lower doses (as a result of their high potency) and tend to be more associated with neurological side effects (see Section 19.5) such as stiffness, restlessness and tremor. Low potency drugs have fewer neurological side effects, but are associated with more side effects such as sedation, dry mouth, constipation, and lowering of blood pressure when the patient arises (postural hypotension). In recent years there has been a strong tendency to prescribe the high-potency drugs since their side effects are usually more manageable. This is particularly true for patients who require relatively high neuroleptic doses since high doses of low-potency drugs can result in intolerable amounts of sedation.

Neuroleptics also differ in their available routes of administration. Athough oral administration of drugs as pills or liquid is most common, there are certain occasions when an intramuscular injectable drug is preferable. For example, patients who refuse to take drugs orally may be administered a short acting injection. An injection may also be used for patients who are dangerously excited since this form of administration has a more rapid onset then the oral form. Although most neuroleptics are available as short-acting injectables, some are not. In addition, a number of neuroleptics

Table 19.1 Classes of neuroleptic compounds

Class	Generic example	Brand name		Usual daily dose acute treatment (mg)
		USA	UK	
Phenothiazines	Fluphenazine	Prolixin	Moditen	5–20
	Chlorpromazine	Thorazine	Cargactil	1000–1000
	Thioridazine	Mellaril	Melleril	100–800
Thioxanthenes	Thiothixene	Navane	Not available	10–50
Butyrophenones	Haloperidol	Haldol	Haldol, Serenace	5–20
Dibenzoxazepines	Loxapine	Loxitane	Loxapac	25–100
Dihydroindolones	Molindone	Moban	Not available	25–100
Dibenzodiazepines	Clozapine	Clozaril	Clozaril	200–900

such as fluphenazine and haloperidol are available as long-acting injectables. This form of drug delivery consists of an injection which is administered once every two to four weeks. The drug is slowly released from the injection site resulting in a reasonably steady drug level for the entire interval between injections. This latter form of drug administration is usually used for patients who have been stabilized and are being maintained in long-term drug therapy.

19.3 DOSAGE OF NEUROLEPTICS

A dose of neuroleptic that causes intolerable side effects in some patients will be insufficient for others. For example, some patients will have an adequate therapeutic response to 2 mg of haloperidol daily while others require 40 mg or more. Similarly, some will experience intolerable side effects on 2 mg while others have no difficulty tolerating 100 mg. Some of this variation can be explained by the fact that different patients will have as much as a 20-fold variation in their blood levels of a drug after receiving the same amount of a neuroleptic. However, this does not explain all of the variation, since patients also differ in the plasma neuroleptic levels that they are able to tolerate without experiencing side effects.

The large differences in dosage requirements presents an obvious dilemma to the clinician who is starting a psychotic schizophrenic patient on a neuroleptic. If no information is available from prior episodes, the decision regarding dosage will usually be made on a trial and error basis. There are some guidelines available from studies that have compared the effectiveness of different doses. In most double-blind studies, a clear difference between neuroleptic drugs and placebo appears when dosages above 300 mg of chlorpromazine daily (or its equivalent for another neuroleptic) are administered. For example, since 100 mg of chlorpromazine is approximately equivalent to 2 mg of haloperidol or fluphenazine, this would represent 6 mg of the more potent drugs. Other studies indicate that only a minority of patients require more than 1000 mg a day of chlorpromazine or 20 mg of haloperidol or fluphenazine (reviewed in Baldessarini *et al.*, 1988). In other words, the range of 300 mg to 1000 mg of chlorpromazine should be sufficient for nearly all acutely psychotic schizophrenic patients. Doses much higher than this may expose patients to unnecessary side effects without increased efficacy.

Some clinicians have proposed that the use of high doses of neuroleptics during the first few days following admission results in a more rapid onset of response. Termed 'rapid neuroleptization', this treatment strategy usually consists of the use of relatively high doses of injectable high potency drugs such as haloperidol or fluphenazine. Drugs are administered until patients demonstrate overt sedation or side effects. A number of carefully designed double-blind studies have tested this strategy. The findings have consistently demonstrated that 'rapid neuroleptization' is no more effective then merely starting patients on a moderate dose such as 10 mg daily of haloperidol (Neborsky *et al.*, 1981).

19.4 MECHANISM OF ACTION OF NEUROLEPTICS

Scientists who are interested in understanding the underlying biology of schizophrenia, have focused on studying the mechanism of action of neuroleptics. Most research in this area has centred around the dopamine hypothesis. This theory proposes that schizophrenia is related to an overactive dopamine system. It is supported by two important lines of evidence. First, drugs that decrease dopamine activity in the brain usually have antipsychotic activity; and second, drugs that increase dopamine activity (including stimulants such as amphetamine or methylphenidate) can either cause psychotic symptoms in normals or will worsen schizophrenic symptoms in patients (reviewed in Stahl and Wets, 1988). The dopamine hypothesis has inspired an enormous amount of research. However, it still remains controversial today largely because there is only weak evidence supporting differences between the dopamine systems of normals and schizophrenic patients.

The strongest evidence supporting dopamine's involvement in the mechanism of action of neuroleptics comes from studies in which different neuroleptic drugs are compared with regard to their affinity for dopamine receptors. These studies have found that the clinical activity of the drugs is closely related to their dopamine blocking activity (Peroutka and Snyder, 1980). This does not mean that schizophrenia is caused by increased dopamine activity. It is common in medicine for illnesses to be treated through mechanisms that are unrelated to the actual cause of the illness. For example, hypertension can be treated by drugs with different biological activities that are far removed from the actual cause of hypertension. In a similar manner, schizophrenic psychosis — or any psychosis — may be attenuated by methods that are unrelated to what causes schizophrenia. The situation is complicated since clozapine, a highly effective antipsychotic drug, has relatively weak affinity for dopamine receptors. One theory about clozapine proposes that it has relatively weak activity at dopamine receptors in the part of the brain — the basal ganglia — that affects movement, but substantial activity in the limbic system. This would explain the drug's relatively weak neurological effects, but strong antipsychotic activity. Another theory proposes that clozapine's activity is related to a balance between dopamine activity and the activity of another neurotransmitter, perhaps serotonin. The observation that clozapine can treat schizophrenia effectively without causing serious neurological side effects opens up new avenues for developing better drugs for schizophrenia.

19.5 SIDE EFFECTS OF NEUROLEPTICS

Neurological side effects, also called extrapyramidal side-effects or EPSs, are the major problem in prescribing neuroleptics. The most common EPS is akathisia, a side effect consisting of a subjective feeling of restlessness. Patients who experience severe akathisia will often pace continuously or move their feel restlessly while they are sitting. Some complain of a feeling that they are unable to feel comfortable, regardless of what they do. Severe akathisia can cause patients to feel anxious or irritable and some reports suggest that severe akathisia can result in aggressive or suicidal acts. Studies from our laboratory indicate that as many as 75% of patients treated with a conventional dose of haloperidol will experience some degree of akathisia (Van Putten *et al.*, 1984).

Acute dystonic reactions are abrupt onset, sometimes bizarre, muscular spasms affecting mainly the musculature of the head and neck, but sometimes the trunk and lower extremities, leading to gait disturbances that may be confused with hysteria. These reactions usually appear within the first few days of therapy when patients are treated with large doses of high-potency neuroleptics such as haloperidol or fluphenazine. They almost always respond rapidly to antiparkinson medications and can usually be prevented by either pretreatment with antiparkinson medications or by limiting the neuroleptic dosage prescribed. Another manifestation of EPS is drug-induced parkinsonism, consisting of stiffness, tremor, and shuffling gait. Often patients with these symptoms will also experience akinesia, a side effect consisting of difficulty initiating movement. In some cases drug-induced parkinsonism can be nearly identical to Parkinson's disease.

For most patients, EPS is treatable. The anticholinergic antiparkinson drugs such as benztropine or trihexiphenidyl are by far the most commonly used drugs for EPS (Table 19.2). Many clinicians will prescribe these drugs routinely for patients who are receiving neuroleptics — particularly potent neuroleptics. A number of studies indicate that prescribing antiparkinson medications before patients demonstrate EPS can prevent dystonias. Unfortunately, these drugs also have side effects of their own including dry mouth, constipation, urinary retention and blurry vision. More recent studies indicate that anticholinergic antiparkinson drugs can also result in some loss of memory (Gelenberg *et al.* 1989). This side

effect is dose dependent and remits when the drug is stopped. Other drugs for treating EPS include amantadine, a drug which is effective against parkinsonism, and propranolol, which is effective in managing akathisia. Both of these drugs can be added to anticholinergic antiparkinson drugs.

There are a number of unfortunate persons who are highly sensitive to EPS — particularly akathisia — at the dose that is necessary to control their psychosis. Some of these patients may agree to tolerate these side effects, at least temporarily, while their most troublesome psychotic symptoms are being treated. For others, the discomfort brought on by medication side effects may seem worse than the illness itself.

Tardive dyskinesia is a movement disorder which may affect the face, mouth, neck, trunk or extremities. Since tardive dyskinesia is relatively rare in patients treated short-term for acute psychosis, it will be discussed in more detail in Section 19.10. At this point it is important to emphasize that tardive dyskinesia should *not* be seen as a risk factor which should concern the clinician who is treating an acutely psychotic individual.

Other side effects that may arise during the course of acute short-term treatment include autonomic effects such as dry mouth, hypotension and sedation. These problems can almost always be managed by a dosage adjustment or by changing to another drug. For example, when patients demonstrate significant daytime sedation on chlorpromazine, changing to a relatively non-sedating drug such as haloperidol will usually solve the problem.

Table 19.2 Examples of antiparkinson drugs

Generic	Brand name	Mechanism	Usual daily dose (mg)
Benztropine	Cogentin	Anticholinergic	1–8
Trihexyphenidyl	Artane	Anticholinergic	4–12
Amantadine	Symmetrel	Dopaminergic	100–300

The neuroleptic malignant syndrome is a potentially fatal, but rare, complication of neuroleptic treatment (reviewed in Guze and Baxter, 1985). It presents initially as muscular rigidity and progresses to elevated temperature, fluctuating consciousness, and unstable vital signs. Mortality in well developed cases has been reported as ranging from 20 to 30% and may be higher when depot forms are used. Clinicians should be concerned about any patient who demonstrates severe muscular rigidity and a rising temperature, since early diagnosis and treatment can be life-saving.

Earlier observations by senior clinicians that drugs might interfere with psychological and social forms of therapy may have resulted from patients being overmedicated — a practice which was probably quite prevalent in the recent past and perhaps still occurs in certain places today. When patients are treated with doses of neuroleptics that result in oversedation or when they appear 'snowed' as the result of akinesia they are likely to respond poorly to psychological treatments. The skill in drug therapy is to find doses that result in therapeutic effects with the minimal amount of side effects.

19.6 MEASURING NEUROLEPTIC BLOOD LEVELS

Finding that best neuroleptic dose for an individual patient often requires weeks or months of treatment. If measuring a patient's plasma (or blood) level were found to be clinically useful, it would make the treatment of schizophrenia more scientific. Early studies of plasma levels indicated that patients who received the same dose of drug had large variations in their plasma levels. These early findings suggested that studying individual differences in plasma levels would provide information that could be useful to clinicians. However, early studies focused on drugs such as chlorpromazine which have a complex metabolism. These drugs are poorly suited for plasma level measurement since some of the

antipsychotic activity in the plasma may result from metabolites of the drug. Because of drug selection and methodological errors (reviewed by May and Goldberg, 1978) early studies failed to find a reliable relationship.

A number of more recent studies have focused on haloperidol and have had more promising results. This may be related to the metabolism of this drug which includes only a single metabolite which may not have significant antipsychotic activity. As a result, measuring the plasma level of haloperidol may provide an accurate representation of the amount of effective drug. Although the measurement of plasma levels should be considered controversial at this stage, there are circumstances — particularly when patients are failing to respond to a neuroleptic — when plasma levels can provide useful information to clinicians.

19.7 WHEN PATIENTS FAIL TO RESPOND

The fact that drugs have been shown to be effective in groups of patients does not mean that they work for every patient. Ten to twenty per cent of schizophrenic patients will fail to demonstrate an adequate response to neuroleptic treatment. When patients fail to respond, clinicians have a number of manoeuvres that will frequently result in an improved response. The most simple is a dosage adjustment — either an increase or a decrease. A reasonable proportion of schizophrenic patients will only respond when their dose is raised to a relatively high level. A relatively small proportion of severely ill patients may require doses as high as 60 to 100 mg each day of haloperidol or fluphenazine. Other evidence suggests that there is a so-called 'therapeutic window' for dose (Van Putten *et al.*, 1989). This means that patients demonstrate their best response in a particular dose range. If patients on too high a dose have their dose reduced they will improve as will patients on too low dose who have their dose increased. When patients fail to respond after an adequate trial of a neuroleptic, the next step is usually to change the patient to another neuroleptic from a different chemical class.

Sometimes adding another drug to a neuroleptic will improve response. Lithium carbonate, a drug usually used for manic-depressive illness, can be helpful for patients with schizoaffective disorders who continue to have an excited or depressed mood despite neuroleptic treatment. Other studies indicate that adding lithium to a neuroleptic is frequently helpful in patients who have no evidence of impaired affect. Other drugs that are sometimes added to a neuroleptic in poorly responsive patients include carbamazepine, an anticonvulsant, and propranolol or other beta adrenergic blockers. For both drugs there is relatively little empirical data supporting this practice, although they are sometimes helpful in desperate situations (Kane, 1989). As noted in section 19.8, clozapine is a new alternative for treatment refractory schizophrenia.

19.8 CLOZAPINE

Clozapine is an unusual neuroleptic that appears to be particularly effective for patients who have not responded to standard drugs. Studies carried out in both Europe and the United States indicate that clozapine appears to be more effective than drugs such as chlorpromazine or haloperidol in the treatment of severely ill drug refractory schizophrenic patients. Moreover, clozapine has the advantage of causing much fewer neurological side effects than conventional drugs. In a recent multicentre trial in the US (Kane *et al.*, 1988) clozapine was compared to chlorpromazine in severely psychotic patients. The trial verified clozapine's clear superiority in this population for treating positive schizophrenic symptoms. In addition, clozapine was significantly more effective than chlorpromazine in treating negative symptoms such as blunted affect and decreased social

interest. This is an extremely important finding since typical neuroleptic drugs are often ineffective in decreasing negative symptoms.

Unfortunately, early clinical trials with clozapine also revealed a serious problem with the drug. Clozapine can cause patients to develop agranulocytosis, an adverse side effect in which the bone marrow stops producing a type of white blood cell that is essential for combating infections. If it is not detected, it can be fatal. Although agranulocytosis can occur with nearly all drugs, it is usually rare. Clozapine, however, has been found to cause agranulocytosis in more than 1% of patients. Fortunately, if this side effect is detected and clozapine is stopped, patients almost always have a full recovery. Due to this serious adverse effect, the US Food and Drug Administration has restricted clozapine to patients who have failed to responded to typical neuroleptics. Patients who receive clozapine should have their blood counts monitored on a weekly basis for as long as they receive the drug. By using this intensive monitoring system, nearly all of the cases of agranulocytosis found in the USA have recovered.

Clozapine is also important because it indicates that schizophrenia may be treatable with a new group of more effective drugs with different range of side effects. The search for a drug with similar therapeutic effects, but without a liability for causing tardive dyskinesia has been intense. It suggests that the drug treatment of schizophrenia will probably undergo dramatic changes during the coming decade.

19.9 MAINTENANCE THERAPY WITH NEUROLEPTICS

Neuroleptic drugs can also be important in managing schizophrenic patients who have stabilized. Treating remitted schizophrenic patients with neuroleptic drugs substantially lowers their rate of relapse. Davis (1975) reviewed 24 double-blind studies of maintenance antipsychotic therapy and found that in all studies many more patients relapsed on placebo than on drug. When the results were pooled, 698 out of 1068 patients on placebo relapsed (65%) in contrast with only 639 out of 2127 patients on drug (30%). Since Davis' review in 1975, numerous double-blind studies have confirmed these results. This very large difference in survival between drug-treated and placebo-treated patients is the main reason why schizophrenic patients are commonly continued on long-term neuroleptic maintenance treatment after a schizophrenic episode. It is interesting to note that clinicians are often tempted to discontinue medications in patients who have been well and stable for prolonged periods of time. Unfortunately, these patients also have high relapse rates when their medications are discontinued (Hogarty *et al.*, 1976).

The decision about when to discontinue maintenance medications is most difficult in patients who have experienced their first-episode of schizophrenia. Relapse rates for first episode patients are somewhat lower than for those who have had multiple episodes. On the other hand, patients early in their illness may have the most to lose. For these patients a relapse may result in a loss of vocational or educational opportunities or in more difficult things to measure such as a loss of self-esteem. Carefully designed double-blind studies indicate that only a relatively small number of first-episode patients will fail to have psychotic episodes in the 3 years that follow an initial psychotic episode (Kane, 1989). A reasonable strategy for most first-episode patients would probably involve continuing drugs for at least a year following an episode with consideration of dosage reduction or observation off drugs during the following year.

The demonstration of maintenance therapy's effectiveness in preventing relapse does not mean that these patients do well. Even when unrelapsed, drug-maintained schizophrenic patients living in the community are often severely impaired. They are likely to be chronically or periodically unemployed, and even when able to work are frequently found in only the lowest paying jobs. In addition, many patients refuse to accept medication, perhaps preferring the delusional world they have created by themselves to the reality associated with being a chronic psychiatric patient. In the USA many of these patients have become homeless and are apparent in major urban centres.

19.10 TARDIVE DYSKINESIA

Tardive dyskinesia (TD) is probably the most serious limitation of long-term neuroleptic therapy. Patients with TD may have any or all of a number of abnormal movements. These frequently consist of mouth and tongue movements, such as lip smacking and puckering as well as facial grimacing. Other movements may include irregular movements of the limbs, particularly piano player-like movements of the fingers and toes and slow, writhing movements of the trunk. Although seriously disabling dyskinesia is uncommon, in a small proportion it may affect walking, breathing, eating and talking. At least 10 to 20% of patients treated with neuroleptics for more than a year develop tardive dyskinesia (Task Force Report, 1980). Certain populations are at a greater risk, than others for developing tardive dyskinesia. Increasing age seems to increase risk with elderly women being particularly vulnerable. Smith and Baldessarini (1980) have reported that tardive dyskinesia in the elderly is less likely to remit when neuroleptics are discontinued. Others have reported that patients with affective disorders may also be at a greater risk for tardive dyskinesia when they are treated with neuroleptics (Rosenbaum *et al.*, 1977). This is important since many patients with affective illness can be maintained with mood stabilizing drugs such as lithium or carbamazepine.

Early observations of the course of tardive dyskinesia suggested that the disorder was inevitably progressive and irreversible. In other words, once patients developed even mild dyskinesias, they were on a dangerous path toward severe TD. More recent evidence indicates otherwise. When neuroleptics are discontinued, a substantial proportion of TD patients will demonstrate a remission. This is particularly likely for those with a rather recent onset of tardive dyskinesia. Sometimes this remission will take several months to occur (reviewed in Marder, 1986).

Tardive dyskinesia does not appear to be a progressive disorder for most patients: TD seems to develop rather rapidly and to then stabilize and often improve. A number of studies have followed the course of TD in patients who were continued on drugs for several years. The consensus of these studies was that most patients improve in the severity of TD even if their neuroleptic drugs are continued (Kane, 1989). Moreover, this improvement can be clinically meaningful in some patients.

These findings suggest a reasonable strategy for following patients who receive chronic neuroleptics. All schizophrenic patients who are receiving neuroleptics for more than a six months should have regular and systematic evaluations for tardive dyskinesia. Although instruments such as AIMS, the Abnormal Involuntary Movement Scale (Task Force Report, 1980) were originally developed as research tools, they also provide a structured system for evaluating and recording abnormal movements. Thus, performing an AIMS test once every three to six months would provide a reasonable strategy for monitoring patients.

Once tardive dyskinesia is diagnosed, the clinician must evaluate the need for continued neuroleptic treatment. This is clearly a complex decision that requires consideration of the dangers of both the schizophrenic illness and the tardive dyskinesia. It is a decision that, whenever possible, should be made in collaboration with the patient and his or her family. The results of this discussion should be docu-mented in the patient's medical record. For most patients with chronic schizophrenia, the best decision will probably involve continuing neuroleptic therapy. If this is the case, there is some evidence that treating patients with the lowest effective neuroleptic dose may minimize the risk of TD (Kane, 1989).

Clinicians have recently begun to appreciate that extrapyramidal side effects have the potential for making schizophrenic patients feel miserable. Two of the most common extra-pyramidal side effects, akathisia and akinesia, have the potential for causing dysphorias by themselves. Akathisia can sometimes be toler-ated for periods of time during the acute stages of treatment. During chronic treatment, even subtle akathisia has the potential for impairing an individual's quality of life. Van Putten (1974) has described the anguish of such patients who live in a world where they have trouble finding any comfort or rest.

Akinesia is an extrapyramidally induced side effect manifest in decreased spontaneous move-ment, diminished conversation, apathy and a disinclination to initiate any activity (Rifkin *et al.*, 1975). Since these symptoms bear a striking resemblance to the flattened affect and decreased motivation that characterize the nega-tive impairments of schizophrenia it is easy to understand why they frequently go unrecog-nized.

It is important to point out that the risk-benefit equation for maintenance therapy can vary for different individuals. For a small proportion of schizophrenic patients, the dis-comforts from the drugs or the risk of tardive dyskinesia may appear greater than the risk of a relapse into psychosis. These are likely to be individuals who have relatively mild schizo-phrenic episodes or whose relapses can be prevented by intervening at the earliest signs that the person is decompensating.

For others — and in our opinion, probably for the majority of schizophrenic individuals — the risks and discomforts of chronic neuro-leptic treatment are justified by the diminished risk of relapse. Extreme examples are individuals who become involved in violent crimes while psychotic or who make serious suicide attempts. Less extreme, the mother who neglects her children whenever she relapses or the mother or father who repeatedly gets fired from a job with each rehospitalization will probably need to be continued on a neuroleptic even when they appear to be symptom-free. Johnson *et al.* (1983) have reported that patients who have their medications discontinued tend to have relapses that are more severe than those who relapse while they are receiving medication. In his study, the relapses occurring in patients who were not receiving drugs were more often associated with antisocial behaviour and violence. Patients who had their medications discontinued actually ended up requiring more neuroleptic in the long run than those who were continued on maintenance treatment. This was because the dose of medication had to be raised substantially to control episodes of psychosis.

19.11 COMPLIANCE

A high proportion of schizophrenic patients either refuse to remain on maintenance neuroleptics or fail to take their medication as prescribed. There are a number of explanations for noncompliance — some directly related to the individual's schizophrenic illness and others unrelated. Some patients appear to be disinterested in the ordinary reality around them. For example they may have grandiose delusions and as a result may prefer their schizophrenic experiences to the harsh realities of their lives, which often include the poverty and humiliation that can be associated with chronic mental illness.

Many schizophrenic patients refuse to take their drugs because of the way these medications make then feel. Side effects of neuroleptics — particularly extrapyramidal side effects — have the potential for making patients feel miserable. Many patients deal with these side effects by failing to take their medication. Patients who experience severe side effects are more likely to refuse drug treatment. This indicates that careful attention to side effects may be an important method for assuring compliance.

Many of the patients who experience side effects — and some who do not — will experiment with stopping their medications for several days or weeks. When they do this, they are likely to feel better — at least for a while. This is because there is usually a lag of several months between drug discontinuation and relapse. And this is the great dilemma for these patients — we recommend that they take a medication which only makes them feel worse. The dilemma for the clinician is that it may be difficult for patients to accept that they need these medications. It is interesting to note that the rates of noncompliance in schizophrenic patients resemble rates in patients with other medical illnesses such as hypertension and penicillin prophylaxis for rheumatic fever. In each of these chronic disorders, the patient is required to take a medication when he or she feels well in order to prevent an unfavourable outcome in the future. An extensive literature on compliance indicates that patients find it difficult to adhere to such a task (reviewed in Kane, 1989).

One of the best methods for assuring compliance is educating both patients and family members about a patient's schizophrenia. A number of investigators have recently developed strategies that include educating patients and their families about schizophrenia and drug treatment (Anderson *et al.*, 1980). In each case, these programmes appear to improve the emotional climate in the patient's family and, at the same time, to improve drug compliance. Educating family members is particularly important in schizophrenia since these patients are more likely to depend on family supervision than most other psychiatric patients. See Chapter 20 for further discussion of strategies to improve compliance.

19.12 DEPOT NEUROLEPTICS

As mentioned previously, some neuroleptic drugs can be administered in an injection which is given once every 2 to 4 weeks. The drug is slowly released from the injection site resulting in a fairly consistent plasma level during the entire interval between injections. There are two possible advantages associated with this route of administration in comparison with oral prescribing. The first advantage is that depot neuroleptics provide a partial solution to the problem of poor compliance in schizophrenic outpatients. Many patients are unable to take pills reliably, but can be convinced to come in regularly for injections. The second advantage is more theoretical. When drugs are administered through injections they result in a more reliable blood level than with oral drugs. This is because oral drugs may vary in the degree to which they are absorbed in the gut. In addition, drugs that are taken orally undergo extensive metabolism in the gut and liver. Both of these obstacles to drug absorption are bypassed by injectable drugs (Marder *et al.*, 1989).

There are some indications that patients who receive depot neuroleptics have a better long-term outcome than patients who receive oral drugs. This advantage is best demonstrated in studies such as those conducted by Johnson *et al.* (1984) under conditions that resemble most closely those that exist in community clinics. In these studies, patients with histories of poor compliance were included in the population and the amount of contact between patients and staff was limited. In the larger, more carefully controlled investigations (Hogarty *et al.*, 1979; Schooler *et al.*, 1980) patients with serious compliance problems — that is, the individuals most likely to benefit from treatment with depot drugs — are commonly not included. In addition, the amount of contact between treating staff and patient usually exceeds that available in community programmes. However, a careful look at the later studies indicates that there may

be advantages for injections even under these carefully controlled conditions. In both the Schooler and Hogarty studies there were no differences in outcome between oral and depot fluphenazine at the end of one year. The Hogarty study also included a second year during which patients receiving fluphenazine decanoate demonstrated a lower risk of relapse than those assigned to oral fluphenazine. Moreover, the best outcomes were found for patients who received fluphenazine decanoate supplemented by a form of social therapy. These results suggest that injected neuroleptics may have advantages over oral drugs for patients who are reasonably reliable as well as for patients who have a history of poor medication compliance.

This author believes that depot neuroleptics are the preferred form of antipsychotic medication for the long-term management of schizophrenic patients living in the community. However, depot drugs are not recommended for the treatment of acute psychosis. This is because these drugs provide little flexibility in dosing on a day-to-day basis. For example, if the dosage prescribed is too high and results in side effects, the patient will suffer the consequences for a longer period of time than with oral drugs. A reasonable management strategy would include treating acute episodes with oral drugs and gradually changing the patient to a depot drug as the patient improves.

19.13 LONG-TERM MAINTENANCE STRATEGIES

Decision-making about drug dosage during the maintenance phase of therapy can be difficult because the patient is usually clinically stable. As a result, drug dose cannot be titrated against clinical response. Therefore, if the dose is too low, this may not be apparent until the patient relapses. If the dose is higher than necessary, the patient may be exposed to unnecessary side effects and may be more vulnerable to developing tardive dyskinesia. For these reasons, there is great interest in methods for determining the lowest effective dose for individual patients.

At the present time, two particular strategies are under active investigation as methods for reducing the amount of medication which patients receive. Some investigators have proposed gradually decreasing the amount of drug that stabilized patients receive until medications are completely discontinued. They are then followed very closely until there are signs that the individual is beginning to relapse. At this time, drugs are reinstituted. To make this strategy work, patients and their families are trained to detect the early signs of impending psychotic breakdown. This makes sense since a number of studies indicate that most schizophrenic patients do not relapse abruptly. There is usually a period of several weeks or even months during which there are signs that the patient is deteriorating. A recent report by Jolley *et al.* (1989) indicates that patients who were assigned to intermittent treatment were more likely to have recurrences of psychotic symptoms. However, these recurrences were relatively mild, and seldom led to a need for hospitalization. Similar findings have been reported by others (Carpenter *et al.*, 1987; Herz *et al.*, 1989).

The second strategy proposes treating patients with much lower doses of depot neuroleptic than usually prescribed. Studies by both Kane *et al.* (1983) and Marder *et al.* (1987) indicate that a substantial number of (but by no means all) 'maintenance' patients do well on doses of fluphenazine decanoate as low as 2.5 or 5 mg every 14 days. This is a substantial lowering of dose since most patients who are prescribed fluphenazine decanoate receive 25 to 50 mg every two weeks. In our studies, we compared patients who were assigned to a double-blind comparison of 5 or 25 mg of fluphenazine decanoate administered every two weeks. Although patients receiving the lower dose had a greater number of psychotic exacerbations, these were usually rather mild and were seldom associated with need for rehospitalization. These minor exacerbations were usually easily controlled by a small dosage adjustment. In addition, patients receiving the lower dose had fewer side effects and complained less of anxiety and depression. Low dose treatment was also associated with a lower drop out rate. Kane *et al.* (1983) has reported that patients on lower doses also had lower dyskinesia ratings, suggesting that the low dose strategy may reduce vulnerability to tardive dyskinesia. These findings suggest that there are likely to be benefits associated with the use of the lowest effective dose of maintenance neuroleptic.

19.14 INTERACTIONS OF DRUGS AND PSYCHOSOCIAL TREATMENTS

It is important to emphasize that maintenance neuroleptics are prescribed to prevent relapse. They should not be expected to do much more than that. When the goals of the clinician and the patient include more that this — perhaps work rehabilitation or improved socialization — the optimal treatment plan will probably include the use of other treatment modalities such as psychotherapy, vocational rehabilitation, family therapy, or social skills training. This is not a matter of any one form of treatment being superior or inferior in general, but rather that different treatments do different things. Drug therapy may have a substantial effect on the severity of psychotic symptoms. It may restore patients to a state where they are able to find a job or prevent a relapse which will result in the loss of a job. It will not provide the social or occupational restoration which the individual may desperately need. Thus, outpatient treatment plans should combine neuroleptic medication with other forms of treatment which attend to the special needs of the patient.

Just to complicate the situation, it appears that psychosocial treatments not only add to the effects of drugs, but the two treatment modalities seem to have complex interactions. For example, in a major collaborative study (Hogarty *et al.*, 1974) patients who received a placebo as opposed to an active drug had a worse outcome when assigned to a form of individual psychotherapy termed Major Role Therapy. This suggested to the investigators that the demands placed on unmedicated patients by the psychotherapists were actually toxic. The psychotherapy, on the other hand, had significant positive effects for patients who were receiving drug treatment. An even more elegant relationship is suggested by a study by Falloon and Liberman (1983). These authors found that patients who received a form of family therapy demonstrated better compliance with drug taking than those in a control group. This may explain why patients in family treatment appeared to require lower doses of neuroleptic. Taken together these findings indicate that during the outpatient phase of treating schizophrenia, patients are likely to benefit from psychosocial therapies or social skills training provided they have been adequately stabilized on drugs.

The art of treating chronic schizophrenia with drugs requires a recognition that drugs are potent forms of treatment that are severely limited. The best clinicians may be those who can set aside fantasies of cure or even dramatic change and accept that limited treatments, delivered to the right patient at the right time, and combined appropriately with other forms of treatment, can have important effects on a devastating illness.

REFERENCES

Anderson, C.M., Hogarty, G.E. and Reiss, D.J. (1980) Family treatment of adult schizophrenic patients: A psychoeducational aproach. *Schizophr. Bull.*, **6**, 490–505.

Baldessarini, R.J., Cohen, B.M. and Teicher, M.H. (1988) Significance of neuroleptic dose and plasma level in the pharmacological treatment of psychoses. *Arch. Gen. Psychiatry*, **45**, 79–90.

Carpenter, W.T., Heinrichs, D.W. and Hanlon, T.E. (1987) A comparative trial of pharma

cologic strategies in schizophrenia. *Am. J. Psychiatry*, **144**, 1466–70.

Cole, J.O. and Davis, J.M. (1969), Antipsychotic drugs. In *The Schizophrenic Syndrome*. L. Bellack and L. Loeb, (eds), Grune & Stratton, New York, pp. 478–568.

Davis, J. (1975) Overview: Maintenance therapy in psychiatry: I. Schizophrenia. *Am. J. Psychiatry*, **132**, 1237–45.

Falloon, I.R.H. and Liberman, R.P. (1983) Interactions between drug and psychosocial treatment of schizophrenia. *Schizophr. Bull.*, **9**, 543–54.

Gelenberg, A.J., Van Putten, T., Lavori, P.W. *et al.* (1989) Anticholinergic effects on memory: Benztropine versus amantadine. *J. Clin. Psychiatry*, **9**, 180–5.

Guze, B.H. and Baxter, L.R. Jr. (1985) Current concepts. Neuroleptic malignant syndrome. *N. Engl. J. Med.*, **18**, 163–6.

Herz, M.I., Glazer, W.M., Mostert, M.A. and Sheard, M.H. (1989) *Intermittent medication in schizophrenia after two years*. Presented at the Annual Meeting, American Psychiatric Assoc. San Francisco, CA.

Hogarty, G.E., Goldberg, S.C., Schooler, N. *et al.* (1974) Drug and sociotherapy in the aftercare of schizophrenic patients II. Two-year relapse rates. *Arch. Gen. Psychiatry*, **31**, 603–8.

Hogarty, G.E., Schooler, N. Ulrich, R.F. *et al.* (1979) Fluphenazine and social therapy in the aftercare of schizophrenic patients: relapse analysis of two year controlled study of fluphenazine decanoate and fluphenazine hydrochloride. *Arch. Gen. Psychiatry*, **36**, 1283–94.

Hogarty, G.E., Ulrich, R.F., Mussare, F. and Aristigueta, N. (1976) Drug discontinuation among long term, successfully maintained schizophrenic outpatients. *Pract. J. Psychiatry/Neurol.*, **9**, 494–503.

Johnson, D.A.W. (1984) Observations on the use of long-acting depot neuroleptic injections in the maintenance therapy of schizophrenia. *J. Clin. Psychiatry*, **5**, 13–21.

Johnson, D.A.W., Pasterksi, J.M. Ludlow, J.M. *et al.* (1983) The discontinuance of maintenance neuroleptic therapy in chronic schizophrenic patients: drug and social consequences. *Acta Psychiatr. Scand.*, **67**, 339–52.

Jolley, A.G., Hirsch, S.R., McRink, A. and

Manchanda, R. (1989) Trial of brief intermittent neuroleptic proxphylaxis for selected schizophrenic outpatients: clinical outcome at one year. *Br. Med. J.*, **298**, 985–90.

Kane, J.M. (1989) Schizophrenia: Somatic Treatment. In *Comprehensive Textbook of Psychiatry/ V.* H.I. Kaplan and B.J. Sadock (eds), Williams and Wilkins, Baltimore, pp. 777–92.

Kane, J.M., Honigfeld, G., Singer, J., Meltzer, H., and the Clozaril Collaborative Study Group (1988) Clozapine for the treatment-resistant schizophrenic: A double-blind comparison versus chlorpromazine/benztropine. *Arch. Gen. Psychiatry*, **45**, 789.

Kane, J.M., Rifkin, A., Woerner, M. *et al.* (1983) Low dose neuroleptic treatment of outpatient schizophrenics: I. Preliminary results for relapse rates. *Arch. Gen. Psychiatry* **40**, 893–6.

Marder, S.R. (1986) Depot Neuroleptics: Side effects and safety. *J. Clin. Psychopharmacol.*, **6**, 24S–29S.

Marder, S.R., Hubbard, J.W., Van Putten, T. and Midha, K.K. (1989) The pharmacokinetics of long-acting injectable neuroleptic drugs: Clinical implications. *Psychopharmacology*, **98**, 433–9.

Marder, S.R., Van Putten, T., Mintz, J. *et al.* (1987) Low and conventional dose maintenance therapy with fluphenazine decanoate: Two year outcome. *Arch. Gen. Psychiatry*, **44**, 518–21.

May, P.R.A. and Goldberg, S.C. (1978) Prediction of schizophrenic patients' response to pharmacotherapy. In *Psychopharmacology: A Generation of Progress*. M.A. Lipton, A. DiMascio and K.F. Killam (eds), Raven Press, New York, pp. 1139–53.

Neborsky, R., Janowsky, D. Munson, E. and Depry, D. (1981) Rapid treatment of acute psychotic symptoms with high- and low-dose haloperidol. Behavioral considerations. *Arch. Gen. Psychiatry*, **38**, 195–9.

Peroutka, S.J. and Snyder, S.H. (1980) Relationship of neuroleptic drug effects on brain dopamine, serotonin, alpha-adrenergic and histamine receptors to clinical potency. *Am. J. Psychiatry*, **137**, 1518–9.

Rifkin, A., Quitkin, F. and Klein, D.F. (1975) Akinesia: a poorly recognized drug induced extrapyramidal behavioral disorder. *Arch. Gen. Psychiatry*, **32**, 672–4.

Rosenbaum, K.M., Niven, R.G., Hanson, N.P. *et al.* (1977) Tardive dyskinesia: Relationship with primary affective disorder. *Dis. Nerv. Syst.*, **38**, 423–7.

Schooler, N.R., Levine, J., Severe, J.B. *et al.* (1980) Prevention of relapse in schizophrenia: An evaluation of fluphenazine decanoate. *Arch. Gen. Psychiatry*, **37**, 16–24.

Smith, J.M. and Baldessarini, R.J. (1980) Changes in prevalence, severity and recovery in tardive dyskinesia with age. *Arch. Gen. Psychiatry*, **37**, 1368–73.

Stahl, S.M. and Wets, K.M. (1988) Clinical pharmacology of schizophrenia. In *Schizophrenia: The Major Issues*. P. Bebbington and P. McGuffin (eds), Heinemann, Oxford, pp. 135–57.

Task Force Report — American Psychiatric Association (1980) Effects of antipsychotic drugs: tardive dyskinesia. *Am. J. Psychiatry*, **37**, 1163–71.

Van Putten, T. (1974) Why do schizophrenic patients refuse to take their drugs? *Arch. Gen. Psychiatry* **31**, 67–72.

Van Putten, T., Marder, S.R., Mintz, J. and Poland, R.E. (1989) Haloperidol plasma levels and clinical response: A therapeutic window relationship. In *Schizophrenia: Scientific Progress*. S.C. Schulz and C.A. Tamminga (eds), Oxford, New York, pp. 325–32.

Van Putten, T., May, P.R.A. and Marder, S.R. (1984) Akathisia with haloperidol and thiothixene. *Arch. Gen. Psychiatry*, **41**, 1036–9.

Chapter 20

Medication — compliance or alliance? A client-centred approach to increasing adherence

OLGA PIATKOWSKA and DOUG FARNILL

20.1 THE CONCEPT AND ETHICS

Therapists routinely expect compliance with treatment. 'Non-compliance' is often attributed to negative personality characteristics. However, the concept of 'compliance' ignores some of the client's rights, difficulties in taking medication, the therapist's responsibility for the interaction, and the possible disadvantages or limitations of treatments. Clients may decide not to 'comply' for many valid reasons, including their activities, values and other situational, social and environmental variables not always explored by health professionals. Research suggests that it is the latter variables, not general personality factors, which lead to non-adherence to medication (Peck and King, 1985). The implicit assumption that professionals are always right is contradicted by the evidence that large proportions of them do not fully carry out their responsibilities regarding patients' medications (Ley, 1982; Peck and King, 1985). In schizophrenia, for example, some studies show problems in prescribing, such as persistent prescription of doses which are no longer appropriate (Clark and Holden,

1987), and rapidly fluctuating over- or under-prescribing at times of organizational stress (Gouse, 1984).

More recent views are replacing 'compliance' with concepts such as 'consensual regimen' (Fink, 1976), 'therapeutic alliance', or at least 'adherence' to medication (a more neutral term). These concepts emphasize respect for patients' rights and needs for information, for two-way communications, and for a sense of control in the treatment situation. By incorporating the ethical ideals of choice, informed consent, mutual understanding and responsibility, these approaches overcome the ethical problems with 'compliance'.

In schizophrenia, the information processing difficulties, symptoms and behaviour problems often pose obstacles to clients' decision-making. There are frequent difficulties in obtaining 'informed consent' (Lidz *et al.*, 1984). A number of legal and clinical dilemmas are involved, such as society's needs for protection, as opposed to patients' rights. One dilemma is a legal ruling on rights to refuse medication even by those legally incarcerated (Appelbaum, 1988). Another is that informed consent can often only be given in the rational state, but in acute schizophrenia, the rational state can only be restored by neuroleptic medication itself. Yet the assumption that decisions by persons with schizophrenia not to take medication are irrational, needs to be further examined. These clients vary greatly in their rationality (Marder *et al.*, 1983) and in the factors which affect their autonomy.

20.2 DEFINING AND DETECTING NON-ADHERENCE TO MEDICATION

One problem in both estimating adherence and evaluating means of improving it, is the wide range of definitions and measures used in the studies (mostly with physically ill groups). Criteria vary from complete cessation or verbal refusal, to any significant deviation from the prescription, including dosage errors or failure to attend for appointments. Some studies used the number of units of medication taken in ratio to the number prescribed. Others used the percentage of patients judged to be 'compliant' according to various standards. 'Compliance' is too often measured by subjective reports or ratings by other patients, doctors or other health professionals, all of whom consistently overestimate the degree of adherence (Babiker, 1986). Clinical judgement has been shown to be a poor predictor of which patients will or will not adhere to medication (Ley, 1986).

The clinician who wishes to detect non-adherence can choose from a number of methods with varying advantages and drawbacks. Sackett (1979) outlines some simple initial steps: (a) identify the patients who have dropped out of treatment — this requires an effective system for 'keeping track' of those who miss appointments; (b) identify patients who have not reached the treatment goal; and (c) assess whether their regimen is vigorous enough to be effective. Then, to determine the sub-group who are not adhering, sympathetic questioning is of first importance, since those

who state they are not taking their medication are most likely to benefit from adherence-increasing strategies (Sackett, 1979). History of previous non-adherence is one useful indicator (Sackett, 1979). Patients should be asked about their feelings and attitudes toward the medication, and the obstacles to adherence that they may be experiencing, such as forgetting. Non-adherence may also be revealed when patients are asked for a description of the specific circumstances and sequence of behaviours when the patient last took the medication, or when they took it on a typical occasion.

If asking the patient is not satisfactory, the clinician may choose from 'indirect' or 'direct' methods of detecting non-adherence (Epstein and Cluss, 1982). Indirect methods include pill counts and reports from the family or significant others. Pill counts are subject to falsification and are best done unannounced, although 'spot checks' can jeopardize the therapeutic relationship. Indirect methods are not very reliable, but may initially suggest some patients who need further monitoring. Many authors, including Epstein and Cluss (1982) and Young *et al.* (1986) recommend more 'direct', objective measures of adherence.

(1) *Blood and serum assays*. These are reliable and accurate in assessing the blood concentration if the person has ingested the medication in the preceding several hours. However unless they are repeated frequently, they cannot determine degrees of usual adherence (Babiker, 1986). Wide individual variations in metabolism and a short assessment 'window' are some of the drawbacks of this method. Random checks are usually suggested.

(2) *Urine assays*. These are more practical, easily obtainable, and less intrusive than blood assays. They are also accurate for assessing recent drug ingestion, but somewhat less reliable than blood assays since they overestimate adherence to drugs with a long half-life, including most neuroleptics (Babiker, 1986).

(3) *Tracer and marker methods*. Substances can be included in the medication

to show traces of the drug, generally in the urine. However, there may be potential dangers in their long-term use (Young *et al.*, 1986).

(4) *Saliva measures*. Drug levels can be reliably measured in saliva, and patients readily accept this measure (Young *et al.*, 1986).

Of all of the 'direct' measures, Young *et al.*, recommend the urine radioreceptor assay, as having the 'ideal combination of sensitivity, specificity, range of application and ease of use' (p. 113). However, all the body-fluid analyses retain limitations in their availability, cost and revealing adherence only for several previous hours. Probably no one measure is sufficient for either research or clinical purposes, and none has replaced the value of a trusting relationship and empathic discussion with clients.

20.3 EXTENT OF NON-ADHERENCE TO MEDICATION

Surveys of the physically ill have shown fairly high rates of non-adherence to medications and other treatments. For example, Peck and King (1985) quote rates of 20–30% of patients not following short-term curative regimes for physical illness, with an average of 50% not adhering to long-term medications. Non-adherence increases the longer the patient is on medication. Consistent with these data, about 50% of chronic psychiatric patients do not take oral neuroleptics (Barofsky and Connelly, 1983). Even highly supervised inpatient settings cannot guarantee adherence (Van Putten *et al.*, 1984). However, averages are misleading, given a reported range of 10–76% non-adherence to oral medication in schizophrenia (Young *et al.*, 1986). This variation may be due to the wide range of definitions of 'non-compliance', to the varying settings in which it is assessed, or to differences within the client populations.

20.4 THE SIGNIFICANCE OF NON-ADHERENCE

Non-adherence is only a problem insofar as it contributes to relapses or poorer functioning or prevents symptom improvement. The effects of neuroleptics in schizophrenia are not all positive.

1. Limitations to the treatment response. Some major symptoms show little relief through neuroleptics. Negative symptoms generally are only partially relieved (Chapter 18). Also, the 'primary' negative symptoms, and the common symptoms of anxiety and depression may be induced or aggravated by neuroleptics (Falloon, 1984; Carpenter *et al.*, 1985). Overall community functioning does not improve in 40–60% of medicated patients (Wallace *et al.*, 1988). Furthermore while relapse rates clearly improve with neuroleptics (Chapter 18), the relationship between non-adherence to medication and schizophrenic relapse is far from perfect. Studies on psychosocial treatments report relapse rates in medicated control groups of 59–83% over two years (Chapter 23), although relapses are less severe if patients continue medication (Young *et al.*, 1986). Conversely, about 20% of patients with schizophrenia appear not to relapse even without maintenance medication (Lehmann *et al.*, 1983). It has now been demonstrated that psychosocial predictors of relapse are at least as powerful as medication adherence, particularly a high 'expressed emotion' environment (Chapter 8), a sign of stress in the family. Psychoeducational family interventions have greatly reduced relapse over 1–2 years (Chapter 23) and it has been found that in a high-stress family environment, medication has only limited protective effects (Falloon and Liberman, 1983).

2. Negative side effects. Phenothiazines often have detrimental side-effects such as drowsiness, apathy, and depression (Carpenter *et al.*, 1985), common extra-pyramidal effects such as akathisia and akinesia, and a risk of tardive dyskinesia (Chapter 18). Less obvious, but highly disturbing to patients, is the 'dysphoric response' (Van Putten *et al.*, 1984). All of these can interfere with rehabilitation and functioning.

The above considerations have led to the question of variations in neuroleptic response, and the predictability of such a response (Goldberg, 1980). A few studies have attempted to classify patients with schizophrenia according to drug responsiveness and to correlate this with other variables. For example, higher levels of information processing ability (Marder *et al.*, 1984; Asarnow *et al.*, 1988), and premorbid social functioning (Goldstein *et al.*, 1978) have been related to neuroleptic response. So also have some neuroendocrine and neurochemical measures (Brown and Herz, 1989), absence of an early dysphoric response and signs of early symptom relief (Hogan *et al.*, 1985). Half of the neuroleptic non-responders gradually withdrawn from drugs either improved or did not deteriorate (Brown and Herz, 1989).

The unclear relationship between adherence and clinical outcome may be due to the common confounding of sub-groups with different drug response. If these sub-groups could be identified, adherence would be important only for the group who respond and function better on neuroleptics. Those concerned about adherence in schizophrenia also have broader problems to consider such as the possibility of non-adherence often being an early symptom of relapse, and the common but often undetected ingestion of street drugs which aggravate symptoms (Ananth *et al.*, 1989). Non-adherence is only a part of the broader problem of long-term outcome and functioning. Psychosocial interventions should play at least as great a role in work with these clients as providing medication and facilitating adherence.

20.5 FACTORS RELATED TO MEDICATION ADHERENCE

A large number of studies have investigated the

relationship between medication adherence and other variables in physical illness. Some studies have also examined the outcome of attempts to increase adherence. Reviews of the literature are available in Sackett and Haynes (1976), Haynes *et al.* (1979), Baum *et al.* (1984), Peck and King (1985) and Meichenbaum and Turk (1987). Epstein and Cluss (1982), and Janis (1984) have discussed studies which attempted to improve medical adherence by changing some of the related variables, and Meichenbaum and Turk (1987) present a practical handbook based on the research literature. The rather meagre literature on medication adherence in schizophrenia has been summarized by Barofsky and Connelly (1983), Babiker (1986), and Young *et al.* (1986).

In this section, some reliance is placed on the results from treatment of physical illness. Haynes *et al.* (1979) used particularly high standards such as randomized trials, random selection and replicable definitions for selecting methodologically sound studies on which to base their conclusions including studies on schizophrenia. However no causation can be deduced, since most studies have been correlational. Nor do conclusions from physical illnesses necessarily apply to schizophrenia, although they may be valuable in describing high-risk groups of patients.

20.5.1 LIVING SITUATION AND FAMILY SUPPORT

A variety of socio-demographic variables have been examined in relation to adherence, with few results. Any relationship is probably mediated by accessibility to and usage of medical services (Haynes, 1976). The few variables associated with higher adherence rates are being married, having a stable family, and perceiving acceptance and support from the family. Clients with schizophrenia living in the community show greater adherence when they live with a concerned family or friend, and the medication is 'supervised' by that person (Barofsky and Connelly, 1983; McEvoy *et al.*, 1989b).

20.5.2 SYMPTOMATOLOGY AND SIDE EFFECTS

In physical disorders, previous episodes or hospitalizations, time of last attack and objective symptom severity do not appear to be related to treatment adherence (Haynes, 1979; Meichenbaum and Turk, 1987). In schizophrenia, symptoms such as anxiety, depression, paranoid ideas and grandiosity have been related to non-adherence (Young *et al.*, 1986), as have hostility or aggression and suspiciousness with thought disorder (Barofsky and Connelly, 1983). Confusion and forgetfulness, which are related directly to non-adherence in physical disorders (Ley, 1979), are also likely to apply in schizophrenia.

The data on the relationship between side-effects and adherence in schizophrenia appears equivocal (Haynes, 1979). One reason may be that patients who complain of side effects are removed from most studies (Barofsky and Connelly, 1983). However Van Putten *et al.*, (1984) claim that an early clear-cut dysphoric response was a nearly fool-proof predictor, not only of non-compliance but of refusal to try out any other antipsychotic drug. Extrapyramidal symptoms such as akathisia and akinesia also appeared to be related to early dysphoric response and to 'drug-reluctance' (Van Putten *et al.*, 1984). However, very broad criteria for 'drug reluctance' and lack of replications by others, limit their conclusions. Nonetheless, more recent authors suggest that side effects are a common reason for non-adherence in schizophrenia (Young *et al.*, 1986). There also appears to be support for a strong negative relationship between early dysphoric response and clinical outcome (Brown and Herz, 1989; Hogan *et al.*, 1985). At the same time, side effects tend to diappear with continuing adherence (Falloon, 1984).

These findings, together with psychological variables discussed below, suggest a complex, circular relationship between adherence and side effects. The degree of symptom relief felt by patients, their interpretation of any dysphoric side effects, knowledge of the long-term benefits and probably their faith in the doctor and the medication, may interact to establish initial adherence. If ongoing adherence reduces side effects, reasons for later non-adherence would be reduced and encourage a positive attitude to medication.

The pattern of relationships also suggests a sub-group in schizophrenia who experience low symptom relief and dysphoric response shortly after receiving neuroleptics, and have poor clinical outcome for neurochemical or non-adherence reasons. Non-adherence would seem a logical decision in the face of such experiences. However, this group may also have poorer information processing and premorbid social functioning (Asarnow *et al.*, 1988) — factors which would not aid adherence, and which probably indicate greater severity of disorder.

Insufficient attention has been paid to subtle internal responses in patients. With recent authors advocating closer attention to patients' reports of their experiences in schizophrenia (Strauss, 1989) and attempts to classify patients according to neuroleptic response (e.g. Asarnow *et al.*, 1988), further research on such subjective predictors seems a priority. For example, patients may not be able to explain dysphoric sensations or drug refusal to clinicians (Marder *et al.*, 1983), but their interpretation of the sensations or lack of relief may be a major determinant of adherence.

20.5.3 DRUG AND TREATMENT VARIABLES

The complexity of the regime and the degree of active behaviour change it requires appear to be related to non-adherence (Haynes, 1976). For example the duration of treatment is negatively correlated with adherence in both physical and mental illness (Haynes, 1976). In physical illness, the frequency of the medication is more often related to non-adherence than is the number of pills taken (Meichenbaum and Turk, 1987).

Some organizational features of treatment related to adherence are continuity of care (i.e. seeing the same therapist), short times before referral and appointment, brief waiting time in the clinic, pleasant atmosphere, regular contacts for supervision of medication, reminders about appointments or rapid follow-up if appointments are missed, and availability of staff in case of side effects (Haynes, 1976). Prospective studies show that increased supervision leads to improved medication adherence (Haynes, 1976).

The perceptual properties of medications have been investigated. Some results suggest that certain colours, larger size and capsule form were seen as more potent, and specific colours were associated with expected physical psychological effects, such as antidepressant or tranquillizing effects (Buckalew and Sallis, 1986).

Other factors of the treatment regime positively related to adherence in schizophrenia include inpatient status (Barofsky and Connelly, 1983), use of a therapy that is consistent with patient expectations (Barofsky and Connelly, 1983) and a vigorous outreach and follow-up programme (McEvoy et al., 1989b).

20.5.4 PATIENT ATTITUDES, BELIEFS AND BEHAVIOUR

In physical illnesses, adherence appears to be greater when patients accept the illness and perceive it as serious (Haynes, 1976). Patients who express a commitment to taking medication and continue to attend therapy also tend to show greater adherence (Haynes, 1976). Most of these factors are included in the 'Health Belief Model', which hypothesizes that individuals reach decisions on health actions based on their perceptions of the seriousness of the illness,

their susceptibility to it, and the benefits and costs of adherence (Becker, 1976). A modified model (Babiker, 1986; Meichenbaum and Turk, 1987; Cochran and Gitlin, 1988) includes further variables such as the patient–therapist relationship, social influence, the process of formulating perceptions, evaluation of care, the structure of the regime and degree of self-efficacy regarding one's ability to perform behaviours needed for adherence. The relevance of these rational processes remains to be tested for schizophrenia. Inaccurate self-reporting, low self-efficacy and problems in decision making (Babiker, 1986) are likely obstacles.

The concept of 'insight' has also been examined in schizophrenia. Some studies have related denial and illness severity to non-adherence (e.g. Nelson et al., 1975; Marder et al., 1983), but McEvoy et al. (1989b) did not find a significant relationship. Most of the studies have had small samples and inadequate measures of 'compliance' and 'insight' such as the Rorschach test (Nelson et al., 1975), the Global Assessment Scale (Bartko et al., 1988) or a single question on 'insight' (Axelrod and Wetzler, 1989). There are no validated measures for most of the factors involved in 'insight'. Attempts at validation have had severe limitations such as using ratings from open interviews of unknown validity and observed compliance as criterion measures for 'insight' (McEvoy et al., 1989a). The difficulties in defining the concept may be resolved by Greenfeld et al. (1989), who defined insight as including views about symptoms, the existence of an illness, aetiology, vulnerability to recurrence and the value of treatment. These are all relevant to the testing of the Health Belief Model and await the development of a reliable, valid measure.

Studies of the Health Belief Model usually show only modest positive relationships between perceptions, beliefs and behaviour (Meichenbaum and Turk, 1987). The relationship between the relevant beliefs and adherence is probably bi-directional, since prospective studies show a weaker correlation than retrospective ones (Becker, 1976; Haynes, 1976). Thus, medication adherence may precede rather than follow perceptions of the severity of disease. This finding is especially relevant to schizophrenia, since neuroleptics assist rational thinking. In the physical illness literature, some writers have found a positive correlation between cooperative behaviours in various aspects of treatment (Haynes, 1976). In schizophrenia, current adherence to medication is partly predicted by a history of non-adherence and failure to attend therapy (Barofsky and Connelly, 1983). However, so far there is insufficient evidence for general treatment 'cooperativeness' in schizophrenia. The correlations may point to a number of other variables such as illness severity and disorganization.

20.5.5 PATIENT–THERAPIST INTERACTIONS

The therapeutic engagement process involves a large number of possible interactions. Only a few guidelines are available as to which are the most significant for obtaining general treatment cooperation or medication adherence. In physical disorders, a consistent finding has been that patients' stated satisfaction with the therapist and clinic is correlated with adherence. Therapists' interpersonal skills, including listening, empathy and eye contact and their belief in the medication, were positively related to adherence (Meichenbaum and Turk, 1987), whereas socio-demographic or cultural differences between patient and therapist were negatively related (Haynes, 1976). Relationship variables such as liking and trusting the doctor also affected adherence, as did patients' participation in the treatment, including discussion of the patient's beliefs, concerns and expectations. Such variables would also increase therapists' influence on patient attitudes to treatment. Patients' interactions with the therapist, including the

process of formulating perceptions, therapist-influence and patient evaluation of the treatment are incorporated into the 'Theory of Reasoned Action' (Cochran and Gitlin, 1988), a more sophisticated model than the Health Belief Model. However the importance of each of these factors remains to be tested.

In psychiatric patients, the average rate of satisfaction with therapists' communications has been found to be 39%, which is similar to satisfaction rates in physical disorders (Ley, 1986). While satisfaction shows some relationship with adherence, the correlation is usually only 0.35 on average (Ley, 1986). In schizophrenia, there is some evidence that adherence is related to the therapist liking the patient and believing in the medication (Barofsky and Connelly, 1983), but this may represent increasing contact with patient. Unresponsiveness to patients' complaints about the side-effects may also be related to non-adherence in schizophrenia (Babiker, 1986).

20.5.6 INSTRUCTIONS AND EDUCATION

A distinction must be made between providing basic instructions about taking medication and broader education about the illness and treatment. Logically, understanding and remembering instructions on taking medication (or other treatments) is basic to being able to carry out the task. Yet even basic instructions often are not given in general health settings (Peck and King, 1985). Even when instructions are given, at least 50% of physically ill patients forget them immediately and frequently misinterpret even simple instructions such as 'take four times a day' (Ley, 1986). Understanding and memory for treatment instructions typically correlate about 0.30–0.34 with adherence (Ley, 1986).

Many studies have shown the most effective ways of communicating instructions to patients, including methods of presentation, providing written information and tailoring it to patients' understanding and circumstances (Ley, 1982).

However, improving information delivery has only a small effect on adherence. Thus, Ley (1986) states that a baseline rate of 52% adherence is increased to 66% by information-giving. Information will only increase adherence if the patient is not intentionally non-compliant and is not already adequately informed. Understanding and remembering instructions is necessary but not sufficient for improving adherence (Ley, 1986).

In physical disorders, 'education' about the illness and treatment has had little relation to compliance, in spite of patients' increased knowledge (Haynes, 1976; Epstein and Cluss, 1982). Similarly no association has been found between intelligence or education and adherence. However the variable quality of educational efforts must be taken into account. D'Onofrio (1988) reported that he had undertaken a re-analysis of Haynes' (1976) data on the basis of stricter criteria for good quality interactive-style education. D'Onofrio claimed that high quality efforts invariably succeeded in improving adherence, but did not report the relevant analyses. A number of papers recommend an interactive method of education rather than just a delivery of information. Meichenbaum and Turk (1987) summarize the requirements of interactive education, including a detailed exploration of beliefs, changing of attitudes and analysis of obstacles. The complexity of this process may explain why it is frequently not carried out. In turn, the apparent absence of effects for education may be explained by inadequate educational methods. In schizophrenia, Soskis (1978), Linden and Chaskel (1981) and Brown et al., (1987) found no relationship between instructions or knowledge of illness or treatment and adherence. Falloon (1984) claimed a relationship but this does not appear in his published evidence. Seltzer et al. (1980) claimed that information-giving improved adherence, but the results of the study were not conclusive because behavioural strategies were included in the same intervention. No well-designed study has shown

a relationship between education alone and adherence in schizophrenia (Hogan et al., 1983). Perhaps the most important point regarding education and adherence is that interoceptive cues are a far more powerful source of information than external sources (Hogan et al., 1983). This is particularly true for the strong, confusing internal experiences of schizophrenia and dysphoric sensations from medication. It remains to be investigated how external information can be made more powerful for patients with schizophrenia, and whether it can relieve distress. In physical disorders, for example, providing information specifically about relevant sensations tends to reduce the distress of symptoms and may accelerate recovery (Ley, 1982). Literature from many sources on 'health education' and behaviour change suggests that education should generally be supplemented by behaviour change and attitude change methods.

20.5.7 BEHAVIOURAL METHODS

Behavioural techniques offer promise for improving adherence. In physical disorders, behavioural methods appear to be more effective than education in increasing adherence (Epstein and Cluss, 1982). These methods include stimulus control techniques and self-control methods such as self-regulating dosages and self-monitoring symptoms and medication. The data suggest that self-control strategies are mainly helpful as adjuncts (Epstein and Cluss, 1982). Reinforcement methods such as contingency contracting have shown some promise (Gerber and Nehemkis, 1986), although methodological problems in some studies preclude firm conclusions (Epstein and Cluss, 1982). Feedback of drug levels which assists self-monitoring and provides reinforcement has also shown some tentative success (Epstein and Cluss, 1982). While behavioural techniques are often powerful, they need to be used in context. Some authors warn of the failures in application of behavioural techniques if patients' internal experiences, values in life, goals and wishes, their lifestyle and those of their support network, are not considered (Gerber and Nehemkis, 1986).

In schizophrenia, Boczkowski *et al.* (1985) carried out a controlled study of behavioural tailoring of the regime to personal routines, as well as self-monitoring. This approach was more effective than psychoeducation, but the small sample and the reliance on pill counts prohibit firm conclusions. The Seltzer *et al.* (1980) study included reinforcement for taking medication. While they used an objective test of adherence, other methodological problems precluded inferences about the impact of the behavioural component.

20.5.8 CRITIQUE OF STUDIES OF FACTORS IN ADHERENCE

Studies of schizophrenia that relate medication adherence to other factors show a number of methodological problems which tend to limit the conclusions. These include the following:

Dropouts. Subjects who drop out from the sample are not always counted within the results.

Definition of 'non-compliance'. The studies show a very wide range of definitions.

Assessment strategies. Measures of 'compliance' are often inadequate. Subjective reports or indirect measures (e.g. pill counts) are often used, in spite of their unreliability (Babiker, 1986). Studies rarely measure clinical outcomes, and measures of some factors that are correlated with adherence are often very inadequate (e.g. Nelson, 1975; Bartko *et al.*, 1988).

Adherence criteria. Many studies simply divide patients into 'compliers' vs. 'non-compliers' on an often arbitrary criterion (e.g. Hogan *et al.*, 1983). Virtually none appear to have related varying degrees of adherence to other variables.

Sample size. Many studies had samples that

were too small to allow adequate statistical power in making group comparisons (e.g. Boczkowski *et al.*, 1985).

Sample heterogeneity. The heterogeneity of patient samples probably masks many of the real relationships by the cancelling out of effects. Most studies obscured major differences, as in the sub-groupings in schizophrenia suggested by Goldberg (1980), Van Putten *et al.* (1984) Asarnow *et al.* (1988) and Brown and Herz (1989), which are probably relevant to both clinical outcome and adherence. Also, some studies included mixed or questionable diagnoses, so that the populations to which the results may be generalized are uncertain.

Confounding of predictor and outcome. Non-adherence to treatment may actually be one of the early signs of an impending relapse itself. Hence, even if cessation of medication precedes symptom relapse, causation cannot be concluded (Curson *et al.*, 1985).

Excessive reliance on cross-sectional designs. There are very few well-controlled prospective studies.

Size of effects. Correlations are almost always low. Even when a relationship is well established, each factor usually accounts for a very small proportion of the variance in adherence. For example, a correlation of 0.3 between 'insight' into illness and self-reported need for medication (McEvoy *et al.*, 1981) represents only 9% of the variance in adherence, which has dubious clinical value. A multiplicity of low correlations points to complex determinants and interactions, yet almost no studies have examined possible interactions. Such interactions might involve neuroleptic response, side effects, information processing and adherence. Complex relationships, together with inadequate control of relevant variables may account for many of the contradictory results.

Generalizability across disorders. Application of results from physical illness to schizophrenia remains uncertain, especially in view of the variable cognitive problems involved.

Failure to build on previous findings. Variables previously found to be related to adherence are rarely described or controlled (e.g. living situation, therapist-patient relationship). Such control to reduce pre-treatment subject variability is important in reducing contradictory results and refining knowledge of outcomes.

20.6 PRACTICAL IMPLICATIONS FOR CLINICIANS

The most comprehensive practical guidelines for clinicians on improving adherence in physical illness are provided by Meichenbaum and Turk (1987). Sackett (1979) also provides a brief summary of a sequence of strategies, relying on those outlined in Haynes *et al.* (1979). Diamond (1983) and Falloon (1984) offer practical strategies for increasing adherence from their clinical experience with schizophrenia, but they do not include extensive literature reviews.

The first, most important step is to establish a trusting relationship with the aim of working together to overcome the effects of the illness. It is the therapist's responsibility to maximize the factors which are conducive to a co-operative alliance. Since many clients will have a fluctuating course regardless of adherence, an important goal within this context is to increase the client's self-efficacy about self-management. The following guidelines describe some major steps required to form an alliance with clients with schizophrenia, and to work towards greater self-management, including medication adherence.

20.6.1 RELATIONSHIP

Establish a relationship of trust, empathy and mutual respect. Elicit and listen to clients' needs and goals in life, concerns, questions and fears about their illness, treatment and medications.

Meichenbaum and Turk (1987) provide a list of therapist behaviours which help to build a participatory, trusting relationship. Perhaps the essential point is to view the treatment situation from the client's standpoint: the helpless confusion of schizophrenia, the fear of change, the low self-efficacy, the dysphoric feelings from medication, the interference with lifestyle, the environmental stresses, and the payoffs for adhering to treatment. Ensure a thorough understanding of the roles and daily tasks demanded of the client and his/her circumstances and habits. Take time to allow the client to feel understood, and to gather information from various sources to find out the client's specific goals or valued activities. These are often not verbalized (Diamond, 1983), but may motivate clients to take medication, if this can facilitate goal attainment.

Allow clients the opportunity to participate in treatment decisions. Check their satisfaction with communications and remedy any problems such as appearing pessimistic about the client. It appears that many 'chronic' patients may make major improvements when they are treated with respect and faith in their capacity for change and are faced with clear choices and consequences (White, 1987).

20.6.2 SELF-REGULATION

Negotiate treatment goals with clients, relating these to their goals and valued activities. Explore a range of approaches to improving self-regulation and reducing relapse, particularly cognitive-behavioural self-management for clients and families (Piatkowska *et al.*, 1989). Within the context of family and self-management training, the client may be suitable for reduced or intermittent doses (Asarnow *et al.*, 1988; Chiles *et al.*, 1989) with regular monitoring of early relapse signs. Self-monitoring alone may be inadequate (Epstein and Cluss, 1982), so it should be embedded within a broader behavioural and family reinforcement approach with regular monitoring by the clinician. Clients and their families can often recognize precipitating stressors and early signs of relapse and take effective action by early help-seeking, stress management, or family support (Herz, 1984). Self-monitoring and medication should be presented as part of a plan of progress towards goals and self-control of symptoms. A number of symptom self-monitoring forms are in use (e.g. Falloon *et al.*, 1988; Piatkowska *et al.*, 1989). Clients' own methods for controlling their symptoms should be explored (Carr, 1988), reinforced and enhanced by teaching of additional methods. Diamond (1983) particularly emphasizes the need to 'look for realistic ways to allow the patient to take control' (p. 8), to explore in concrete detail how medication improves symptoms and desired activities, and to embed the regime in an overall rehabilitation programme to meet the patient's needs.

20.6.3 CONTINUITY AND EFFICIENCY OF FOLLOW-UP CARE

Ensure continuity of care, through providing the same therapist regularly, assertive follow-up, an easy transition from hospital to community care, short times between contacts, and convenient appointment times. Appointments should be arranged immediately, with telephone calls or cards as reminders. Presenting a rationale for attendance, clear instructions on how to get there, and asking about the client's expectations of treatment, should enhance attendance.

The service needs to be easily accessible and the staff available in case of side effects or other stresses. The clinic atmosphere should be friendly, and non-threatening. Avoid chaotic, crowded or depressing waiting rooms (Falloon, 1984) or lengthy waiting periods. If the client misses an appointment, prompt assertive follow-up through home visits is important. If appointments are repeatedly broken or the client is unwilling to be visited, an exploration of their reasons, fears and feeling is useful, together with problem solving. A family member or significant others may provide reminders or unobtrusive supervision without aversive nagging.

20.6.4 IDENTIFYING CLIENTS MOST PRONE TO RELAPSE

Clients most vulnerable to relapse in schizophrenia include those with poorer information processing or premorbid social functioning, early dysphoric responses, and particularly those experiencing high levels of stress in their family or other environment with low social support. Special attention is needed by this group, including psychoeducational family intervention and closely supervised rehabilitation programmes.

20.6.5 SIMPLIFYING AND TAILORING THE REGIME

The regime should be as simple as possible, to facilitate understanding and memory. Long-acting injections are simple and effective, increasing adherence to 80% (Falloon, 1984). However, some patients find them unacceptable, or develop excessive side effects. With oral medications, doses should be once daily unless there are good reasons otherwise (Diamond, 1983). The regime should be tailored to suit individual needs and characteristics, including adequate dosage for the person's weight, and allow for the person's sensitivities (e.g. allergies or fears of a specific side effect) or activities (e.g. outside sports). Questions about symptoms, adherence and side effects should be raised regularly and the regime should be responsive to the client's reactions. It is more likely to be followed if it is tailored to daily habits and needs, e.g. associating it with a meal or tooth-brushing. This stimulus control method is simple to apply, but may require a careful behaviour analysis to determine whether the person has regular habits that are appropriate to link with medication taking.

20.6.6 INSTRUCTIONS AND EDUCATION

The main steps in giving effective instructions include grouping statements together, stating the most essential point first, emphasizing its importance, speaking simply and avoiding jargon (Ley, 1982). Both clinician and client should repeat the instructions, check for understanding of even the simplest instructions and make specific, not general statements (e.g. 'Take two tablets straight after dinner' instead of 'Take the tablets with food'). The instructions are also more likely to be remembered if they are backed up with written instructions and easy-to-read labels. Educate patients about the rationale and expected benefits of the medication, when any changes may be felt, the possible consequences of not taking it, likely side-effects and what to do about these. The evidence suggests that participatory rather than didactic education, is much more likely to be effective. This includes exploring clients' knowledge, beliefs and fears about the illness, medication and side effects, and involving them in goal setting and decision making. Clinicians should explore patient expectations, probing for questions and concerns, discuss possible problems in medication taking and address ways of handling these. They need to provide reassurance, and teach patients how to implement the regime in their own circumstances. When clients are included in experimenting with medication and monitoring concurrent changes, they are more likely to see connections between medication taking or cessation and the effects on their feelings and behaviour (Diamond, 1983). The family or significant others generally should be involved in this educative process and be taught to support the client's learning and attempts at self-monitoring.

20.6.7 REDUCING FORGETFULNESS

Reminders and cues are useful behavioural methods if clients have problems with confusion or forgetting, Using daily routines as cues, prominent stickers, cards with instructions, or pictorial labels (e.g. clock faces with the appropriate time circled) can all be helpful, and there is now an increasing range of memory aids such as alarm watches and buzzing pill boxes. Personal reminders can also be effective if they are not aversive. Communication training for significant others may be needed to prevent 'nagging'.

20.6.8 COGNITIVE RESTRUCTURING

There has been little rigorous testing of cognitive methods of changing adherence, especially in schizophrenia. Since interoceptive cues such as dysphoric responses to neuroleptics may lead to non-adherence, efforts to reinterpret or restate the negative sensations are worth testing (e.g. 'this is a sign that the medication is working'). The questioning of negative beliefs and use of positive, realistic self-statements has been applied to clients with depression who were reluctant to take medication. Beck *et al.* (1979) provide a number of such examples. Reminder cards with any positive statements the client can make may be useful (e.g. 'the tablets help me to think clearly').

Training clients to notice success is important because of the low self-efficacy often associated with schizophrenia. The steps include eliciting and reinforcing successful efforts by the client such as attending a programme, or taking medication. They also include reinforcing attribution of the success to self rather than external circumstances, and eliciting clients' conclusions about themselves (Meichenbaum and Turk, 1987). It is essential to separate the symptoms and problems of schizophrenia from the person and reduce blame and labelling, by presenting schizophrenia as an objective, externalized stress against which therapist and client are aligned. It is essential to focus on and reward any successes by clients in overcoming symptoms, adhering to treatment and achieving steps towards their goals in spite of the obstacles that they encountered. Some clients may also be taught to reward themselves for successes or for thinking positive, realistic thoughts. Self-efficacy in coping with side effects may also facilitate adherence and may be increased through education and skills training (Falloon *et al.*, 1988).

The fact that clients have choices in behaviours should be highlighted and explored, as should the cumulative effects of choices over time. For example, clients may be asked to describe the consequences at times when they sought medication after detecting early symptoms, as opposed to family chaos when they ignored early signs. The long-term consequences of such choices can be made more immediate by a 'time collapsing' procedure (White, 1987), as part of a structured plan for progress. Language is an important factor in attitude change. The therapist should avoid labelling people as 'schizophrenics' since this stereotypes people with the illness. Instead, they should enhance clients' awareness of their own potential for change and for developing control (White, 1987).

20.6.9 SOCIAL SUPPORT

The family or significant others should be involved in education on the illness and treatment, negotiating goals, behaviour change, monitoring, reducing forgetfulness by non-aversive reminders, rewarding and contracting for adherence. Enhancing treatment cooperation and medication adherence thus becomes part of an educational and skills training programme for client and family. Chapter 23 reviews family psychoeducational approaches which may also be used with significant others. Hostel managers, clients living together, or other change agents may provide reinforcement for cooperation, and supervise medication taking. They may also accompany the client to programmes if necessary.

20.6.10 BEHAVIOURAL STRATEGIES

Self-monitoring of medication taking through ticks or tear-off calendar sheets provides feedback to clients. However its effects tend to be small unless it is accompanied by other strategies. Objective measures of adherence should be followed by feedback to the client. Reinforcement procedures have been used successfully in improving medication or programme adherence and appointment keeping. Some authors have used payments of money (Diamond, 1983), others used lottery tickets or response cost procedures such as loss of a deposit (Meichenbaum and Turk, 1987). Contracting is a powerful procedure which may be used by clinicians and significant others. Meichenbaum and Turk (1987) set out specific guidelines on contracting. Behavioural skills training in techniques of coping with side effects has been suggested by Falloon (1984). A recent study that taught skills such as identifying side effects, obtaining information and negotiating with therapists, showed a positive effect on adherence in schizophrenia (Eckman and Liberman, 1990).

20.7 MAINTAINING ADHERENCE AND INTEGRATING APPROACHES

A short-term increase in cooperation does not necessarily imply that it will be maintained. Adherence to medication often declines in the long term and additional strategies to maintain it are required. Continuing a long-term trusting relationship is central to the success of these strategies. Ongoing incentives include praise and material rewards which can be delivered by the therapist and family or by the client. Reminding clients about the benefits of treatment is important, along with ongoing self-monitoring and regular reviews of progress. Problems can be addressed by re-contracting and re-examining beliefs and attitudes that are interfering with continued adherence. Generally more than one strategy is required in order to increase cooperation. Haynes *et al.* (1979) recommend using a sequence of adherence-improving strategies beginning with the simplest and proceeding up the hierarchy until they are successful. Meichenbaum and Turk (1987) describe ways of integrating various adherence methods. Liberman's (1986) Medication Management Module, is an example of a programme which combines education with training in multiple skills relating to medication effects and communication with therapists. The programme has recently been shown to increase adherence from 60% to 79% at 3 months after training (Eckman and Liberman, 1990).

The following is a case example of integrated strategies. The therapist developed a relationship of trust over five years with Mrs A, a middle-aged lady with schizo-affective disorder, agitated anxiety and depression. Initially, multiple side effects caused Mrs A to cease medication. After a second episode the medication was changed, resulting in fewer side effects. She agreed to contract to take medication in return for temporary accommodation. However after months of feeling well, she again ceased medication and experienced a further relapse.

The therapist educated her about her illness, warning her honestly about likely further episodes. She helped Mrs A to identify her early signs of illness and its precipitating factors, to observe her own behaviours after ceasing medication as compared with when she was taking medication, and repeatedly discussed the consequences of not taking medication. She taught her to monitor the early symptoms and to detect the stresses that may be linked with them. After some months, Mrs A detected early signs of poor sleep, confused thoughts and exaggerated sensations which were precipitated by financial stresses and marital conflict. She requested help and received a temporary increase in medication, stress management plans, together with a referral for marital counselling. Since then she has been working

and functioning well for two and a half years.

This case highlights the gradual, often fluctuating course of educating the client in the context of continuity of care and a trusting, honest relationship. It also shows the value of the therapist's persistence and faith in the client's ability to work towards self-management. This approach and many of the practical suggestions outlined above, may require attitude change on the part of some therapists. Many therapists have been trained to attribute non-adherence or failures in therapy to supposed personality characteristics or 'chronicity' of the client, rather than re-examining their own methods, their relationship with the client, or the meaning of the treatment for the client. Such a re-examination, together with a more equal treatment alliance, is likely to yield significant benefits to clients.

ACKNOWLEDGEMENT

The case example was provided by Tina Philip, Clinical Nurse Specialist, Bateman's Bay Community Health Centre.

REFERENCES

Ananth, J., Vandewater, S., Kamal, M. *et al.* (1989) Missed diagnosis of substance abuse in psychiatric patients. *Hosp. Community Psychiatry*, **40**, 297–9.

Appelbaum, P.S. (1988) The right to refuse treatment with antipsychotic medications: Retrospect and prospect. *Am. J. Psychiatry*, **145**, 413–9.

Asarnow, R.F., Marder, S.R., Mintz, J. *et al.* (1988) Differential effect of low and conventional doses of fluphezanine on schizophrenic outpatients with good or poor information processing abilities. *Arch. Gen. Psychiatry*, **45**, 822–6.

Axelrod, S. and Wetzler, S. (1989) Factors associated with better compliance with psychiatric aftercare. *Hosp. Community Psychiatry*, **40**, 397–401.

Babiker, I.E. (1986) Noncompliance in schizophrenia. *Psychiatr. Dev.*, **4**, 329–37.

Barofsky, I. and Budson, R.D. (eds) (1983) *The Chronic Psychiatric Patient in the Community: Principles of Treatment.* S.P. Medical and Scientific, New York.

Barofsky, I. and Connelly, C.E. (1983) Problems in providing effective care for the chronic psychiatric patient. In *The Chronic Psychiatric Patient in the Community: Principles of Treatment.* I. Barofsky and R.D. Budson (eds), SP Medical and Scientific, New York, pp. 83–119.

Bartko, G., Herczeg, I. and Zador, G. (1988) Clinical symptomatology and drug compliance in schizophrenic patients. *Acta Psychiatr. Scand.*, **77**, 74–6.

Baum, A.R., Taylor, S.E. and Singer, J.E. (eds), (1984) *Handbook of Psychology and Health, Vol IV, Social Psychological Aspects of Health.* Lawrence Erlbaum, NJ, Hillsdale.

Beck, A.T., Rush, A.J., Shaw, B.F. and Emery, G. (1979) *Cognitive Therapy of Depression.* Guilford Press, New York.

Becker, M.H. (1976) Sociobehavioral determinants of compliance. In *Compliance with Therapeutic Regimens.* D.L. Sackett, and Haynes, R.B. (eds), Johns Hopkins University Press, Baltimore, pp. 40–50.

Boczkowski, J.A., Zeichner, A. and De Santo, N. (1985) Neuroleptic compliance among chronic schizophrenic outpatients: an intervention outcome report. *J. Consult. Clin. Psychol.*, **53**, 666–71.

Brown, C.S., Wright, R.G. and Christenson, D.B. (1987) Association between type of medication instruction and patients' knowledge, side effects and compliance. *Hosp. Community Psychiatry*, **38**, 55–60.

Brown, W.A. and Herz, L.R. (1989) Response to neuroleptic drugs as a device for classifying schizophrenia. *Schizophr. Bull.*, **15**, 123–8.

Buckalew, L.W. and Sallis, R.E. (1986) Patient compliance and medication perception. *J. Clin. Psychol.*, **42**, 49–53.

Carpenter, W.T., Heinrichs, D.W. and Alphs, L.D. (1985) Treatment of negative symptoms. *Schizophr. Bull.*, **11**, 441–52.

Carr, V. (1988) Patients' techniques for coping with schizophrenia: An exploratory study. *Br. J. Med. Psychol.*, **61**, 339–52.

Chiles, J.A., Sterchi, D., Hyde, T. and Herz, M.I. (1989) Intermittent medication for schizophrenic outpatients: Who is eligible? *Schizophr. Bull.*, **15**, 117–21.

Clark, A.F. and Holden, N.L. (1987) Persistence of prescribing habits: A survey and follow up of prescribing to chronic hospital in-patients. *Br. J. Psychiatry*, **150**, 88–91.

Cochran, S.D. and Gitlin, M.J. (1988) Attitudinal correlates of lithium compliance in bipolar affective disorders. *J. Nerv. Ment. Dis.*, **176**, 457–64.

Curson, D.A., Barnes, T.R.E., Bamber, R.W., Platt, S.D., Hirsch, S.R. and Duffy J.C. (1985) Long-term depot maintenance of chronic schizophrenic outpatients: The seven year follow-up of the Medical Research Council fluphenazine/placebo trial. *Br. J. Psychiatry*, **146**, 464–80.

Diamond, R.J. (1983) Enhancing medication use in schizophrenic patients. *J. Clin. Psychiatry*, **44**, 7–14.

D'Onofrio, C.N. (1988) Patient compliance and patient education: Some fundamental issues. In *Patient Education: An Inquiry into the State of the Art.* W.D. Squyres (ed), Springer-Verlag, NY pp. 271–9.

Eckman, T.A. and Liberman, R.P. (1990) A large-scale field test of a medication management skills training program for people with schizophrenia. *Psychosoc. Rehab. J.*, **13**, 31–5.

Epstein, L.H. and Cluss, P.A. (1982) A behavioural medicine perspective on adherence to long-term medical regimens. *J. Consult. Clin. Psychol.*, **50**, 950–71.

Falloon, I.R.H. and Liberman, R.P. (1983) Interactions between drug and psychosocial therapy in schizophrenia. *Schizophr. Bull.*, **9**, 543–54.

Falloon, I.R.H. (1984) Developing and maintaining adherence to long-term drug taking regimens. *Schizophr. Bull.*, **10**, 412–7.

Falloon, I.R.H., Mueser, K., Gingerich, S. *et al.* (1988) *Behavioural Family Therapy: A Workbook.* Buckingham Mental Health Service, Buckingham, UK.

Fink, D.L. (1976) Tailoring the consensual regimen. In *Compliance with Therapeutic Regimens.* D.L. Sackett and R.B. Haynes (eds), Johns Hopkins University Press, Baltimore, p. 115.

Gerber, K.E. and Nehemkis, A.M. (eds) (1986) *Compliance: The Dilemma of the Chronically Ill.* Springer-Verlag, New York.

Goldberg, S.C. (1980) Drug and psychosocial

therapy in schizophrenia: current status and research needs. *Schizophr. Bull.*, **6**, 117–21.

Goldstein, M.S., Rodnick, E.M., Evans, J.R. *et al.* (1978) Drugs and family therapy in the after-care of acute schizophrenics. *Arch. Gen. Psychiatry*, **35**, 1169–77.

Gouse, A.S. (1984) The effects of organisational stress on inpatient psychiatric medication patterns. *Am. J. Psychiatry*, **141**, 878–81.

Greenfeld, D., Strauss, J.S., Bowers, M.G. and Mandelkern, M. (1989) Insight and interpretation of illness in recovery from psychosis. *Schizophr. Bull.*, **15**, 245–52.

Haynes, R.B. (1976) A critical review of the 'determinants' of patient compliance with therapeutic regimens. In *Compliance with Therapeutic Regimens*. D.L. Sackett and R.B. Haynes (eds), Johns Hopkins University Press, Baltimore, pp. 26–39.

Haynes, R.B. (1979) Determinants of compliance: The disease and the mechanics of treatment. In *Compliance in Health Care*. R.B. Haynes, D.W. Taylor and D.L. Sackett (eds), Johns Hopkins University Press, Baltimore, pp. 49–62.

Haynes, R.B., Taylor, D.W. and Sackett, D.L. (eds) (1979) *Compliance in Health Care*. Johns Hopkins University Press, Baltimore.

Herz, M.I. (1984) Recognizing and preventing relapse in patients with schizophrenia. *Hosp. Community Psychiatry*, **35**, 344–9.

Hogan, T.P., Awad, A.G. and Eastwood, M.R. (1983) A self-report scale predictive of drug compliance in schizophrenics: Reliability and discriminative validity. *Psychol. Med.*, **13**, 177–83.

Hogan, T.P., Awad, A.G. and Eastwood, M.R. (1985) Early subjective response and prediction of outcome to neuroleptic drug therapy in schizophrenia. *Can. J. Psychiatry*, **30**, 246–8.

Janis, I.L. (1984) Improving adherence to medical recommendations: Prescriptive hypotheses derived from recent research in social psychology. In *Handbook of Psychology and Health, Vol IV: Social Psychological Aspects of Health*. A.R. Baum, S.E. Taylor and J.E. Singer (eds), Lawrence Erlbaum, Hillsdale, NJ, pp. 113–148.

Lehmann, H.E., Wilson, W.H. and Deutsch, M. (1983) Minimal maintenance medication: Effects of three dose schedules on relapse rates and symptoms in chronic schizophrenic outpatients.

Compr. Psychiatry, **24**, 293–301.

Ley, P. (1979) The psychology of compliance. In *Research in Psychology and Medicine*. D.J. Oborne, M.M. Gruneberg, and F.R. Eiser, (eds), Academic Press, London, pp. 187–195.

Ley, P. (1981) Professional non-compliance: A neglected problem. *Br. J. Clin. Psychol.*, **20**, 151–4.

Ley, P. (1982) Giving information to patients. In *Social Psychology and Behavioral Medicine*. J.R. Eiser (ed), Wiley, New York, p. 49–62.

Ley, P. (1986) *Obtaining Compliance in Medication Taking*. Lecture presented on May 16 at Manly District Hospital, Sydney.

Liberman, R.P. (1986) *Social and Independent Living Skills: Medication Management Module*. Rehabilitation Research and Training Center in Mental Illness, UCLA School of Medicine, California.

Lidz, C.W., Meisel, A., Zerubavel, E. *et al.* (1984) *Informed Consent: A Study of Decision Making in Psychiatry*. Guilford, New York.

Linden, M. and Chaskel, R. (1981) Information and consent in schizophrenic patients in long-term treatment. *Schizophr. Bull.*, **7**, 372–8.

McEvoy, J.P., Aland, J., Wilson, W.H. *et al.* (1981) Measuring chronic schizophrenic patients' attitudes toward their illness and treatment. *Hosp. Community Psychiatry*, **32**, 856–8.

McEvoy, J.P., Apperson, L.J., Appelbaum, P.S. *et al.* (1989a) Insight in schizophrenia. Its relationship to acute psychopathology. *J. Nerv. Ment. Dis.*, **177**, 43–7.

McEvoy, J.P., Freter, S., Everett, G. *et al.* (1989b) Insight and the clinical outcome of schizophrenic patients. *J. Nerv. Ment. Dis.*, **177**, 48–51.

Marder, S.R., Mebane, A., Chien, C. *et al.* (1983) A comparison of patients who refuse and consent to neuroleptic treatment. *Am. J. Psychiatry*, **140**, 470–2.

Marder, S.R., Asarnow, R.F. and Van Putten, T. (1984) Information processing and neuroleptic response in acute and stabilized schizophrenic patients. *Psychiatry Res.*, **13**, 41–9.

Meichenbaum, D. and Turk, D.C. (1987) *Facilitating Treatment Adherence: A Practitioner's Guidebook*. Plenum Press, New York.

Nelson, A.A., Gold, B.H., Hutchinson, R.A. and Benezra, E. (1975) Drug default among schizophrenic patients. *Am. J. Hosp. Pharm.*, **32**, 1237–42.

Peck, C.L. and King, N.J. (1985) Compliance and the doctor–patient relationship. *Curr. Ther.*, **26**, 46–52.

Piatkowska, O., Kavanagh, D.J., Manicavasagar, V. and O'Halloran, P. (1989) *Prevention of Relapse in Schizophrenia: Family Intervention Manual*. Department of Psychology, University of Sydney, Sydney.

Sackett, D.L. and Haynes, R.B. (eds) (1976) *Compliance with Therapeutic Regimens*. Johns Hopkins University Press, Baltimore.

Sackett, D.L. (1979) A compliance practicum for the busy practitioner. In *Compliance in Health Care*. R.B. Haynes, D.W. Taylor and D.L. Sackett (eds), Johns Hopkins University Press, Baltimore, pp. 286–294.

Seltzer, A., Roncari, I. and Garfinkel, P. (1980) Effect of patient education on medication compliance. *Can. J. Psychiatry*, **25**, 638–45.

Soskis, D.A. (1978) Schizophrenic and medical inpatients as informed drug consumers. *Arch. Gen. Psychiatry*, **35**, 645–7.

Strauss, J.S. (1989) Subjective experiences of schizophrenia: Toward a new dynamic psychiatry – II. *Schizophr. Bull.*, **15**, 179–87.

Van Putten, T., May, P.R.A. and Marder, S.R. (1984) Response to antipsychotic medication: The doctor's and the consumer's view. *Am. J. Psychiatry*, **141**, 16–9.

Wallace, C.J., Donahoe, C.P. and Boone, S.E. (1988) Schizophrenia. In *Pharmacological and Behavioral Treatment: An Integrative Approach*. M. Hersen, (ed), Wiley, New York.

White, M. (1987) Family therapy and schizophrenia: Addressing the 'in-the-corner' lifestyle. *Dulwich Centre Newsletter*, Spring, 14–21. Dulwich Centre, 345 Carrington St. Adelaide, South Australia.

Young, J.L., Zonana, H.V. and Shepler, L. (1986) Medication noncompliance in schizophrenia: Codification and update. *Bull. Am. Acad. Psychiatry Law*, **14**, 105–22.

355

Chapter 21

Psychological treatment of positive schizophrenic symptoms

NICHOLAS TARRIER

Despite major advances in pharmacological treatments there is considerable evidence that a significant number of sufferers of schizophrenia continue to experience psychotic symptoms, though possibly less severely than during their acute episode. For example, in a recent survey of all patients in a London psychiatric hospital Curson et al. (1988) found that just under half experienced delusions or hallucinations despite long standing and frequently 'energetic' pharmacological treatment. Results of community surveys indicate a similar picture. In a three-year follow-up study 47% of patients continued to experience psychotic symptoms (Harrow and Silverstein, 1977; Silverstein and Harrow, 1978) and in a seven-year follow-up study 23% of patients were found to have florid symptoms (Curson et al., 1985). Besides being extremely distressing in themselves and a frequent cause of anxiety and depression (Breier and Strauss, 1983; Tarrier, 1987), persistent symptoms also contribute to more general disabilities and handicaps (Falloon, 1986). There is also a high risk of suicide amongst patients experiencing persistent symptoms (Falloon and Talbot, 1981).

These studies provide compelling evidence for the need to formulate and evaluate psychologically-based treatment methods to be used as an adjunct to medication in the management of persistent and refractory psychotic symptoms. Besides being used in combination and as an adjunct to neuroleptics to treat residual psychotic symptoms there are occasions when psychological treatments could be used as an alternative to medication. An example is when severe and undesirable medication side effects, notably tardive dykinesia, develop or when patients refuse or poorly adhere to medication regimens (Baskett, 1983; Chapter 20). Furthermore, psychological treatments could be implemented in combination with minimal dosage and targeted-medication pharmacological programmes (Chapter 19). However, as yet little attention has been paid to investigating these latter possibilities. The purpose of this chapter is to examine the literature on psychological treatments of specific positive psychotic symptoms to evaluate whether such intervention strategies as mentioned above would be viable and warrant further investigation.

21.1 ASSESSMENT ISSUES

Before reviewing the treatment literature itself it is necessary to comment on some of the issues relating to the assessment of positive symptoms. This is important because it relates not only to the recognition and measurement of symptoms but also to the evaluation of outcome in treatment studies.

21.1.1 POSITIVE AND NEGATIVE SYMPTOMS

There has been extensive debate concerning the relationship between positive or florid symptoms and negative or deficit symptoms and their relationship to the schizophrenic illness (e.g. Crow, 1980; Andreasen, 1985). The focus in this chapter is upon the treatment of positive symptoms, however, patients with residual positive symptoms frequently also suffer negative symptoms and experience deficits in functioning. The situation is further compounded by the effects of neuroleptic drugs which can impair functioning especially when used in high doses. Patients experiencing persistent symptoms are more likely to receive high doses of medication and thus suffer such side effects (Falloon, 1986). The relationship between positive symptoms, negative symptoms, general deficits in functioning and the effects of medication is complex and has yet to be resolved. Although negative symptoms may be a result of an underlying schizophrenic psychopathology and exist in their own right, there is also the possibility that deficits in functioning, especially at an interpersonal and social level, are the result of, or exacerbated by, persistent delusions, hallucinations or thought interference. For example, social withdrawal may be a consequence of experiencing positive symptoms in social situations, and inactivity and avolition the result of a preoccupation with persistent symptoms. This possibility argues for the clear definition of symptoms and impairments and for the analysis of their covariation. Furthermore, assessment should not be restricted to specific impairments (i.e. symptoms) but should include multiple measures of broader and generalized disability

and handicap. In this way the functional relationship between measures of positive symptoms and these other measures may be elucidated. For further discussion see Harvey and Walker (1987) and for a psychological explanation of positive and negative symptoms see Frith (1987).

The relationship between positive symptoms themselves also appears unclear. For example, how are hallucinations and secondary delusional elaborations linked? What processes underlie primary (i.e. delusional perceptions) and secondary delusions (i.e. delusional explanations) and are they the same? At the present there are no satisfactory answers to these questions, there are few empirical data and a dearth of a rigorous psychological theory with which to conceptualize the problems. (For more extended discussion of the nature of hallucinations and delusions see Winters and Neale, 1983; Slade and Bentall, 1988; Oltmanns and Maher, 1988.)

21.1.2 THE BEHAVIOURIST'S DILEMMA

Traditionally behaviourists and behaviour therapists have had difficulty accommodating private events such as thoughts and beliefs, and the importance of the assessment and measurement of observable behaviours has been emphasized (e.g. see Nelson and Hayes, 1986). However, with schizophrenia, which is essentially a disorder of the experience of the disruption to thought and perceptual processes, the behaviour therapist is posed with the dilemma that the defining characteristics of the disorder are not available to public observation. There are a number of possible strategies to address this problem. For example, we could maintain that schizophrenia as an entity does not exist, or focus on a wide range of behaviours that are typical but not exclusive to schizophrenia or restrict our attention to a narrower range of behaviours which are thought to be correlated with the experiential symptoms. These latter two approaches are exemplified in Wallace's (1976) chapter on the assessment of psychotic behaviour in the second edition of Hersen and Bellack's *Behavioural Assessment* (1976).

Both these approaches have problems, focusing on a wide range of behaviours such as social skills and self-care skills which are important in their own right and may not directly reflect the presence of positive symptoms. Similarly, the assessment of the behavioural correlates of symptoms, such as the spontaneous emission of delusional talk or gestures and grimaces that are possibly associated with hallucinations, may not be a reliable measure of the patient's experience. Comparisons of the patient's subjective report of symptoms and observer ratings of behavioural correlates suggests poor reliability between these measures (Patterson *et al.*, 1976). Furthermore, any relationship between the patient's experience of symptoms and their spontaneous behavioural correlates may not be linear. This lack of concordance between experience and behaviour is especially true in contingency management treatment approaches where the use of rewards and punishments to modify overt behaviour may actually decrease this concordance.

Having accepted that the experience of hallucinations, delusions or thought interference are a legitimate focus of assessment and treatment the problem of measurement is still present.

21.2 MEASUREMENT

The problems of reliability and diagnostic validity are discussed elsewhere in this volume (Chapters 1, 2 and 10; Neale *et al.*, 1983). It is obviously necessary to be able to describe individual symptoms adequately, however this apparently simple task is fraught with major difficulties. Furthermore, the accurate definition and measurement of symptoms is mainly for the purpose of diagnosis or alternatively the monitoring of symptoms may be used to identify relapse, in which a marked

worsening of symptoms occurs. Much less interest has been given to monitoring symptoms because they are of interest in themselves. This has meant that issues of symptom assessment and measurement are not well developed. A number of methods are potentially of use and these are briefly reviewed below.

The Present State Examination (Wing *et al.*, 1974) includes a scoring system which involves a judgement on whether the symptom is present or not, and if so a rating of either 1 or 2 is given depending on severity. Such a narrow range of measurement is not suitable for assessing the variation in any symptom. However, Tress *et al.* (1987) have produced a scale of PSE change scores which greatly assists the re-assessment of symptoms. This consists of an 8-point scale (0 to 7) where 4 indicates no change, 5 to 7 an increasing worsening, 3 to 1 an increasing improvement and 0 indicates that the symptom has completely remitted.

The BPRS, Brief Psychiatric Rating Scale, (Overall and Gorham, 1962; Lukoff *et al.*, 1986) in its latest version consists of 18 items. Each item is rated on a 1 to 7 scale increasing with severity. Those items of greatest importance for assessing symptomatology are: hallucinations, unusual thought content (including delusions) and conceptual incoherence. The Comprehensive Psychopathological Rating Scale (Asberg *et al.*, 1978) covers a wide range of symptomatology. Items are rated on a 4-point scale (0 to 3) increasing with severity. The rating of idiosyncratic individual symptoms has been used in a number of studies, including a 100-point scale (May, 1980) and a 1 to 7 point scale similar to the BPRS (Falloon *et al.*, 1984). For a more detailed review see Lukoff *et al.* (1986).

In a series of papers Garety and her colleagues (Garety, 1985; Brett-Jones *et al.*, 1987) have discussed the problems in measuring delusions. They have criticized the tendency in modern psychiatry to regard delusions as an all-or-none phenomena principally important in diagnosis. These workers have assessed delusions by taking into account their complexity and multidimensional nature, especially in relation to the properties of intensity and fixity of the delusional belief (Garety, 1985). Brett-Jones *et al.* (1987) describe a delusional rating scale which consists of three ordinal scales: conviction (a 6-point scale); preoccupation (a 6-point scale) and interference (a 4-point scale); and two categorical measures: reaction to hypothetical contradiction and accommodation of the delusional belief to contradiction. Interestingly they report that there was little correlation between the different measures. In a similar vein, Kendler *et al.* (1983) suggested five important dimensions to delusions: conviction, extent, disorganization, preoccupation and bizarreness. All except the last had good interobserver reliability. They also found that the intercorrelations between the different dimensions were uniformly low. The low correlations between these different dimensions emphasizes the need for multidimensional assessment. Other workers have also attempted to measure different aspects of delusions such as: the subjects' control over the sypmtoms (Fowler and Morley, 1989), the strength of belief (Watts *et al.*, 1973; Hole *et al.*, 1979; Alford, 1986; Fowler and Morley, 1989), encapsulation (Hole *et al.*, 1979) and emotional distress caused by the symptom (Tarrier, 1987; Fowler and Morley, 1989).

Similar difficulties are encountered in the assessment of hallucinations. Junginger and Frame (1985) describe five characteristics of auditory hallucinations which can be measured using analogue scales. These were frequency, loudness, clarity, location and reality. Subjects experienced some difficulty assessing the reality dimension and the reliability of this parameter was lower than the other four.

These are much-needed attempts at a multidimensional assessment of psychotic phenomena. However, these ratings of different dimensions are still largely dependent on patient self-report. Although self-report is clearly of clinical importance, future research should also be directed at more objective methods of assessment. For example, laboratory-based methods have been used to assess reality testing (e.g. Bentall and Slade, 1985; Johnson and Raye, 1981) and although these methods have more frequently attempted to measure dispositional traits they could potentially be applied to the assessment of symptom variation and clinical status. An innovative attempt to objectively detect hallucinations was reported by Gould (1948). Following the suggestion that hallucinations may be the result of covert speech he measured the EMGs of subjects' lips and chin. There was an increase in EMG activity in a far higher percentage of hallucinating subjects than in control subjects. Following a similar line of enquiry, Green and Preston (1981) report on a case in which throat microphones were used to amplify the unintelligible utterings of a patient suffering from auditory hallucinations. The content of these vocalizations corresponded with what the voices were reported to say. It is unclear whether this finding would generalize to all schizophrenic patients experiencing auditory hallucinations or how hallucinations in other sensory modalities could be explained.

Delusions and hallucinations can be understood in terms of faults in the cognitive process of reality testing (Spaulding *et al.*, 1986). A closer understanding of the cognitive processes involved in this activity is clearly required. Hemsley and Garety (1986) have argued that an understanding of the testing of normal beliefs would provide a normative model against which a deviation could be used to assess abnormal beliefs. The challenge to experimental cognitive psychology is to produce theoretical models of such processes that have an assessment and treatment utility.

The comprehensive assessment of psychotic phenomena is at the present in its infancy and research efforts need to be channelled into producing multidimensional assessment methods. Not only will this provide important measures for assessing the evolution and treatment of symptoms but it may also provide information about the elusive nature of psychotic experience.

21.2.1 COGNITIVE BEHAVIOURAL ASSESSMENT

The aims of a cognitive–behavioural assessment are to elucidate the determinants of symptom occurrence in terms of their antecedent conditions and consequences. The rationale here is that although psychotic symptoms may have a biological origin, their occurrence and maintenance may be determined by environmental factors such as increased levels of stress or over-stimulation, or the patient's ability to cope with the symptoms, or the resulting distress. A number of studies have used such an analysis to investigate the contingencies surrounding persistent psychotic symptoms with a view to a better understanding of their maintenance and hence management. Falloon and Talbot (1981) investigated strategies used by 40 chronic schizophrenic outpatients to cope with auditory hallucinations. A wide range of coping methods were reported which were classified into three categories: (a) behavioural, (b) sensory/affective, and (c) cognitive. The three most cited first choice strategies were increased interpersonal contact, relaxation or sleep and reduced attention to the hallucinations. These accounted for two-thirds of the strategies considered to be effective by the better adapted patients. However, these strategies were also used more often by poorly adapted patients. Patients who were least handicapped by their symptoms used fewer coping strategies but found specific methods that proved effective for them. They appeared to apply these strategies more consistently and had a greater understanding of the discriminative stimuli associated with symptom onset. In a similar study, Tarrier (1987) used a semi-structured interview to assess identifiable antecedents, the emotional or disruptive

consequences of residual delusions or hallucinations and the presence and effectiveness of any coping strategies in 25 schizophrenic out-patients. Fifty-two per cent of patients reported that they could identify antecedent stimuli to the onset of their symptoms and 92% reported that their symptoms were distressing or had unpleasant consequences for them. Coping strategies were reported as being used by 72% of the sample and could be categorized as (a) cognitive, (b) behavioural, (c) sensory and (d) physiological. A surprising result was that, contrary to the findings of Falloon and Talbot (1981), there did not appear to be an association between the success of coping and the identification of antecedents. Patients who did report their coping strategies as more effective were more likely to use multiple strategies. However, the vast majority of coping strategies were at best only moderately successful.

Breier and Strauss (1983) investigated the coping methods of 20 patients within a self-control framework. This refers to a closed loop model of self-control consisting of three phases: self-monitoring, self-evaluation and self-reinforcement (Kanfer, 1980). All patients were suffering from psychotic illness and just over half were diagnosed as schizophrenic or schizoaffective. Seventeen patients (85%) reported that they attempted to control their symptoms and all of them described a capacity to observe behaviour in themselves that they considered to antecede psychotic symptoms. Three main coping stategies were used: self-instruction, decreased involvement in activity and increased involvement in activity. The use of the latter two strategies appears contradictory at first sight but agrees with the findings of Tarrier (1987) who found that patients did report the use of these different strategies. Presumably a decrease in activity or withdrawal serves a stress or arousal decreasing function, whereas increasing activity levels serves as a distraction or increases the number of stimuli competing with the psychotic phenomena.

360

These results were supported by a brief report by Kanas and Barr (1984), except that they found self-instruction less common. These self-control studies appear to support Falloon and Talbot's assertion that patients need to be able to monitor their symptoms and the conditions under which they occur to successfully bring them under control. It also suggests that the patient's amount of insight into their illness is an important factor.

Two other studies have also investigated coping strategies in schizophrenic patients, but they have examined coping with both psychotic and non-pyschotic symptomatology (Cohen and Berk, 1985; Carr, 1988). This makes direct comparisons with the previous studies difficult.

Brenner and his colleagues have adopted a different approach (e.g. Brenner *et al.*, 1987) and investigated patients' ability to cope with subjectively experienced attentional dysfunctions (termed basic disorders). These basic disorders derive from disorders of information processing and it is hypothesized that they can develop into psychotic symptomatology. These authors report that 75% of patients make coping efforts. Basic disorders are not unique to schizophrenic patients however, and are also reported in a neurotic and normal control sample, albeit at a lower frequency.

Comparisons of these studies are hampered by the use of varying methodologies and different classifications of coping. Notwithstanding these problems it appears well established that patients do use various methods to cope with their symptoms and there is general agreement that coping strategies could have great importance in symptom management. Studies using a coping strategy approach to treatment will be discussed later.

21.3 TREATMENT

This section will review the literature on psychological treatment methods. The majority of studies, with a few exceptions, contain treatment methods derived from general psychological theories applied to clinical problems rather than being directly formulated from specific psychological theories of schizophrenic psychopathology. Furthermore, there is a dearth of group controlled studies with the majority of published reports describing uncontrolled comparisons or single cases. This fact must clearly limit the generalizability of any positive results. The studies will be categorized within the general approach that characterizes the treatment method.

21.3.1 CONTINGENCY MANAGEMENT

The success of manipulating external contingencies in decreasing maladaptive behaviours and increasing a wide range of appropriate and adaptive behaviours through token economy programmes is well known (e.g. Paul and Lentz, 1977). Operant methods have also been used to modify psychotic symptoms or at least their behavioural expression. Early laboratory attempts to bring such behaviour under control were disappointing (Lindsley, 1963). Subsequent studies usually carried out in psychiatric institutions were more successful. Ayllon and Haughton (1964) used the reactions of ward staff to modify their symptomatic verbal behaviour in three patients. It was demonstrated that both psychotic and non-psychotic talk could be increased or decreased depending on contingent social reinforcement. A subsequent anecdotal report supported these results and also suggested that improvements could be long lasting (Kennedy, 1964). However, Liberman *et al.* (1973) reported on four well-controlled case studies in which a multiple baseline design was used. Although 200 to 600% increases in rational speech were produced, delusional talk was not completely eliminated. There was also a considerable increase in delusional talk when conversation focused on topics that were more likely to evoke the patients' delusions. Furthermore, there was little evidence of generalization to other settings. Similarly, Bulow *et al.* (1979) manipulated social contingencies and decreased, but did not eliminate delusional verbalizations. However the effect was not resistant to extinction. Davis *et al.* (1976) used a time-out procedure to reduce delusional and hallucinatory speech in a chronic schizophrenic patient, but there was poor generalization and inappropriate speech returned to baseline as time-out was faded out.

Interference of hallucinatory behaviour through social engagement has been demonstrated to eliminate such behaviour, but the effect is short lived (Alford and Turner, 1976; Turner *et al.* 1977; Alford *et al.*, 1982).

Turner *et al.* (1977) reported that successful and stable elimination of hallucinatory behaviour could be produced by faradic aversive conditioning. However, other reports had failed to produce similar results (Butcher and Fabricatore, 1970; Anderson and Alport, 1974). Weingaertner (1971) carried out a controlled study of the efficacy of self-administered shock contingent on the onset of symptoms. Although patients improved there was no superiority of this treatment over placebo and no treatment. Fonagy and Slade (1982) investigated the relative efficacy of punishment and negative reinforcement on hallucinations in three schizophrenic patients. They presented white noise either following the hallucination or during the hallucination. Since patients indicated when they were hallucinating, the procedure included aspects of self-monitoring. At least two patients showed considerable decreases in the time hallucinating and improvement appeared to be maintained. Negative reinforcement appeared more effective than punishment. Belcher (1988) reported the success of a mild aversive contingency programme (exercise) in reducing aggressive hallucinatory behaviour. Treatment gains were maintained at 12 months.

The literature on contingency management is somewhat equivocal and has a number of difficulties. First, the evidence suggests that although delusional and hallucinatory behaviour can be reduced by changing the contingencies, these changes are not resistant to extinction. Whereas it may be possible to control contingencies within an institutional setting this is much more difficult, if not impossible, within a community setting. Second, there is little evidence that generalization occurs across settings. This provides a similar difficulty for community management as does the lack of resistance to extinction. Even if it were possible to manipulate contingencies in one part of the patient's environment, there is little to suggest any benefit would transfer to other aspects. Third, because manipulations have focused on the behavioural correlates of hallucinations and delusions there is no guarantee that a successful reduction of the behaviour also decreases the experience of hallucinations or delusions. In effect the patient has learnt not to talk about the symptoms. Finally, since many of the contingency management programmes were designed for a chronic institutionalized population, they may not be appropriate outside of that setting. It is possible that the natural contingencies operating in such institutions encourage much of the 'mad' behaviour in the first place, so rearranging the contingenices merely reduces the situational or artificial 'mad' behaviour and would be ineffective with true residual symptoms. Although the evidence suggests that contingency management alone would not be suitable for the treatment of residual psychotic symptoms it is probably an important part of all treatment programmes.

21.4 STIMULUS CONTROL

A number of studies have focused on the role of antecedents in maintaining psychotic symptoms. Slade (1972) reported a case study in which a patient's hallucinations were experienced in situations in which he found anxiety provoking or arousing. The patient was then successfully treated with systematic desensitization (SD) to reduce the situational anxiety, and there was a concomitant reduction in hallucinations. In a second report SD failed to result in a reduction of the frequency of hallucinations, however subsequent treatment with *in vivo* desensitization was successful (Slade, 1973). The author suggests that the initial failure of SD in this case study was due to the patient's inability to accurately identify high levels of internal arousal. Two points are salient here: first, successful symptom control requires the accurate identification of the antecedents (see above); second, there may be a low correlation between physiological states of arousal and the patient's self-report. This latter point has been demonstrated empirically (Tarrier *et al.*, 1988). Such poor discrimination of internal stimuli is not exclusive to schizophrenic patients and may be rectified through further training of the patient in discrimination of internal arousal cues or through emphasis on situational control.

In a frequently cited study, Nydegger (1972) reported the case of a young inpatient diagnosed as suffering from paranoid schizophrenia. The patient reported experiencing visual and auditory hallucinations, had paranoid ideation and was passive and withdrawn. An analysis of the situations in which the symptoms occurred and the implementation of assertive training and verbal conditioning procedures resulted in a cessation of symptom-related behaviour within two months and no recurrence within two years. However, it appeared as though the patient's verbal behaviour, that is reporting symptoms as being present, may have had a functional value in avoiding difficult or stressful situations. Hence it is difficult to ascertain whether these interventions reduced actual symptoms or their report. Moreover, a report by Serber and Nelson (1971) failed to demonstrate any benefits of SD and assertion training in a group of 24 hospitalized schizophrenic patients. Watts *et al.* (1973) also found relaxation and *in vivo* desensitization to be ineffective in reducing the strength of patient's delusional beliefs.

21.4.1 CONTROL OF AUDITORY INPUT

An integral part of a number of theories of auditory hallucinations has been the relationship between external (physical) stimuli and the perception of internal (mental) phenomena (e.g. West, 1962; Horowitz, 1975; Slade, 1976). Feder (1982) predicted from these theories that increased external stimuli would decrease auditory hallucinations. This prediction receives some support from two sources: a study on the manipulation of auditory input (Margo *et al.*, 1981) and the use of increases in sensory (auditory) input as a coping strategy (Tarrier, 1987). In a case study, Feder (1982) reported that auditory hallucinations were dramatically reduced when the patient listened to the radio through stereo headphones. However, only temporary success using a similar method was reported by Morley (1987).

Green *et al.* (1983) advanced the theory that due to a primary dissociation in function of the cerebral hemispheres any verbal activity in the non-dominant hemisphere would be perceived as alien by the dominant hemisphere. A prediction from this theory would be that, a reduction in auditory input to the non-dominant hemisphere and an increase in incompatible (dominant hemisphere) verbalizations should disrupt hallucinations (Birchwood, 1986). A number of case studies have used earplugs to reduce auditory input in the non-dominant side in conjunction with the patient naming objects in their environment as an incompatible activity (Green *et al.*, 1979; James, 1983; Birchwood, 1986; Morley, 1987). These case studies have demonstrated a decrease in auditory hallucinations, but whether the mechanisms support Green *et al.*'s theory is less clear. Following from Birchwood's prediction, one test of the theory would be to increase the auditory input to the non-dominant hemisphere by means of a hearing aid or similar device and demonstrate an increase in hallucinations. This has yet to be done.

21.4.2 BIOFEEDBACK

Biofeedback has rarely been used with schizophrenic patients, however Schneider and Pope (1982) report on an intriguing use of EEG biofeedback. They attempted to effect changes in the EEGs of nine schizophrenic patients similar to those associated with neuroleptic-induced clinical improvement. Significant within-session changes were observed but there were no session-to-session changes. Unfortunately no assessments were made of any dimension of psychopathology so it is impossible to assess the clinical utility of such a procedure.

21.4.3 COGNITIVE MODIFICATION

21.4.3.1 Self-instructional training (SIT)

Meichenbaum observed that a number of schizophrenic patients instructed themselves to emit 'healthy talk'. This has been confirmed by a number of studies investigating the use of coping strategies (Falloon and Talbot, 1981; Breier and Strauss, 1983; Tarrier, 1987). Meichenbaum later synthesized this serendipitous observation into a training procedure, self-instructional training (SIT) (Meichenbaum and Cameron, 1973). In this procedure patients learn to evaluate the demands of a task, focus their attention on the relevant demands, apply self-instruction in the form of self-guidance whilst performing the task and use self-reinforcement to maintain task performance. In a series of experiments, Meichenbaum and Cameron (1973) demonstrated that SIT procedures improved the performance of hospitalized patients on a number of tasks and also reduced the amount of 'sick' talk. These results were supported by a report of two case studies (Meyers *et al.*, 1976). However, other researchers have failed to replicate these findings (Margolis and Shemberg, 1976; Gresen, 1974). Bentall *et al.* (1987) demonstrated that SIT did improve task per-

formance in chronic inpatients compared with controls, but there was little generalization to other tasks unless they closely resembled the training task. Furthermore, SIT did not prove superior to general problem solving.

21.4.3.2 Belief modification

Cognitive therapy methods, in which the patient's thoughts and beliefs are thought to underlie the disorder, have now been developed for a wide range of psychiatric conditions (Hawton *et al.*, 1989). These methods typically focus not on confronting the belief itself but on the evidence on which it is based. Although Beck is well known for developing these methods in depression he also described an early case study in which cognitive therapy was successfully used to treat delusions in a chronic schizophrenic patient (Beck, 1952). A similar approach was adapted by Watts *et al.* (1973). In a series of controlled case studies they demonstrated that belief modification significantly reduced the strength of the abnormal belief in less than six hours of treatment, whereas relaxation and *in vivo* desensitization to social situations had little effect. In this treatment approach, Watts and his colleagues avoided the direct confrontation of the abnormal belief, since they reasoned that this might maintain or even increase the strength of the belief (they termed this process, 'psychological reactance'). To test this hypothesis, Milton *et al.* (1978) performed a small controlled trial of confrontation versus belief modification. Both treatments produced improvements, but at six week follow-up those of the belief modification group were significantly greater. There was also evidence that confrontation did result in psychological reactance in some patients and their symptoms worsened. Changes in BPRS scores and social anxiety were less clear cut.

The use of cognitive therapy to treat eight patients in an uncontrolled study is described by Hole *et al.* (1979). Of these eight patients, four showed only slight improvements in delusional conviction and pervasiveness, while two had moderate improvement and two showed marked improvement. Hartman and Cashman (1983) report in three cases in which cognitive therapy was used to reduce delusional thinking. The results are equivocal and there is doubt whether these patients would receive a diagnosis of schizophrenia. Alford (1986) in a well-controlled case study demonstrated decreases in frequency and strength of delusional belief in a schizophrenic patient. Chadwick and Lowe (1990) used a multiple baseline design to demonstrate the efficacy of verbal challenge and reality testing. In three patients who received a verbal challenge alone, two showed marked decreases on conviction in the delusional belief. Reality testing markedly decreased conviction in two other patients who had not responded to verbal challenge and moderately reduced it in a third. There were considerable decreases in preoccupation with the delusions in four patients and a similar reduction in anxiety in the five patients who experienced it. These improvements were largely maintained at six-month follow-up.

The technique of belief modification would appear promising and it is a pity that the initial research of Beck (1952), Watts *et al.* (1973), and Milton *et al.* (1978) has not stimulated more extensive research.

21.4.3.3 Modification of cognitive processes

In schizophrenia disorders of cognitive processing are taken to mean deficits in attention, discrimination, information processing and retrieval. Since schizophrenia is frequently considered a disorder of cognitive processes a logical treatment approach is to modify these processes. A distinction is made between an approach that attempts to address cognitive deficits and cognitive therapy (Adams *et al.*, 1981). The latter is characterized by attempts to modify conscious thoughts and beliefs,

although the distinction between the two is now becoming much less clear cut (Brewin, 1988; Ingham, 1986).

A considerable amount has been written, (especially in the American and German literature) about the potential for treating the cognitive or basic disorders which are thought to underlie schizophrenia (e.g. Spaulding *et al.*, 1986; Magaro *et al.*, 1986; Gross, 1986; Brenner, 1986). However this literature does not seem to have generated many treatment studies. Although it is eminently plausible that disorders of attention and information processing result in the characteristic symptoms of schizophrenia, it is not at all clear how this would happen or what mechanisms would be involved. The lack of progress in producing such explanations probably indicates that the relationship between cognitive processes and experiential symptoms is very complex. Furthermore, it is difficult to demonstrate that poor performance on cognitive tests is not a result of generalized schizophrenic deficits rather than an index of underlying processes (i.e. a consequence rather than a cause). The large body of knowledge on information processing has yet to exert considerable clinical influence.

Treatment approaches that utilize training in cognitive tasks to rectify basic deficits need to show that such training reduces symptoms as well as improving task performance. Olbrich and Mussgay (1988) demonstrated improvements in some cognitive functions in an experimental group compared with a control group. However, there was no indication that this treatment was decreasing psychopathology or ameliorating symptoms or that any group differences could not be explained by a non-specific training effect. Adams *et al.* (1981) reported a case study in which a multifaceted programme aimed to improve the patient's attentional skills. Performance on a number of cognitive tasks increased over treatment and there was also a dramatic increase in the self-reported frequency of 'crazy thoughts'. This improvement was maintained at six-month follow-up. In a series of studies carried out by Brenner and his colleagues in Bern (Brenner *et al.*, 1990) a treatment programme which integrated training in cognitive, communication and social skills has been evaluated. Patients showed significant improvements on a variety of psychological tests and on measures of general psychopathology when they were compared with placebo and control groups. These improvements were maintained at 18 months. However, in the previous studies there were serious methodological problems in establishing treatment processes.

21.5 SELF-MANAGEMENT

A number of studies have utilized what can loosely be termed as self-management procedures, in which the patient is taught various management procedures which they then have to apply themselves in order to bring their symptoms under self-control. This requires an ability to selectively attend to the occurrence of symptoms and monitor their presence. In one case study self-monitoring alone was reported as sufficient to eliminate hallucinations (Baskett, 1983), but it is improbable that this finding could be reproduced with most patients.

21.5.1 THOUGHT STOPPING (TS)

In a controlled study, 20 patients were randomly allocated to TS with medication or medication alone (Lamontague *et al.*, 1983). Some improvements were found in a decrease in frequency of persecutory thoughts, but these differences were only significant at six months. There were no differences in duration of persecutory thoughts nor in the frequency or duration of hallucinations. Similarly, Erickson *et al.* (1978) failed to demonstrate that TS was effective in reducing hallucinations. Therefore the evidence for the efficacy of TS in minimal, although it may have use as part of a treatment package.

21.5.2 SELF-CONTROL

In a well-controlled case study the efficacy of a ward-based self-control programme was demonstrated (Alford *et al.*, 1982). However, improvements gradually reversed once the patient was discharged. The authors speculate that the reversal was because the patient viewed her symptoms as positive and such a view served a reinforcing function to re-establish and maintain symptom-related behaviour. For self-control procedures to be effective it would seem that patients need to be able to reinforce their own self-management behaviour.

21.5.3 COPING STRATEGIES

The naturalistic studies on the use of coping strategies have suggested that symptoms such as delusions may not be completely impervious to non-pharmacological intervention and systematic training in coping methods could be a productive method of management. Coping implies a cognitive or behavioural effort by the patient to master, reduce or tolerate their symptoms. This approach clearly has features in common with self-management and also includes other methods such as self-instruction. Three characteristics distinguish this approach. First, there is an attempt to use and build on coping methods already used by the patient so that the patient's current coping repertoire is assessed and utilized. Second, *in vivo* practice is encouraged, that is during training in coping the patient is encouraged to simulate or even bring on the symptoms and practice the coping strategies. Third, training in coping is not restricted to the application of a single technique but may include an array or combinations of individual coping strategies.

Fowler and Morley (1989) report on five case studies in which patients were asked to continually monitor their mood states, the frequency of their symptoms and three aspects of psychotic experience: the extent to which they could control their symptoms, the extent to which they believed their symptoms to be true and the extent to which they were distressed by their symptoms. One patient showed a marked overall improvement and three others showed improvements on their perceived ability to control their symptoms.

Tarrier *et al.* (1990) reported two case studies who received what the authors termed Coping Strategy Enhancement (CSE). This involved the careful behavioural analysis of the patient's symptoms and their antecedents and consequences. The patient was first given a detailed rationale of the approach. If the patient lacked insight then the alleviation of any distress caused by their symptoms was emphasized. One symptom was then chosen and a strategy selected to cope with it. The strategy was then systematically practised under increasingly more difficult conditions in the treatment session and as homework. Cognitive strategies were first demonstrated overtly by the therapist, then the patient practised them overtly and covertly. Training in behavioural strategies was through role playing or guided practice. If the strategy was successful another symptom was selected for treatment, if not then the patient was trained in a further coping strategy and so on. The two patients treated in this manner both showed considerable improvements in the severity, conviction, preoccupation and interference of their symptoms. At six-month follow-up one patient had continued to improve while the second had shown some deterioration from post-treatment but still showed an improvement from pre-treatment. For more extensive details of this treatment method see Tarrier (1990).

21.6 CASE EXAMPLE

One of the subjects treated in the Tarrier *et al.* (1990) study was a 47-year-old married man who lived with his wife. He had a 28-year history of schizophrenia and since his last admission seven years previously he had been unable to work and had attended a day hospital intermittently over this period. When he was recruited into the treatment programme the subject was experiencing nine identifiable psychotic symptoms including thought broadcast, thought echo, delusions of his thoughts being read, auditory hallucinations (both in the third person and directly hostile voices) and delusional explanations (e.g. telepathy). He reported that thought echo, delusions about his thoughts being read and auditory hallucinations occurred one to three times each day for a duration of between one to six hours, most frequently during the evening. These symptoms were selected as target symptoms as he could accurately identify their occurrence and because they seemed sufficiently frequent and disruptive to engage him in the proposed intervention. He coped with them in a number of ways: by trying to sleep, by listening to music drown them out and by singing to himself.

He was taught to carefully monitor his symptoms, and then instructed to cognitively relabel them as illness phenomena and to distract himself. This was then combined with environmental distractions guided by self-talk. Training was given in not responding to auditory hallucinations by exposure to increasingly hostile voices (simulated by the therapist) whilst the subject engaged in coping strategies taught in the earlier sessions. He was then taught progressive muscle relaxation over two sessions as a further coping strategy. At the seventh session he reported that he had been symptom free for a number of days but that he felt depressed. He was instructed over the next two sessions in methods to cope with low moods including goal setting to increase his activity level. During the final session discussion focused in how he could cope if the symptoms returned.

21.7 A CONTROLLED EVALUATION OF CSE

In an ongoing controlled trial presently being carried out by the author and his colleagues

(Tarrier *et al.* 1991) [1] CSE is being compared with problem solving (PS). CSE follows the same procedure as described in the case study above. In PS (which is used as the control treatment) the patient is given the rationale for the approach, and the procedure is initially practised on a neutral task (e.g. a simple game such as draughts or noughts and crosses) with the therapist first modelling the use of overt self- instruction to problem-solve the possible moves and their consequences. This procedure is practised by the patient overtly and then covertly. A similar procedure is then applied to a standard problem (e.g. how to make new friends). Finally, the patient is asked to apply the PS method to problems he is experiencing at that time.

Patients are recruited into the study if they have a diagnosis of schizophrenia (including first rank symptoms), they are still experiencing psychotic symptoms which are not responding to medication, they have been ill for at least six months, they are living in the community and are between the ages of 16 and 65. Patients are randomly allocated to CSE or PS. Both groups receive 10 sessions of the appropriate treatment over a 5-week period. Fifty percent of subjects in each limb are first entered into a 5-week waiting/no treatment period before treatment starts. In each treatment limb 50% of patients are allocated to high expectancy, in which the positive benefits of the treatment are continually emphasized and the remainder are allocated to neutral expectancy. Assessment is carried out before the waiting period (if appropriate), at pre-treatment, post-treatment and at six month follow-up. The assessment battery includes:

(a) *Symptom measurement*. Psychotic symptoms are elicited using the PSE and then rated on severity, and on conviction, pre-occupation and interference (Brett-Jones, 1987). At post-treatment and follow-up the PSE is repeated and change scores (Tress *et al.*, 1987) produced for any psychotic symptom that had been present at pre-treatment.

(b) *Global psychopathology*. This is assessed by the Psychiatric Assessment Scale (PAS) (Krawieka *et al.*, 1977).

(c) *Social functioning*. This is assessed by means of the Social Functioning Scale (SFS) (Birchwood *et al.*, 1990).

(d) *The frequency and efficacy of any coping strategies*.

(e) *The problem solving abilities*. This is measured on a standardized task. The credibility of the treatment and the patient's expectancy of its success are assessed after the first session during which the rationale had been given. The subjective estimate of the perceived benefit of the treatment is assessed at post-treatment.

At the time of writing 43 patients have been assessed as suitable for the study. Of these 9 (21%) refused to participate. Thirty-four patients have been allocated, 14 to PS and 20 to CSE. Of these 21 have completed treatment, 13 have completed follow-up and 13 have completed a waiting period. This study is as yet incomplete and any results presented at this stage should be viewed with a certain amount of caution. However, preliminary analyses indicate that if the symptom severity score is aggregated across symptoms, the CSE group show significant improvements in symptom severity, whereas no significant change is seen in the PS group or during the waiting period. Two (22%) patients in the PS limb show a complete remission of symptoms at post-treatment; however no other patients show a greater than 50% improvement. In the CSE limb 7 (58%) patients show an improvement of 50% or more; 2 (17%) of these show a complete remission of symptoms. Patients in the CSE limb show a decrease in preoccupation, conviction and interference from their symptoms but only the latter reaches significance. Patients receiving PS show a decrease in conviction and preoccupation of which the latter reaches significance. Both treatments show a non-significant decrease in depression and CSE patients show a significant decrease in anxiety. There are no changes over the waiting period on any of these measures. Neither treatment appears to affect social functioning. Patients receiving neutral expectancy show a decrease in symptom severity that just reaches significance, whilst the high expectancy group just fails to reach significance. Hence expectancy does not appear an influential factor.

The results at this point indicate a superiority of CSE over PS and no treatment and we await the completed study to see if these improvements are maintained.

21.8 CONCLUSIONS

The results on psychological treatment methods for individual symptoms are mixed. Single techniques seem to have a weak effect and there is frequently a lack of maintenance of any improvements. The absence of large controlled trials makes generalizations difficult and patient selection for psychological treatment may be a crucial variable in the treatment effects seen in case studies. Methods of cognitive therapy, self-management and coping all appear to hold some promise and are worth investigating further. It is probable that combinations of techniques are more likely to succeed and contingency manipulation, self-instruction, thought stopping and other methods may all be a useful part of a treatment package.

Emphasis should be placed both in research and clinical endeavours to find out why patients do not improve. This may mean investigating the value and the meaning of symptoms to the patient. The elimination of symptoms which may be a considerable factor in a patient's daily life could result in the patient feeling depressed and empty even though their experiences were illness related. These patients are also most likely to be without the resources to replace their illness with positive alternatives. Therefore in clinical practice symptom management should not be thought of in isolation but as a part of an integrated approach which might include family management (Chapter 24) and social and living skills (see Chapter 23).

In conclusion, there is no evidence that psychologically based treatment methods would provide a viable alternative to neuroleptic medication. However these methods are certainly worth pursuing with patients who continue to experience psychotic symptoms. At the present time there needs to be a development in symptom assessments and investigations into patient selection criteria which could predict who would benefit from these methods.

NOTE

1. Tarrier, N., Harwood, S., Yusopoff, L., Beckett, R., Baker, A. and Ugarteburu, I. The Salford Symptom Project: unpublished data.

REFERENCES

Adams, H.E., Malatesta, V., Brontley,P.J. and Turkat, I.D. (1981) Modification of cognitive processes: A case study of schizophrenia. *J. Consult. Clin. Psychol.*, **49**, 460–4.

Alford, B.A. (1986) Behavioural treatments of schizophrenic delusions: A single-case experimental analysis. *Behav. Ther.*, **17**, 637–44.

Alford, G.S., and Turner, S.M. (1976) Stimulus interference and conditioned inhibition of auditory hallucinations. *J. Behav. Ther. Exp. Psychiatry*, **7**, 155–60.

Alford, G.S., Fleece, L., and Rothblum, E. (1982) Hallucinatory-delusional verbalizations: Modification in a chronic schizophrenic by self-control and cognitive restructuring. *Behav. Mod.*, **6**, 421–35.

Anderson, L.T. and Alpert, M. (1974) Operant analysis of hallucination frequency in a hospitalized schizophrenic. *J. Behav. Ther. Exp. Psychiatry*, **5**, 13–8.

Andreasen, N.C. (1985) Positive vs. negative symptoms: A critical evaluation. *Schizophr. Bull.*, **11**, 380–9.

Asberg, M., Montgomery, S.A., Perris, C., Shalling, D. and Sedvall, G. (1978) A comprehensive psychopathology rating scale. *Acta Psychiatr. Scand.*, **Suppl. 271**, 5–69.

Ayllon, T. and Haughton, E. (1964) Modification of symptomatic verbal behaviour of mental patients. *Behav. Res. Ther.*, **2**, 87–97.

Baskett, S.J. (1983) Tardive dyskinesia and treatment of psychosis after withdrawal of neuroleptics. *Brain Res. Bull.*, **11**, 173–4.

Beck, A.T. (1952) Successful out-patient psychotherapy of a chronic schizophrenic with a delusion based on borrowed guilt. *Psychiatry*, **15**, 305–12.

Belcher, T.L. (1988) Behavioural reduction of overt hallucinatory behaviour in chronic schizophrenics. *J. Behav. Ther. Exp. Psychiatry*, **19**, 69–71.

Bentall, R.P., and Slade, P.D. (1985) Reality testing and auditory hallucinations: A signal detection analysis. *Br. J. Clin. Psychol.*, **24**, 159–69.

Bentall, R.P., Higson, P. and Lowe, C.F. (1987) Teaching self-instruction to chronic schizophrenic patients: Efficacy and generalization. *Behav. Psychother.*, **15**, 58–76.

Birchwood, M. (1986) Control of auditory hallucinations through occlusion of monoaural auditory input. *Br. J. Psychiatry*, **149**, 104–7.

Birchwood, M., Smith, J., Cochrane, R., Wetton, S., and Copestake, S. (1990) The social functioning scale: The development and validation of a scale of social adjustment for use in family intervention programmes with schizophrenic patients. *Br. J. Psychiatry*, **157**, 853–9.

Breier, A. and Strauss, J.S. (1983) Self-control in psychotic disorders. *Arch. Gen. Psychiatry*, **40**, 1141–5.

Brenner, H.D. (1986) On the importance of cognitive disorders in treatment and rehabilitation. In *Psychosocial Treatment of Schizophrenia*. J. Strauss, W. Boker and H.D. Brenner (eds), Hans Huber, Bern, pp. 136–51.

Brenner, H.D., Boker, W., Muller, J., Spichtig, L. and Wurgler, S. (1987) On autoprotective efforts of schizophrenics, neurotics and controls. *Acta Psychiatr. Scand.* **75**, 405–14.

Brenner, H.D., Kraemer, S., Hermanutz, M. and Hodel, B. (1990) Cognitive treatments in schizophrenia. In *Schizophrenia: Concepts, Vulnerability and Intervention*. E.R. Straube and K. Hahlweg (eds), Springer-Verlag, Berlin, pp. 161–92.

Brett-Jones, J., Garety, P. and Hemsley, D. (1987) Measuring delusional experience: A method and its application. *Br. J. Clin. Psychol.*, **26**, 257–65.

Brewin, C.R. (1988) *Cognitive Foundations of Clinical Psychology*. LEA, London.

Bucher, B. and Fabricatore, J. (1970) Use of patient self-administered shock to suppress talk. *Behav. Ther.*, **1**, 382–5.

Bulow, H., Oei, T.P.S., and Pinkey, B. (1979) Effects of contingent social reinforcement with delusional chronic schizophrenic men. *Psychol. Rep.*, **44**, 659–66.

Carr, V. (1988) Patients' techniques for coping with schizophrenia: An exploratory study. *Br. J. Med. Psychol.*, **61**, 339–52.

Chadwick, P. and Lowe, F.L. (1990) The measurement and modification of delusional beliefs. *J. Consult. Clin. Psychol.* (in press).

Cohen, C.I. and Berk, B.S. (1985) Personal coping styles of schizophrenic outpatients. *Hosp. Community Psychiatry*, **36**, 407–10.

Crow, T.J. (1980) Molecular pathology of schizophrenia. More than one disease process. *Br. J. Psychiatry*, **145**, 303–24.

Curson, D.A., Barnes, T.R.E., Bamber, R.W. *et al.* (1985) Long-term depot maintenance of chronic schizophrenic outpatients. *Br. J. Psychiatry*, **146**, 464–80.

Curson, D.A., Patel, M., Liddle, P.F. and Barnes, T.R.E. (1988) Psychiatric morbidity of a long stay hospital population with chronic schizophrenia and implications for future community care. *Br. Med. J.*, **297**, 819–22.

Davis, J.R., Wallace, C.J., Liberman, R.P. and Finch, B.E. (1976) The use of brief isolation to suppress delusional and hallucinatory speech. *J. Behav. Ther. Exp. Psychiatry*, **7**, 269–75.

Erickson, E., Darnell, M.H. and Labeck, I. (1978) Belief treatment of hallucinatory behaviour with behavioural techniques. *Behav. Ther.*, **9**, 663–5.

Falloon, I.R.H. (1986) Cognitive and behavioural interventions in the self-control of schizophrenia. In *Psychosocial Treatment of Schizophrenia*. J. Strauss, W. Boker and H.D. Brenner (eds), Hans Huber, Bern, pp. 180–90.

Falloon, I.R.H. and Talbot, R.E. (1981) Persistent auditory hallucinations: Coping mechanisms and implications for management. *Psychol. Med.*, **11**, 329–39.

Falloon, I.R.H., Boyd, J.L. and McGill, C. (1984)

Family Care of Schizophrenia. Guilford Press, New York.

Feder, R. (1982) Auditory hallucinations treated by radio headphones. *Am. J. Psychiatry*, **139**, 1188–90.

Fonagy, P. and Slade, P. (1982) Punishment vs negative reinforcement in the aversive conditioning of auditory hallucinations. *Behav. Res. Ther.*, **20**, 483–92.

Fowler, D. and Morley, S. (1989) The cognitive-behavioural treatment of hallucinations and delusions: A preliminary study. *Behav. Psychother.*, **17**, 267–82.

Frith, C.D. (1987) The positive and negative symptoms of schizophrenic reflect impairment in perception and initiation of action. *Psychol. Med.*, **17**, 631–48.

Garety, P. (1985) Delusions: Problems in definition and measurement. *Br. J. Med. Psychol.*, **58**, 25–34.

Gresen, R. (1974) The effects of instruction and reinforcement on a multifaceted self-control procedure in the modification and generalization of behaviour in schizophrenia. Unpublished Ph.D. thesis, Bowling Green University (cited by Margolin and Shemberg, 1976).

Gould, L.N. (1948) Verbal hallucinations and activity of vocal musculature: An electromyographic study. *Am. J. Psychiatry*, **105**, 362–72.

Green, W.P. and Preston, M. (1981) Reinforcement of vocal correlates of auditory hallucinations by auditory feedback: A case study. *Br. J. Psychiatry*, **139**, 204–8.

Green, W.P., Glass, A. and O'Callaghan, M.A. (1979), Some implications of abnormal hemisphere interaction in schizophrenia. In *Hemisphere Asymmetries of Function in Psychopathology*. J. Gruzelier and P. Flor-Henry (eds), Macmillan, London, pp. 431–8.

Green, W.P., Hallett, S. and Hunter, M. (1983) Abnormal interhemispheric specializations in schizophrenic and high risk children. In *Laterality and Psychopathology*. P. Flor-Henry and J. Gruzelier (eds), Elsevier, Amsterdam, pp. 443–70.

Gross, G. (1986) Basic symptoms and coping behaviour in schizophrenia. In *Psychosocial Treatment of Schizophrenia*. J. Strauss, W. Boker and H.D. Brenner (eds), Hans Huber, Bern, pp. 126–35.

Harrow, M. and Silverstein, M.L. (1977) Psychotic symptoms in schizophrenia after the acute phase. *Schizophr. Bull.*, **3**, 608–16.

Hartman, L.M. and Cashman, F.E. (1983) Cognitive-behavioural and psychopharmacological treatment of delusional symptoms: A preliminary report. *Behav. Psychother.*, **11**, 50–61.

Harvey, P.D. and Walker, E.F. (1987) *Positive and Negative Symptoms of Psychosis*. LEA, New Jersey.

Hawton, K., Salkovskis, P.M., Kirk, J. and Clark, D.M. (1989) *Cognitive Behaviour Therapy for Psychiatric Problems*. Oxford University Press, Oxford.

Hemsley, D.R. and Garety, P.A. (1986) The formation and maintenance of delusions: a Bayesian analysis. *Br. J. Psychiatry*, **149**, 51–6.

Hersen, M. and Bellack, A.S. (eds) (1976) *Behavioural assessment: A Practical Handbook*, Pergamon, Oxford.

Horowitz, M.J. (1975) A cognitive model of hallucinations. *Am. J. Psychiatry*, **132**, 789–95.

Hole, R.W., Rush, A.J. and Beck, A.T. (1979) A cognitive investigation of schizophrenic delusions. *Psychiatry*, **42**, 312–9.

Ingram, R.E. (1986) *Information Processing Approaches to Clinical Psychology*. Academic, New York.

James, D. (1983) The experimental treatment of two cases of verbal hallucinations. *Br. J. Psychiatry*, **143**, 515–16.

Johnson, M. and Raye, C. (1981) Reality monitoring. *Psychol. Rev.*, **88**, 67–85.

Junginger, J. and Frame, C.L. (1985) Self-report of the frequency and phenomenology of verbal hallucinations. *J. Nerv. Ment. Dis.*, **173**, 149–55.

Kanas, N. and Barr, M.A. (1984) Self-control of psychotic productions in schizophrenia. *Arch. Gen. Psychiatry*, **41**, 919–20.

Kanfer, F.H. (1980), Self-Management Methods. In *Helping People Change*, 2nd Edition. F. Kanfer and A. Goldstein. (eds), Pergamon, New York, pp. 334–89.

Kendler, K.S., Glazer, W.M. and Morgenstein, H. (1983) Dimensions of delusional experience, *Am. J. Psychiatry*, **140**, 466–9.

Kennedy, T. (1964) Treatment of chronic schizophrenia by behaviour therapy. case reports. *Behav. Res. Ther.*, **2**, 1–6.

Krawieka, M., Goldberg, D. and Vaughan M. (1977) A standardized psychiatric assessment scale for rating chronic psychotic patients. *Acta Psychiatr. Scand.*, **55**, 299–308.Lamontagne, Y., Audet, N. and Elie, R. (1983) Thought stopping for delusions and hallucinations: A pilot study. *Behav. Psychother.*, **11**, 177–84.

Liberman, R.P., Teigan, J., Patterson, R. and Baker, V. (1973) Reducing delusional speech in chronic paranoid schizophrenics. *J. Appl. Behav. Anal.*, **6**, 57–64.

Lindsley, O. (1963) Direct measurement and functional definition of vocal hallucinatory symptoms, *J. Nerv. Ment. Dis.*, **136**, 293–7.

Lukoff, D., Nuechterlein, K.H. and Ventura, J. (1986) Manual for expanded Brief Psychiatric Rating Scale (BPRS). *Schizophr. Bull.*, **12**, 594–602.

Magaro, P.A., Johnson, M. and Boring, R. (1986) Information processing approaches to the treatment of schizophrenia. In *Information Processing Approaches to Clinical Psychology.* R.E. Ingram (ed), Academic, London, pp. 295–305.

Margo, P., Hemsley, D.R. and Slade P.D. (1981) The effects of varying auditory input on schizophrenic hallucinations. *Br. J. Psychiatry*, **139**, 122–7.

Margolis, R. and Shemberg, K. (1976) Use of self-instruction for the elimination of psychotic speech. *Behav. Ther.*, **7**, 668–71.

Meichenbaum, D. and Cameron, R. (1973) Training schizophrenics to talk to themselves: A means of developing attentional control. *Behav. Ther.*, **4**, 515–34.

Meyers, A., Mercatons, M. and Sirota, A. (1976) Use of self-instruction for the elimination of psychotic speech. *J. Consult. Clin. Psychol.*, **44**, 480–2.

Milton, F., Patwa, V.K. and Hafner, J. (1978) Confrontation vs belief modification in persistently deluded patients. *Br. J. Med. Psychol.*, **51**, 127–30.

Morley, S. (1987) Modification of auditory hallucinations: Experimental studies of headphones and earplugs. *Behav. Psychother.*, **15**, 240–51.

Nelson, R.O. and Hayes, S.C. (1986) *Conceptual Foundations of Behavioural Assessment.* Guilford Press, New York.

Nydegger, R.V. (1972) The elimination of hallu

cinatory and delusional behaviours by verbal conditioning and assertive training: A case study. *J. Behav. Ther. Exp. Psychiatry*, **3**, 225–7.

Olbrich, R. and Mussgay, L. (1988) Reduction of schizophrenic deficits by cognitive training: An evaluation study. Unpublished manuscript.

Oltmanns, T.F. and Maher, B.A. (1988) *Delusional Beliefs.* Wiley, New York.

Overall, J.E. and Gorham, D.R. (1962) The Brief Psychiatric Rating Scale. *Psychol. Rep.* **10**, 799–812.

Patterson, R.L., Liberman, R.P. and Baker, V. (1976) A problem in behavior assessment of the frequency of hallucinations. Unpublished report (cited by Falloon and Talbot, 1981).

Paul, G. and Lentz, R. (1977) *Psychological Treatment of Chronic Mental Patients. Milieu versus Social Learning Programs.* Harvard University Press, Cambridge, MA.

Schneider, S.J. and Pope, A.T. (1982) Neuroleptic-like electroencephalographic changes in schizophrenics through biofeedback. *Biofeedback Self-Regulation*, **7**, 479–90.

Serber, M. and Nelson, P.(1971) The ineffectiveness of systematic desensitisation and assertive training in hospitalised schizophrenics. *J. Behav. Ther. Exp. Psychiatry*, **7**, 107–9.

Slade, P.D. (1972) The effects of systematic desensitisation on auditory hallucinations. *Behav. Res. Ther.*, **10**, 85–91.

Slade, P.D. (1973) The psychological investigation and treatment of auditory hallucinations: A second case report. *Br. J. Med. Psychol.*, **46**, 293–6.

Slade, P.D. (1976) Towards a theory of auditory hallucinations: outline of an hypothetical four-factor model. *Br. J. Soc. Clin. Psychol.*, **15**, 415–23.

Slade, P.D. and Bentall, R.P. (1988) *Sensory Deception: Towards Scientific Analysis of Hallucinations.* Croom Helm, London.

Silverstein, M.L. and Harrow, M. (1978) First-rank symptoms in the post acute schizophrenic: A follow-up study. *Am. J. Psychiatry*, **135**, 1481–6.

Spaulding, W.D., Storms, L., Goodrich, V. and Sullivan, M. (1986) Application of experimental psychopathology in psychiatric rehabilitation. *Schizophr. Bull.*, **12**, 560–77.

Tarrier, N. (1987) An investigation of residual

psychotic symptoms in discharged schizophrenic patients. *Br. J. Clin. Psychol.*, **26**, 141–3.

Tarrier, N. (1990) Management and modification of residual psychotic symptoms. In *Innovations in the Psychological Management of Schizophrenia*. M. Birchwood and N. Tarrier (eds), Wiley, Chichester, in press.

Tarrier, N., Barrowclough, C., Porceddu, K. and Watts, S. (1988) The psychophysiological reactivity to the expressed emotion of the relatives of schizophrenic patients. *Br. J. Psychiatry*, **152**, 618–24.

Tarrier, N., Harwood, S., Yusopoff, L., Beckett, R. and Baker, A. (1990) Coping Strategy Enhancement (CSE): A method of treating residual schizophrenic symptoms. *Behav. Psychother.*, **18**, 283–93.

Tress, K.H., Bellenis, C., Brownlow, J.M., Livinston, G., and Leff, J.P. (1987) The Present State Examination Change rating scale. *Br. J. Psychiatry*, **150**, 201–7.

Turner, S., Herson, M., and Bellack, A. (1977) Effects of social disruption, stimulus interference and aversive conditioning on auditory hallucina-tions. *Behav. Mod.*, **1**, 249–58.

Wallace, C.J. (1976) Assessment of psychotic behavior. In *Behavioural Assessment*. M. Herson and A.S. Bellack (eds), Pergamon, Oxford, pp. 261–304.

Watts, F.N., Powell, G.E. and Austin, S.V. (1973) The modification of abnormal beliefs. *Br. J. Med. Psychol.*, **46**, 359–63.

Weingaertner, A.H. (1971) Self-administered aversive stimulation with hallucinating hospit-alized schizophrenics. *J. Consult. Clin. Psychol*, **36**, 422–9.

West, L.J. (1962) A general theory of hallucinations and dreams. In *Hallucinations*. L.J. West (ed), Grune & Stratton, New York, pp. 275–90.

Wing, J.K., Cooper, J.E. and Sartorius, N. (1974) *Measurement and Classification of Psychiatric Symptoms: An Instruction Manual for the PSE and Catego Programme*. Cambridge University Press, Cambridge.

Winters, K.C. and Neale, J.M. (1983) Delu-sions and delusional thinking in psychotics: A review of the literature. *Clin. Psychol. Rev.*, **3**, 227–53.

Chapter 22

Social skills training with schizophrenic patients

W. KIM HALFORD and ROBYN L. HAYES

Deficits in interpersonal and social functioning are key characteristics of schizophrenia, as defined by DSM–III-R (American Psychiatric Association, 1987). These deficits seem to be particularly persistent, pervasive problems as many adult schizophrenic patients have been socially isolated and withdrawn from childhood (Lewine *et al.*, 1978, 1980). Deficits in social functioning are a significant source of stress for persons with schizophrenia, have a negative impact on their community functioning, and contribute to relapse (Anthony and Liberman, 1986; Falloon *et al.*, 1984). Such deficits in schizophrenic patients are more than a consequence of positive and negative schizophrenic symptoms. Schizophrenic patients exhibit social skills deficits, even with positive symptoms in remission and in the absence of a manifest negative syndrome (Wallace, 1984; Jackson, 1988; Bellack *et al.*, 1989).

Social skills training (SST) has been employed with schizophrenic patients for over two decades in an attempt to remediate poor social functioning (Herson and Bellack, 1976; Liberman *et al.*, 1989; Wallace *et al.*, 1980) This chapter is a review of SST with schizophrenic patients, focused on the impact of SST on schizophrenic individuals' functioning in the community.

22.1 THE PRINCIPLE OF SOCIAL SKILLS TRAINING

The key assumption underlying SST is that many schizophrenic patients either have never learned, or have forgotten, socially skilled behaviours for coping with important interpersonal situations (Goldsmith and McFall, 1975). These skills deficits are seen as the key reason for patients' poor social functioning and social isolation, and it is presumed that acquisition and utilization of skills will improve patient functioning. From within this theoretical framework, therapy is an active, directive process designed to teach patients skills. Implicitly it is presumed that use of skills will be prompted and reinforced in the patients' environment sufficiently to maintain the behaviours (i.e. patients will have people with whom they interact who respond positively to the use of social skills; and patients will feel little anxiety, or will achieve desired goals, when using the skilled behaviours in their day-to-day lives).

The numerous attempts to define social skill vary greatly in their emphasis (Bellack, 1983). Wallace *et al.* (1980) suggested there are four major elements commonly included in definitions of social skills:

(1) patients' internal states, i.e., their feelings, attitudes, and perceptions of interpersonal contexts;

(2) the topography of patients' behaviour — the rates of behaviours such as eye contact, hand gestures, body posture, speech dys-fluencies, voice volume and latency of verbal response;

(3) the outcomes of interactions, as reflected in the achievement of patients' goals; and

(4) the outcomes of interactions as reflected in the attitudes, feelings, behaviours, and goals of other participants.

Elements 3 and 4 are the most important components of the definition of social skills as they reflect the adaptiveness of the person's social behaviour. Element 1 is important, though it is inappropriate to overemphasize the subjective perceptions and feelings of schizo-phrenic patients. For example, lying around in bed for prolonged periods may feel comfortable for the patient in the short term, but may be maladaptive. Element 2 is important in so far as it is possible to define the specific behaviours which are adaptive on criteria 3 and 4.

Anthony and Liberman (1986) provide a representative example of a definition used in SST which focuses on elements 3 and 4. They define social skills as those skills which allow the individual to: 'Promote problem solving, engage others in successful affiliative and instrumental relationships, mobilize supportive networks and engage in work' (p. 544). This definition (and most others like it) lack detail about exactly what these social skills are. This lack of specificity reflects the large variations in what constitutes social skill in different situations, which is an issue reviewed in detail by Mueser and Douglas (Chapter 11).

Early SST programmes with schizophrenic patients conceptualized social skill as a relatively stable set of overt responses, and targeted changes in topographical features of those behaviours. For example, Bellack *et al.* 1976, targeted appropriate speech duration, intonation and gestures. Kale *et al.* (1968)

taught just one discrete behaviour, a simple greeting, 'Hello'. Serber and Nelson (1971) trained patients in assertive responses. However, it became evident that a simple list of overt behaviours was not an adequate conceptualization of social skill.

Two fundamental changes have occurred in the social skills targeted in SST. First, in more recent reports of SST, interpersonal communication has been taught within a context of life skills, focusing on general classes of behaviour viewed as adaptive (Brown and Munford, 1983; Wallace and Liberman, 1985; Liberman *et al.*, 1989). Definition of specific therapeutic targets usually relies on the therapist applying principles underlying these classes of behaviour to specific situations problematic for patients. For example, assertion has widely assumed to be an adaptive means of responding to interpersonal conflict (Lange and Jakubowski, 1976), though it is clear this is not universally so (St. Lawrence *et al.*, 1985). SST therapists need to guide clients as to when assertion is appropriate, and help them formulate appropriate assertive responses to specific problem situations.

Second, recent SST programmes also focus on a more comprehensive range of social skills incorporating social perception and social problem-solving skills, as well as overt behaviours. The comprehensive model of social skills adopted in many recent SST programmes was first described by Argyle and Kendon (1967), and is presented schematically in Figure 22.1. Essentially social skill is argued to be a analogous to any serial motor skill. The individual first must be able to accurately perceive the social situation. That input has to be translated into the definition of achievable personal goals, the identification of a range of possible responses, and selection of an appropriate response. Finally, the selected response has to be made skilfully.

Representative examples of SST programmes which incorporate this more comprehensive range of social skills, including social

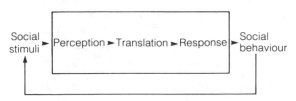

Figure 22.1 Schematic representation of a model of social skill.

perception, problem solving and overt response skills, have been described by Trower *et al.* (1978) Beidel *et al.* (1981); Wallace (1982); Liberman *et al.* (1989); Hayes and Halford (1990). In each of these programmes SST involves structured behavioural training of interpersonal competencies (Liberman *et al.*, 1985) and the training is conducted in small groups. Patients' social skills in the areas of social perception, social problem solving, and overt behaviour are assessed systematically, and specific areas of assets and deficits identified.

The process used to train social skills is the same, regardless of the specific skills targeted. The whole process throughout SST relies on the therapist and clients defining specific interpersonal situations which are examples of identified interpersonal problems. The selection of appropriate examples is crucial. In the early stages of therapy it is particularly important to select situations of immediate relevance to clients' current life situations, in which the clients are maximally likely to be reinforced for small changes in their interpersonal behaviour. It also is important to define the situation as precisely as possible in terms of the other people present, the setting, and the patient's goals.

Once an appropriate situation is defined the therapist has the patient role play the situation. The more realistic the role play the better, so the setting of an appropriate mood and arranging the physical environment to simulate the setting are important. The therapist needs

to decide if the patient's behaviour is appropriate to the situation. Some higher functioning schizophrenic patients can accurately self-evaluate social behaviour, but therapists need to be wary of using patients' notions of normative social behaviour to establish training goals. If the behaviour is appropriate, then the therapist can proceed to setting a behavioural assignment to deal with the interpersonal problem. If the behaviour is inappropriate, then further assessment is required.

The first step of further assessment is to evaluate the patient's social perception. One method for achieving this is to ask the patient a series of questions about the identified target situation such as 'What is your short-term goal in this situation?' 'What is your long-term goal?' 'How is the other person feeling?' 'What is the other person's goal?' The appropriateness of the patient's answers can be used to gauge the patient's assets and deficits in social perception. If social perception is deficient then training is required. Methods of social perception training have not been described as extensively in the literature as other elements of SST. In our approach we videotape patients role-playing interpersonal situations they find problematic. We use questions and answers based on the videotape to shape realistic perceptions of these social situations.

The need for training social perception is demonstrated by the findings that schizophrenic persons often misperceive the behaviour of others. In particular they often cannot recognize the affect of persons they are interacting with, and this can lead to inappropriate responding (Morrison *et al.*, 1988).

The next step in SST is social problem solving. Typically social problem solving training utilizes the same procedures of assessment, modelling, instructions, role play practice, feedback and homework tasks as other aspects of SST. However, social problem solving focuses on training subjects, when confronted with difficult social situations, to follow through a series of steps including goal definition, generation and evaluation of

Table 22.1 Responding to patients' failure to complete assignments

Reason for failure to complete the task	*Recommendation for overcoming problem*
1. Patient lacks the necessary knowledge or skills to complete task	1. Ensure what is to be done, and when, can be described by patient. 2. Check patient can demonstrate required behaviour, and do skill training if required. 3. Have patients cognitively rehearse behaviours before undertaking them.
2. Patient's cognitions interfere with completion of the assignment.	1. Check the patient understands the rationale for the task. 2. Have the patient make a public statement of intent to complete the task. 3. Develop the patients' private commitment to task completion by strongly reinforcing attempts to complete, remind patient of past successes from completion of tasks, highlight the association of current tasks with achievement of current goals.
3. The patient's environment elicits non-compliance	1. The therapist should use multiple cues to elicit the behaviour, e.g. use of 'buddies', reminder cards and telephone calls. 2. Ensure as far as possible that the targeted skills will be reinforced, e.g. cue significant others in the patient's life to reinforce targeted behaviour, try to anticipate and reduce the negative effects of compliance. 3. The therapist should monitor compliance from multiple sources, and reinforce compliance strongly. 4. The therapist should start with brief simple assignments and build to more complex tasks.

Adapted from Shelton and Levy (1981)

alternative solutions, and selection of the most effective solution (Wallace, 1982; Hansen *et al.*, 1985). One training procedure is for therapist and patient to generate a range of alternative responses to a defined situation, and then have the patient identify the advantages and disadvantages of each option. The therapist assists the patient to select the option they wish to use to solve the problem. Once the desired response is defined, instruction, coaching, modelling, behaviour rehearsal and feedback are used to train the patient to skilfully make the targeted overt response. This can involve multiple role plays until the patient is able to demonstrate a response that is judged likely to be reinforced in the target setting.

Homework tasks are assigned between treatment sessions to enhance transfer of training effects to community settings (Brady, 1984a). Such tasks involve applying the skills learnt to the target setting. The outcome of the tasks provides feedback to the patient and therapist about the appropriateness of the skills acquired to patients' life situations. Patients sometimes partially or totally fail to complete assignments between sessions, and this can present a significant difficulty in SST. Shelton and Levy (1981) proposed three primary reasons why patients fail to complete behavioural assignments. Table 22.1 presents their typology, and some suggestions we have generated for overcoming these problems.

22.2 CONTENT OF SOCIAL SKILLS TRAINING

A typical SST programme includes components on interpersonal communication and community living skills (Beidel *et al.*, 1981; Curran *et al.*, 1982; Wallace *et al.*, 1985). The interpersonal communication component typically includes skills to initiate, maintain and terminate conversations; positive assertion skills such as extending invitations, giving and receiving praise and compliments; and the skills of negative assertion such as refusing unreasonable requests, and expressing and responding to negative statements (Beidel *et al.*, 1981; Wallace *et al.*, 1985). Community living skills include areas such as job seeking, interviewing and job maintenance skills, medication self-management, dating skills, self-care, home-making, money management, public transportation, and leisure and recreation skills (Beidel *et al.*, 1981; Wallace *et al.*, 1985).

Covering all of the possible skill areas identified above would be very time-consuming and unnecessary, as many patients have deficits in only some of these areas. Consequently, the content of a number of SST programmes has been divided into modules (e.g. Liberman *et al.*, 1989; Hayes and Halford, 1990). Modularization allows individual patients to be directed into content areas of relevance to them, while providing some degree of standardization of programme content needed for the delivery of group therapy. At the same time the use of standardized modules aids dissemination of SST. Table 22.2 lists examples of the modules which might be included within a broad ranging SST programme.

Each module within a SST programme consists of a number of training sessions. Tables 22.3 and 22.4 summarize the content of typical SST sessions. These sessions are typical in that the first parts are devoted to the review of assignments set in previous sessions. As noted earlier, such assignments routinely are set to encourage patients to practice the targeted skills in the targeted social situations.

The sessions described in Tables 22.3 and 22.4 then proceed on to the introduction and practice of some additional skills, followed by the setting of further behavioural assignments. We see SST as being assignment driven, in the sense that patients who are successfully completing well-designed assignments are achieving the goals of altering their social behaviour in their day-to-day lives. An example of a behavioural assignment is presented in Table 22.5.

22.3 STUDIES EVALUATING SOCIAL SKILLS TRAINING WITH SCHIZO-PHRENIC PATIENTS

Many of the studies of SST with schizophrenic patients from the past 15 years have been reviewed previously (Hersen, 1979; Wallace *et al.*, 1980; Curran *et al.*, 1982; Brady, 1984a, b). The earlier reviewers generally agreed that SST had been effective in increasing participants' feelings of ability and comfort in social situations. Reviewers also agreed that, in nearly all of the SST within-subject and group-design intervention studies, the researchers have been able to make a significant impact on the topographical elements of social skills (e.g. Goldsmith and McFall, 1975; Bellack *et al.*, 1976; Finch and Wallace, 1977; Monti *et al.* 1979, 1980). However, this was only the case when the assessment situation was very similar to the training setting. Often the generalization of

Table 22.2 An example of the content of social skills training programme modules

1. Introduction

   Introduction of group members
   Feedback of assessment data
   Negotiating individual goals

2. Conversation skills

   Starting a conversation
   Using open-ended questions and expanded replies
   Generating conversation content
   Nonverbal communication
   Ending a conversation

3. Assertion and conflict management

   Discrimination of assertion
   Nonassertion and aggression
   Negative assertion
   Conflict resolution
   Positive assertion
   Empathic assertion

4. Medication self-management

   Knowledge of medication
   Self-monitoring of medication
   Knowledge of symptoms and side-effects
   Self-monitoring and management of symptoms and side-effects
   Discussing symptoms and medication with health professionals
   Relapse warning sign identification

5. Time use and recreational skills

   Assessment of time use and recreational activity
   Identification of recreational activities to increase
   Using the telephone to obtain information
   Gathing information on recreation
   Planning the use of free time

6. Survival skills

   Budgeting and money management
   Banking
   Seeking and establishing accommodation
   Knowledge of and interaction with community resources and welfare agencies
   Asking for help

7. Employment skills

   Job seeking strategies
   Gathering information on jobs
   Interview skills
   Job maintenance skills

Table 22.3 An example of a therapist's social skills training session outline

Session/objectives

On completion of this session and associated activities participants should be able to:
1. Devise a range of possible topics to discuss when starting a conversation.
2. Demonstrate making 'small talk' with a stranger.

1. *Introduction to session*

In today's session we will look at how people went starting a conversation for their Take Home Task. After reviewing the Take Home Task we will concentrate more on some conversational skills looking at how to keep a conversation going. This will also help people get more out of the communication they have with others.

2. *Take Home Task – review: starting a conversation*

Ask each client individually whether they were able to complete their homework assignment. Ask each client to say:

   (a) who they spoke to
   (b) where they were when they spoke to them
   (c) each question they asked them followed by the response they received to that question
   (d) what they felt was good about the way they interacted, in particular the questions/statements they asked/made
   (e) what they would do differently next time

N.B. If a client has difficulty describing what happened, set up a role play to assess their response.

Give positive feedback about specific aspects of each subject's attempt at the task.

Give specific feedback about a maximum of one or two aspects that each subject could change next time. This might just be a summary of points identified by the subject. Use behaviour rehearsal and modelling as required.

3. *Generating conversation content*

Provide a brief rationale, e.g.: When we have conversations we need to find something to talk about. Now I would like to look at something to talk about. Ask for suggestions.

Discuss topics people can talk about:

   The situation
   The other person or their interests — especially things you know about the person already
   Yourself or your interests

Generate a couple of specific situations (e.g. sitting at the Day Hospital) and ask the clients to generate suggestions of topics, write the ideas on the whiteboard under the headings:

   The situation
   The other person
   Yourself

Discuss areas you do not talk about with people you do not know very well because the other person might be embarrassed or offended. Ask people to identify areas e.g. sex, religion, politics, money, your illness/problems/medication or invitations to people you do not know very well.

Role play/practice exercise

Identify situations which group member would like to initiate conversations and have them role play having conversations with each other in those situations.

Set homework task of starting conversation with someone they want to get to know better.

Table 22.4 Another example of a therapist's social skills training session outline

Session objectives

On completion of this session and associated activities participants should be able to:

1. Describe the short- and long-term consequences of assertive, non-assertive and aggressive responses to an unreasonable request.
2. Demonstrate assertive, non-assertive and aggressive responses to an unreasonable request.

Introduction

Today we are going to start working on an area of skills that come under the heading of 'Assertion'. Does anyone know what I mean by assertion? Try and attempt to draw group members suggestions/points together to give a definition based on the practical application of assertiveness: — e.g.:

Assertion is used in: (give examples and generate members personal examples where possible).

- standing up for ourselves
- expressing our opinions
- letting others know what we think and feel
- letting others know how their behaviour affects us
- making reasonable requests of other people

Take Home Task — Review

The different outcomes of aggressive, passive and assertive responses

One group member role plays making an unreasonable request of the therapist. The group member asks the therapist if they could have a dollar for a can of Coke.

The group member is told to be persistent. The role play is conducted three times. The first time the therapist gives an aggressive reply, the second time a passive reply and the third time an assertive reply.

After each vignette the therapist asks the group to describe the outcome for each member of the role play (appropriate responses are summarized and written on the white board) — e.g.:

	Outcome
● AGGRESSIVE	Therapist feels angry
	Person making request feels angry
	Future friendship put at risk

- PASSIVE (gives in and gives the person a dollar)

    Therapist feels bad because they did not want to do it.
    Person thinks therapist is an 'easy target' and will continue to do this.
    Person does not need to be responsible with own money.
    Person could ask others and get self into trouble.

- ASSERTIVE   Therapist feels OK

    Person making the request might not be very happy with the result but is not stirred up or angry as they would be with the aggressive response.

    Person is less likely to ask for money again.

    Person might be more responsible with their own money if they cannot use other people's money.

Situations where group members have difficulty saying 'No'

Ask group members to think of as many situations as possible where they have difficulty saying 'No'. Model, prompt and reinforce as appropriate. Write appropriate responses on the whiteboard.

Table 22.4 (cont'd)

e.g.: People asking: for money or cigarettes, borrow things, for help when you don't have time or just don't want to help. Collectors for charities, telephone sales people, door to door sales people, door to door religious callers, invitations to places you do not want to go to.

Introduction to the concept of rights

Ask the group if they can describe what is meant by rights. Prompt them by giving examples of some rights. e.g.: the right of people 17 years and over to drive a car or the right to social security if you are unable to work for a legitimate reason. After the group's suggestions have been exhausted, give a definition which incorporates group members' suggestions if possible, e.g.:

'Rights are the things in life that you are entitled to as a member of a fair society'.

Individual's rights in relation to others' requests

Refer to the list of requests on the whiteboard and get group members to identify what they think their rights are in relation to each one — e.g.: in relation to people asking for money, your right is to spend your money how you want to.

In relation to invitations to places you do not want to go, your right is to be able to decide where you do and don't want to go.

Rules for saying 'No' to requests

- Decide if the request is reasonable *or* whether you want to comply with it.
- Decide if there are any other conditions which might be applied to make you want to comply with the request e.g. another time might suit but not now.
- Give a simple 'No'
- Only give a reason if you want to. If you do, keep it honest and simple.
- If you just do not want to fulfil the request simply say ''I prefer not to . . . ' don't argue the point, just continue to say 'No' and the reason.
- If the person persists you can say, 'I understand but . . . '
- Keep a pleasant tone of voice.

Role playing — Saying 'No' to requests.

If possible use scenes which are of importance to the individual involved.

If an individual cannot identify a situation in which they have difficulty saying 'No' when they want to, the therapist should select a situation which they feel might be relevant to the person.

Take Home Task — Saying 'No'' to an unreasonable request.

The group is instructed that each member will be asked to make an unreasonable request of another group member. Each person will be told what request it is they have to make and that they are to persist a little. Group members are told to say 'No' to any unreasonable requests which are made of them and to write down the outcome on their Take Home Task sheet.

It should be stressed that the unreasonable request is just a practise exercise which everyone is expected to do, so no one should be upset by the request.

On the Take Home Task sheet the therapist should fill in the person receiving the request's name, their telephone number if they are agreeable, and the unreasonable request. The therapist should attempt to match people who are not likely to aggravate each other. The therapist should also select requests which are appropriate to the person, unreasonable but not ridiculous, e.g. asking to borrow a car or asking someone to accompany them to somewhere they wouldn't particularly like going to or could not afford. The therapist should use the knowledge they have accumulated about the participants to guide them in their judgement.

Table 22.5 An example of a Take Home assignment to promote the positive assertion skills of expressing praise and compliments

---

NAME: DATE:

TAKE HOME TASKS: POSITIVE ASSERTION

Think of someone you know you will see before the next session. There should be something about them that you think deserves complimenting or praising.

Who is the person?

....

What compliment would you like to give that person?

....

....

When and where are you likely to see them?

....

Before the next session pay the person a compliment and record their response below.

What was the person's response?

....

....

If you cannot get to compliment that person, find someone else you would like to compliment.

Please fill in this form and bring it with you to the next session.

---

changes in social behaviour to natural settings was not assessed. The broader clinical impact of SST on factors such as relapse and social functioning were not assessed in most studies.

Over the last six years there has been the publication of five well-controlled group comparison studies of SST with schizophrenic patients, which have included assessment of the generalization of training effects and/or the clinical significance of treatment effects (Brown and Munford, 1983; Spencer *et al.*, 1983; Bellack *et al.*, 1984; Wallace and Liberman, 1985; Hogarty *et al.*, 1986). These studies were published after the earlier reviews cited above, and are reviewed in some detail below.

Bellack *et al.* (1984) randomly assigned 64 patients to either day hospital treatment only (DH), or one of two day hospital plus SST groups. The two SST groups differed in that one had directed *in vivo* practice of social skills and the other did not. Bellack *et al.* (1984) reported that there were no significant differences between the outcome of the two SST groups, so results for these two groups were reported jointly. This resulted in 20 DH patients and 44 SST patients.

The DH programme was described by Bellack *et al*. (1984) as highly structured, having an educative-rehabilitative focus, and involving approximately five hours per day of small group activity three to five days per week over 12 weeks. SST consisted of three hours per week of instructions, modelling, behaviour rehearsal, feedback and homework assignments conducted in small groups. SST focused on social skills considered necessary for establishing a social network, and reducing stress in interpersonal encounters. Skills targeted in training included initiating and maintaining conversations, assertion skills and social perception.

Outcomes of the two interventions were assessed at post-treatment and at six-month follow-up. Less than half of the subjects were able to be located for assessment at follow-up. A planned 12-month follow-up was abandoned due to inability to locate sufficient patients for reassessment. Multiple *t*-tests were reported contrasting change scores between the two treatment conditions from pre- to post-treatment on a series of outcome measures. Bellack *et al*. (1984) reported these tests 'were almost uniformly nonsignificant, reflecting a consistent lack of differences in degree of improvement' (p. 1025). Further statistical analyses were reported on the significance of multiple *t*-tests of differences between pre- and post-treatment and follow-up measures for each group. Bellack *et al*. (1984) concluded that these analyses showed 'the effect of social skills training were discernable over and above the core treatment programme' (p. 1027). This conclusion is questionable. The repeated use of univariate statistical analysis on measures that are likely to covary probably inflated the type one error rate. The larger sample size in the SST gave the *t*-test in this group greater power, which might in part explain the slightly larger number of significant score changes reported in this group over time. The attrition of over 50% of subjects by follow-up also raises doubts about the results. The only measures available for all

subjects were rehospitalization rates over the next year, which were approximately 50% of subjects in each group. Thus the two treatments appeared essentially the same in their effects.

Brown and Munford (1983) randomly assigned 28 male inpatients meeting the DSM criteria for chronic schizophrenia to either a life skills training programme or a traditional rehabilitation programme. The life skills training consisted of six training modules: interpersonal skills, health, nutrition, time management, finance and community networks. Transfer of training to the community was encouraged by training activities in naturally occurring social situations. The comparison condition was a traditional veterans' administration rehabilitation programme consisting of activities such as recreation, art, and occupational therapies. Both programmes were conducted four hours per day, five days a week for seven weeks. Treatment and control groups were compared pre- and post-treatment on four self-report questionnaires relating to depression social anxiety, and optimism about the future; the Hamilton Rating Scale for Depression (HRSD) and the Life Skills Inventory (LSI). The LSI was developed by the authors and comprised a self-report questionnaire, and a behavioural role-play test, assessing targeted life skills. The treatment group improved significantly more than the control group on seven of the 25 measures derived from the 6 instruments. Of the six life skills evaluated in the LSI, four had improved significantly more in the life skills training than the control condition. However, life skills were not assessed in a natural social setting, and no follow-up evaluation was conducted to assess the durability of change. Significantly more improvement was found on the HRSD in the life skills condition than in the comparison condition. The failure to assess generalization of the new skills to naturalistic social settings and the lack of follow-up precluded demonstration of the effectiveness of life skills training with schizophrenic patients in this study.

Spencer *et al.* (1983) assigned 24 chronic hospital in-patients, 22 of whom were diagnosed as chronic schizophrenic on unspecified criteria, to one of three treatment conditions: SST, remedial drama, or group discussion. Assignment was based on matching of social skill level as assessed by a role-play test. SST was based on Trower *et al.*'s (1978) manual, and targeted modifying verbal and nonverbal behaviours across a range of social settings. Remedial drama incorporated role-playing interactions in problematic social situations, but no instructions, modelling or feedback were provided by therapists. In this condition debriefings of role-plays were conducted focusing on patients' feelings during interactions. In the discussion group patients discussed problems in communication, with the leader taking a non-directive, facilitative role in developing group consensus about how to improve conversational skills. All groups had eight weeks of twice-weekly one hour sessions.

Spencer *et al.* (1983) assessed the effects of treatment with a battery of measures at pre- and post-treatment, and at two-month follow-up. Measures used included a social skills role-play test, standardized nursing staff observations of patients' social behaviour, time sampling of patient social activity during free time and global ratings of behavioural adjustment. Only SST produced a significant improvement on social skills in the role-play tests which was maintained at follow-up. Both SST and remedial drama produced significant increases in levels of patient social interaction on the wards. Results for the control group were not reported. There was little evidence of change on the broader measures of clinical status for any of the treatment groups.

The unspecified subject diagnostic selection criteria, and the inclusion of nonschizophrenic patients, admittedly only 2 out of 24, limit the interpretability of the Spencer *et al.* (1983) study. The comparison conditions of remedial drama and group discussion are good choices for controlling for nonspecific treatment effects of SST. Clearly SST produced a specific effect on social skills, however there was little evidence of a generalized effect on social functioning. Subjects were inpatients throughout the study, so generalization to non-institutional settings could not be evaluated.

Wallace and Liberman (1985) randomly assigned 28 male inpatients, who met the CATEGO criteria for schizophrenia, and who were at high risk for relapse by living with relatives high in expressed emotion (EE), to either behavioural SST or Holistic Health Therapy (HHT). All members from both groups participated in a standard inpatient programme which included a three-tier token economy system intended to improve all subjects' activities of daily living. Family education, training to improve grooming and eating skills, and interventions to reduce assault and property destruction also were included. In addition all participants received carefully monitored medication.

SST was based on a problem-solving model which emphasized the receiving, processing, and sending skills of interpersonal communication. The SST groups were conducted two hours per morning, five days a week. In these groups, three patients led by two therapists were trained to improve interpersonal problem solving. Skill generalization was encouraged through thrice-weekly practice sessions conducted in the community with different interpersonal partners. Twice-weekly homework assignments were designed to encourage the use of newly learnt skills in the community with new locations, situations and people.

The HHT had the same number and duration of sessions as the SST group, but the HHT sessions consisted of jogging, meditation, yoga, group discussion of stress control techniques, and the development of positive beliefs and expectations relating to recovery. Instead of undertaking homework tasks the HHT group simply accompanied the social skills group members on their trips into the community. Overall each group received approximately 200 hours of treatment above the standard inpatient programme.

Programme evaluation was both extensive and intensive. Nineteen measures were used at pre-test, post-test and follow-up; and assessed the broad areas of social skills, social adjustment, and psychopathology. The social skills measures included a role-play test of social competence and a series of self-report inventories. An unobtrusive test of social skills was used in a contrived interaction with a confederate. Three psychiatrist-administered measures of psychopathology were used, and two self-report measures assessed global psychopathology. Rehospitalization data also were collected.

Both groups showed statistically significant improvements on all measures of schizophrenic psychopathology following treatment, and gains were maintained at the nine- and twelve-month follow-ups. The SST group was significantly more improved after treatment than the HHT group on the social adjustment measures, 'sending' skills (as assessed by a role-play test), and were significantly less hostile, less mistrusting, less detached, less inhibited and less submissive in conversations with strangers. During the two-year follow-up the HHT members were rehospitalized almost twice as many times as the SST group (30 versus 16 rehospitalizations) but this difference did not reach acceptable levels of statistical significance (Liberman *et al.*, 1986).

Hogarty *et al.* (1986) assessed the impact on medicated schizophrenic outpatients of family treatment (FT) alone, SST alone, FT combined with SST, and a control group involved in supportive individual therapy. Participants met the Research Diagnostic Criteria (RDC) for schizophrenia or schizoaffective disorder. All subjects resided in households rated high in EE. Twenty-two subjects received FT, 23 SST, 23 combined FT and SST, and 35 were controls. Two-thirds of the patients were male.

SST was based on the treatment techniques of Liberman *et al.* (1975), Hersen and Bellack

1976), Wallace (1982) and combined behavioural instruction, modelling, role-play, feedback and homework tasks. Subjects were trained first in family related interaction, and then later in wider social and vocational interpersonal relations. FT was intended to decrease the level of expressed emotion within the family and establish realistic expectations of the patient's behaviours. Families were taught about the disorder, and trained in strategies to help them manage their schizophrenic family member. The control group received weekly supportive individual counselling. The active treatment groups were seen weekly during the acute phase of treatment, biweekly for three to four months after that, and then monthly for the duration of the one year follow-up period. The SST + FFT combined group received more face-to-face treatment than the other groups.

Relapse rates were the only form of programme evaluation reported. Schizophrenic relapse was judged to have occurred if the subject, according to the RDC criteria had changed from being nonpsychotic to psychotic or if a severe clinical exacerbation of persistent psychotic symptoms had occurred (Hogarty *et al.*, 1986 p. 636). There was a statistically significant effect of SST and FT on relapse. At 12 months after discharge relapse rates were 41% of the controls, 20% of the SST only group, 19% of the FT only group, and 0% of the SST + FT group. Unfortunately, there was no measure of the subjects' level of social or problem-solving skills to compare with their likelihood of relapse. At two-year follow-up there were still significant effects of treatment, though relapse rates in all groups had increased and now were 66% for the controls, 42% for the SST group, 32% for the FT group and 25% for the SST + FT group (Hogarty *et al.*, 1987). The amount of therapy time was not consistent across the groups, which precludes demonstration of a specific effect of particular treatment components in this study.

In the three studies which evaluated positive symptomatology (Bellack *et al.*, 1984; Wallace and Liberman, 1985; Hogarty *et al.*, 1986) SST had significantly more impact than the control group in two studies. The day hospital group in Bellack *et al.*'s (1984) study were found to have improved on positive schizophrenic symptomatology to an approximately equal extent as the SST group. No studies to date have measured negative symptomatology. However, Brown and Munford (1983) found SST produced significant improvement on a depression scale, as well as optimism for the future. In the four studies in which specific social skills were measured, SST produced significant improvements (Brown and Munford, 1983; Spencer *et al.*, 1983; Bellack *et al.*, 1984; Wallace and Liberman, 1985). Generalization of social skills was assessed in three of the studies (Spencer *et al.*, 1983; Bellack *et al.*, 1984; Wallace and Liberman, 1985), though only the Wallace and Liberman (1985) study used a naturalistic non-institutional setting. Their SST group subjects were significantly more successful conversing with a stranger, and were more likely to retain the skills at follow-up than the control group. Only in the Hogarty *et al.* (1986, 1987) study were the relapse rates in the SST group statistically significantly lower than the control. There was a trend in this direction in the Wallace and Liberman (1985) study, but not in the Bellack *et al.* (1984) study.

22.4 CONCLUSIONS

The methodology of studies of SST and schizophrenia have been refined over the past two decades. However, recent studies do not substantially change the conclusions that can be drawn: SST produces behaviour change in the treatment setting, but the transfer of training effects to patients' behaviour in the community has not been assessed adequately. The only studies to demonstrate a clinical effect of SST were the Hogarty *et al.* (1986) and Wallace and Liberman (1985) studies. Neither study

produced clear evidence of a change in patients' social behaviour in the community.

The observed changes in topographical features of social behaviour occurring in response to SST are insufficient to justify use of this intensive treatment. Unless these skills are generalized to interactions with different people in the home, workplace and community, the training serves little purpose. Even in the Hogarty *et al.* (1986) study which reported the clearest clinical effects of SST the authors noted that: 'The failure of earlier acquired social skills seems to suggest an inability of patients to generalize skills to novel situations or to environments beyond the control of clinicians' (Hogarty *et al.*, 1987, p. 13). Generalization of social skills training has not been routinely assessed, and this needs to be done in future studies.

Implicit in the use of SST is the assumption that, once new behaviours are acquired, these improved social skills will be maintained by reinforcement in the natural environment (Goldsmith and McFall, 1975). As noted elsewhere (Payne and Halford, 1990), the social environments of many schizophrenic patients, (e.g. day hospitals and hostels with large numbers of fellow chronic psychiatric patients), probably do not reinforce much of the social behaviour acquired in SST. Social environments within the broader community in which socially skilled behaviour is reinforced (e.g. paid employment, recreation in general community facilities), may demand entry levels of social skill beyond many chronic schizophrenic patients.

Reinforcement and maintenance of socially skilled behaviour in schizophrenic patients may be enhanced with the use of transitional environments. Transitional environments are structured to provide a systematic shift in the criteria for reinforcement of social skills over time, so they eventually approximate reinforcement contingencies in the targeted social environment. For example, vocational rehabilitation has been conducted with schizophrenic patients across a hierarchy of settings in which the level of skill required is increased gradually to approximate normal employment conditions (Jacobs, 1988). In addition naturally occurring social environments can be identified which provide reinforcers salient to individual patients, and which will reinforce and maintain socially skilled behaviour. For example, in ongoing work the current authors have had schizophrenic patients identify active recreation they wish to pursue. We have conducted functional analyses of the social skills required to take part in these activities, selected activities which require skills not much beyond the patients' current level of functioning, and then trained these skills as participation is prompted and reinforced. It is hypothesized that the natural reinforcers within these recreational environments will maintain use of the targeted socially skilled behaviours.

Even if generalized change in social behaviour is achieved and maintained, the impact of that change on patients' quality of life and clinical status is undemonstrated. In the use of SST with schizophrenic patients it is presumed that improved social skills will enable the patient to develop and maintain a social network from which to draw support, and also will enable the patient to cope better with life stress (Anthony and Liberman, 1986). The impact of social skills on either the size or availability of the patient's social networks, or on the patient's ability to cope with stress, have not been demonstrated (Halford and Hayes, 1991).

SST is a complex multi-component treatment, and the crucial elements in treatment are unclear. It is notable that in some recent studies, both the social skills groups and the comparison groups improved to a point where there were few significant differences between them on the outcome measures (e.g. Bellack *et al.*, 1984). It is likely that staff and group support are responsible for at least some of the change experienced in both treatment and control groups. Bellack *et al.*'s (1984) control group participated in a day hospital programme

only. They did not specify in detail what this entailed. Wallace and Liberman's (1986) HHT group received the same amount of treatment time as the SST group but with different activities including yoga, jogging, and community outings. Other researchers have not matched control and treatment groups for duration of intervention and staff involvement. Brown and Munford's (1983) control group received a 'traditional rehabilitation programme', Finch and Wallace's (1977) 'normal hospital routine' and Monti *et al.*'s (1979) bibliotherapy requiring minimal staff attention. In future research SST and comparison condition subjects should receive comparable amounts of time spent in positive activities with staff expressing care and concern, to control for nonspecific treatment factors. Spencer *et al.* (1983) provide a good model of such matching.

Aside from the nonspecific treatment effects, the relative contributions of training in social perception, social problem solving, and overt social behaviour are unclear. Bellack *et al.* (1989) argued that social problem solving has not been shown to be appropriate for schizophrenic patients, while Liberman *et al.* (1985) argue it is the most appropriate intervention for higher cognitive functioning schizophrenic patients. No research as yet allows resolution of this issue, though the two most successful SST intervention studies published thus far have utilized social-problem solving (Liberman *et al.*, 1985; Hogarty *et al.*, 1986). A specific effect of social perception training has not yet been demonstrated, though recent evidence suggests that social perception deficits are a major problem in schizophrenia (Morrison *et al.*, 1988).

The heterogeneity in patients' responses to SST has been noted previously (e.g. Bellack *et al.*, 1984; Liberman *et al.*, 1986), and this variability makes it difficult to demonstrate treatment effects. Liberman *et al.* (1985) suggested some low functioning schizophrenic patients with severe cognitive deficits are unlikely to benefit from traditional SST. They described use of an 'attention focusing' strategy which focused on training very specific skills in a highly repetitive manner. This approach improved social skills in patients previously unresponsive to SST. Similarly Payne and Halford (1990) reported successful use of a highly structured board game to train social skills to low functioning schizophrenic patients who seemed unlikely to benefit from traditional SST. Brenner (1987) has reported interventions in which training to overcome the cognitive disorders prevalent in schizophrenia are combined with more standard SST. Almost all of the work is published in the German language, but Brenner (1987) claims those procedures improve the efficacy of SST. Procedures remediating cognitive deficits are likely to become of increasing importance in SST with schizophrenic patients.

Different aspects of schizophrenic symptomatology and behaviour may respond to different aspects of SST. For example, the impact of SST on negative symptomatology has not been assessed, but it is possible that cognitive rehabilitation efforts may be particularly relevant to patients with predominant negative symptoms. Some authors have suggested that the presence of predominately negative symptoms in schizophrenia predicts a chronic course unresponsive to psychological or other treatment (Crow, 1985). Others argue that patients with negative symptoms are most in need of psychosocial interventions (Anthony and Liberman, 1986). Research is needed to assess which aspects of schizophrenia respond to SST.

SST with schizophrenic patients shows potential to improve patients' coping in the community, increase their quality of life, and decrease the cost of hospitalization for the community. The most recent studies offer some limited evidence of the benefits, but the most successful programmes have involved very extensive therapeutic intervention.The future use of SST depends upon clarification of the extent of generalization of training effects to community settings, whether changes are durable over time, and whether these changes improve the broad clinical status of the patient. There is a need to examine the impact of particular types of social skills training on patients with different levels of functioning, and different patterns of positive and negative symptoms. Particular attention needs to be paid to treating the cognitive deficits evident in schizophrenic patients. It is only by matching treatment goals and procedures to patients' needs more carefully that we can hope to be more helpful to our patients.

22.5 SUMMARY

Deficits in social and interpersonal functioning are central in most definitions of schizophrenia. Social skills training (SST) has been utilized over the past two decades in attempts to remediate these interpersonal skill deficits. SST uses a structured behavioural approach including instructions, modelling, behaviour rehearsal, structured feedback, and structured homework exercises, to teach schizophrenic patients appropriate ways of dealing with difficult social situations. These skill training procedures do improve patients' interpersonal skills. However, the extent to which these effects transfer from the training environment to the patient's day-to-day social life is questionable. Furthermore, there is very limited evidence of the specific effects of social skills training on the broader clinical status of schizophrenic patients. Development of more effective social skills training requires further research assessing the effects of cognitive deficits and intrusive symptomatology on social behaviour, and evaluating the utility of adding cognitive rehabilitation strategies to SST. It also is necessary to better assess the transfer of training effects to a patient's every day life, and to promote such generalization by ensuring there is sufficient reinforcement in a client's environments to maintain acquired social skills.

ACKNOWLEDGEMENT

The authors thank Beverley Raphael, Roger Dooley, Matt Sanders and Frank Varghese for helpful comments on an earlier draft of the paper, and Jill Faddy and Janet Dupree for manuscript preparation.

REFERENCES

American Psychiatric Association (1987) *DSM-III-R: Diagnostic and Statistical Manual of Mental Disorders* (3rd ed. Revised). American Psychiatric Association, Washington, DC.

Anthony, W.A. and Liberman, R.P. (1986) The practice of psychiatric rehabilitation: Historical, conceptual, and research base. *Schizophr. Bull.*, 12, 542–59.

Argyle, M. and Kendon, A. (1967) The experimental analysis of social behaviour. In *Advances in Experimental Social Psychology Vol. 3*. L. Berkowitz (ed), Academic Press, New York, pp. 55–98.

Beidel, D.C., Bellack, A.S., Turner, S.M. *et al.* (1981) *Social Skills Training for Chronic Psychiatric Patients: A Treatment Manual*. Western Psychiatric Institute and Clinic. Pittsburg, PA.

Bellack, A.S. (1983) Recurrent problems in the behavioural assessment of social skill. *Behav. Res. Ther.*, 21, 29–41.

Bellack, A.S., Hersen, M. and Turner, S.M. (1976) Generalization effects of social skills training in chronic schizophrenics: An experimental analysis. *Behav. Res. Ther.*, 14, 391–8.

Bellack, A.S., Turner, S.M., Hersen, M. and Luber, R.F. (1984) An examination of the efficacy of social skills training for chronic schizophrenic patients. *Hosp. Community Psychiatry*, 35, 1023–8.

Bellack, A.S., Morrison, R.L. and Mueser, K.T. (1989) Social problem solving in schizophrenia. *Schizophr. Bull.*, 15, 101–16.

Brady, J.P. (1984a) Social skills training for psychiatric patients, I: Concepts, methods, and clinical results. *Occup. Ther. Ment. Health*, 4, 51–68.

Brady, J.P. (1984b) Social skills training for psychiatric patients, II: Clinical outcome studies. *Am. J. Psychiatry*, 141, 491–8.

Brenner, H.D. (1987) On the importance of cognitive disorders in treatment and rehabilitation. In *Psychosocial Treatment of Schizophrenia*. J.S. Strauss, W. Boker and H.D. Brenner (eds), Hans Huber, Toronto, pp. 136–51.

Brown, M.A. and Munford, A.M. (1983) Life skills training for chronic schizophrenics. *J. Nerv. Ment. Dis.*, 171, 466–70.

Crow, T. (1985) The two-syndrome concept: Origins and current status. *Schizophr. Bull*, 11, 471–85.

Curran, J.P., Monti, P.M. and Corriveau, D.P. (1982) Treatment of schizophrenia. In *International Handbook of Behavior Modification and Therapy*. A.S. Bellack, M. Hersen and A.E. Kazdin (eds), Plenum, New York, pp. 433–66.

Falloon, I.R.H., Boyd, J.L. and McGill, C.W. (1984) *Behavioral Family Management of Mental Illness: Enhancing Family Coping in Community Care*. Guilford, New York.

Finch, B.E. and Wallace, C.J. (1977) Successful interpersonal skills training with schizophrenic inpatients. *J. Consult. Clin. Psychol.*, 45, 885–90.

Goldsmith, J.B. and McFall, R.M. (1975) Development and evaluation of an interpersonal skill-training programme for psychiatric inpatients. *J. Abnorm. Psychol.*, 84, 51–8.

Halford, W.K. and Hayes, R.L. (1991), Psychological rehabilitation of schizophrenia: Recent findings on social skills training and family psychoeducation. *Clin. Psychol. Rev.*, 11, 23–44.

Hansen, D.J., St Lawrence, J.S. and Cristoff, K.A. (1985) Effects of interpersonal problem-solving training with chronic aftercare patients on problem-solving component skills and effectiveness of solutions. *J. Consult. Clin. Psychol.*, 53, 167–74.

Hayes, R.L. and Halford, W.K. (1990) *Social Skills Training for Chronic Schizophrenic Patients: A Therapist's Manual*. Unpublished manuscript, Department of Psychiatry, University of Queensland.

Hersen, M. (1979) Modification of skill deficits in psychiatric patients. In *Research and Practice in Social Skills Training*. A.S. Bellack and

M. Hersen (eds), Plenum Press, New York, pp. 189–236.

Hersen, M. and Bellack, A.S. (1976) Social skills training for chronic psychiatric patients: Rationale, research findings, and future directions. *Compr. Psychiatry*, **17**, 559–80.

Hogarty, G.E., Anderson, C.M. and Reiss, D.J. (1987) Family psychoeducation, social skills training, and medication in schizophrenia: The long and the short of it. *Psychopharmacol. Bull*, **23**, 12–13.

Hogarty, G.E., Anderson, C.M., Reiss, D.J. *et al.* (1986) Family psychoeducation, social skills training and maintenance chemotherapy in the aftercare treatment of schizophrenia. *Arch. Gen. Psychiatry*, **43**, 633–42.

Jackson, K.J. (1988) *Social Skills and Negative Symptoms in Schizophrenia*. Unpublished M.A. Thesis, University of Melbourne.

Jacobs, H.E. (1988) Vocational rehabilitation. In *Psychiatric Rehabilitation of Chronic Mental Patients*. R.P. Liberman (ed), American Psychiatric Press, Washington, DC, pp. 245–84.

Kale, R.J., Kaye, J.H., Whelan, P.A. and Hopkins, B.L. (1968) The effects of reinforcement on the modification and generalization of social responses of mental patients. *J. Appl. Behav. Anal.*, **1**, 307–14.

Lange, A. and Jakubowski, P. (1976) *Responsible Assertive Behavior*. Research Press, Champaign, Illinois.

Lewine, R.R.J., Watt, N.F. and Fryer, J.H. (1978) A study of childhood social competence, adult premorbid competence, and psychiatric outcome in three schizophrenic subtypes. *J. Abnorm. Psychol.*, **87**, 294–302.

Lewine, R.R.J., Watt, N.F., Prentky, R.A. and Fryer, J.H. (1980) Childhood social competence in functionally disordered patients and in normals. *J. Abnorm. Psychol.*, **89**, 132–8.

Liberman, R.P., King, L.W., De Risi, W.J. and McCann, M. (1975) *Personal Effectiveness*. Research Press, Champaign, Illinois.

Liberman, R.P., Massel, A.K., Mosk, M.D. and Wong, S.E. (1985) Social skills training for chronic mental patients. *Hosp. Community Psychiatry*, **36**, 396–403.

Liberman, R.P., Mueser, K.T. and Wallace, C.J. (1986) Social skills training for schizophrenic individuals at risk for relapse. *Am. J. Psychiatry*, **143**, 523–6.

Liberman, R.P., De Risi, W.J. and Mueser, K.T. (1989) *Social Skills Training with Psychiatric Patients*. Pergamon, New York.

Monti, P.M., Curran, J.P., Corriveau, D.P. *et al.* (1980) Effects of social skills training groups and sensitivity training groups with psychiatric patients. *J. Consult. Clin. Psychol.*, **48**, 241–8.

Monti, P.M., Fink, E., Norman, W. *et al.* (1979) Effects of social skills training groups and social skills bibliotherapy with psychiatric patients. *J. Consult. Clin. Psychol.*, **47**, 189–91.

Morrison, R.L., Bellack, A.S. and Mueser, K.T. (1988) Deficits in facial-affect recognition and schizophrenia. *Schizophr. Bull.*, **14**, 67–83.

Payne, P. and Halford, W.K. (1990). Generalization of social skills training with schizophrenic patients living in the community. *Behav. Psychother.*, **18**, 49–64.

Serber, M. and Nelson, P. (1971) The ineffectiveness of systematic desensitization and assertive training in hospitalized schizophrenics. *J. Behav. Ther. Exp. Psychiatry*, **2**, 107–9.

Shelton, J.L. and Levy, R.L. (1981) *Behavioural Assignments and Treatment Compliance: A Handbook of Clinical Strategies*. Research Press, Champaign, Illinois.

Spencer, P.G., Gillespie, C.R. and Ekisa, E.G. (1983) A controlled comparison of the effects of social skills training and remedial drama on the conversational skills of chronic schizophrenic inpatients. *Br. J. Psychiatry*, **143**, 165–72.

St. Lawrence, T.S., Hansen, D.J., Cutts, T.F. *et al.* (1985) Situational context: Effects on perceptions of assertive and unassertive behaviour. *Behav. Ther.*, **16**, 51–62.

Trower, P., Bryant, B. and Argyle, M. (1978) *Social Skills and Mental Health*. Methuen, London.

Wallace, C.J. (1982) The social skills training project of the Mental Health Clinical Research Center for the study of schizophrenia. In *Social Skills Training*. J.P. Curran and P.M. Monti (eds), Guilford, New York, pp. 57–89.

Wallace, C.J. (1984) Community and interpersonal functioning in the course of schizophrenic disorders. *Schizophr. Bull.*, **10**, 223–57.

Wallace, C.J. and Liberman, R.P. (1985) Social skills training for patients with schizophrenia: A controlled clinical trial. *Psychiatry Res.*, **15**, 239–47.

Wallace, C.J., Boone, S.E., Donohue, C.P. and Foy, D.W. (1985) The chronically mentally disabled: independent living skills training. In *Clinical Handbook of Psychological Disorders*. D. Barlow (ed), Guilford, New York, pp. 462–501.

Wallace, C.J., Nelson, C.J., Liberman, R.P. *et al.* (1980) A review and critique of social skills training with schizophrenic patients. *Schizophr. Bull.*, **6**, 42–63.

Chapter 23

Training life skills

SHIRLEY M. GLYNN and SALLY MacKAIN

23.1 HISTORICAL TRENDS IN THE TREATMENT OF SCHIZOPHRENIA

Our conceptualizations of schizophrenia and other major psychiatric disorders have gone through revolutionary changes in the past 40 years. Prior to the advent of anti-psychotic medications in the mid-1950s, patients suffering with schizophrenia were thought to be caught in an unremitting downward spiral, with little hope for recovery or rehabilitation (Kraepelin, 1919, 1921). In light of this poor prognosis, it is not surprising that treatment efforts typically involved trying to keep patients comfortable, calm, and occupied while they were sequestered away from the stresses and strains of everyday living situations. Persons suffering from schizophrenia frequently resided in asylums or institutions for many years, or lived sheltered lives at a relative's or friend's home.

The discovery that antipsychotic medications could often reduce or eliminate symptoms such as hallucinations, delusions and formal thought disorder brought a new spirit of hope to mental health professionals working with patients in schizophrenia. This enthusiasm for new treatment innovations and more active interventions for patients with severe mental illness culminated with legislative acts both in the USA and Europe to decentralize care for the mentally ill and to base it in the community. Rather than being considered intractable, schizophrenia was re-conceptualized as a serious, but temporary, disorder which could be controlled and even eradicated by proper care and medication. Massive efforts were made to discharge patients from hospitals and return them to their communities, where they would presumably thrive (Bachrach, 1983).

Thirty years later, the vigour with which mental health professionals embraced the idea that the availability of psychotropic medications would permit most patients to be reintegrated into society seems almost embarrassingly naive. As we now know, while the benefits of neuroleptic medication are very real, they are also limited. Three factors contribute to this less optimistic appraisal of the positive aspects of anti-psychotic agents. First, these medications offer little of no benefit for 20–30% of all patients with schizophrenia (Gardos and Cole, 1976; Chapter 19). Second, even among patients who do obtain relief fom their psychotic symptoms with the medications, continued compliance is a problem. Reasons for this non-compliance include denial of the illness and dislike of the particularly noxious side effects resulting from neuroleptic medications (Van Putten, 1974; Chapter 20). Finally, even when these medications are effective in reducing hallucinations and the other positive symptoms of schizophrenia, they frequently do little to reduce negative symptoms such as anhedonia, apathy, social isolation, and alogia (Kane and Meyerhoff, 1989). In addition, neuroleptic side effects such as sedation and akinesia may actually make these negative symptoms worse.

The failure of neuroleptic medications to 'cure' schizophrenia is beginning to have a profound influence on our newer models of the disorder. As Bellack and Mueser note, the conceptualization of schizophrenia as a circumscribed, short-lived disturbance in functioning which is highly responsive to pharmacological intervention, which was prevalent in the 1960s and 1970s, has not been confirmed by clinical experience (Bellack and Mueser, 1986). Certainly, up to 25% of patients with schizophrenia do have extended periods of high social and vocational functioning interrupted only briefly and very infrequently by psychotic episodes (Stephens, 1978). These patients typically have had high levels of premorbid functioning, and are able to return to these levels; some require anti-psychotic medications, while others do not.

Most patients with schizophrenia have a less benign illness course. A substantial number (approximately 25%) obtain little benefit from anti-psychotic agents and require ongoing supervision in a protected setting such as a psychiatric hospital or locked residential facility. The remaining 50% typically do not require extended hospitalizations, but their overall level of functioning between psychotic episodes is impaired, and they may need supervision and case-management support, in addition to psychiatric intervention. For them, schizophrenia is a chronic incurable illness which is exacerbated by stress, analogous to juvenile diabetes or kidney disease. They require training in coping with the disorder by managing symptoms effectively and instruction in ways to live as full and independent a life as possible.

It is important to note, however, that training and support in successful living is to be distinguished from intensive psychotherapy or excessively demanding psychosocial programmes. Schizophrenia seriously impairs the patient's ability to tolerate stress, whether it is from intensive introspection or from participation in an over-stimulating, confrontative milieu (Drake and Sederer, 1986). Given their own state of hyperarousal (Dawson and Nuechterlein, 1984), most patients with schizophrenia benefit most from structured programmes with clear, explicit expectations of attainable performance levels. These comprehensible, reasonable expectations help reduce environmental stimulation to manageable levels. Confusing, overstimulating therapy programmes are generally to be avoided for these patients, as they can have toxic effects on participants (Mueser and Berenbaum, 1990).

23.2 THE IMPORTANCE OF LIFE SKILLS IN TEACHING COPING WITH SCHIZOPHRENIA

Living a full and independent life raises many challenges for the person with schizophrenia. Analogous to those for physical illness, rehabilitation approaches to psychiatric illness conceptualize the disorder as proceeding in four stages: (1) pathology; (2) impairment; (3) disability; and (4) handicap (Anthony and Liberman, 1986). The stress-vulnerability model of mental illness embraces these concepts in positing that biological abnormalities, or 'pathologies' interact with an increased vulnerability to stress. This interaction results in diverse constellations of symptom 'impairments', associated with social and vocational 'disabilities' and 'handicaps' in role functioning. The goal of psychiatric rehabilitation is to increase the mentally ill individual's repertoire of social and instrumental skills in order to improve his or her ability to cope with a stressful world.

These coping skills, together with social support and psychotropic medications protect, or serve as a buffer in guarding against relapse.

Skills training for individuals or whole families significantly reduces psychiatric symptoms in schizophrenic patients already stabilized on medication (Falloon *et al.*, 1982; Liberman *et al.*, 1984; Wallace and Liberman, 1985; Chapter 24). For example, in one study of schizophrenic patients, 41% of the subjects who received medications alone relapsed after one year, whereas only 21% of subjects relapsed during the same time period if they received medications *and* individual skills training to help reduce family conflict. None of the patients who received medication, the individual skills training *and* psychoeducational family sessions relapsed (Hogarty *et al.*, 1986).

In the interpersonal realm, many persons with schizophrenia have reduced social networks and heightened social anxiety (Pattison *et al.*, 1979). By using *social skills*, these persons can increase their social networks and reduce anxiety, thereby buffering the noxious effects of life stress. There is now a large body of literature suggesting that social skills training can have a beneficial impact on at least short-term prognosis in schizophrenia, and the reader is referred to Chapter 22 for a more thorough discussion of this topic.

Adequate social skills alone are not enough to live an effective life, however. There is a range of other activities and areas which must be mastered for successful living. These include personal hygiene and grooming, attention to medical and physical needs, clothes care, money management and budgeting, nutrition and food preparation, housekeeping, transportation, and the development of vocational and avocational competencies. Taken together, these can all be subsumed under the label life skills. Surveys indicate that persons with schizophrenia, especially those residing in supervised or hospital settings, frequently have serious skills deficits in these areas (Sylph *et al.*, 1977; Brewin *et al.*, 1988).

When patients resided for extended periods in hospitals or were under close observation by family members, competence in these skills was not a necessary component of successful living. Hospital staff or family members were typically available to prepare meals, do laundry, prompt patients to care for their personal hygiene, and help manage or supervise the hundreds of other details of life. In contrast, patients discharged to the community, especially those residing with relatives or in supervised settings, must typically assume more responsibility for these types of activities. If they do not budget their money well enough to buy food, they may go hungry. If they are unable to use the public transportation system, they may be unable to get to the clinic to see the physician and obtain their medication.

Achieving and maintaining satisfactory work functioning is among the most challenging of the life skills for persons with schizophrenia. The low employment rate among patients with serious psychiatric difficulties highlights the difficulty of this challenge. Only about 25–30% of patients return to work within six months of their discharge from the hospital, and only about half of these are still employed one year later (Anthony *et al.*, 1978). This fact is particularly disturbing, given the central aspect that vocational training plays in the part of most (non-psychotic) individuals' judgments of their self-worth, and the findings that structured activities tend to reduce bizarre, inappropriate behaviours among psychiatric patients (Rosen *et al.*, 1981). Vocational rehabilitation, including the development of literacy if it is lacking, should clearly be a critical component of treatment plans for most patients with schizophrenia.

Prognostic studies reveal the importance of adequate life skills in predicting successful community adjustment. Presley *et al.* (1982) found that only baseline self-care skills such as money management and care of clothes discriminated long-stay psychiatric patients in a new rehabilitation programme who were subsequently discharged to more independent settings from those who were not. In a large-scale sample of chronically mentally ill patients participating in the National Institute of Mental Health Community Support Program, Tessler and Mandersheid (1982), found that levels of basic living skills was more strongly related to community work adjustment and involvement in positive social activity than either amount of behavioural problems or somatic complaints. In a five-year outcome study of 100 English patients with schizophrenia, Prudo and Blum (1987) found that social functioning at baseline, including vocational achievement, social relationships, and residence adequacy and stability, significantly predicted both symptomatic status and social functioning at follow-up. Importantly, in predicting both social and symptom outcome, baseline vocational and social functioning improved predictions of follow-up status made based on initial symptom level alone. These three studies highlight the influence of vocational and living skills on successful community adjustment.

Until recently, most treatment programmes for persons with schizophrenia have placed relatively little emphasis on developing life skills. When schizophrenia was considered an intractable illness and patients resided for extended periods in hospitals, there was little reason or motivation to teach the skills necessary for independent or semi-independent living. During the first decade of the deinstitutionalization movement, when the prevailing model of schizophrenia was a temporary disorder which would remit and allow a premorbid level of functioning, there was an implicit assumption that, once their symptoms were under control, patients would be able to return to independent functioning. It has only been by witnessing the high number of patients who fail in community placements that their deficits in living skills have become painfully apparent to all concerned.

23.3 CAUSES OF LIFE SKILLS DEFICITS

In retrospect, the pervasiveness of these deficiencies should not have been unexpected.

Schizophrenia typically develops during young adulthood, often as the individual is making his or her first strides towards independence. The psychotic episode may interupt college attendance, military enlistment, or initial vocational activities, as well as early attempts to live separately from one's family of origin. The brevity of this premorbid independent functioning may prohibit the individual from learning to navigate many of the more difficult aspects of life (e.g. budgeting and money management, succeeding vocationally). Even after the psychotic episode is over, this inexperience can result in a living skills deficit.

Schizophrenic symptomatology can also have a direct influence on the adequate performance of living skills. Certainly, experiencing distressing hallucinations can reduce interest and motivation in the more basic aspects of life, such as grooming and nutrition. Many persons with schizophrenia also suffer from cognitive difficulties such as distractibility and memory impairments (Nuechterlein and Dawson, 1984). These problems frequently impede the patient's ability to form a plan of action and follow it to conclusion. This reduction in goal setting and planned activity can result in an inability to complete necessary tasks such as shopping, cleaning, and seeking and keeping employment. Finally, negative symptoms such as apathy, anhedonia, and amotivation are integral aspects of the schizophrenic illness for many patients. Unfortunately, these deficit symptoms may be more impervious to treatment with neuroleptic medication (Kane and Mayerhoff, 1989), and in fact may be worsened by pharmacological interventions. Needless to say, persons experiencing apathy and amotivation will typically not pursue life activities with enthusiasm and vigour.

23.4 MODELS OF TRAINING LIFE SKILLS

Twenty-five years of experience with deinstitutionalization have highlighted the need to support persons with schizophrenia as they try to master the skills necessary to live a satisfying life. There are currently three primary approaches to improving the life skills of patients with schizophrenia and other serious psychiatric illnesses: (1) the token economy, (2) the community support model, and (3) the modular skills training approach. All three approaches use a thorough life skills assessment, as discussed in Chapter 12, as their foundation. These models are similar in that they emphasize skills development and de-emphasize insight as a treatment goal, they focus on helping patients develop as much autonomy as possible, and they often include at least some formal instruction in relevant skills. These programmes differ, however, in whether they are situated in inpatient facilities or outpatient settings, or both, the importance they place on utilizing professional staff to train life skills, and whether the programme provides time-limited instruction or more long-term support. The basic principles of each approach and research supporting their efficacy are discussed in more detail below.

23.4.1 THE TOKEN ECONOMY

Carlson *et al.* (1972) have provided a succinct description of the actual workings of a token economy for psychiatric patients. According to the authors, token economy programmes share a variety of common characteristics, regardless of their setting. The fundamental component of the token economy is the use of operant learning principles, including developing and maintaining life skills, to yield a positive impact on patient functioning. Target behaviours must be clearly operationalized. Behaviours can be either pro-social, appropriate ones (e.g. brushing teeth, having a conversation) or inappropriate ones (e.g. assaulting someone, lying on the floor). Many of the behaviours targeted for intervention involve basic life skills. For example, patients may earn tokens for taking a thorough shower. Consequences for each of these behaviours are defined, using

tokens or points as secondary reinforcements. Typically, tokens are provided as positive reinforcements for appropriate behaviours (e.g. patient earns three tokens for getting up on time in the morning) or are withheld (extinction) or even taken away (response cost, e.g. the patient is fined five tokens for writing on the wall) for inappropriate behaviours. Other behavioural techniques, such as chaining, modelling, time-out, prompting, and differential reinforcement for other behaviour, are often included in the treatment programme. Frequently, shaping procedures can be utilized through the payment of partial token amounts for approximations to the operationalized appropriate behaviour.

Tokens can be used to purchase a variety of desirable reinforcements, such as access to grounds or preferred snacks. Tokens are usually awarded immediately when earned, resulting in more rapid learning of contingencies, although patients may have to wait to purchase desired back-up reinforcers. Tokens may actually be tangible plastic or metal chips, or may be tallied on logs kept on individual cards. Typically, at least some aspects of the token economy will be applied to the entire treatment unit or facility, resulting in a standard set of rules with specified consequences by which all patients are expected to abide (e.g. each patient is expected to clean up his or her meal area, for which he or she will earn a specified number of tokens). In addition, individualized behavioural treatment programmes that address specific problems for each patient are often embedded in the more general token economy programme and include additional positive reinforcements, extinction, instruction, or response cost procedures; for example, John earns five extra tokens each night at 8 p.m. if he has not used foul language in the past 24 hours (Butler, 1979).

Lindsley and Skinner (Lindsley and Skinner, 1954; Lindsley, 1956, 1960) were among the first behaviourists to demonstrate that operant learning principles could be used to modify the discrete, motoric behaviours of psychotic individuals. Their positive results met with enthusiasm and influenced many investigations with psychiatric patients in the 1960s and 1970s. For example, using reversal and multiple-based designs, Ayllon and Azrin (1965, 1968) found that tokens increased work performance among a group of chronic female psychiatric patients. These authors and their colleagues also demonstrated that other behavioural techniques such as extinction and differential reinforcement for other behaviour could be used by nursing staff to increase the frequency of appropriate behaviours (e.g. polite mealtime behaviour) and decrease inappropriate behaviours (e.g. hoarding, stealing). Atthowe and Krasner (1968) extended this work by developing a token economy which was developed 'to cover all aspects of the patient's life' (p. 38) rather than just specific behaviours. Since that time, hundreds of studies have demonstrated the benefits of participation in a token economy for psychiatric patients (see Kazdin, 1977 and 1982 for a thorough review)

The most dramatic evidence of the benefits of the token economy on subsequent life functioning can be seen in the results of a study conducted by Paul and Lentz (1977). These investigators randomly assigned 84 long-term schizophrenic patients to state hospital units using social learning, milieu therapy, or traditional custodial care approaches. Additional subjects were added to replace discharged patients, yielding a final sample size of 102. The social learning programme employed a highly specific token economy with many hours of structured educational activities throughout the day. The milieu programme was based in a therapeutic community structure wherein all patients were members of a 9- or 10-person living group. Living groups were assigned the tasks of identifying problems and promoting change among individual members by exerting social and group pressure. As in the social learning group, milieu patients were scheduled to spend the majority of their time in structured life skills or academic classes. Patients in both programmes were scheduled to be in formal treatment 85% of the time.

In evaluating the results of this study, it is important to note that self-care and instrumental role training classes, with the latter including the development of literacy, housekeeping, and marketable vocational skills, were embedded in the overall treatment for the two active treatment groups.

An extensive battery of assessments, including behavioural observations, clinical event recording, and more traditional measures of symptomatology and discharge status established the social learning approach as the most efficacious. By the end of the study, social learning patients had spent less time in the hospital, achieved greater discharge rates, were maintained longer in the community, and required less psychotropic medication than either the milieu or traditional care comparison groups. Self-care skills improved over three times as much in the social learning as in the milieu groups Instrumental role functioning improved over twice as much in the social learning group as in the milieu group. All differences were statistically significant, and suggest that while formal instruction helped in skill development, actually using these skills in the token economy was also integral to attaining mastery and competence.

Curran *et al.* (1985) have noted that token economy approaches to the development and maintenance of life skills may be especially important for patients who function at low levels and must struggle with persistent psychotic symptoms. These patients are frequently labelled treatment refractory; they typically obtain little benefit from psychiatric medications and require intensive supervision and structure. Poor premorbid functioning and/ or years of hospitalization have often resulted in extreme skills deficits in these patients. By providing structured rules and tangible reinforcement over repeated trials, token economies frequently provide the best opportunities for these patients to develop at least minimal skills.

The primary criticism of token economy approaches focus on issues of maintenance and generalization (Kazdin, 1982, 1985). It seems clear that token economies can be used to develop basic life skills. However, data are still generally lacking regarding whether these changes are maintained once the patient has made a transition to another, typically more independent, living situation which does not utilize a token economy.

23.4.2 THE COMMUNITY SUPPORT MODEL

Token economy programmes have most often been based in inpatient settings. Unfortunately, gains achieved in the hospital are not always maintained post-discharge (Kazdin, 1982, 1985). In addition, successful adaptation to the community often requires an entirely new set of skills which are not critical in the hospital. Community support programmes have been developed to bolster patient functioning after discharge. These programmes typically see themselves as providing ongoing support over extended periods of time, frequently years, rather than being brief, time-limited interventions.

One of the most critical variables differentiating types of community support programmes is the relative emphasis placed on the use of professional staff versus recovering patients in supporting the rehabilitation of other patients. At one extreme are programmes such as the Training in Community Living (TCL) Model (Stein and Test, 1985) in Wisconsin and the Bridge Program (Witheridge and Dincin, 1985) in Chicago. These programmes utilize aggressive professional community based case-management teams. Treatment teams assume responsibility for making certain that all patient needs are met, including coordinating other services such as welfare payments, work training programmes, and medical treatment. Meetings between case managers and patients are usually held in the community, at the

patient's residence or some public gathering place such as a coffee shop or library, rather than in an office. When patients need to utilize community services or resources with which they are unfamiliar or with which they anticipate difficulties, case managers typically accompany them to provide 'hands on' training and guidance in navigating the system. For example, if a patient needs to go to the telephone company office to discuss a dispute about a bill, a case manager may also attend to act as the patient's advocate and coach.

The results of the initial Wisconsin studies on the TCL programme were very encouraging. In a sample of 130 patients scheduled for hospitalization (50% with schizophrenia), Stein and Test (1980) found the random assignment to the TCL programme yielded significant benefits at 12 months follow-up, compared with assignment to the standard county-sponsored outpatient services. At follow-up, TCL subjects had spent significantly less time in the hospital, were less symptomatic, and had better social and vocational functioning, compared to controls.

This model of comprehensive community-based service delivery is currently being investigated in a large-scale prospective study involving random assignment of schizophrenic subjects to modified TCL or customary care over a 12-year period. One objective of the TCL programme is to help patients learn and use coping and living skills to achieve successful community tenure. Test *et al.* (1985) note that the concept of teaching living skills has evolved as the TCL programme has progressed. They assert that many patients can recover dormant skills or learn new ones by the extensive staff use of prompts, modelling, and reinforcement in the community setting itself. In their assessment, formal instruction is often not required. Results of their study are not yet available, but a recent description of their preliminary two-year findings are positive (Test *et al.*, 1989). Especially germane to the topic of training in living skills is their report that the majority of TCL subjects resided in low supervision settings (primarily independent apartments), while the majority of the customary care subjects lived in high-supervision settings, most typically with their families.

A contrasting community support model emphasizes the importance of developing a therapeutic milieu by encouraging patients to help each other and by minimizing (although not eliminating) the role of professional staff. This model, labelled the clubhouse model, was pioneered at Fountain House in New York City (Anthony and Liberman, 1986). Here, ex-psychiatric patients joined together to provide mutual aid, support, and vocational encouragement by becoming club 'members'. This model flourished, giving birth to comprehensive rehabilitation treatment programmes such as Thresholds in Chicago and Portals House in Los Angeles. Typically, these programmes are based in large community facilities, where members are provided with educational and vocational training, psychiatric evaluation and medication, meals, opportunities for social and leisure activities, living skills classes, and supportive group therapy. Insight as a therapeutic goal is minimized, while training and support in achieving functional independence, especially regarding vocational goals, is highlighted.

To meet career training needs, clubhouses frequently organize member work teams who, under the supervision of a paid staff person, contract with a local business for janitorial or clerical work. In meeting the terms of these contracts, members develop many critical vocational skills, such as setting and meeting deadlines, soliciting and responding appropriately to supervisorial feedback, and working cooperatively with others. Clubhouses frequently own a series of apartment buildings or homes in which members can reside, under decreasing levels of staff supervision, for specified periods of time. Members typically make a transition from sharing a room in an almost dormitory-like setting to living independently and assuming complete responsibility for bill payment, apartment upkeep, and food preparation, through a series of progressive steps. Both vocationally and residentially, the clubhouse model strives to move members from a high level of dependence and supervision to functional autonomy.

As the clubhouse model was developed as a service system rather than part of a research programme, rigorous evaluations of its effects have not been conducted. While research does suggest that participating in a clubhouse programme has a beneficial impact on community tenure (Beard *et al.*, 1978), methodological difficulties with self-selection, non-randomly assigned control groups, and lack of diagnostic clarity limit the conclusions that can be drawn from this work. In addition, the relatively small numbers of clubhouses reduces the availability of these services, especially for psychiatric patients in non-urban areas. Nevertheless, clubhouses appear to provide excellent training in necessary life skills for participating members.

23.4.2 MODULE TRAINING PROGRAMMES

An innovative method of teaching skills for independent living has been developed through the collaborative efforts of Dr Robert Liberman and colleagues at the UCLA Department of Psychiatry, Brentwood Veterans Administration Medical Center, and Camarillo State Hospital. The Social and Independent Living Skills (SILS) Modules comprise a highly structured, cohesive set of teaching tools based on behavioural learning principles which are designed to meet the specific needs of people with serious, chronic mental illness. In contrast to the interventions mentioned previously, the modules are designed to be time-limited training programmes but can be used in all phases of an individual's treatment, in inpatient, daycare or outpatient treatment, in residential care facilities, clinics, or in the community on a continuing case management basis. Completion of a module can take three to four months, and 'booster sessions' are recommended in the following weeks and months to reinforce the skills and information that are acquired in the modules.

The modules can be taught by people with a wide variety of backgrounds and interests. Although no formal training is necessary to teach a module, trainers must be able to follow printed instructions and be willing to adapt the module to the needs of their patients. Trainers need to create a positive, non-threatening learning environment and utilize modelling and shaping procedures that focus on each person's successes, no matter how small. This approach also involves a great deal of repetition and is designed to combat negative symptoms associated with long-term mental disorders, including poor memory, low motivation, and social withdrawal.

As can be seen in Table 23.1, modules are available to help provide support for and training in many diverse aspects of patient's lives. The modules most pertinent to independent living will be described in some detail below. First, however, a brief description of how the modules are organized will help clarify how they are implemented.

Table 23.1 Module content areas

Social and independent living skills modules*
Recreation for leisure
Symptom self-management
Medication management
Grooming and personal hygiene
Job-finding
Interpersonal problem-solving
Basic conversational skills

*These modules are currently available or in development

23.4.2.1 How the modules are organized

Each SILS module consists of a trainer's manual, patient workbook and a videotape that models the skills to be learned. [1]. The trainer's manual describes in detail, session-by-session, exactly what is to be taught on any given day. Patient workbooks provide group participants with self-monitoring materials, worksheets, and printed information relevant to the skills being taught. SILS groups may consist of anywhere from 1 to 15 patients, depending on the trainer's personal style and preference, the needs of the patients, and the requirements of the particular setting. Optimally, groups should be conducted a minimum of twice a week, for one hour per session. Given this schedule, about three or four months are needed to complete a module with a group of about 10 participants. The very disruptive positive symptoms of the mental illness should be under sufficient control so that the individual can at least sit with the group and not disrupt the training. The modules are highly adaptable and are appropriate for patients of a wide variety of functioning levels.

Skill areas. Each module is divided into a number of skill areas, or content areas. The *Recreation for Leisure* module has four skill areas: (1) How to identify the benefits of recreational activities; (2) Getting information about recreational activities; (3) Finding out what's needed for participating in recreational activities; and (4) Making a commitment, evaluating, and maintaining a recreational activity.

In conjunction with classroom work, weekly field trips or other recreational activities are recommended. These outings give participants opportunities to use and practice newly acquired skills.

The *Grooming and Personal Hygiene* module is divided into eight skill areas, although more could be added: (1) Bathing; (2) Dental care; (3) Hair care; (4) Shaving; (5) Foot care; (6) Women's issues; (7) Clothing care; (8) Buying clothing. In addition, personal appearance checklists are provided and completed during the group. Participants are also asked to keep self-monitoring sheets in their room or locker and to complete these daily.

Training of Interpersonal Problem Solving Skills (TIPSS) teaches patients how to recognize and solve problems they may encounter in everyday life. A videotape models for patients and for trainers the techniques for conducting sessions and using social problem-solving skills, and another tape of supplementary exercises provides the stimulus for discussion and practive. A trainer's manual, patient workbooks, and a method for assessing interpersonal problem solving skills (AIPSS) are also included.

The *Job-Finding* module arose from the Job-Finding Club, a vocational programme at the Brentwood VA (Veterans Administration) in California (Jacobs *et al.*, 1984). The concept of working with groups of psychiatric patients to help them support each other and develop skills for job seeking and maintenance was developed by Azrin and Besalel (1980). The Job-Finding module involves two phases, job seeking skills, and the job search. In the first phase of the programme, members are given instruction in completing job applications and are taught how to identify and manage resources needed to find a job such as transportation and advertisements for employment opportunities. Patients also learn how to present themselves effectively in an interview situation and are taught how to solve job-related problems.

Once participants have learned these job-finding skills, they participate in phase two of the programme and actively seek employment with the help of trainers. If a member loses his or her job or wants to find additional or alternative employment, he or she may rejoin the group. A job maintenance group is also held once a week, where employed participants can work on solving problems, role play problem situations, and can obtain feedback from other members and trainers. For most participants, the job-finding module takes considerably less time to complete than the others.

Learning activities. Each skill or content area of the modules is taught using seven learning activities, or teaching steps. Although the content or skills differ from module to module, the **process** by which the skills are taught is relatively the same. All seven learning activities are used in the *Grooming and Personal Hygiene modules*, while the *Interpersonal Problem Solving* and *Job-Finding modules use* various combinations of them:

(1) *Introduction to the skill area.* The trainer defines key terms and encourages group members to identify ways in which learning the skills might benefit them.

(2) *Videotaped questions and answers.* To **model** the skill, a videotape is shown in which actors successfully perform a set of behaviours. The trainer pauses the tape periodically to ask the group members questions that are specified in the trainer's manual, in order to increase patients' attention and to assess comprehension.

(3) *Role played exercises.* Next, members are asked to **practise** the skills they have recently viewed in the video, and to learn effective communication skills. Group members are encouraged to repeat their role plays until they can demonstrate that they have learned the information and skills that were demonstrated on the video. The group leader, or trainer, uses shaping and modelling techniques, may choose to videotape role plays, and offers specific, positive feedback.

(4) *Resource management problems.* To teach patients how to anticipate and solve problems they may encounter when using the skill outside the group, members learn to identify the resources they will need (e.g. money, transportation) and to evaluate various methods of obtaining these resources.

(5) *Outcome problems.* In this learning activity, participants learn a seven-step method for solving problems that may arise when trying to use the skill.

(6) *In vivo exercise.* To increase the chances that patients will use a skill effectively outside the group, participants practice the newly learned skill in situations outside the training

environment. The trainer accompanies the patient in order to provide moral support, prompts, and feedback.

(7) *Homework exercises*. Finally, group members perform the skill on their own in the community or other non-group setting. Members return to the group to discuss how the exercises went, and the group may help an individual problem-solve if he or she had difficulty with it.

The first three learning activities focus on skill acquisition, while (4) and (5) teach the individual how to prepare him or herself and teach him or her how to solve problems that may arise while using the skills. The last two activities help increase the chances that the skills will be generalized to settings outside the module group. Each learning activity builds on information learned in previous activities and takes into consideration the cognitive characteristics of people with serious mental illness.

Evidence for efficacy. The SILS modules have been field tested extensively at state hospitals, residential treatment facilities, and community health centres around the country, and the initial results are encouraging (MacKain and Wallace, 1988; Wallace, 1988) To date, the Medication Management Module has been most thoroughly evaluated; the findings are promising. For example, a recent study revealed that, compared to their baseline scores, 160 patients in 28 field-sites who completed the Medication Management module, achieved statistically significant improvements in the four knowledge areas comprising this module (obtaining information about anti-psychotic information, administration of medication and evaluation of its benefits, identifying medication side-effects, and negotiating medication issues with health care providers). In addition, their psychiatrists reported a significant increase in patients' actual use of these skills as well as a significant increase in medication compliance (Eckman *et al.*, 1990). Importantly, leaders who had been unable to attend a two-day training session in Los Angeles on how to use the modules still

facilitated groups which lead to significant patient changes, indicating that the modules are user-friendly and well-supported by written documentation.

Preliminary results of another study using the Medication Management and Symptom Self-Management modules currently ongoing at the Brentwood VA Medical Center are also encouraging. In this study, patients with schizophrenia are randomly assigned to participate in either the module or group psychotherapy, and to receive either an oral neuroleptic supplement or placebo when they demonstrate early evidence of decompensation, in a 2×2 design. While outcome data are not yet available, patients who participated in the modules demonstrated statistically significant gains in knowledge and behaviour, as compared with the group psychotherapy subjects (Marder *et al.*, 1989).

Quality assurance and programme evaluation. One of the advantages of using the skills training modules is that documentation and evaluation of patient progress is built in to the modules' structure. Progress checklists to be completed by group leaders follow each skill area, and pre-and post-tests are available in the patient workbooks. To assess how closely the SILS leader follows the module, a fidelity measure (Alexander and MacKain, 1987) can be admininstered by an observer or SILS co-leader. Results of studies of module implementation at a variety of settings indicate that the less the trainer deviates from the module *structure* (e.g. skips or rearranges activities), the more patients learn. The fidelity measure can also serve as a helpful feedback tool to help the trainer improve his/her teaching skills.

The modules are limited in that they have been designed specifically to meet the needs of the chronically mentally ill. In addition, the greatest emphasis has been placed on validating the efficacy of the Medication Management module; further tests of the other living skills modules are needed. Therapists who are uncomfortable taking a very directive role in working with patients may be uncomfortable with the structured and active nature of module activities. Nevertheless, the availability of modules to teach life skills can be expected to have a beneficial impact on the functioning of many patients with schizophrenia.

23.5 CONCLUSION

Unfortunately, training life skills has been of low priority for most mental health professionals working with persons with schizophrenia. It is of course not surprising that many clinicians have emphasized the control of hallucinations and delusions or the reduction of formal thought disorder in developing and implementing suitable treatment plans. It is now apparent, however, that failure to remediate deficits in the patient's living skills in tandem with reducing psychotic symptoms has a profound, negative impact on prognosis in the majority of patients with schizophrenia. We must continue to develop, implement and support new models of teaching living skills if we are ever to make community treatment a reality and increase the quality of life of our patients.

NOTE

1. More information on the Modules can be obtained by writing to the Training Dissemination Co-ordinator, Camarillo-UCLA Research Center, Camarillo State Hospital, Box 6022, Camarillo, CA 93011.

REFERENCES

Alexander, J.M. and MacKain, S.J. (1987) *Module Fidelity Measure*. Unpublished manuscript. UCLA-NPI Clinical Research Center for Psychiatric Rehabilitation and the Study for Schizophrenia, Los Angeles.

Anthony, W.A., Cohen, M.R. and Vitalo, R. (1978) The Measurement of Rehabilitation Outcome. *Schizophr. Bull.*, **4**, 365–83.

Anthony, W.A. and Liberman, R.P. (1986) The Practice of Psychiatric Rehabilitation. *Schizophr. Bull.*, **12**, 542–59.

Atthowe, J.M. and Krasner, L. (1968) Preliminary report on the application of contingent reinforcement procedures (token economy) on a 'chronic' psychiatric ward. *J. Abnorm. Psychol.*, **73**, 37–43.

Ayllon, T. and Azrin, N. (1965) The measurement and reinforcement of behavior of psychotics. *J. Exp. Anal. Behav.*, **8**, 357–83.

Ayllon, T. and Azrin, N. (1968) *The Token Economy: A Motivation System for Therapy and Rehabilitation*. Appleton-Century-Crofts, New York,

Azrin, N.H. and Besalel, V.A. (1980) *Job Club Counselor's Manual*. University Park Press, Baltimore,

Bachrach, L.L. (1983) An overview of deinstitutionalization. In *New Directions for Mental Health Services: Deinstitutionalization*. L. Bachrach (ed), Jossey-Bass, San Francisco, pp. 5–14.

Beard, J.H., Malamud, T.J. and Rossman, E. (1978) Psychiatric rehabilitation and long-term rehospitalization rates: The findings of two research studies. *Schizophr. Bull.*, **4**, 622–35.

Bellack, A.S. and Mueser, K.T. (1986) A comprehensive treatment programme for schizophrenia and chronic mental illness. *Community Ment. Health J.*, **22**, 175–89.

Brewin, C.R., Wing, J.K., Mangen, S.P., Brugha, T.S., McCarthy, B. and Lesage, A. (1988) Needs for care among the long-term mentally ill: Report from the Camberwell high contact survey. *Psychol. Med.*, **18**, 457–68.

Butler, R.J. (1979) An analysis of individual treatment on a token economy for chronic schizophrenic patients. *Br. J. Med. Psychol.*, **52**, 235–43.

Carlson, C.G., Hersen, M. and Eisler, R.M. (1972) Token economy programmes in the treatment of hospitalized adult psychiatric patients. *J. Nerv. Ment. Dis.*, **155**, 192–204.

Curran, J.P., Faraone, S.V. and Dow, M.G. (1985) Schizophrenia and other psychotic disorders. In *Practice of Inpatient Behaviour Therapy: A Clinical Guide*. M. Hersen (ed), Grune & Stratton, New York, pp. 113–39.

Dawson, M.E. and Nuechterlein, K.H. (1984)

Psychophysiological dysfunctions in the developmental course of schizophrenic disorders. *Schizophr. Bull.*, **10**, 204–32.

Drake, R.E. and Sederer, L.I. (1986) The adverse effects of intensive treatment of chronic schizophrenia. *Compr. Psychiatry*, **27**, 313–26.

Eckman, T.A., Liberman, R.P., Phipps, C.C. and Blair, K.E. (1990) Teaching medication management skills to schizophrenic patients. *J. Clin. Psychopharmacol.*, **10**, 33–8.

Falloon, I.R.H., Boyd, J.L., McGill, C.W. *et al.* (1982) Family management in the prevention of exacerbation of schizophrenia: A controlled study. *N. Eng. J. Med*, **306**, 1437–40.

Gardos, G. and Cole, J.O. (1976) Maintenance antipsychotic therapy: Is the cure worse than the disease? *Am. J. Psychiatry*, **133**, 32–6.

Hogarty, G.E., Anderson, C.M., Reiss, D.J. *et al.* (1986) Family psychoeducation, social skills training and maintenance chemotherapy in the aftercare treatment of schizophrenia: I. One-year effects of a controlled study on relapse and expressed emotion. *Arch. Gen. Psychiatry*, **43**, 633–42.

Jacobs, H.E., Kardashian, S., Kreinbring, R.K., Ponder, R. and Simpson, A.S. (1984) A skills oriented model for facilitating employment among psychiatrically disabled persons. *Rehabilitation Couns. Bull.*, **28**, 87–96.

Kane, J.M. and Mayerhoff, D. (1989) Do negative symptoms respond to pharmacological treatment? *Br. J. Psychiatry*, **155**, 115–8.

Kazdin, A.E. (1977) *The Token Economy: A Review and Evaluation*. Plenum, New York.

Kazdin, A.E. (1982) The token economy: A decade later. *J. Appl. Behav. Anal.*, **15**, 431–45.

Kazdin, A.E. (1985) The token economy. In *Evaluating Behavior Therapy Outcome*. R. Turner and L.M. Asher (eds), Spring Publishing Co, New York, pp. 225–53.

Kraepelin, E. (1919) *Dementia Praecox and Paraphrenia*. Translated and edited by R.M. Barclay and G.M. Robertson, E. and S. Livingstone, Edinburgh.

Kraepelin, E. (1921) *Manic Depressive Insanity and Paranoia*. Translated and edited by R.M. Barclay and G.M. Robertson., E. and S. Livingstone, Edinburgh.

Liberman, R.P., Falloon, I.R.H., and Wallace, C.J. (1984) Drug-psychosocial interactions in the treatment of schizophrenia. In *The Chronically Mentally Ill: Research and Services*. M. Marabi (ed), Spectrum, New York, pp. 175–212.

Lindsley, O.R. (1954) Operant conditioning methods applied to research in chronic schizophrenia. *Psychiatry Res. Rep.*, **5**, 118–53.

Lindsley, O.R. (1960) Characteristics of the behavior of chronic psychotics as revealed by free-operant conditioning methods. *Dis. Nerv. System*, **21**, 66–78.

Lindsley, O.R. and Skinner, B.F. (1954) A method for the experimental analysis of psychotic patients. *Am. Psychol.*, **9**, 419–20.

MacKain, S. and Wallace C.J. (1988) *Evaluation of Social and Independent Living Skills*. Unpublished manuscript. UCLA-NPI Clinical Research Center for Psychiatric Rehabilitation and the Study of Schizophrenia, Los Angeles.

Marder, S.R., Van Putten, T., Eckman, T. *et al.* (1989) Low dose pharmacotherapy and skills training. *Schizophr. Res.*, **2**, 211.

Mueser, K.T. and Berenbaum, H. (1990) Editorial: Psychodynamic treatment of schizophrenia: Is there a future? *Psychol. Med.*, **20**, 253–62.

Nuechterlein, K. and Dawson, M. (1984) Information processing and attentional functioning in the developmental course of schizophrenic disorders. *Schizophr. Bull.*, **10**, 160–203.

Pattison, E.M., Llamas, R. and Hurd, G. (1979) Social network mediation of anxiety. *Psychiatr. Ann.*, **9**, 474–82.

Paul, G.L. and Lentz, R.J. (1977) *Psychosocial Treatment of Chronic Mental Patients: Milieu Versus Social-Learning Programs*. Harvard University Press, Cambridge, MA.

Presley, A.S., Grubb, A.B. and Semple, D. (1982) Predictors of successful rehabilitation in long-stay patients. *Acta Psychiatr. Scand.*, **66**, 83–8.

Prudo, R. and Blum, H.M. (1987) Five-year outcome and prognosis in schizophrenia: A report from the London Field Research Centre of the International Pilot Study of Schizophrenia. *Br. J. Psychiatry*, **150**, 345–54.

Rosen, A.J., Sussman, S.Y., Mueser, K.T., Lyons, J.S. and Davis, J.M. (1981) Behavioural assessment of psychiatric inpatients and normal controls across different environmental contexts. *J. Behav. Assess.*, **3**, 25–36.

Stein, L.I. and Test, M.A. (1980) An alternative to mental hospital treatment I: Conceptual model treatment programme, and clinical evaluation. *Arch. Gen. Psychiatry*, **37**, 392–7.

Stein, I. and Test, M.A. (eds) (1985) *The Training in Community Living Model: A Decade of Experience*. Jossey-Bass Inc., San Francisco.

Stephens, J.H. (1978) Long-term prognosis and follow-up in schizophrenia. *Schizophr. Bull.*, **4**, 25–47.

Sylph, J.A., Ross, H.E. and Kedward, H.B. (1977) Social disability in chronic psychiatric patients. *Am. J. Psychiatry*, **134**, 1391–4.

Tessler, R.C. and Manderscheid, R.W. (1982) Factors affecting adjustment to community living. *Hosp. Community Psychiatry*, **33**, 203–7.

Test, M.A., Knoedler, W.H. and Allness, D.J. (1985) The long-term treatment of young schizophrenics in a community support program. In *The Training in Community Living Model: A Decade of Experience*. L.I. Stein and M.A. Test (eds), Jossey-Bass Inc., San Francisco, pp. 17–27.

Test, M.A., Knoedler, W.H. and Allness, D.J. (1989) Long-term community care through an assertive continuous treatment team. *Schizophr. Res.*, **2**, 230.

Van Putten, T. (1974) Why do schizophrenic patients refuse to take their drugs? *Arch. Gen. Psychiatry*, **31**, 67–72.

Wallace, C.J. (1988) *Adoption of Innovations in Mental Health: Progress Report to the Department of Mental Hygiene, State of California*. UCLA-NPI Clinical Research Center for Psychiatric Rehabilitation and the Study of Schizophrenia, Los Angeles.

Wallace, C.J. and Liberman, R.P. (1985) Social skills training for patients with schizophrenia: A controlled clinical trial. *Psychiatry Res.*, **15**, 239–47.

Witheridge, T.F. and Dincin, J. (1985) The bridge: An assertive outreach program in an urban setting. In *The Training in Community Living Model: A Decade of Experience*. L.I. Stein and M.A. Test (eds), Jossey-Bass, San Francisco, pp. 65–76.

Chapter 24

Family interventions for schizophrenia

DAVID J. KAVANAGH

24.1 OUTCOMES OF FAMILY INTERVENTION (FI)

Family relationships seem to play an important part in the course of schizophrenia (Chapter 8). The concept of expressed emotion (EE) (Brown *et al.*, 1972) has proved particularly influential, although it continues to attract controversy among scientific commentators and family advocates (Hatfield *et al.*, 1987; Parker *et al.*, 1988). When schizophrenia sufferers live in a setting that is critical, overprotective or overconcerned, they have a nine-month relapse rate that is more than twice the level in low EE environments (Kavanagh, 1992). Inspired by the research on EE and schizophrenic relapse, a number of treatment teams have developed family interventions (FI) to reduce relapse (e.g. Falloon *et al.*, 1982; Anderson *et al.*, 1986).

The effect of family interventions on schizophrenic relapse is summarized in Table 24.1. Readers are also referred to reviews by Tarrier and Barrowclough (1990) and Smith and Birchwood (1990). There are four controlled trials of single-family FI and routine or individual treatments, which have a total sample size of 76 in each condition. Schizophrenia sufferers from high EE environments who receive routine treatment including neuroleptic

medication have a median relapse rate of 49% over nine months. In contrast, similar subjects who receive FI have a median relapse rate of only 8% over the same period. This treatment effect compares favourably with the median differences between high EE and low EE in the naturalistic outcome studies (48% vs. 21%: Kavanagh, 1992). Despite relatively low subject numbers, all four of the studies that compared individual or routine treatment with a FI that included the patient showed a statistically significant effect at either nine or twelve months. Relapse rates from a relatives group lay between those of FI and control treatments and did not significantly differ from either.

Over 24 months, statistical significance for F1 was only retained by Falloon *et al.* (1985), but the outcomes of the family and control conditions (33% and 72%) still paralleled the ones from low and high EE environments — 27% and 66% (Kavanagh, 1992). As well as impacting on the sufferer's symptoms, the family approach has a sustained differential effect on employment, performance of house-hold tasks and decision making (Falloon *et al.*, 1985, 1987). It also affects the well-being of other members: Falloon and Pederson (1985) found that families who received FI had less disruption of their activities, fewer

Table 24.1 Relapse data from treatment studies that preselected for high EE

Study	Family intervention (%)	Relatives' groups (%)	Individual or routine treatment (%)
0–9 month relapses			
Leff *et al.* (1982)	8	—	50*
Falloon *et al.* (1982)[1]	6	—	44**
Köttgen *et al.* (1984)	—	33[2]	50 n.s.
Hogarty *et al.* (1987, 1991)[3]	10	—	28 n.s.
Tarrier *et al.* (1988)	12	—	48[4]*
Leff *et al.* (1989)	8	36 n.s.[5]	—
Vaughan *et al.* (1989)	—	41	65 n.s.[6]
Median across studies	8	36	49
0–24 month relapses			
Leff *et al.* (1985)	40	—	78 n.s.[7]
Falloon *et al.* (1985)[1]	17	—	83***
Hogarty *et al.* (1987)[8]	32	—	66 n.s.
Tarrier *et al.* (1989)	33	—	59 n.s.
Leff *et al.* (1990)	33	36 n.s.	—
Median across studies	33	36	72

Recomputed significance of the group comparison using Fischer z or X^2 tests:
n.s. $p > 0.05$ * $p < 0.05$ ** $p < 0.01$ *** $p < 0.001$

1. Households were either high in EE or showed significant problems.
2. The intervention consisted of separate groups for relatives and sufferers.
3. At 12 months the relapse rates were 19% (FI), 41% (controls), $p < 0.05$. Social skills training to individual clients (SST) resulted in 20% relapses in 9 months, and there were no relapses for FI + SST.
4. The control group included families who received a brief education programme. There were no significant differences between the outcomes of education and routine treatment.
5. Only 6/11 families attended the group at all: These subjects had 17% relapses.
6. Relapse rates include subjects who were symptomatic at discharge. If these subjects were excluded, the rates were: 25% (relatives group), 65% (control group).
7. These figures count suicides as relapses but exclude subjects who stopped medication. The rates across the full sample were 50%(FI) and 75% (routine), n.s.
8. SST gave 42% relapses and there were 25% in FI + SST.

health problems, and less subjective burden than those who did not.

Table 24.1 excludes studies that did not preselect for high EE (Goldstein *et al.*, 1978;

Hogarty *et al.*, 1973, 1974, 1979). Consistent with the EE hypothesis, these studies have typically achieved less powerful results than the ones in the table. For example, Goldstein *et al.* (1978) evaluated the effect of six weekly sessions of crisis-oriented family therapy. Over six months there were no relapses among family therapy subjects who received a moderate dose of fluphenazine, but the main effect for family therapy was only marginally significant (11%, vs. 28% for controls) and the results may be contaminated by access to other therapies. Similarly, Hogarty *et al.* (1979) failed to obtain a significantly superior outcome from a combination of family and individual casework than from routine surveillance.

There are substantial similarities between the family programmes in the successful studies. They all begin during an episode of schizophrenia, when the whole family is most under stress and is most highly motivated to begin treatment. Programmes that begin at other times have substantial difficulty in engaging families (e.g. McCreadie *et al.*, 1991). The successful programmes are also based on the idea that relapse risks are reduced when everyone in the household is more informed about schizophrenia and has improved skills in dealing with the problems it poses. Accordingly, they all include some education about the disorder and provide practical suggestions for its management within the family, so that relatives can control their own stress and avoid high EE responses. Usually families are trained in systematic goal setting and problem-solving procedures. Typically the majority of sessions with individual families are held in the home, although some positive results have been obtained with inpatient variants of the approach (Liberman *et al.*, 1981; Glick *et al.*, 1985). Most sessions include the sufferer, but often supportive groups for relatives are also provided. In contrast, (Köttgen *et al.*, 1987) used a more psychodynamic approach which included less skills training. Treatment was delivered in the clinic to separate groups of

Table 24.2 Contact time in family treatments

	Family sessions[1]			
	0–9 months		9 months to 2 years	
	Mean or median number	Total hours	Mean or median number	Total hours
Leff *et al.* (1982)	15	19	2	3
Falloon *et al.* (1982)	25	25	15	15
Tarrier *et al.* (1988)	13	20	0^2	0^2
Leff *et al.* (1989)	17	17	—	—
Median across studies	16	20	2	3

1. Includes single or group family sessions, but excludes telephone contacts and crisis intervention. Contact time is rounded to the nearest hour.
2. From 9 months to 2 years, 17% families had additional sessions, and the maximum contact was once every 6 months.

sufferers and relatives. These differences in their intervention could have contributed to the relatively weak effects from their intervention.

The impact of FI can be achieved with a relatively low intensity of treatment (Table 24.2). For example, Tarrier *et al.* (1988) reduced the nine-month relapse rate to 12% with an intervention of only 13 sessions, or around 20 hours of contact. The most intensive intervention, by Falloon *et al.* (1982), had 25 one-hour sessions over the first nine months. However, there is little evidence that FI results in a sustained drop in relapse rates once sessions stop altogether (Goldstein and Kopeiken, 1981; Hogarty *et al.*, 1987). For example, in the Vaughan *et al.* (1990) study the intervention was restricted to ten weekly sessions for relatives, and no significant impact on nine-month relapse rates was observed. The Falloon *et al.* (1985) study, which best maintained the initial treatment effects, had monthly sessions with families throughout the follow-up period. At this stage we do not know whether family sessions need to continue indefinitely, but the evidence suggests that some contact is required for at least two years.

24.1.1 ALTERNATIVE EXPLANATIONS FOR FI EFFECTS

Sampling and dropouts. Sample characteristics of the outcome studies are shown in Table 24.3. The samples are predominantly males with repeated admissions, and are likely to be representative of schizophrenia sufferers encountered by most treatment centres. There were no systematic sample differences between treatment groups that could explain the superior results of family approaches. For example, routine treatment clients did not have more intractable problems. The median refusal rate of 13% (Table 24.4) was well within acceptable limits. Nor were the outcomes of FI inflated by greater dropout rates from that condition. The significant studies had a median dropout rate of only 7% for FI. Leff *et al.* (1982) had no dropouts, and Falloon *et al.* (1982) had no withdrawals after the first month of treatment. Tarrier *et al.* (1988) included the partially treated subjects in the main analysis, and Hogarty *et al.* (1986) found that a 12-month FI effect was retained whether partially treated subjects were included or not.

Assessment bias. Not all of the outcome studies have used symptom assessors who were unaware of the treatment group (e.g. Type 2 relapses in Leff *et al.*, 1982). However the outcomes in Falloon *et al.* (1982, 1985), Tarrier *et al.* (1988), and Leff *et al.* (1989) were confirmed by blind assessments.

Medication and symptom monitoring. Neither medication compliance nor dosage can account for the differential effects from FI (Leff *et al.*, 1982; Hogarty *et al.*, 1986; Tarrier *et al.*, 1988). Falloon *et al.* (1985) showed that subjects in the FI condition actually received a lower dose of medication, whether prescribed dosage or ingested dosage was examined. However it remains possible that the family approach resulted in better communication between the family and clinicians, so that medication side effects were more quickly treated and there was earlier administration of medication for

Table 24.3 Subject characteristics

	% Male	Mean age	Mean age of onset	Mean number of previous admissions	% First admission
Leff *et al.* (1982)	50	35	30	1.8	33
Falloon *et al.* (1982)	67	26	22	3.0	36
Hogarty *et al.* (1986)	67	27	21	2.7	23
Tarrier *et al.*(1988)	35	35	29	2.8	30
Leff *et al.* (1989)	57	27	21	2.2	44
Vaughan *et al.* (1990)	83	26	21	4.3	25
Median across studies	62	27	22	2.8	32

Table 24.4 Refusals and dropout rates

	Rates of refusals and dropouts			
	Refusals of assessment or treatment		Dropouts from single family sessions over 9–12 months	
	%	(n)	%	(n)
Leff *et al.* (1982)	18	(49)	0	(12)
Falloon *et al.* (1982)	5	(41)	10	(20)
Hogarty *et al.* (1986)	13	(118)	5	(22)
Tarrier *et al.* (1988)	15	(86)	12	(25)
Leff *et al.* (1989)	4	(24)	8	(12)
Vaughan *et al.* (1990)	—	—[1]	6	(18)
Median rates	13		7	

1. The refusal rate was not provided.

symptomatic crises. This variable has not been specifically tested, but it is unlikely to have mediated effects in Falloon *et al.* (1982), since there was a high level of information exchange with families in the control condition.

Nonspecific controls. Contact time was confounded with FI effects in some of the outcome studies (Leff *et al.*, 1982; Hogarty *et al.*, 1986; Tarrier *et al.*, 1988). However, clients in Falloon *et al.* (1982) received equal contact time across treatments. None of the studies equalized for contact time with the whole family, although therapist contact with one or more relatives may actually be higher in some individual treatments (Falloon, 1989). Current studies also fail to exclude effects of

other factors such as the family's participation in a special treatment or the provision of social support. Existing controls for social support are confounded with specific treatment effects, such as information and modelling of skills by other participants (Rosenthal and Bandura, 1978).

Home delivery. Delivery of treatment in the home was confounded with a family approach in some of the studies (Leff *et al.*, 1982, 1989; Falloon *et al.*, 1982). Home treatment may result in better generalization and maintenance of training than if sessions are conducted in a therapy room. It is unlikely that this factor accounts for all of the short-term effects of FI, since significant effects on symptoms can be obtained for a brief FI that is delivered in the hospital (Glick *et al.*, 1985). An ongoing study by Kavanagh *et al.* (1988) is testing the long-term effects of FI effects and a comparable individual treatment when both interventions are delivered in the home. Results from that study are still to come.

Content of the intervention. Unfortunately, the current comparisons of FI with individual or routine treatment are confounding the specific content and skill focus of the interventions with family vs. individual delivery. As a result, the current evidence is consistent with the idea that an individual intervention with similar behavioural targets as the FI could achieve similar effects. There is some evidence supporting this idea. In Hogarty *et al.* (1986) FI had almost identical effects as individual social skills training for clients which aimed at reducing family conflict by targeting specific behaviours that were initiating conflict and by training clients in negotiation. However the FI does not seem to have emphasized training these skills, so even this study did not equalize content across the conditions.

24.2 HOW DO THE FAMILY INTERVENTIONS ACHIEVE THEIR RESULTS?

While some questions remain, the FI studies are standing up well on methodological grounds. We know much less about how they might be reducing relapse.

24.2.1 INCREASES IN KNOWLEDGE AND SKILLS

The successful interventions all aim to convey information and skills that will improve the family's ability to deal with schizophrenia. A series of education sessions increases the family's knowledge (Smith and Birchwood, 1987), but has little impact on relapse unless it describes specific management techniques in detail (Tarrier *et al.*, 1988). Similarly, the outcome studies have presented little data that families do acquire the targeted skills, or that skill acquisition produces the improved patient outcomes. The FI approach in Falloon *et al.* (1982) had a greater impact on constructive problem solving than did individual treatment (Doane *et al.*, 1986), but the correlation between problem solving and relapse was not reported. It is plausible that FI achieves its impact by increasing the family's knowledge and skills, but the evidence is incomplete at the moment.

24.2.2 REDUCTION IN EE

A similar situation applies to the status of EE as a mechanism for reductions in relapse. A family approach results in greater reductions in EE than routine treatment (Tarrier *et al.*, 1988), although the differential changes are mainly in criticism rather than emotional over-involvement (EOI) (Leff *et al.*, 1982, 1989; Tarrier *et al.*, 1988). In cases where EE is low at post-treatment there are particularly low relapse rates (Hogarty *et al.*, 1986; Leff *et al.*, 1989).

However these data do not necessarily mean that reductions in EE are responsible for improvements in schizophrenic symptoms. FI may directly affect symptoms by increasing the family's skills in problem solving, goal setting and symptom management. Differences in EE could be a consequence of symptomatic improvement from these skills or may be an index of the family's general response to the intervention rather than the primary mechanism for its effects. Improvements in negative symptoms or social functioning do not have an immediate effect on family attitudes (Tomaras *et al.*, 1988), but there is evidence that EE is higher when positive symptoms are worse (Kavanagh, 1992). The issue would be resolved if we could alter EE without increasing the family's skills, and could show that the changes occurred before any differences in symptomatic outcome. No one has demonstrated this yet.

Furthermore, data from Hogarty *et al.* (1986) suggested that reductions in EE may not be essential for positive outcomes when a family intervention is combined with training for patients in avoiding conflict and settling disputes. While this observation needs replication in a larger sample, it does cast doubt on a unidirectional model of the treatment effects.

24.2.3 REDUCTION IN FAMILY CONTACT

When EE remains high, sufferers may be able to moderate its effects by reducing contact with their relatives (Vaughn and Leff, 1976). However, any lower contact time after FI is usually associated with increased involvement by sufferers or their relatives in leisure activities, employment or day programmes (Leff *et al.*, 1982). This increased activity may reflect improvements in functional skills: improvements that could

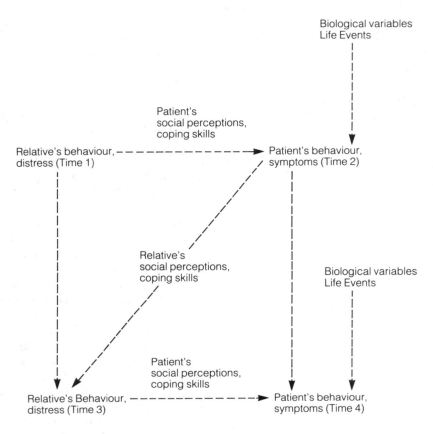

Figure 24.1 A model of relapse in schizophrenia.

independently affect the risk of relapse. Activities also offer a number of benefits apart from time out of family conflict. For example, they can help to maintain positive moods (Lewinsohn and Graf, 1973), give opportunities to build skills and self-efficacy (Bandura, 1982), or supply alternate sources of social support. The contact data would be more persuasive if they were not confounded with these other potential effects.

24.2.4 EARLY TERMINATION OF SYMPTOMATIC EXACERBATIONS

A mechanism for the FI effects is suggested by Falloon *et al.* (1982). In their study the overall rate of symptom exacerbations was similar across treatments, but subjects in the FI programme had a greater proportion of minor or aborted episodes of schizophrenic symptoms. This suggests that FI may help sufferers head off exacerbations before they become severe. When the underlying biological process puts sufferers through a period of greater vulnerability, the FI subjects' resources may be greater (e.g. they may have greater social support from their family) or their social context may present them with fewer concurrent demands. Further investigation of recovery from minor episodes may shed light on the mechanisms involved.

24.3 TOWARDS AN INTERACTIVE MODEL OF FAMILY INTER-ACTIONS AND RELAPSE

A simple unidirectional model from EE to symptoms or from skills to symptoms is probably inadequate to explain FI effects, and does not capture the true conceptual basis of the current interventions. Elsewhere I have argued that the data on EE and schizophrenia are poorly described by models such as these (Kavanagh, 1992) and suggest that EE and patient behaviours are reciprocally determined (Bandura, 1986). Both schizophrenia symptoms and EE are seen as problems in coping that become entrapped in a feedback loop.

An interactive model is reproduced in Figure 24.1. The model represents a 'stress-vulnerability' approach to schizophrenic relapse (Zubin and Spring, 1977), which incorporates biological vulnerability and background stressors as well as social behaviours (including EE). When patients experience a high level of critical or intrusive behaviour from other people, they often experience distress, their confidence in their functional capabilities is undermined and their risk of relapse is increased (Patient's behaviour and symptoms, Time 2) (Brown et al., 1972; Mintz et al., 1987a). This risk is highest when they are biologically vulnerable to symptoms and they are under challenge from life events outside the household (top right of the figure). In turn, the patient's behaviours and symptoms often provoke frustration and criticism from other people (bottom left of figure), or result in overprotective and intrusive behaviour. The cycle is potentially repeated (bottom right).

Individual interactions are terminated by one or more parties suppressing negative responses or leaving the field, or by the intervention of other people. However the cycle may be maintained across a series of separate interactions

when participants ruminate about the events and worry about recurrences. These cognitions maintain the emotional reaction over time. To break the cycle, a marked change is required in one or more of the factors in the model. For example, a significant reduction of symptoms is likely to impact strongly on the reactions of other people.

The model predicts that the reactions of both patients and their relatives are moderated by their social perceptions and their skills in coping with stressful situations. For example, relatives' emotional reactions to the problematic behaviours of the patient are affected by their attributions of the behaviour to the disorder or to other factors such as the patient's deliberate intentions or personality features (Brewin et al., 1991). The behavioural responses of relatives will also be determined by their skills and self-efficacy in such areas as anger control, negotiation and behaviour management (Bandura, 1986). Similar processes affect patients' reactions, but the risks of misunderstandings and dysfunctional responses are magnified by the disorder.

There are two factors in the model that entrench existing ways of interacting to similar situations. One involves the establishment of behavioural expectations from previous events, so that current social perceptions are coloured by recollections of the past. Repeated behaviours also tend to become automatic (Bandura, 1986), so that little cognitive processing is invested in evaluating the appropriateness of the response or considering alternatives. As a result, one person's attempt to break out of the cycle or prevent it recurring is often met with unchanged responses fronm others (Hubschmid and Zemp, 1989). Sustained changes in a person's behaviour may often be required before other people's expectations are changed and their habitual reactions extinguish (Tomaras et al., 1988; Tarrier, 1989).

While the model in Figure 24.1 can be described in terms of negative influences, each factor can also be seen as a potentially positive effect. The household is an important source of social support for the patient — -support that may moderate the impact of other stressful events (Katschnig, 1986). Similarly, medication decreases the immediate biological risk of symptoms (Davis, 1975), and positive events help to reduce depressive mood (Lewinsohn and Graf, 1973).

The model in Figure 24.1 is consistent with current evidence on EE (Kavanagh, 1992) and with the outcomes of FI. It also provides a theoretical basis for an effective intervention. A successful strategy to alter the interactional cycle could focus either on the interpersonal behaviours of sufferers or their relatives (Hogarty *et al.*, 1986). However an intervention that simultaneously altered the behaviour of all the family members might be more effective (Hogarty *et al.*, 1986), since it reduces the difficulty in initiating changes and increases the probability that improvements are rewarded. For example, if everyone is applying less intrusive and more coping strategies, each person will experience fewer problems in maintaining the behaviour. If the entire household is testing the accuracy of their social perceptions, members will be more likely to notice attempts to change by another person. Similarly, an approach which has an impact on several of the risk factors in Figure 24.1 should be more successful than a method which only alters one. For example, behaviour changes by patients will be easier when their symptoms are being adequately controlled by neuroleptic medication (Goldstein *et al.*, 1978).

A study by Hogarty *et al.* (1986) provides evidence in favour of a combined approach. The authors compared FI with individual social skills training (SST) for the sufferer. SST was focused on accurately perceiving family interactions and learning how to avoid conflict. At an early stage sufferers attempted to reduce behaviours that formerly evoked criticism from other members. As the training progressed, they were trained to handle more difficult tasks such as responding to criticism and helping the

family resolve conflict. The FI attempted to modify the survival skills of both relatives and sufferers, but it placed less emphasis on communication training or conflict resolution. Thus FI and SST both focused on aspects of the model in Figure 24.1, but with significantly different emphases. Each had a 10% relapse in the first nine months and 19–20% in the first year (Table 24.1). When the two approaches were combined the 12-month relapse rate dropped to zero. While the combined intervention had more therapist contact, the results could also mean that: (a) the combined intervention contributed features that were omitted by FI and SST alone, and/or (b) individual sessions may sometimes augment the impact of FI. As predicted from the model, the most powerful intervention had multiple skill targets and simultaneously altered the behaviour of both sufferers and their relatives.

24.4 COMPONENTS OF SUCCESSFUL FI APPROACHES

Although there are substantial similarities between family interventions from different treatment centres, individual teams have focused on different aspects. Falloon *et al.* (1984) used a highly structured programme for individual families that emphasized problem solving and included behaviour management. Tarrier *et al.* (1988) featured systematic goal setting, while Hogarty *et al.* (1986) initially focused on developing family tolerance for the schizophrenia symptoms and strengthening supportive relationships. The intervention in Leff *et al.* (1982) was less structured and included components from a number of theoretical apporoaches. Most of the methods incorporated a group for relatives, but the group had different functions in each one. In Hogarty *et al.* (1986) relatives met in groups for a one-day educational workshop, while in Leff *et al.* (1982) the groups provided ongoing support for relatives and allowed members to model functional skills to other participants. Falloon *et al.* (1982) did not have separate groups for relatives, but delivered the follow-up sessions to multiple family groups.

Some of the differences between methods may be more semantic than real: for example effective goal setting usually incorporates some type of problem solving. Furthermore the differences between research teams are probably far outweighed by variations in the strategies that each team applies to meet the needs of different families. While this variation reduces the precision of the treatment descriptions it may be an important feature of an effective intervention. Overall, it is noteworthy that a range of FI programmes seem to produce substantially similar effects. Consistent with the interactive model, this suggests that there may be many alternate skill targets that will prove effective.

24.4.1 EVALUATION OF COMPONENTS

Up to now, there has been little evaluation of component intervention strategies. The interactive model would predict that interventions would only be successful if they had a sustained impact on the behaviour of participants, and would emphasize a skills training and social support approach. The limited evidence that is currently available is consistent with these predictions.

Education. Several studies have examined the impact of education about schizophrenia and its treatment. Information is delivered in one to four sessions that total two to six hours, usually with a lecture/discussion format that is supplemented by leaflets about the disorder. These sessions produce an immediate increase in knowledge (e.g. McGill *et al.*, 1983; Barrowclough *et al.*, 1987) that is maintained for up to six months (Smith and Birchwood, 1987; Cozolino *et al.*, 1988). However a short-term impact on the relatives' distress is not maintained and there is no significant correlation between gains in knowledge and reductions in distress (Smith and Birchwood, 1987). Nor does the programme have a significant impact

on the client's symptoms (Smith and Birchwood, 1987; Tarrier *et al.*, 1988). These results suggest that a brief didactic programme is insufficient to impact on the critical treatment aims, although it may provide an informational basis for other strategies.

Education within a family intervention is not confined to the one or two formal sessions at the beginning of the programme. It continues throughout the programme and is explicitly related to the current concerns of the family. The repetition and current relevance may be critical elements of the education component that are poorly tested within the brief educational paradigm. When educational material extends over nine months and includes specific behavioural management strategies, it may be as effective as enactive behavioural skills training (Tarrier *et al.*, 1988).

Support groups. The only other component that has been separately evaluated is the use of support groups for relatives. Leff *et al.* (1989) found that these groups resulted in a nine-month relapse rate of 36%, but only 55% of the families attended a single meeting. Among the six families who attended one or more sessions the relapse rate (17%) was comparable to results from the single-family intervention (8% relapse). This result confounds treatment effects with self-selection, but it suggests that relatives groups may be effective for those who wish to attend them (cf. Abramowitz and Coursey, 1989). A pilot study by Kuipers *et al.* (1989) suggests that attendance can be substantially improved if a session at home is held to initiate engagement and the group is held in the local mental health facility.

24.5 A COGNITIVE BEHAVIOURAL INTERVENTION FOR CLIENTS AND RELATIVES

The model in Figure 24.1 and the evidence on effective components provide the basis for the specific objectives and content of an intervention that is described in detail by Piatkowska *et al.* (1992) and is currently being evaluated by Kavanagh *et al.* (1988). The broad components are similar to ones in Falloon *et al.* (1982), but the intervention has a greater emphasis on cognitive–behavioural assessment and management, on self-control and on addressing the current concerns of family members. Detailed manuals on alternate FI programmes are provided by Anderson *et al.* (1986) and Falloon *et al.* (1984).

24.5.1 OBJECTIVES AND FEATURES

While households showing high EE behaviours are likely to derive special benefits from our intervention, it is not restricted to these families (Smith and Birchwood, 1990). Nor are its aims confined to decreasing EE and preventing relapse (Falloon and Pedersen, 1985), although these remain key objectives. The programme encourages members to give each other non-intrusive support, and attempts to improve the quality of life for all the family (Packenham and Dadds, 1987). It emphasizes the mutual influences between sufferers and other members and specifically avoids blaming any individual (Hatfield *et al.*, 1987; Mintz *et al.*, 1987b). Instead it builds a coalition of the trainer and all the family members against the schizophrenia symptoms and supports the client's attempts at self-control. Special attention is paid to ensuring that the family sessions themselves do not prove to be excessively demanding on clients, by assisting them to express their views, discouraging labelling and blaming, and providing rest breaks as necessary.

The approach applies cognitive and behavioural strategies that are tailored to the specific schizophrenia symptoms and to the capabilities and concerns of family members as they are identified in behavioural analyses. It emphasizes their current knowledge and achievements, encourages them to model functional behaviours (Rosenthal and Bandura, 1978), and fosters realistic optimism about the future. To increase maintenance and generalization, the concepts are applied to a range of

issues and progressive steps to self-management are encouraged. The programme in Kavanagh *et al.* (1988) consists of approximately 10 sessions over the first six months, which are initially held weekly and are gradually reduced in frequency. They are followed by three-monthly sessions for at least another 18 months, which review the material in the programme and apply it to new issues. Each session is 1.5 hours long, plus time for rest breaks. Two family trainers participate in the sessions and provide peer consultation and ensure continuity when one is unable to attend.

Whenever possible sessions are held in the home and everyone in the household, including the sufferer, is encouraged to attend. Some other FIs have sessions without the patient (e.g. Leff *et al.*, 1982; Anderson *et al.*, 1986): These may be especially useful when the patient is highly symptomatic and is unable to tolerate a family session. Where possible, members of the extended family are also included in sessions, since they may be more tolerant of withdrawal and eccentric behaviour (El-Islam, 1982).

The programme is intended to fit into a comprehensive rehabilitation treatment plan for each client, and encourages the family to use other community resources as well. Families and sufferers are offered crisis intervention sessions by the trainers (Langsley *et al.*, 1968, 1971) that are supplemented by 24-hour community crisis services if they are available (Hoult, 1986). While the family intervention in Kavanagh *et al.* (1988) excludes individual treatment for the sufferer, supplementary individual sessions may further increase the impact of FI (Liberman *et al.*, 1981; Hogarty *et al.*, 1986). These sessions could focus on SST or on behavioural self-management of symptoms, drug abuse or aggression.

The approach in Piatkowska *et al.* (1992) is delivered to individual families, but the method can also be adapted to multiple family groups. These groups form the basis for mutual support and positive modelling of skills (Leff *et al.*, 1989) and may be especially useful for delivering introductory information about the disorder and its management (Anderson *et al.*, 1986).

24.5.2 COMPONENTS OF THE INTERVENTION

Segments are usually presented in the order that they appear below, where each one builds on the previously trained skills and represents a theme that continues throughout the rest of the programme. Skills are demonstrated in the context of current family issues, and the concepts are discussed afterwards. This method allows a full range of strategies to be applied to issues that emerge early in the programme, while preserving the sequence of concept development. The approach minimizes didactive teaching: wherever possible, participants are assisted to discover the concepts from their experience and current knowledge. When the material conflicts with current beliefs (e.g. that the sufferer is 'lazy' or is not making an effort), the trainers avoid confrontation and encourage members to test the evidence for their ideas (Beck *et al.*, 1979). It may be necessary for relatives to experience repeated disconfirmations before they relinquish firmly held beliefs (Smith and Birchwood, 1987; Abramowitz and Coursey, 1989).

Engagement. Families usually begin the programme immediately after an episode of schizophrenia, when they are most highly motivated to participate. The trainers explore the effects of the disorder on family members, their current attempts to cope, and the consequences of their efforts. They help the family to derive a set of behavioural goals for the immediate future and relate these goals to the intervention. Throughout the programme, family members are reminded of the benefits they are receiving from it, and costs of their attendance and participation in the sessions are minimized.

Education. The education sessions focus on current interests of the family, and are supplemented by leaflets on schizophrenia and its management. Patients are as recognized as experts on the subjective experience of the disorder, and are encouraged to discuss this experience with the family. The information emphasizes the symptom pattern of the particular client, in order to establish credibility and increase the relevance of the material (Cozolino and Nuechterlein, 1986). To ensure that members understand and recall the information, the trainers revise the main points and return to them in later sessions as relevant issues arise (Tarrier and Barrowclough, 1986). Sometimes the educational material induces grief over the losses that schizophrenia has produced, and strategies to resolve the grief may be required (Kavanagh, 1990). If there is difficulty in accepting a diagnosis of schizophrenia the label is not forced on the client, but symptoms and diagnostic questions are discussed. Key objectives of the educational sessions are to underscore the importance of medication and review the early warning signs that the sufferer experiences before a major episode. Families are asked to help the patient monitor these signs and obtain treatment quickly (Chapter 17).

Communication training. Hostile or critical communication cycles within the early sessions may reflect the current emotional climate in families rather than deficiencies in elementary social skills. These problems can often be addressed by setting some rules for interactions in the family sessions (such as excluding verbal abuse) and resolving some the contentious family issues. The sufferer's social performance may also improve dramatically when residual symptoms are better controlled. However sometimes family members have such major deficiences in social skills that progress is impeded. If so it may be necessary to train skills such as attention and social perception, expressing agreement and praise, offering suggestions, or making requests for behavioural change. Standard SST methods are applied, where: (a) alternative responses are discussed, (b) the trainers describe and model the appropriate behaviours, (c) family members rehearse the skill, (d) trainers praise the attempt and suggest improvements, and (e) members practise the skill as homework (Chapter 22). During the remainder of the programme the trainers praise attempts to apply the skills and give additional training as required.

Goal setting. Criticisms that families express about clients often reflect unrealistic expectations and goals (Cozolino *et al.*, 1988). One of the major aims of the intervention is to modify these expectations and thereby reduce the family's distress and dissatisfaction. Goal setting is also important for the client. Overly ambitious or intensive interventions are known to increase the risk of positive symptoms, but if the goals are too low the client's progress is slow and negative symptoms may be seen (Wing and Brown, 1970). In this phase of the programme clients and their families develop medium-term objectives and convert one of them into an achievable daily goal. During later sessions attempts to reach the goal are rewarded and the goals are revised. The goal setting procedure is applied to each of the later segments of the programme.

Problem solving. The training in problem solving is based on the approach of D'Zurilla and Goldfried (1971). The method involves family members defining the problem and developing a set of possible solutions by a brainstorming technique. All members are encouraged to participate in generating ideas, recording suggestions or summarizing the discussion so that their understanding and retention are maximized. After several alternatives are generated they discuss the relative merits of each one and make a selection. Then the strategy is implemented and they evaluate its effectiveness. To ensure that the sufferer's information processing abilities are not overloaded (Bellack *et al.*, 1989), problem solving is first applied to a relatively simple, non-emotive issue. Once the family is proficient at applying problem-solving to neutral issues the techniques are applied to issues of family

conflict. Trainers help members to focus on the objective problem and make constructive proposals rather than criticizing individuals. If members become distressed or confused the trainers cut short the discussion and later they assist the family to clarify the difficulty and reduce their distress.

As Bellack *et al.* (1989) point out, many of the important problems faced by the families are ill-defined, and often the difficulty is not so much in the problem-solving skills as in the way the original problem was defined. A critical part of this segment is encouraging members to exchange their views of the problem, test their accuracy and decide on a tentative joint definition. For example, the client's parents may initially describe a problem as: 'our daughter deliberately refuses to talk to our friends when they visit'. She on the other hand may have difficulty talking to outsiders or may think they are laughing about her. Each description invites a different set of possible solutions. Once the family agrees on a definition of the problem, these solutions often fall into place.

Cognitive–behavioural self-management. This segment targets some behaviours that are producing special difficulties for the sufferer or other members. The trainers assist family members to assess the behaviour, its situational cues and the consequences that maintain it. Behavioural interviews are supplemented by observation and monitoring between sessions, although self-monitoring records are used sparingly and are adapted to the capabilities of the members. The family applies problem-solving skills to develop alternative behaviours, exert situational control and apply alternative consequences. The aim is for all members to manage their own behaviours and help others to apply cognitive–behavioural methods. There is a special focus in strategies to improve self-control of schizophrenia symptoms by increasing medication adherence (Chapter 20) and applying strategies such as attention diversion, stimulus control and reality testing

(Falloon and Talbot, 1981; Breier and Strauss, 1983; Chapter 21).

Increasing family well-being. Family members are all encouraged to develop enjoyable leisure activities to help maintain a positive mood. Joint activities that each person finds enjoyable can provide an opportunity to build positive relationships in the family. When members are in daily contact with the sufferer, time away from interactions may also be important and should include both daily activities and vacations. Not only does 'time out' reduce the risk of conflict, but it expresses confidence in the sufferer's ability to function without the relative's assistance. The programme also emphasizes building a wider social network for the patient and family (Chapter 16). This is assisted by offering support groups as part of the intervention (e.g. Hogarty *et al.*, 1986; MacCarthy *et al.*, 1989) or encouraging members to join community groups.

Maintenance of skills. Many schizophrenia sufferers have difficulty in generating rules from specific instances (Bellack *et al.*, 1989). Accordingly, the family is offered regular sessions to reward attempts to apply the skills, revise the material in the programme and encourage members to apply it to new situations. In Falloon *et al.* (1982) these sessions were delivered to multiple family groups, but individual family sessions may ensure a higher level of attendance and allow the family to discuss private concerns more easily.

24.6 CONTINUING QUESTIONS

Are FI programmes effective within standard clinical settings?

These recommendations are predicated on FI being applicable outside the research centre, yet the published evaluation studies have all used a narrowly-based treatment team. To establish wider applicability, we need to assess its impact within the constraints of a standard field setting. An ongoing study by Kavanagh *et al.* (1988) is attempting to do this at the moment.

Practising clinicians from community health centres across Sydney and surrounding cities receive 35 hours of formal training as well as ongoing supervision (cf. McCreadie *et al.*, 1991, where one reason for weak effects of family intervention could have been inadequate training in delivering the intervention). The current project evaluates the relative effects of individual and FI versions of the programme that are administered to clients of the centres. It is expected to provide a rigorous field test of the family approach.

Can family strategies be applied to other living environments?

Up to now these interventions have focused on families, but around one-third of patients are discharged to live in non-familial settings (MacMillan *et al.*, 1986). It is plausible that EE-related behaviours may be important in these settings as well. Intensive supervision by professional staff, which is analogous to EOI, is associated with a higher relapse risk (Wing, 1978; Drake and Sederer, 1986). Staff or co-residents can also be highly critical (Herzog, 1988), and informal observations suggests that increased symptoms are often preceded by an interpersonal crisis within the residence.

If the EE results are generalizable to other living groups, perhaps we could apply a strategy like FI to moderate relapse risks. A preliminary study by Higson and Kavanagh (1988) showed that a 10–12 session programme did have a short-term impact on criticism within hostels for schizophrenia sufferers. While a more extensive evaluation is required, the study suggested that modified FI programmes might be productively applied to hostels or group homes. Modifications are likely to include: (a) simplifying the material, with briefer sessions, frequent repetitions, and more assistance in applying techniques to new situations; (b) a greater emphasis on basic SST and rewarding postive communication; (c) a special focus on coping with changes in group membership and with fluctuations in the symptoms of other residents; and (d) extensive training on resolving disputes with the hostel. Staff are trained to consistently model the central skills and prompt the residents to apply them daily. With modifications such as these, an FI approach is likely to have a wide implication to other living environments as a strategy to control symptoms and improve the satisfaction of residents and staff alike.

REFERENCES

Abramowitz, I.A. and Coursey, R.D. (1989) Impact of an educational support group on family participants who take care of their schizophrenic relatives. *J. Consult. Clin. Psychol.* 57, 232–6.

Anderson, C.M., Reiss, D.J., and Hogarty, G.E. (1986) *Schizophrenia in the family: A practitioner's guide to psychoeducation and management.* Guilford, New York.

Bandura, A. (1982) Self-efficacy mechanism in human agency. *Am. Psychol.*, 37, 122–47.

Bandura, A. (1986) *Social foundations of thought and action: A social cognitive theory.* Prentice-Hall, Englewood Cliffs, NJ.

Barrowclough, C., Tarrier, N., Watts, S. *et al.*, (1987) Assessing the functional value of relatives' knowledge about schizophrenia: A preliminary report. *Br. J. Psychiatry*, 151, 1–8.

Beck, A.T., Rush, A.J., Shaw, B.F. and Emery, G. (1979) *Cognitive therapy of depression.* Guilford, New York.

Bellack, A.S., Morrison, R.L., and Mueser, K.T. (1989) Social problem-solving in schizophrenia. *Schizophr. Bull.*, 15, 101–16.

Breier, A. and Strauss, J.S. (1983) Self-control in psychotic disorders. *Arch. Gen. Psychiatry*, 40, 1141–5.

Brewin, C., McCarthy, B., Dida, K. and Vaughn, C. (1991) Attribution and expressed emotion in the relatives of patients with schizophrenia. *J. Abnorm. Psychol.* in press.

Brown, G.W., Birley, J.L.T. and Wing, J.K. (1972) Influence of family life on the course of schizophrenic disorders: A replication. *Br. J. Psychiatry*, 121, 241–58.

Cozolino, L.J., Goldstein, M.J., Nuechterlein, K.H. *et al.*, (1988) The impact of education about schizophrenia on relatives varying in levels of expressed emotion. *Schizophr. Bull.*, 14, 675–85.

Cozolino, L.J. and Nuechterlein, K.H. (1986) Pilot study of a family education program on relatives of recent-onset schizophrenic patients. In *Treatment of schizophrenia: Family assessment and intervention.* M.J. Goldstein, I. Hand and K. Hahlweg, (eds), Springer-Verlag, Berlin, pp. 129–44.

Davis, J. (1975) Overview: Maintenance therapy in psychiatry: I. Schizophrenia. *Am. J. Psychiatry*, 132, 1237–45.

Doane, J.A., Goldstein, M.J., Miklowitz, D.J. and Falloon, I.R.H. (1986) The impact of individual and family treatment on the affective climate of families of schizophrenics. *Br. J. Psychiatry*, 148, 279–87.

Drake, R.E. and Sederer, L.I. (1986) The adverse effects of intensive treatment of chronic schizophrenia. *Compr. Psychiatry*, 27, 313–26.

D'Zurilla, T.J. and Goldfried, M.R. (1971) Problem solving and behavior modification. *J. Abnorm. Psychol.* 78, 107–26.

Falloon, I.R.H. (1989) Personal communication. Perth, Australia.

Falloon, I.R.H. and Talbot, R.E. (1981) Persistent auditory hallucinations: coping mechanisms and implications for management. *Psychol. Med.*, 11, 329–39.

Falloon, I.R.H. and Pedersen, J. (1985) Family management in the prevention of morbidity of schizophrenia: The adjustment of the family unit. *Br. J. Psychiatry*, 147, 156–63.

Falloon, I.R.H., Boyd, J.L. and McGill, C.W. (1984) *Family care of schizophrenia.* Guilford Press, New York.

Falloon, I.R.H., Boyd, J.L., McGill, C.W. *et al.*, (1982) Family management in the prevention of exacerbations of schizophrenia: A controlled study. *N. Engl. J. Med.*, 306, 1437–40.

Falloon, I.R.H., Boyd, J.L., McGill, C.W. *et al.* (1985) Family management in the prevention of morbidity of schizophrenia: Clinical outcome of a two-year longitudinal study. *Arch. Gen. Psychiatry*, 42, 887–96.

Falloon, I.R.H., McGill, C.W., Boyd, J.L. and Pedersen, J. (1987) Family management in the prevention of morbidity of schizophrenia: Social outcome of a two-year longitudinal study. *Psychol. Med.*, 17, 59–66.

Glick, I.A., Clarkin, J.F., Spencer, J.H. *et al.* (1985) A controlled evaluation of inpatient family education. *Arch. Gen. Psychiatry*, **42**, 882–6.

Goldstein, M. and Kopeikin, H. (1981) Short- and long-term effects of combining drug and family therapy. In *New developments in interventions with families of schizophrenics*. M. Goldstein (ed), Jossey-Bass, San Francisco, pp. 5–26.

Goldstein, M.J., Rodnick, E.H., Evans, J.R. *et al.* (1978) Drug and family therapy in the after care of acute schizophrenics. *Arch. Gen. Psychiatry*, **35**, 1169–77.

Hatfield, A.B., Spaniol, L. and Zipple, A.M. (1987) Expressed emotion: A family perspective. *Schizophr. Bull.*, **13**, 221–35.

Herzog, T. (1988) Nurses, patients and relatives: A study of family patterns on psychiatric wards. In *Family intervention in schizophrenia: Experiences and orientations in Europe*. C.L. Cazzullo and G. Invernizzi (eds), Proceedings of a conference held in Milan; November 18–19.

Higson, M. and Kavanagh, D.J. (1988) A hostel-based psychoeducational intervention for schizophrenia: Programme development and preliminary findings. *Behav. Change*, **5**, 85–9.

Hogarty, G.E., Anderson, C.M. and Reiss, D.J. (1987) Family psychoeducation, social skills training and medication in schizophrenia: The long and the short of it. *Psychopharm. Bull.*, **23**, 12–3.

Hogarty, G.E., Anderson, C.M., Reiss, D.J. *et al.* (1986) Family psychoeducation, social skills training, and maintenance chemotherapy in the aftercare treatment of schizophrenia. I. One-year effects of a controlled study on relapse and Expressed Emotion. *Arch. Gen. Psychiatry*, **43**, 633–42.

Hogarty, G.E., Anderson, C.M., Reiss, D.J. *et al.* (1991) Family psychoeducation, social skills training, and maintenance chemotherapy in the aftercare treatment of schizophrenia. II. Two-year effects of a controlled study on relapse and adjustment. *Arch. Gen. Psychiatry*, **48**, 340–7.

Hogarty, G.E., Goldberg, S. and Collaborative Study Group. (1973) Drug and sociotherapy in the aftercare of schizophrenic patients. *Arch. Gen. Psychiatry*, **28**, 54–64.

Hogarty, G.E., Goldberg, S., Schooler, N.R., Ulrich, R. and Collaborative Study Group (1974) Drug and sociotherapy in the aftercare of schizophrenic patients: II. Two-year relapse rates. *Arch. Gen. Psychiatry*, **31**, 603–8.

Hogarty, G.E., Schooler, N.R., Ulrich, R. *et al.* (1979) Fluphenazine and social therapy in the aftercare of schizophrenic patients: Relapse analyses of a two-year controlled study of fluphenazine decanoate and fluphenazine hydrochloride. *Arch. Gen. Psychiatry*, **36**, 1283–94.

Hoult, J. (1986) The community care of the acutely mentally ill. *Br. J. Psychiatry*, **149**, 137–44.

Hubschmid, T., and Zemp, M. (1989) Interactions in high- and low-expressed emotion families. *Soc. Psychiatry Psychiatr. Epidemiol.*, **24**, 113–9.

Katschnig, H. (ed), (1986) *Life Events and Psychiatric Disorders: Controversial Issues.* Cambridge University Press, Cambridge.

Kavanagh, D.J. (1992) Toward a cognitive-behavioural intervention for adult grief reactions. *Br. J. Psychiatry*, **157**, 373–83.

Kavanagh, D.J. (1990) *Recent developments in expressed emotion and schizophrenia Br. J. Psychiatry*, in press.

Kavanagh, D.J., Tennant, C.C., Rosen, A. *et al.* (1988) *Prevention of relapse in schizophrenia.* Research and Development Grant, Australian Department of Health, University of Sydney (unpublished.)

Köttgen, C., Sonnichsen, I., Mollenhauer, K., and Jurth, R. (1984) Group therapy with families of schizophrenic patients: Results of the Hamburg Camberwell Family Interview Study III. *Int. J. Fam. Psychiatry*, **5**, 83–94.

Kuipers, L., MacCarthy, B., Hurry, J. and Harper, R. (1989) Counselling the relatives of the long-term mentally ill. II. A low-cost supportive model. *Br. J. Psychiatry*, **154**, 775–82.

Langsley, D.J., Machotka, P. and Flomenhaft, K. (1968) Family crisis therapy. *Family Process*, **7**, 145–58.

Langsley, D.J., Machotka, P., and Flomenhaft, K. (1971) Avoiding mental hospital admission: A follow-up study. *Am. J. Psychiatry*, **127**, 1391–4.

Leff, J., Berkowitz, R., Shavit, N. *et al.* (1989) A trial of family therapy v. a relatives group for schizophrenia. *Br. J. Psychiatry*, **154**, 58–66.

Leff, J., Berkowitz, R., Shavit, N. *et al.* (1990) A trial of family therapy versus a relatives group for schizophrenia: Two-year follow-up. *Br. J. Psychiatry*, **157**, 571–7.

Leff, J., Kuipers, L., Berkowitz, R. *et al.* (1982)

A controlled trial of intervention in the families of schizophrenic patients. *Br. J. Psychiatry*, **141**, 121–34.

Leff, J., Kuipers, L., Berkowitz, R. and Sturgeon, D. (1985) A controlled trial of social intervention in the families of schizophrenic patients: Two year follow-up. *Br. J. Psychiatry*, **146**, 594–600.

Lewinsohn, P.M. and Graf, M. (1973) Pleasant activities and depression. *J. Consult. Clin. Psychol.*, **41**, 261–8.

Liberman, R.P., Wallace, C.J., Falloon, I.R.H. and Vaughn, C.E. (1981) Interpersonal problem solving therapy for schizophrenics and their families. *Compr. Psychiatry*, **22**, 627–30.

MacCarthy, B., Kuipers, L., Hurry, J. *et al.* (1989) Counselling the families of the mentally ill: I. Evaluation of the impact on relatives and patients. *Br. J. Psychiatry*, **154**, 768–75.

MacMillan, J.F., Gold, A., Crow, T.J. *et al.* (1986) The Northwick Park study of first episodes of schizophrenia. IV. Expressed emotion and relapse. *Br. J. Psychiatry*, **148**, 133–43.

McCreadie, R.G., Phillips, K., Harvey, J.A. *et al.* (1991) The Nithsdale schizophrenia surveys. VIII. Do relatives want family intervention – and does it help? *Br. J. Psychiatry*, **158**, 110–13.

McGill, C.W., Falloon, I.R.H., Boyd, J.L. and Wood-Siverio, C. (1983) Family educational intervention in the treatment of schizophrenia. *Hosp. Community Psychiatry*, **34**, 934–8.

Mintz, J., Mintz, L. and Goldstien, M. (1987a) Expressed emotion and relapse in first episodes of schizophrenia: A rejoinder to MacMillan *et al.* (1986), *Br. J. Psychiatry*, **151**, 314–20.

Mintz, L.I., Liberman, P., Miklowitz, D.J. and Mintz, J. (1987b) Expressed emotion: A call for partnership among relatives, patients, and professionals. *Schizophr. Bull.*, **13**, 227–35.

Packenham, K.I. and Dadds, M.R. (1987) Family care and schizophrenia: The effects of a supportive educational programme on relatives' personal and social adjustment. *A .N.Z. J. Psychiatry*, **21**, 580–90.

Parker, G., Johnston, P. and Hayward, L. (1988) Parental 'expressed emotion' as a predictor of schizophrenic relapse. *Arch. Gen. Psychiatry*, **45**, 806–13.

Piatkowska, O., Kavanagh, D., Manicavasagar, V. and O'Halloran, P. (1988) *The 'Living with Schizophrenia' (LWS) programme: Self-management training for clients and families.* University of Sydney.

Rosenthal, T.L., and Bandura, A. (1978) Psychological modeling: Theory and practice. In: *Handbook of psychotherapy and behavior change: An empirical analysis.* S.L. Garfield and A.E. Bergin (eds), Second edition, Wiley, New York, pp. 621–58.

Smith, J.V. and Birchwood, M.J. (1987) Specific and non-specific effects of educational intervention with families living with a schizophrenic relative. *Br. J. Psychiatry*, **150**, 645–52.

Smith, J.V. and Birchwood, M.J. (1990) Relatives and patients as partners in the management of schizophrenia: The development of a service model. *Br. J. Psychiatry*, **156**, 654–60.

Tarrier, N. (1989) Arousal levels and relatives' expressed emotion in remitted schizophrenic patients. *Br. J. Psychiatry*, **28**, 177–80.

Tarrier, N. and Barrowclough, C. (1986) Providing information to relatives about schizophrenia: Some comments. *Br. J. Psychiatry*, **149**, 458–63.

Tarrier, N. and Barrowclough, C. (1990) Family interventions for schizophrenia. *Behav. Mod.*, **14**, 408–40.

Tarrier, N., Barrowclough, C., Vaughn, C. *et al.* (1988) The community management of schizophrenia: A controlled trial of a behavioural intervention with families to reduce relapse. *Br. J. Psychiatry*, **153**, 532–42.

Tarrier, N., Barrowclough, C., Vaughn, C. *et al.* (1989) Community management of schizophrenia: A two-year follow-up of a behavioural intervention with families. *Br. J. Psychiatry*, **154**, 625–8.

Tomaras, V., Vlachonikolis, I.G., Stefanis, C.N. and Madianos, M. (1988) The effect of individual psychosocial treatment on the family atmosphere of schizophrenic patients. *Soc. Psychiatry Exp. Epidemiol.*, **23**, 256–61.

Vaughan, K., Doyle, M., McConaghy, N. *et al.* (1990) The Sydney intervention trial: A controlled trial of relatives' counselling to reduce schizophrenic relapse. Under editorial review.

Vaughn, C. and Leff, J. (1976) The influence of family and social factors on the course of psychiatric illness. *Br. J. Psychiatry,* **129**, 125–37.

Wing, J.K. (1978) The social context of schizophrenia. *Am. J. Psychiatry*, **135**, 1333–9.

Wing, J.K. and Brown, G.W. (1970) *Institu-tionalism and schizophrenia.* Cambridge University Press, Cambridge.

Zubin, J., and Spring, B. (1977) Vulnerability: A new view of schizophrenia. *J. Abnorm. Psychol.*, **86**, 103–26.

Chapter 25

Community care: an evaluation

MATTHIJS MUIJEN

25.1 INTRODUCTION

Major changes have taken place during the last decades in the structure of psychiatric care of many developed countries. Mental hospitals have been closed or drastically reduced in size. In the USA the state hospital population declined from 559 000 in 1955 to 138 000 in 1980 (Brown, 1985) and in the UK from 148 100 in 1954 to 64 800 in 1985 (Audit Commission, 1986). This reduction can partly be explained by shorter admissions, but more important is an ideological shift in the principles of psychiatric care, moving away from the 19th century belief that mentally ill patients required long-term protection in asylums towards the conviction that users of mental health services could function in the community, provided support was available.

The move towards community care has been enforced by a rare coalition between public, professionals and legislators, although each of these groups had its own motives. Scandals in mental hospitals received much publicity, shaping public opinion against the perceived abuse inherent in a system which reminded people of human suffering during the war. From a sociological perspective, Goffmann (1961) pointed out the characteristics of total institutions. All aspects of patients' lives are conducted in the same place under the same

authority, patients receive the same treatment often together, days are structured with explicit rules and activities are designed from an institutional perspective. This was followed by insights into the individual sufferings of patients made understandable by psychiatrists such as Laing (1960) in the UK and Foudraine in Holland (1971), and the remarkable response of these patients to more personal forms of treatment. In Italy, Basaglia (quoted in Jones and Poletti, 1985) went further, claiming that the diagnosis of mental illness is a political decision leading to the isolation of the individual in mental hospitals. 'But', he states, 'health and recovery are in society'.

A second factor leading to changes in care was the lack of efficacy found in traditional forms of treatment. Studies showed that community adjustment of patients after discharge was not correlated to functioning in hospital (Erickson, 1975), and that about 50% of discharged patients could expect to be readmitted within a year (Anthony et al., 1972). Clinicians began to experiment with alternative forms of care, often based on the beliefs of charismatic leaders (Marx et al., 1973), and a range of radical projects appeared to provide more effective forms of treatment than standard hospital care (Braun et al., 1981).

After two decades opinions on community care are as strong and divided as ever. Although it is recognized that groups of patients have benefited, critics have accused governments and mental health services in many countries of patchy developments and neglect of the most vulnerable groups. These are the deinstitutionalized patients, discharged after having lived in hospital for years and the young mentally ill, often from deprived backgrounds, who in the past would have been admitted to hospital but are now at risk of neglect, slipping through the net of community care (Bassuk and Gerson, 1978; Pepper *et al.*, 1981; Jones and Poletti, 1985; Weller, 1989).

25.2 NEED FOR EVALUATION

The similarities between the problems of community care in countries with such differences in the structure of their health services as Italy, the UK and the USA is striking. Underfunding, inequity, scarcity of housing and day centres, poor coordination of services, absence of follow-up care and neglect of the long-term mentally ill (Stern and Minkoff, 1979) are not confined by frontiers. However, the advantages of good quality community care have also been illustrated by the improvements in quality of life that can be achieved (Kiesler, 1982). The strengths and weaknesses of community care need to be compared with our experiences of standard hospital care, the practice of which can vary as much as that of community care. Rather than rushing into a radical reform based on potentially inappropriate examples, careful stepwise evaluation of model programmes and regular services seems preferable, accepting the limited external validity of any single experience (Bachrach, 1982). So far evaluations of services have often been *post hoc*, following changes in national or local policies which affected large numbers of patients, relatives and staff (Tansella, 1986; Audit Commission, 1986).

A large number of programmes, services, and specific interventions have been studied, offering some indications about the potential of various models of care. A division can be drawn between the evaluation of hospital care, day care, and home care. These are reviewed in the following sections.

25.3 EVALUATIONS OF HOSPITAL USE

Since the principle of community care is to provide comprehensive and continuing care in the least restrictive environment (Bachrach, 1981), it is not surprising that a major objective of many projects has been to minimize hospital use. Although many different alternatives to standard hospital care have succeeded in minimizing the use of hospital beds, no model of care has managed to show that a service can be run without any psychiatric beds (Braun *et al.*, 1981).

Studies seemed to support the idea that hospital admissions do not benefit patients. A consistent finding of retrospective studies is that admissions predict readmissions, and that length of admissions are correlated to previous duration of stay (Mendel, 1966; Erickson, 1975; Strauss and Carpenter, 1977). The possibility has often been ignored that patients with frequent and long admissions were very disturbed prior to admission and thus required frequent intensive care rather than developing chronicity as a consequence of admission. However some evidence suggests that the association between length of initial hospital care and of readmission may be real. A study comparing the efficacy of long (about 150 days) with short (about 90 days) admissions (Rosen *et al.*, 1976; Mattes *et al.*, 1977a, b) found at follow-up that the long admission group had required longer readmissions than the shorter admission group. Unfortunately their design was pseudo-random, possibly allowing for the selection of the most severely ill patients in the longer treatment group. This can explain the poorer cognitive level of functioning of this group at baseline. Another potential source of bias in this study were differences in follow-up care between the groups, which may have confounded the association between length of admission and readmission.

Endicott *et al.* (1979) found that duration of community stay before readmission was correlated to previous number of admissions. Three groups had been randomized to standard care (50 days in hospital) with regular outpatient care or to either of two forms of short admissions (about 10 days), where the admission was followed by outpatient care or by day care. For each past admission the standard care group spent 26 days more in hospital during the year of follow up, the brief day care group 2 days more and the brief outpatient 8 days less, this effect being particularly strong for patients with a diagnosis of schizophrenia. No differences were found between the groups for patients with no previous admissions. What these *post hoc* results fail to address is whether standard patients spent more time in hospital because they were offered long admissions or whether standard care caused dependency leading to long periods of care in hospital. The fact that the same proportion of patients from each group required readmission and that patient functioning at follow-up was the same in each group suggests that clinical decisions based on research demands may have been as important as patient needs.

It is clear, however, that hospital stay can cause 'an institutional neurosis' characterized by dependency, apathy, lack of initiative and withdrawn behaviour, similar to the negative symptoms of schizophrenia (Barton, 1966; Gruenberg, 1967), which leads to long stays in hospital. This dependency syndrome is at least partly the result of institutional processes (Goffman, 1959), and is correlated to duration of hospital stay (Wing, 1962), although an interaction between organic and social factors seems likely (Ciompi, 1983). In a survey of chronic patients in mental hospitals (Mann and Cree, 1976), 30% of patients wanted to leave (some unrealistically so), 30% preferred to stay and the other 40% did not mind. Some of this

apathy and dependence, however, can respond to rehabilitiation. Wing and Brown (1970) observed wards in three hospitals, some of which changed patient care to rehabilitation orientated models. Improvement of patient functioning was correlated with the intensity of the programmes, although some caution is required because of an increase in psychopathology in some patients due to overstimulation.

In conclusion, it appears that long admissions can lead to dependency and long readmissions, but few studies unaffected by bias or confounding variables have been conducted on the effect of relatively brief periods in hospital. An important factor is the point in time at which hospitalization can induce dependency. It is unlikely that a simple answer can be offered as chronicity is multifactorial, not only caused by time in hospital, but also by factors such as disease process, treatment model and social interaction.

25.4 HOSPITAL CARE AND COMMUNITY ADJUSTMENT

A reason for minimizing admissions is the evidence that hospital treatment does not lead to improved community functioning (Anthony *et al.*, 1972, 1978). Several studies indicate that good hospital adjustment is not related to community adjustment, and can indeed prolong further hospitalization (Fontana and Corey, 1970; Ellsworth, 1971; Erickson, 1975). An example is given of chronic patients assuming the role of patient leaders, negotiating 'a status quo which simultaneously gave the staff an active programme and preserved group members as patients' (Fontana and Corey, 1970). Few specific ward variables predict functioning after discharge, and with less power than patient variables such as symptomatology and instrumental role behaviour (Fontana and Dowds, 1975). Consistent findings are that units with good results have highly motivated, involved, non-dominant staff, and emphasize skills and independence in their patients. Duration of stay was not found to be important (Ellsworth *et al.*, 1971; Moos *et al.*, 1973). These results are non-specific, and it is unclear how these open studies controlled for treatments and aftercare. Nevertheless, staff motivation appears to be a powerful predictor in any programme (Erickson, 1975). This may also contribute to the good outcome of community adjustment in programmes which offer intense behaviourally orientated care, although success is difficult to assess without the use of a control group, a frequent problem in descriptions of services (Jacobs and Trick, 1974; Becker and Bayer, 1975).

Although hospital care is not strongly related to community adjustment, non-specific ward variables and behavioural interventions seem to be of importance, in particular for patients at high risk of institutionalization.

25.4.1 DURATION OF STAY AND IMPROVEMENT FOR THE ACUTE MENTALLY ILL

A logical next step is to investigate whether short admissions have any advantages as compared to standard admissions on psychopathology, social functioning and family burden by preventing the development of a dependency syndrome. If so, this means better care at lower cost.

Several controlled studies randomized patients to different treatment groups on admission, and followed these patients up for at least a year. Unfortunately, the various projects are difficult to compare due to variations in patient selection, duration of admission in short and standard care and type of treatment offered. Particularly confusing are the differences in mean admission durations. Short and standard care can respectively be 85 and 150 days (Rosen *et al.*, 1976), 25 and 80-120 days (Caffey *et al.*, 1971; Glick *et al.*, 1975), 10 and 50 days (Herz *et al.*, 1977) and 22 and 28 days (Hirsch *et al.*, 1979). This

implies that during the 1970s standard admissions have been reduced to much shorter periods than experimental brief admissions in earlier studies, possibly as a result of the findings in those earlier studies.

This would have made any interpretation impossible, were it not for the result that no differences in psychopathology, social functioning and family burden have been found for either form of treatment in these studies. Improvements in the short admission group occurred earlier, although the standard group had made up for this difference at the time of their discharge. The reason for this seems to have been that experimental groups had a concentration of therapeutic interventions within their short admission period, while the standard patients received the same amount of treatment over a longer period (Glick *et al.*, 1975; Herz *et al.*, 1977).

Where differences have been reported confounding variables may have played an important role. For example, Glick *et al.* (1976) reported that schizophrenic patients in the long-term hospital group performed better at one and two years follow-up than the short-term hospital group. However, long-term patients had a better pre-admission level of functioning and had received more medication and psychotherapy during follow-up. Schizophrenic patients with poor pre-hospital functioning and non-schizophrenic patients showed no difference in outcome. It is interesting to compare this with Mattes *et al.* (1977a, b), who found that patients with brief admission had been given more medication and group therapy at follow up, and had required fewer readmissions than the long admission group.

Cost-wise, short hospital stay offers a saving, although some of this is offset by a more intense use for alternative services such as day hospitals (Hirsh *et al.*, 1979). Not only direct treatment costs are lower, but also costs to patients and relatives are reduced due to an earlier return to work (Endicott *et al.*, 1978), without added burden to relatives (Herz *et al.*, 1979).

The impression from the hospital admission studies is that duration of stay is not a significant variable of long-term outcome, but that brief hospital admissions are preferable for most patients in the short term. Also taking into account the economic advantages for everyone concerned, a strong argument for limiting the duration of stay can be made. It also appears that the alternative care given to compensate for early discharge often improves functioning. This has led to studies investigating the use of day care and home care as alternatives to hospital care.

25.5 DAY CARE

Day care is a term used for all services providing interventions in a structured setting for less than 24 hours. An alternative term used in the USA is partial hospitalization, but this may be emphasizing too strongly the clinical side of day care. This vague and all-encompassing definition covers a wide range of services for many types of psychiatric patients. A global distinction can be made (Rosie, 1987) between day hospitals, day treatment programmes and day centres. Day hospitals, funded in the UK by the health services, are intended for active time-limited treatment of the seriously mentally ill, ideally providing an alternative or being complementary to hospitals. Day treatment programmes are mostly considered to be part of day hospitals, but can be identified as offering time-limited interventions to specific groups of patients. These can include detoxification programmes, assertiveness training or family groups. Day centres, funded by social services, aim to maintain the chronically mentally ill, if necessary providing support for life.

In practice many similarities exist between highly staffed, expensive day hospitals and the cheaper day centres with their more basic facilities. Both tend to care for the long-term mentally ill, about 70% of whom suffer from schizophrenia. Patients attend between a day a month and five days a week. A national survey in the UK (Edwards and Carter, 1980) reported that turnover is higher in day hospitals; more than half the patients at day centres but less than one-third of day hospital patients continued to attend for more than two years.

The characteristics of clients referred to or accepted for day care seems to depend largely on the setting of the centre (Gath *et al.*, 1973). Day hospitals connected to large mental hospitals treat older and more chronic patients, while day hospitals at district general hospitals care for more younger patients with neurotic conditions. It is unclear whether this represents differences in patient populations between the two types of hospitals, or whether differences in staff attitudes lead to the selection of these groups.

A concern about day care is the high dropout rate. This can be as much as 50% after the first visit (Baekland and Lundwall, 1975), and may be due to service or patient characteristics. If day care does not offer the interventions or support patients expect they are unlikely to return. Patient characteristics which predict dropout from day care are depression, low self-esteem, a diagnosis of personality disorder, living in a hostel and poor employment history. Age, sex, psychosis and chronicity of illness are not related (Bender and Pilling, 1985). The implications of patients withdrawing from treatment can be serious, since follow-up and outreach is not always included in the programmes.

25.5.1 EFFICACY OF DAY CARE

The variety of care offered under the heading of day care means that a general evaluation is not possible. It has to be considered which patient groups are targeted with what objective. Three groups of studies are distinguished here: day hospital care as an alternative to inpatient treatment, day hospital care as an alternative to outpatient care and the efficacy of day care in the maintenance of the long-term mentally ill in the community.

25.5.2 DAY CARE AS AN ALTERNATIVE TO HOSPITAL CARE

The first studies evaluating the use of day hospitals were conducted as early as the late 1950s, coinciding with the emergence of psychotropic drugs (Smith and Cross, 1957; Craft, 1958). Patients suffering from neurotic conditions who were not considered to be a risk to themselves or others were allocated to day care. A matched inpatient group was selected as controls. Little difference in outcome was found between the two groups after 12 months' follow-up, although the day care group had a slightly better social adjustment. Michaux *et al.* (1974), compared patients with a serious mental illness suitable for day care facilities. They found more psychopathology but better social functioning in the day care group after two months, and after a year the functioning had remained superior. However, the matching procedure in these studies may have biased the groups. For example, more inpatients came from a low social class (Michaux *et al.*, 1974).

Studies randomizing patients to either day or standard hospital care report that day care patients had longer community stays (Wilder *et al.*, 1966) and fewer readmissions (Herz *et al.*, 1971). Day patients showed less psychopathology and functioned better after four weeks' follow up, but after a year only a small advantage in social functioning could be detected (Herz *et al.*, 1971).

These studies indicate that day care is a valid alternative to hospital care, but not for all patients. It was found that about 40% of all seriously mentally ill patients admitted to an inpatient unit could be cared for in a day hospital setting without the further need of inpatient care (Wilder *et al.*, 1966; Herz *et al.*, 1971). Half of these patients were diagnosed as suffering from schizophrenia. In the UK the emphasis has been on the potential of day care in the treatment of neurotic disorders. Again, about 50% of emergency admissions could be transferred to day care (Dick *et al.*, 1985a).

Both patients (Dick *et al.*, 1985a) and their relatives (Michaux *et al.*, 1974) preferred day care to hospital care. This is likely to lead to higher compliance and may be a factor in achieving good treatment results. Cost-effectiveness studies indicate that day care is considerably cheaper than hospital care (Fink *et al.*, 1978; Dick *et al.*, 1985a).

Such results argue in favour of an expanded role for day treatment in the care of many seriously mentally ill patients, but have to be interpreted cautiously. For many patients day care is not suitable due to behavioural, physical or social problems and not all patients benefit equally from day care. Patients suffering from schizophrenia may gain from an initial period in hospital care following by day care, suggesting that day care should be considered as complementary.

25.5.3 DAY CARE AS AN ALTERNATIVE TO OUTPATIENT CARE

Day hospitals can provide more intensive treatment than an outpatient clinic, and if this leads to a faster and more persistent improvement in symptoms and functioning, the gains may balance the inherently higher costs of day care. However, this is often not the case (Weldon *et al.*, 1979; Tyrer *et al.*, 1987). Thirty patients suffering from schizophrenia were randomly allocated to day hospital treatment or outpatient care following discharge from hosptial, and no differences between groups were found after three months on clinical symptomatology and community adjustment, although the low number of patients warrants caution about this negative finding. Employment status was considerably better in the day hospital group. No information was given on the interventions offered in either setting (Weldon *et al.*, 1979).

The role of outpatient care is largely unevaluated. It is possible that specific conditions can benefit from outpatient care rather than day care, and further work is required in this field.

25.5.4 DAY CARE IN THE MAINTENANCE OF CHRONIC MENTALLY ILL PATIENTS

The majority of people attending day centres and also many day hospitals are the long-term mentally ill living in the community. Unfortunately, facilities for this group are often poorly coordinated and lacking in provisions. A survey of day care in London found a lack of emphasis on rehabilitation, deficiencies in leisure activities and inadequate support of relatives (Wing, 1982). Individualized treatment programmes are required, but are difficult to implement because of poor levels of staffing. This leads to a lack of flexibility in the activities of many facilities, often demanding either a high degree of assertiveness from users or providing them with a low level of stimulation, resulting in a high dropout rate with the risk of neglect. Some day centres allow patients to use the centre as a social meeting place, and the appreciation of this by patients is expressed by an improvement in attendance.

Programmes not only affect attendance, but also outcome, although little research has been done in this area. Milne (1984) compared two neighbouring day hospitals with similar staffing levels and chronicity of patients. One centre offered directive, behavioural interventions, the other a non-directive, social interaction programme. Only the problem-solving behavioural programme led to improvements. In a retrospective analysis of good outcome day centres as compared with relatively poor outcome day centres in the treatment of schizophrenia, good outcome characteristics appeared to be a low patient turnover, more behavioural and fewer psychotherapeutic interventions, the use of care plans and a key worker system (Linn *et al.*, 1979). Differences existed between the patient groups, with the good outcome centres having older patients and more men, although the effects of these variables on outcome are unclear.

Home care has been evaluated against day care. Patients were randomized to an assertive outreach programme, where they were visited on average twice weekly, or to a drop-in centre (Bond, 1987). Patients in the outreach project had significantly fewer readmissions and days in hospital. Outreach alone did not improve quality of life, in spite of the very basic provisions and the lack of follow up care in the drop-in centre.

The combination of day and home care could be of benefit to the long-term mentally ill, and it is surprising that this has not been studied. Many of the skills acquired in day centres do not transfer to the home, and some additional sessions at home might compensate for this. Home visits can increase the attendance at day care facilities, with resulting reduction in relapse and improvements in community adjustment (Beard *et al.*, 1978).

25.6 HOME CARE

Home care is the most radical form of community care, aiming to treat and rehabilitate patients in their own environments with the intent to maximize independent functioning and minimize handicaps. The objective is that patients receive comprehensive treatment and support based on each individual's needs. The teaching of daily living skills *in vivo* is thought to minimize the need of generalization (Marx *et al.*, 1973) and resulting improvements in instrumental behaviour and coping skills are more likely to persist than those taught in a clinical setting (Anthony and Buell, 1972).

A distinction can be made between the needs of the acute mentally ill without a history of hospital stay and long-term dependent patients who may have stayed in institutions for years. Home care aims to prevent the development of a hospital dependency syndrome in the first group, while the aim for the second group is to alleviate this dependency with rehabilitation in the least restrictive setting. In practice teams will often care for a mixed client group, requiring a large number of skills.

Unless community care is comprehensive, patients are at risk of neglect. Community care has to accept responsibility not only for the mental well-being of patients but also for components of care that are not traditionally part of the role of psychiatric services. These include the functions of the Community Support Programme (Turner and Ten Hoor, 1978) such as continuity of care, case management and regular medical check-ups, but also the organization of material resources, assertive support and follow-up, and active involvement of relatives in treatment and education (Stein and Test, 1980).

25.6.1 EFFICACY OF HOME CARE FOR THE SEVERELY MENTALLY ILL

Studies comparing home-based care with standard hospital care have been conducted since the early 1960s (Pasamanick *et al*; Grad and Sainsbury, 1968), evaluating the feasibility and outcome of this type of care. Six controlled studies randomized seriously mentally ill patients who were due to be hospitalized and followed these patients up for a year or more (Pasamanick *et al.*, 1967; Langsley *et al.*, 1969; Test and Stein, 1980; Fenton *et al.*, 1982a; Hoult and Reynolds, 1983).

The project by Pasamanick *et al.* (1967) is remarkable in that it anticipates future developments, both in service ideology and study design, by about 20 years. The study was instigated in 1957, but patient intake started in Louisville in 1961, delayed by the reluctance of state hospitals to cooperate. Inclusion criteria were a diagnosis of schizophrenia, the absence of suicidal or homicidal intent, and a supportive family. The 152 patients were randomized into three groups: a standard hospital control and two home treatment groups. Both home treatment groups received identical community support, but in one of these groups psychotropic medication was replaced with placebo. Patients stayed in the programme for two years. The seven staff members visited home patients weekly during the initial three months, fortnightly the next three-month period and monthly thereafter. Home care was considered to be a failure if patients required admission, and at this point they were taken out of the study. Regular

ratings were completed by the staff members.

Fenton *et al.* (1982a) used the same entry criteria in Montreal, and only 19% of all hospital admissions were eligible for randomization into home or hospital treatment. The home care team consisted of a half-time psychiatrist and social worker and a full-time nurse, caring for 78 patients. On average patients were visited 17 times during the year of follow-up, most of these contacts taking place in the first month.

Family therapy was compared with hospital admission in Denver (Langsley *et al.*, 1969, 1971). An unknown number of family therapists conducted an average of just over five sessions during the month of entry. Each group accommodated 150 patients, but the only entry criteria specified were expected hospital admission and living with a family. Follow-up ratings were completed by independent clinicians.

The most comprehensive studies were conducted in Madison, Wisconsin (Stein and Test, 1980) and Sydney (Hoult and Reynolds, 1983). The Sydney study replicated the Madison project, so many features were similar. Patients were randomized if they were deemed to require admission for serious mental illness (schizophrenia and affective psychosis) in the absence of brain damage or primary addiction. Patients presenting with aggression, no fixed abode or no social support were excluded. The projects employed 10 staff for 65 patients in Madison and 8 staff for 60 patients in Sydney. Both projects used an approach integrating crisis intervention and rehabilitation, visiting patients as often as required during the year of follow-up. The research teams worked strictly independent from the clinical teams.

In spite of the considerable differences between the projects, outcomes were very similar. No study found an advantage for hospital care in any area, but home care had led to significantly better functioning in several studies. Patients in home care had fewer and shorter admissions than standard care patients. Between 18% (Stein and Test 1980) and 40% (Fenton *et al.*, 1982a; Hoult and Reynolds, 1983) of home care patients required hospitalization, and average admission duration of these patients was about 70% shorter than those of the hospital care groups. Only in the Louisville study (Pasamanick *et al.*, 1967) were hospitalized patients from the home treatment group institutionalized for a longer period than the control group. This was the only project not offering continuity of care, and it is possible that the clinical responsibility of the other community projects even during admission permitted early discharge because of an awareness of the resources in the community (Fuller Torrey, 1986). The transfer of responsibility to the hospital team on admission can easily lead to prolonged stays due to differences in approach and priorities, such as an emphasis on symptomatology rather than social functioning in hospital.

Fewer psychotic symptoms were displayed by patients in the home care groups in Sydney and Madison, but not in other projects. No difference were found in self-esteem and leisure time activities, but experimental patients in Madison had spent more time in sheltered employment, resulting in higher earnings. In Montreal (Fenton *et al.*, 1982a), a higher proportion of home care patients employed at entry had resumed work after 12 months' follow up (50%) than hospital patients (33%).

Satisfaction with home care was higher for both patients and relatives than with hospital care in Sydney (Reynolds and Hoult, 1984). Family and community burden, measured by police contacts and suicide attempts, was not affected by type of care in any of the projects (Test and Stein, 1980; Fenton *et al.*, 1982; Reynolds and Hoult, 1984). Amount of interaction with staff in the community has been established in other studies as the major variable contributing to family satisfaction (Grad and Sainsbury, 1967; Grella and Grusky, 1989), and home treatment is a model of care which can provide this well.

More evidence of the efficacy of home care is given by the gradual deterioration of patients from the experimental groups who were returned to standard care at the end of home treatment (Stein and Test, 1980; Davis *et al.* 1972). Eventually all the gains accomplished in home care had eroded and no differences between the original groups could be detected.

An important objective is to determine those patient groups which would benefit most from this model of care. Hoult and Reynolds (1983) separated their patient population retrospectively into those with a diagnosis of schizophrenia, patients with no previous admissions and chronic patients. The group responding best to community care as compared with standard care were the first admissions. Chronic patients showed relatively smaller gains with home care, but even for this group hospital use had been reduced substantially with some clinical improvements over the year.

25.7 COSTS

Cost of community care has been reported as lower than hospital care, saving from 5% (Weisbrod *et al.*, 1980) to 25% (Hoult and Reynolds, 1983) and even 61% (Fenton *et al.*, 1982b). However, these variations reflect differences in both methods of cost calculation and treatment models. The various projects used a cost-benefit analysis (Weisbrod *et al.*, 1980), cost-efficiency analyses (Fenton *et al.*, 1982b; Hoult *et al.*, 1983) and comparisons of direct treatment costs only (Pasamanick *et al.*, 1967; Langsley *et al.*, 1968). In Madison (Weisbrod *et al.*, 1980) the 26% higher treatment cost of community care was compensated for by societal benefits such as earnings of patients. Their analysis included capital costs, but the high starting costs of community care were disregarded. Pasamanick *et al.* (1967) and Langsley *et al.* (1968) only measured costs of inpatient stay and community services, while Fenton *et al.* (1982) and Hoult and Reynolds (1983) also calculated cost incurred by public and private agencies. Since all studies included the main cost components, such as total hospital expenditure, and the relative costs and usage of these components were similar, the large differences in savings seem to be related to variations in the model of care, such as staff-patient ratios and intensity of care.

The consistent finding that home care costs less than hospital care suggests that some savings can be expected after an initial capital investment in areas such as staff training and small scale community developments, making community care an attractive option. Caution is advisable for several reasons. First, savings in hospital expenditure can lead to higher costs elsewhere, such as day care, hostels or social services (Borland *et al.*, 1989), with an unpredictable result. A second problem is posed by marginal costs; closure of half a ward or half a hospital does not save half the cost because of fixed overheads. This means that a gradual implementation of community services can be disproportionately expensive, encouraging the notion of rapid closures of hospitals without the necessary evaluation of the impact of such change.

25.8 VALIDITY

Even though individual projects have demonstrated that many alternatives to standard hospital care are effective, this in itself does not mean that these programmes can confidently be implemented elsewhere (Bachrach, 1980). The external validity of model programmes can be limited (Bachrach, 1982) due to their experimental and time-limited nature. Unless evaluative and clinical methods are revealed in detail, the repeatability and relevance of the results of individual model programmes cannot be relied on, and replication is unlikely to be successful. Many of the projects have identical aims, and are based on similar principles, which appear to reinforce the power of evidence in favour of alternatives to standard care. However, differences do exist between studies which may be affecting results, and these are too often ignored. Nevertheless, the evidence seems strongly in favour of the efficacy of community care.

5.9 CONTINUITY OF CARE

The consistency in good outcome from home care and day care programmes is surprising, considering the differences in variables between model programmes such as treatment methods, patient groups and staff-patient ratios. This may suggest a commonality between studies that is responsible for their efficacy other than a structural variable such as setting. A process variable which appears to be present in different proportions in experimental projects and control treatments is continuity of care. This is defined by Bachrach (1981) as the orderly, uninterrupted movement of patients among the diverse elements of the service delivery system. Aftercare is part of continuity of care, but is an inappropriate term for patients never receiving the inpatient care.

Continuity of care has been a component of treatment models in several of the controlled studies described under hospital care, day care or home care. The contradictory results of Mattes *et al.* (1977) and Glick *et al.* (1976), respectively reporting better outcomes of short admissions and long admissions, can be reconciled by the presence of more aftercare in each of the better functioning groups. Caffey (1971), compared standard hospital care followed by regular outpatient care with standard- and short-stay hospital care which offered continuity of care by the treatment teams. There was no difference between patients in either of the groups providing continuity of care and both outperformed standard care. The home-care studies found that community teams using continuity of care did better than standard care. However when continuity of care was withdrawn the differences disappeared. In contrast, projects not offering continuity of care in either of the treatment groups could not detect differences in outcome at follow-up (Wilder *et al.*, 1966;

Herz *et al.*, 1971). Several uncontrolled studies confirm the value of continuity of care, especially for schizophrenic patients (Winston *et al.*, 1977), although the attribution of results to continuity of care has to be cautious. Patients may have been selected for continuing care on the grounds of likely benefits, or patients at risk of relapse may have selectively withdrawn from care.

Not all studies found that aftercare protected against relapse (Purvis and Miskimins, 1970; Mayer *et al.*, 1973). Globally, patients receiving no or regular care seem to function better than patients obtaining only a few sessions. Kirk (1976) found that 31% of patients who had not received aftercare were rehospitalized as compared with 41% of patients who had been followed-up. When the group receiving aftercare was further analysed, it showed that 55% of those receiving between one and ten visits relapsed, but only 20% of patients attended to more than ten times during the two to three years of follow-up. The effect of after care only seemed to benefit chronic patients. Patients with good premorbid functioning suffered a relapse rate of 30%, independent of follow up. For chronic patients aftercare reduced the relapse rate from 50% to 30%. This was confirmed in a controlled study by Beard *et al.* (1978), who found a significant positive correlation in the care of chronic patients between continuous outreach, regular attendance at a rehabilitation centre and lower relapse rates with shorter hospital stays.

In conclusion, it appears that continuity of care is an important, and possibly essential component of community care. It is effective in preventing loss of functioning, especially for patients suffering from a severe mental illness.

25.9.1 CASE MANAGEMENT

Continuity of care requires the coordination of all available resources to ascertain the optimal care for this dependent group of patients. This is the task of the case manager, who has a central position in community care (Intaglata, 1982; Harris and Bachrach, 1988). The responsibilities of case management are patient assessment, formulation of a care plan, implementation of interventions, coordination of services, monitoring of quality of care and regular evaluation. In addition the administration of budgets is sometimes included. This multiplicity of tasks cannot be expected from a single mental health worker, but the case manager is responsible for quality of care. Advantages to patients are accountability and accessibility. Patients know who to approach for help, and a supportive relationship may develop between patient and professional (Harris and Bergman, 1988). Although staff tend to appreciate this model because of the continuing involvement with familiar patients, case management can also lead to demoralization as a consequence of the intensity of this involvement, especially if patients do not improve or deteriorate. 'Burn-out' needs to be prevented by means of training, clinical supervision, flexible hours and regular holidays (Harris and Bergman, 1988).

25.10 CONCLUSION

The consistent finding that experimental programmes are superior to standard care is promising, and implies that improvements in standard patient care can be expected. The efficacy of short admissions, day care and home care for groups of patients suffering from serious mental illness has been illustrated repeatedly. By now the beneficial results on social functioning of community care can be accepted, although concerns remain about the long-term effects of this form of care, the extent of reliance on the enthusiasm of staff and relatives and the stability of patient functioning. The comprehensive, long-term demands on a regular service are distinct from those of well-defined, short-lived projects (Bachrach 1980).

A limitation of model programmes is the frequently narrow scope of service evaluations. A comparison of home care and standard care cannot quantify the relative impact of many other services such as day hospitals, housing, social services and relatives and friends. Model programmes have an important role to play because variables are easier controlled for, but more attention should be given to the evaluation of standard services. Descriptions of the planning and running of new services (Gudeman *et al.*, 1983; Dean and Gatt, 1989) can indicate the potential of innovations.

It is questionable whether more studies are required on the general feasibility of brief admissions, day hospital care or home care. More specificity is required, such as research into the best interventions in the various settings for sub-groups of patients. These sub-groups should not only be based on diagnosis, but also on social handicaps, such as the studies on expressed emotion (Leff *et al.*, 1985) and environmental stress (Falloon *et al.*, 1982).

The most important determinant of type of care is frequently the habit of the practitioners (Platt *et al.*, 1980) or the availability of services (Dick *et al.*, 1985b). Evidence on the efficacy of a new form of care cannot be expected to produce changes in routine practice without strong advocacy and the provision of training and resources.

Innovations in psychiatric care are taking place everywhere in the world. It is to be hoped that these changes will be carefully evaluated, and that successful forms of care will be disseminated and implemented.

REFERENCES

Anthony, W.A., Buell, G.J., Sharratt, S. and Althoff, M.E. (1972) The efficacy of psychiatric rehabilitation. *Psychol. Bull.*, **78**, 447–56.

Anthony, W.A., Cohen, M.R. and Vitalo, R. (1978) The measurement of rehabilitation outcome. *Schizophr. Bull.*, **4**, 365–83.

Audit Commission for Local Authorities in England and Wales. (1986) *Making a Reality of Community Care.* HMSO, London.

Bachrach, L.L. (1980) Overview: Model Programs for Chronic Mental Patients. *Am. J. Psychiatry*, **137**, 1023–131.

Bachrach, L.L. (1981) Continuity of care for chronic mental patients: A conceptual analysis. *Am. J. Psychiatry*, **138**, 1449–55.

Bachrach, L.L. (1982) Assessment of outcomes in community support systems: results, problems and limitations. *Schizophr. Bull.*, **8**, 39–60.

Baekland, F. and Lundwell, L. (1975) Dropping out of treatment, a critical review. *Psychol. Bull.*, **82**, 738–83.

Barton, R. (1966), *Institutional Neurosis.* John Wright and Sons, Bristol.

Bassuk, E.L. and Gerson, S. (1978) Deinstitutionalization and mental health services. *Sci. Am.*, **238**, 46–53.

Beard, J.H., Malamud, T.J. and Rossman, E. (1978) Psychiatric rehabilitation and long term rehospitalization rates: the findings of two research studies. *Schizophr. Bull.*, **4**, 622–35.

Becker, P. and Bayer, C. (1975) Preparing chronic patients for community placement: a four-stage treatment programme. *Hosp. Community Psychiatry*, **26**, 448–50.

Bender, M.P. and Pilling, S. (1985) A study of variables associated with under-attendance at a psychiatric day centre. *Psychol. Med.*, **15**, 395–401.

Bond, G.R., Witheridge, I.F., Setae, P.J. *et al.* (1985) Preventing rehospitalization of clients in a psychosocial rehabilitation agency. *Hosp. Community Psychiatry*, **36**, 993–5.

Borland, A., McRae, J. and Lycan, C. (1989) Outcomes of five years of continuous intensive case management. *Hosp. Community Psychiatry*, **40**, 369–76.

Braun, P., Kochansky, G., Shapiro, R. *et al.* (1981) Overview: deinstitutionalization of psychiatric patients, a critical review of outcome studies. *Am. J. Psychiatry*, **136**, 736–49.

Brown, P. (1985) *The Transfer of Care. Psychiatric Deinstitutionalization and its Aftermath.* Routledge, New York.

Caffey, E.M., Galbrecht, C.R., Klett, C.J. and Point, P. (1971) Brief hospitalization and aftercare in the treatment of schizophrenia. *Arch. Gen. Psychiatry*, **24**, 81–6.

Ciompi, L. (1983), Schizophrenic deterioration. *Br. J. Psychiatry*, **142**, 79–80.

Craft, M. (1958) An evaluation of treatment of depressive illness in a day hospital. *Lancet*, **ii**, 149–51.

Davis, A.E., Dinitz, S. and Pasamanick, B. (1972) The prevention of hospitalization in schizophrenia: Five years after an experimental programme. *Am. J. Orthopsychiatry*, **42**, 375–88.

Dean, C. and Gadd, E. (1989) An inner city home treatment service for acute psychiatric patients. *Psychiatr. Bull. Royal Coll. Psychiatr.*, **13**, 667–9.

Dick, P., Cameron, L., Cohen, D., Barlow, M. and Ince, A. (1985a) Day- and full-time psychiatric treatment — a controlled comparison. *Br. J. Psychiatry*, **147**, 246–249.

Dick, P., Ince, A. and Barlow, B. (1985b) Day treatment: suitability and referral procedure. *Br. J. Psychiatry*, **147**, 250–3.

Edwards, C. and Carter, J. (1980) *The Data of Day Care*. National Institute for Social Work, London.

Ellsworth, R., Maroney, R., Klett, W. *et al.*, (1971) Milieu characteristics of successful psychiatric treatment programs. *Am. J. Orthopsychiatry*, **41**, 427–40.

Endicott, J., Cohen, J., Nee, J. *et al.*, (1979) Brief vs. standard hospitalization; For whom? *Arch. Gen. Psychiatry*, **36**, 706–12.

Endicott, J., Herz, M.I. and Gibbon, M. (1978) Brief vs. standard hospitalization: the differential costs. *Am. J. Psychiatry*, **135**, 707–12.

Erickson, R.C. (1975) Outcome studies in mental hospitals: a review. *Psychol. Bull.*, **82**, 519–40.

Falloon, I.R.M., Boyd, J.L., McGill, C.W. *et al.* (1982) Family management in the prevention of exacerbations of schizophrenia. *N. Engl. J. Med.*, **43**, 633–42.

Fenton, F.R., Tessier, L., Struening, E.L. *et al.* (1982a) *Home and Hospital Psychiatric Treatment*. Croom Helm, London.

Fenton, F.R., Tessier, L., Contandriopolous, A.P. *et al.* (1982b) A comparative trial of home and hospital psychiatric treatment: financial costs. *Can. J. Psychiatry*, **27**, 177–87.

Fontana, A.F. and Corey, M. (1970) Culture conflict in the treatment of 'mental illness' and the central role of the patient leader. *J.*

Consult. Clin. Psychol., **34**, 244–9.

Fontana, A.F. and Dowds, B.N. (1975) Assessing treatment outcome. 2, The prediction of re-hospitalization. *J. Nerv. Ment. Dis.*, **161**, 231–8.

Foudraine, J. (1971) *Not Made of Wood*. Macmillan, New York.

Fuller Torrey, E. (1986) Continuous treatment teams in the care of the chronic mentally ill. *Hosp. Community Psychiatry*, **37**, 1243–7.

Gath, D., Hassal, C. and Cross, K.W. (1973) Whither psychiatric day care? A study of day patients in Birmingham. *Br. Med. J.*, **i**, 94–8.

Glick, I.D., Hargreaves, W.A., Drues, J. and Showstack, J.A. (1976) Short vs long hospitalization: a prospective controlled study. iv. One year follow-up results for schizophrenic patients. *Am. J. Psychiatry*, **133**, 509–14.

Glick, I.D., Hargreaves, W.A., Raskin, M. and Kutner, S.J. (1975) Short versus long hospitalization: a prospective controlled study. ii. Results for schizophrenic inpatients. *Am. J. Psychiatry*, **132**, 385–90.

Goffman, E. (1961) *Asylums*. Pelican, Harmondsworth.

Grad, J. and Sainsbury, P. (1986) The effects that patients have on their families in a community care and a control psychiatric service — a two year follow-up. *Br. J. Psychiatry*, **114**, 265–78.

Grella, C.E. and Grusky, O. (1989) Families of the seriously mentally ill and their satisfaction with services. *Hosp. Community Psychiatry*, **40**, 831–5.

Gruenberg, E. (1967) The social breakdown syndrome – some origins. *Am. J. Psychiatry*, **123**, 1481–9.

Gudeman, J.E., Dickey, B., Evans, A. and Shore, M.F. (1985) Four year assessment of a hospital inn program as an alternative to inpatient hospitalization. *Am. J. Psychiatry*, **142**, 1330–3.

Harris, M. and Bachrach, L.L. (1988) Clinical case management. *New Dir. Ment. Health Serv.*, **40**, 1–96.

Harris, M. and Bergman, H.C. (1988) Clinical case management for the chronically mentally ill: a In Clinical case management, M. Harris and L.L. Bachrach (eds), *N. Dir. Ment. Health Service.*, **40**, Jossey-Bass, San Francisco, pp. 1–14.

Herz, M.I. , Endicott, J. and Gibbon, M. (1979) Brief hospitalization. A two-year follow-up. *Arch. Gen. Psychiatry*, **36**, 701–5.

Herz, M.I., Endicott, J. and Spitzer, R.L. (1977) Brief hospitalization: a two-year follow-up. *Am. J. Psychiatry*, **134**, 502–7.

Herz, M.I., Endicott, J., Spitzer, R.L. and Mesnikoff, A. (1971) Day versus inpatient hospitalization: a controlled study. *Am. J. Psychiatry*, **127**, 1371–81.

Hirsch, S.R., Platt, S., Knights, A. and Weyman, A. (1979) Shortening hospital stay for psychiatric care: effect on patients and their families. *Br. Med. J.*, **i**, 442–6.

Hoult, J. and Reynolds, I. (1983) *Psychiatric Hospital versus Community Treatment: A Controlled Study*. New South Wales, Department of Health.

Intagliata, J. (1982) Improving the quality of community care for the chronically mentally disabled: the role of case management. *Schizophr. Bull.*, **8**, 655–74.

Jacobs, M.K. and Trick, O.L. (1974) Successful psychiatric rehabilitation using an in-patient teaching laboratory. *Am. J. Psychiatry.*, **131**, 145–8.

Jones, K. and Poletti, A. (1985) Understanding the Italian experience. *Br. J. Psychiatry*, **146**, 341–8.

Kiesler, C.A. (1982) Mental hospitals and alternative care. *Am. Psychol.*, **37**, 349–60.

Kirk, S.A. (1976) Effectiveness of community services for discharged mental hospital patients. *Am. J. Orthopsychiatry*, **46**, 646–59.

Laing, R.D. (1960) *The Divided Self*. Penguin, London.

Langsley, D.G., Pittman, F., Machotka, P. and Flomenhaft, K. (1968) Family crisis therapy — results and implications. *Fam. Process, 7*, 145–58.

Langsley, D.G., Flomenhaft, K. and Machotka, P. (1969) Follow-up evaluation of family crisis therapy. *Am. J. Orthopsychiatry*, **39**, 753–9.

Langsley, D.G., Machotka, P. and Flomenhaft, K. (1971) Avoiding mental hospital admission, a follow-up study. *Am. J. Psychiatry*, **127**, 1391–4.

Leff, J., Kuipers, L., Berkowitz, R. and Sturgeon, D. (1985) A controlled trial of social intervention in the families of schizophrenic patients: two-year follow-up. *Br. J. Psychiatry*, **146**, 594–600.

Linn, M.W., Caffey, E.M., Klett, C.J. *et al.* (1979) Day treatment and psychotropic drugs in the aftercare of schizophrenic patients. *Arch. Gen. Psychiatry*, **36**, 1055–66.

Mann, S.A. and Cree, W. (1976) 'New' long-stay psychiatric patients: a national sample survey of fifteen mental hospitals in England and Wales 1972/3. *Psychol. Med.*, **6**, 603–16.

Marx, A.J., Test, M.A. and Stein, L.I. (1973) Extrahospital management of severe mental illness. *Arch. Gen. Psychiatry*, **29**, 505–11.

Mattes, J.A., Rosen, B. and Klein D.F. (1977a) Comparison of the clinical effectiveness of 'short' versus 'long' stay psychiatric hospitalization. II. Results of a 3-year posthospital follow-up. *J. Nerv. Ment. Dis.*, **165**, 387–94.

Mattes, J., Rosen, B., Klein, D.F. and Milan, D. (1977b) Comparison of the clinical effectiveness of 'short' versus 'long' stay psychiatric hospitalization. III. Further results of a 3-year posthospital follow-up. *J. Nerv. Ment. Dis.*, **165**, 395–402.

Mayer, J., Hotz, M. and Rosenblatt, A. (1973) The readmission patterns of patients referred to aftercare clinics. *J. Bronx State Hosp.*, **1**, 4.

Mendel, W.M. (1966) Effect of length of hospitalization on rate and quality of remission from acute psychotic episodes. *J. Nerv. Ment. Dis.*, **143**, 226–34.

Michaux, M.H., Chelst, M.R., Foster, S.A. *et al.* (1974) Post release adjustment of day- and full-time psychiatric patients. *Arch. Gen. Psychiatry*, **29**, 647–51.

Milne, D. (1984) A comprehensive evaluation of two psychiatric day hospitals. *Br. J. Psychiatry*, **145**, 533–7.

Moos, R., Shelton, R. and Petty, C. (1973) Perceived ward climate and treatment outcome. *J. Abnorm. Psychol.*, **82**, 291–8.

Pasamanick, B., Scarpitty, F.R. and Dinitz, S. (1967) *Schizophrenics in the Community*. Appleton-Century-Crofts, New York.

Pepper, B., Kirshner, M. and Rylewics, H. (1981) The young adult chronic patient: overview of a population. *Hosp. Community Psychiatry*, **32**, 463–9.

Platt, S.D., Knights, A.C. and Hirsh, S.R. (1980) Caution and conservatism in the use of a psychiatric day hospital: evidence from a research project that failed. *Psychiatry Res.*, **3**, 123–32.

Purvis, S.A. and Miskimins, R.W. (1970) Effects of community follow-up on post-hospital adjustment fpr psychiatric patients. *Community Ment. Health J.*, **6**, 374–82.

Reynolds, I. and Hoult, J.E. (1984) The relatives of the mentally ill, a comparative trial of community oriented and hospital oriented psychiatric care. *J. Nerv. Ment. Dis.*, **172**, 480–9.

Rosen, B., Katzoff, A., Carillo, C. and Klein, D. (1976) Clinical effectiveness of 'short' vs 'long' psychiatric hospitalization. *Arch. Gen. Psychiatry*, **33**, 1316–22.

Rosie, J.S. (1987) Partial hospitalization: a review of recent literature. *Hosp. Community Psychiatry*, **38**, 1291–9.

Smith, S. and Cross, E.G.W. (1957) Review of 1000 patients treated at a psychiatric day hospital. *Int. J. Soc. Psychiatry*, **2**, 292–8.

Stein, L.J. and Test, M.A. (1980) Alternative to mental hospital treatment. 1, Conceptual model, treatment program and clinical evaluation. *Arch. Gen. Psychiatry*, **37**, 392–7.

Stern, R. and Minkoff, K. (1979) Paradoxes in programming for chronic patients in a community clinic. *Hosp. Community Psychiatry*, **30**, 613–17.

Strauss, J.S. and Carpenter, W.T. (1977) Prediction of outcome in schizophrenia. iii. Five year outcome and its predictors. *Arch. Gen. Psychiatry*, **34**, 159–63.

Tansella, M. (1986) Community psychiatry without mental hospitals; the Italian experience: a review. *J. Royal Soc. Med.*, **79**, 664–9.

Test, M.A. and Stein, L.I. (1980) Alternative to mental hospital treatment. 3 Social cost. *Arch. Gen. Psychiatry*, **37**, 409–12.

Turner, J.C. and Ten Hoor, W.J. (1978) The NIMH support program: Pilot approach to a needed social reform. *Schizophr. Bull.*, **4**, 319–48.

Tyrer, P., Remington, M. and Alexander, J. (1987) The outcome of neurotic disorders after out-patient and day hospital care. *Br. J. Psychiatry*, **151**, 57–62.

Weisbrod, B.A., Test, M.A. and Stein, L.I. (1980) Alternative to mental hospital treatment. 2. Economic benefit-cost analysis. *Arch. Gen. Psychiatry*, **37**, 400–5.

Weldon, E., Clarkin, J.E., Hennesy, J.J. and Frances, A. (1979) Day hospital versus out-patient treatment: a controlled study. *Psychiatr. Quart.*, **59**, 144–50.

Weller, M.P.I. (1989) Mental illness — who cares? *Nature*, **39**, 249–52.

Wilder, J.F., Levin, G. and Zwerling, I. (1966), A two year follow-up evaluation of acute psychotic patients treated in a day hospital. *Am. J. Psychiatry*, **122**, 1095–101.

Wing, J.K. (1962) Institutionalism in mental hospitals. *Br. J. Clin. Soc. Psychol.*, **1**, 38–51.

Wing, J.K. (ed) (1982) Long-term community care: experience in a London borough. *Psychol. Med. Monogr. Suppl.*

Wing, J.K. and Brown, G.W. (1970) *Institutionalism and Schizophrenia*. Cambridge University Press, Cambridge.

Chapter 26

Preventive interventions in the community

MARC LAPORTA and IAN R.H. FALLOON

26.1 A GENERAL FRAMEWORK FOR PREVENTIVE INTERVENTIONS IN THE COMMUNITY

In contrast to services that are primarily geared to acute or rehabilitative treatment, the key aim of all health services to communities is the prevention of morbidity. However, in practice few mental health services achieve this objective, most functioning as crisis intervention resources that deal with mental disorders in their most florid phases. While prevention of mental disorders has been viewed with extreme scepticism, there is accumulating evidence that modern approaches to mental health may contribute to a more benign course of several major mental disorders. This chapter outlines some of the principles and methods that embody prevention of the morbidity associated with schizophrenic disorders.

Raeburn and Seymour (1977) have described a straightforward approach to the development of mental health services that address the specific needs of the communities they serve (Figure 26.1).

In the initial assessment stage, the more thoroughly defined are the needs, the easier it is to articulate the service's active role in

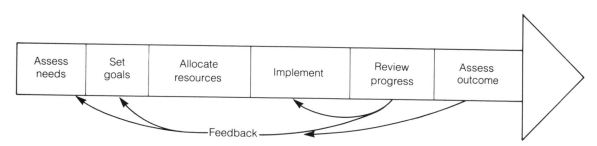

Figure 26.1 Steps in the development of preventive interventions.

prevention. In assessing population needs (Price and Smith, 1985), the target population is described demographically, and major stresses affecting it are carefully identified. A survey of the perceived stresses and needs of the people who are to utilize services forms part of this assessment. Careful assessment enhances the understanding of the problems related to specific stresses that are experienced by the target population. In schizophrenia, not only are episodes precipitated by stressful events, but the illness itself acts as a potent stressor to contribute to many complicating symptoms and problems.

In planning interventions, specific, short-term objectives are established and a constructive feedback process that allows for adjustments is initiated. Symptomatic impairments are not the exclusive focus of prevention. Some of the general objectives of preventive interventions in schizophrenia are summarized in Table 26.1.

Health care professionals are often portrayed as experts who provide highly specialized remedial skills and competencies to individuals. However, Rappaport (1981) has proposed that

Table 26.1 Objectives of preventive interventions for schizophrenia

Illness-related objectives
    Preventing episodes and relapse
    Managing symptoms and impairments
    Treatment of ancillary symptoms
    Long-term management planning

Stressors, precipitants and complications
    Identifying and managing stressors
    Fostering social and interpersonal reintegration
    Managing family and carer symptomatology
    Reducing handicap

Other objectives
    Enhancing self-help and generalization skills
    Mobilizing extra-familial support
    Liaison and cooperation with other helping
        agencies
    Maximizing cost-efficiency
    Research and evaluation
    Influencing social policy toward preventive work

natural carers (families, residential facilities and self-help groups) be empowered to solve their problems with the clinician acting as an educator and resource provider. Identifying and organizing community resources includes thinking through ways of securing motivation, cooperation and interest of relevant groups. It is crucial that intervention strategies be framed in terms of supplying the targeted population with skills that can be used to cope with stresses and crises, and to foster community-based preventive skills and strategies. Taking care not to duplicate existing community resources and manpower is a cost-efficient way of providing needed expertise.

In choosing interventions, ease of implementation in the community is an important consideration. Interventions that have a high likelihood of achieving goals at the lowest cost to the service should be preferred. When they are relevant to the target population's needs and stresses, these interventions are likely to be developed by patients and carers into self-help skills.

As the prevention programme is implemented, the effectiveness of its methods is continuously renewed, enabling rapid adjustment of strategies to adapt to changing problems and needs as they arise. Physical and financial resources of the service deserve detailed elaboration, and specific steps are often required to secure their adequacy.

26.2 PREVENTION: CONCEPTS AND APPROACHES

26.2.1 PRIMARY, SECONDARY AND TERTIARY PREVENTION

A useful general conceptual orientation for community preventive work is the distinction made in public health between primary, secondary and tertiary prevention (Cowen, 1983). **Secondary prevention** is aimed at reducing the prevalence of cases of a disorder in a population. These efforts seek to shorten the duration

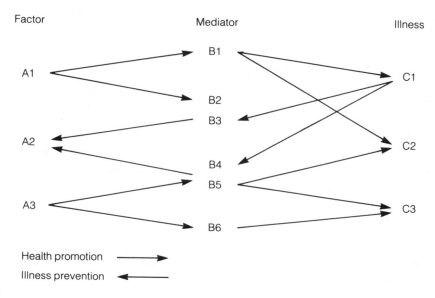

Factor   Mediator   Illness

Health promotion ⟶

Illness prevention ⟵

Figure 26.2 Primary prevention.

and lessen the negative consequences of early identified symptoms of impairment. Most of our interventions in modern psychiatry are at a secondary prevention level since they are focused on dysfunctions that are already evident. As prodromal signs and symptoms become better defined, secondary prevention can be initiated earlier. An example of this is the identification of disturbed sleep as an indication for early secondary intervention in someone previously diagnosed as having bipolar affective disorder. **Tertiary prevention efforts** are designed to reduce the disability associated with a fully developed illness. Many consider this term to be a misnomer, as it is only very remotely 'preventive'. **Primary prevention** has become an increasingly important focus of preventive service implementation. It differs from the two other aspects of prevention in that it aims at reducing the incidence of disorder and is directed to members of a population who are as yet unaffected. Primary prevention in psychiatry can be looked at from two perspectives (Newton, 1988): illness prevention and health promotion (Figure 26.2). Illness prevention aims to establish specific treatments for specific disorders, using strategies derived from the analysis of risk factors. Health promotion aims at forward-directed effects, instigating general health-promoting factors to prevent the onset of illness. An example of this in modern psychiatry is the teaching of stress-management skills. These are relatively non-specific interventions to deal with a variety of stressors such as life events, and may help prevent stress-related disorders such as burnout, anxiety disorders, some forms of depression, and even marital breakdown. The health perspective focuses less on illness than on maintaining well-being. In health promotion, any given intervention need not follow a 'one illness-one treatment' model, but will at best contribute to the prevention of many illness-related problems. In practice, the demarcation between these two perspectives is not always so clearcut. For schizophrenia, inadequate information about early markers and risk factors limits our ability to target the high-risk population and implement primary prevention interventions.

26.2.2 THE STRESS-VULNERABILITY MODEL OF SCHIZOPHRENIA

In attempting to understand schizophrenia, it is important to realize that there is not a single unified concept of the disorder, and that its definition is not straightforward (Black *et al.*, 1988). From the aetiological point of view, schizophrenia probably represents a heterogeneous group of disorders with varying aetiologies (Chapter 2); it is unlikely to stem from a single disease process. Genetic factors are clearly involved in its aetiology (Chapter 7). They are relatively weak, and probably expressed as a propensity to develop the disorder, where environmental factors then play an important role in its onset, manifestations and course (Day, 1981; Leff and Vaughn, 1985; Chapter 8). Nevertheless, in our present state of knowledge about the illness, the identification and diagnosis of schizophrenia still relies upon detecting specific symptom clusters.

Current theories of aetiology, symptom expression and complications can advantageously be integrated into a simple model that helps organize interventions. The stress-vulnerability model of schizophrenia integrates biological and environmental influences to explain symptomatic outbreaks (Zubin and Spring, 1977; Nuechterlein and Dawson, 1984; Neuchterlein, 1987). This model posits that each individual has a biologically determined stress threshold, which interacts with various biological, social and psychological stresses, be they ambient or emergent and circum-scribed. When stresses exceed the threshold, certain physiological responses are triggered that bring on symptoms.

One of the most significant advances in refining the notion of psychosocial stress in schizophrenia has been the research on expressed emotion (EE: Chapter 8). EE is a construct representing types of familial attitudes toward schizophrenic family members. In a series of publications the EE was predictive of outcome for patients with schizophrenia. Family attitudes labelled as being critical, hostile or emotionally over-involved correlated with higher rates of relapse in the patient (Leff and Vaughn, 1985). These attitudes have been translated into observable family interactional descriptors, and grouped into the construct of affective style (Miklowitz *et al.*, 1989). This research has focused largely on negative family attitudes and interactions: better outcome was associated with the absence of negative attitudes. Such concepts are advanced as risk factors or mediators of illness. Clinicians seeking to enhance protective factors and mediators of health such as efficient family coping, have not found satisfactory concepts in the EE literature.

A large body of research has shown that a variety of life events can act as important psychosocial stressors as well. It has been found that there is a greater likelihood of significant life events in the three to four-week period preceding the onset of an episode of schizophrenia (Brown and Birley, 1968; Day *et al.*, 1987; Ventura *et al.*, 1989). While this supports the stress-vulnerability hypothesis, a significant proportion of patients have no such identifiable events prior to relapse.

In an attempt to define coping strengths that may be important mechanisms for dealing with stress, Doane *et al.* (1985) compared the number of problem-solving statements made by families trained to solve problems with those not trained, and observed important differences favouring trained families. The schizophrenic members in trained families had better outcomes than those in untrained families. This points to a

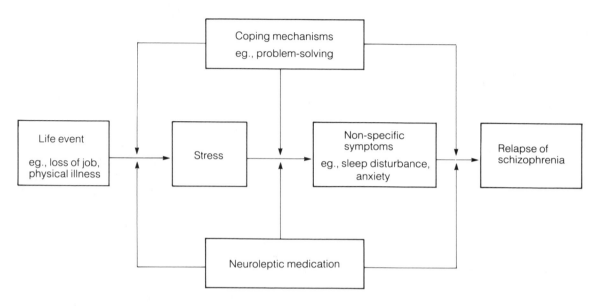

Figure 26.3 Therapeutic modifiers of life event stress (from Falloon, Boyd and McGill, 1984).

significant moderating factor in the stress-vulnerability model. Other therapeutic modifiers of schizophrenia can also be integrated into the stress-vulnerability model (Figure 26.3).

Psychosocial stresses may include the accumulation of household, interpersonal and work stresses, as well as independent life events. The threshold of vulnerability seems to be modifiable through appropriate management strategies. The stress-vulnerability model suggests a variety of possible interventions that would involve the patient, the family and the social network in a comprehensive preventive approach.

26.2.3 A FRAMEWORK FOR DEFINING AND UNDERSTANDING SCHIZOPHRENIA

Liberman (1988) has suggested a framework

for understanding the nature and consequences of schizophrenia (see also Chapter 12). The disorder can be conceptualized as proceeding in four stages: (a) pathology; (b) impairment; (c) disability; and (d) handicap. The pathology of the illness is the biological substrate of the illness. The pathological basis of schizophrenia is far from being elucidated, though much promising work is under way. The second element of this model, the impairments, result from the intrusion of symptoms and the impairment of basic perceptual, cognitive and emotional processes in the patient. It has become clear that in prevention work, this notion of impairment must be expanded to include early warning signs, as well as some negative and residual symptoms, all of these being important impairments to target in management planning. Disability, the limited ability to perform ordinary social and vocational tasks, typically stems from impairments that are

443

not being compensated for by adequate coping mechanisms. Disability may be apparent as lack of motivation, or as deficits in conversation skills or in social skills. Handicap refers to roles and tasks which cannot be fulfilled by the patient because of the illness. The mismatch between the abilities of the patient and the expectations of friends, family, and society may place the patient at a clear disadvantage relative to others in terms of employment, satisfying interpersonal relations and access to pleasurable activities.

26.2.4 THE IMPACT OF SCHIZOPHRENIA ON FAMILY AND CAREGIVERS

An important complication associated with schizophrenia is the effect of the illness on involved carers. A survey by Hatfield (1983) highlights this point. A group of families was receiving professional services relating to a family member with mental illness. The most frequently reported needs of relatives were, in order of importance: (1) reduction of anxiety about the patient; (2) understanding appropriate expectations; (3) learning to motivate patients to do more; and (4) assistance during times of crisis.

Clearly, a response to the needs of both patient and carers is an essential responsibility of community services. The needs of the carers and patients must be carefully evaluated in terms of minimizing the morbidity of all concerned, preferably in a mutually satisfying manner. In the years since deinstitution- alization, families have increasingly assumed the role of caregivers. About two-thirds of patients with schizophrenia are discharged from the hospital to families (Talbott, 1978), and around half live with one relative or more (Goldstein and Caton, 1983). Relatives are faced with the longer term disabilities and consequences of the illness. It has been esti- mated that half the relatives feel that they have developed severe or very severe personal problems due to the fact that someone with

schizophrenia is living within the household (Creer and Wing, 1974). Some of these problems include a sense of powerlessness, self- blame, fear of the unpredictability of symptoms as well as resentment (Kreisman and Joy, 1974). Among married couples where one develops the illness, there is a high divorce and separation rate (Brown *et al.*, 1966).

People in a patient's network may have strengths that could be a true asset in the management of the illness. The analysis of all aspects of the context of the patient is more likely to yield relevant data about the problems, and about important areas of intervention (Falloon, 1985). Carers are both affected by the illness and sometimes may unwittingly affect its course. This issue is still rarely addressed in traditional service settings (Group for the Advancement of Psychiatry Committee on the Family, 1989). There is ample evidence to suggest that the family and interpersonal contexts can significantly contribute to effective clinical management of schizophrenia.

26.3 THE ASSESSMENT OF PREVENTIVE NEEDS

26.3.1 PREVENTION OF PATHOLOGY

Efforts to delineate factors that could be clinically relevant in the primary prevention of schizophrenia have met with limited success. Recent family linkage studies, although excit- ing, have not contributed significantly to the treatment of the disorder. Certain personality characteristics are termed premorbid because they seem to predict a greater risk of developing schizophrenia. People with a diagnosis of 'schizotypal personality disorder', for example, are more likely to develop schizophrenia than the general population (Fenton and McGlashan, 1989). Other work has attempted to identify premorbid stress markers that could predict the development of schizophrenia. Goldstein (1987) and his group have followed a small group of families over a 15-year period, who had originally applied for help because of a mildly to moderately disturbed teenager. Data indicated that certain interactive styles in the family, coupled with early signs of maladjustment in an adolescent, weakly predict the development of 'schizophrenia-spectrum disorders'. Where support for the stress-vulnerability model of schizophrenia comes mostly from studies looking at patients with an established diagnosis, this work loosely supports the importance of stress in vulnerable individuals prior to their developing an overt disorder, and implicates family stresses as a possible contributor to the development of such disorders.

If we assume that the stress-vulnerabilty model applies to the onset of illness, we might attempt to foster 'health-promoting' coping attitudes in at-risk populations as means of preventing the development of schizophrenia. Health-promoting approaches using communication and problem-solving skills training, have been used to prevent marital dissatisfaction in controlled studies (Hahlweg and Markman, 1988). This may serve as a model of the preventive potential of stress-management approaches. Similarly, stress-management techniques, when effectively targeted to populations at risk for the development of schizophrenia, may conceivably reduce the incidence of the illness (Shanahan *et al.*, 1989). A family-based stress-management approach in families where one individual has a diagnosis of schizophrenia extends the benefits of treatment to the whole family, the unaffected members of which are presumably at a higher risk for developing the disorder. In clinical settings it has been very difficult to evaluate the effects of general interventions on primary prevention. However the emphasis of health services has slowly been shifting from the treatment of full-blown episodes to managing earlier manifestations of the illness in the hope of curtailing the complications of florid impairments, disabilities and handicaps. This focus on early secondary prevention has been

given impetus by the research on early warning signs of schizophrenia.

26.3.2 ASSESSMENT OF IMPAIRMENTS IN SCHIZOPHRENIA

26.3.2.1 Early warning signs and acute impairments

A key element in an effective preventive service is early and accurate detection of potentially disabling disorders. Prognosis is almost always related to early recognition followed by effective intervention. The first step in the preventive process is detecting impairments in the primary care setting, and making a provisional diagnosis. In the absence of biological markers for schizophrenia (Flach, 1988), clinical markers assume critical importance in this process. Adequate coordination of all the levels of health care will result in earlier case finding. General nurses, GPs and health workers can be trained to detect important signs of impairment. After this initial screening, the mental health team should be rapidly involved in a more specific assessment using standardized measures. Such assessment may find that patients referred for possible schizophrenia may actually be suffering from another problem. Stress responses can present like schizophrenia, as may certain drug-related responses and some symptoms of depression and obsessive-compulsive disorders. Abrupt changes of neuroleptic or of anticholinergic medication dosage can result in a supersensitivity psychosis (Chouinard and Jones, 1980), or in akathisia-related psychosis (Van Putten *et al.*, 1974). These must be distinguished from signs of relapse, and treated accordingly. All too frequently, a patient with schizophrenia is diagnosed only after the family notices an intolerable change in behaviour. Family and friends initially show a surprising tolerance for a wide range of symptoms before seeking professional help. In fact, even effective psychosocial intervention programmes cannot completely prevent the occurrence of relapses (Hogarty *et al.*, 1987).

Early on in the evolution of schizophrenia, patients may experience low grade impairments. These may escape clinical attention because often they do not fit neatly into any syndromal category. Sensitivity to these represents a crucial aspect of preventive work: there is evidence now that these 'early warning signs' (EWS) are impairments that often precede florid symptoms (Chapter 17). Herz and Melville (1980) in a retrospective study, found that over 90% of family members and 70% of patients were able to remember EWS occurring most often in the week preceding a relapse. In a prospective study, Heinrichs and Carpenter (1985) investigated the early symptoms of patients with an established diagnosis of schizophrenia. Emergent symptoms were sought in widely defined symptom categories. It was found that at least one symptom out of ten occurred in 90% of all the patients before florid exacerbations. These studies indicate that it is possible to identify an impending episode of schizophrenia and point to the possibility of mounting early interventions in the crucial time prior to full relapse. Table 26.2 lists the most common EWS in each study.

Table 26.2 Early warning signs in schizophrenia

Heinrichs and Carpenter	Herz and Melville
Hallucinations	Tense and nervous
Suspiciousness	Trouble concentrating
Change in sleep	Depression
Anxiety	Restlessness
Cognitive inefficiency	Trouble sleeping
Anger/hostility	Loss of interest in things
Somatic symptoms/ delusions	Enjoy things less
Thought disorder	Eating less
Depression	Preoccupied with one or two things
Disruptive/inappropriate behaviour	Cannot remember things

The full-blown impairments of an acute exacerbation of schizophrenia are most often characterized by hallucinations, delusions and formal thought disorders. These are sometimes called 'positive' symptoms or impairments, and are contrasted with the 'negative' impairments that are more apparent in the prodromal and in the non-acute phases of the illness. Florid symptoms account only for a fraction of the morbidity associated with schizophrenia, and must be understood in the context of the course of this disorder. Although these symptoms are absent for most of the illness' course, they are a constant source of worry to patients and relatives alike. In one recent study, recurrences of first rank symptoms occurred in nearly 80% of index patients within five years (Shepherd *et al.*, 1989). On the shorter term, however, the acute symptoms will have abated completely within three months of an episode for most patients.

26.3.2.2 Ancillary impairments

Ancillary symptoms of impairment are less specific to schizophrenia, but can take on a greater importance in the period following the florid episode (Wing, 1978). They may include a range of anxiety and affective symptoms, including obsessive-compulsive symptoms, major depressive episodes and suicidal ideation. These frequently need treatment independently from schizophrenic symptoms.

Depressive symptoms. One frequent ancillary syndrome in the course of schizophrenia is depressive symptomatology. It is thought to occur following a quarter of episodes or more. These symptoms can be very difficult to differentiate from the negative syndrome of schizophrenia, and from neuroleptic-induced akinesia.

Negative syndrome. Another commonly observed impairment in schizophrenia is the negative syndrome. The use of the term negative or deficit syndrome refers to a state characterized by a lack of ambition, initiative and energy. Cognitive and emotional responses are blunted. The patient often feels that he is not able to get into gear. This state can precede, coexist with, or follow the florid or positive syndrome, and may be of long duration (Andreasen and Olsen, 1982). One difficulty in identifying this impairment is that it resembles depressive impairments, or may be caused by side effects of neuroleptic medications. Very low-stress environments are understimulating and can also contribute to the syndrome (Carpenter *et al.*, 1985). Other possible diagnoses that could account for the negative symptoms must be ruled out prior to diagnosing a deficit syndrome.

Acute and ancillary impairments, because they occur as a dramatic change in the patient's usual mode of functioning, beckon for immediate attention. As dramatic and disruptive as these symptoms are, preventive principles demand that resources be carefully organized so as not to be completely absorbed by the treatment of acute symptoms. The complications of schizophrenia include social disabilities and their psychological sequelae. Such complications affect all the members of the patient's network. Furthermore, attention must be paid to identifying the likely stresses that can bring on another episode, and means of coping with them can become a productive focus of intervention.

26.3.3 ASSESSMENT OF DISABILITY AND HANDICAP IN SCHIZOPHRENIA

Disabilities in performing social and vocational skills are evaluated in functional situations as patients are seen interacting with family and peers. Common social contexts such as the workplace or supermarket may represent important areas of disability for patients. Disabilities are frequently transient and arise as a consequence of acute or subacute impairments. A patient with auditory hallucinations may have very deficient attention and conversation skills that will abate as the impairment

improves. Other disabilities such as poor hygiene may require focused interventions over a longer period of time, while some disabilities may be persistent despite intervention. Older reports on the long-term outcome of schizophrenia concluded that only about 50% of patients had a social recovery (Brown *et al.*, 1966; Bleuler, 1978). This proportion has improved with the introduction of psychosocial rehabilitation services and long-term neuroleptic drug therapy, although it remains low (Shepherd *et al.*, 1989).

In the subacute and chronic phases of the illness, persistent impairments and disabilities can be accompanied by severe handicap. Many patients lose their jobs, and in the course of the illness, they may also lose friendships, suffer marital difficulties or become homeless. Patients' sense of self-esteem suffers, and they often feel stigmatized. Handicaps may be minimized by management efforts, community support programmes and government policies that meet the patients' basic needs.

26.3 PREVENTIVE INTERVENTIONS

26.3.1 PLANNING INTERVENTIONS

Once the impairments and disabilities have been clearly identified, a plan of intervention can be worked out, based on a detailed analysis of the stresses and coping strategies that modulate the illness, as well as the particular strengths and weaknesses of the patient and carers. Factors that may reinforce or reduce problem behaviours are an important aspect of this analysis. The resulting intervention strategy is tailored to the people seeking help, and invariably consists of a psychosocial intervention, with specific drug therapy if indicated. The caregivers are included in the treatment plan, both to assist in the management of the patient and to identify and work toward their own personal goals that will maximize their quality of life in the face of the burden that the illness imposes on them.

447

26.3.2 IMPLEMENTATION OF PREVENTATIVE INTERVENTIONS

26.3.2.1 Where to implement interventions

The traditional venue for treating people suffering episodes of schizophrenia has been the hospital. As discussed in Chapter 25, recent research supplies information that helps evaluate this tradition. There is some evidence that patients who are hospitalized for shorter periods of time tend to preserve role functioning better than those hospitalized for longer periods. They do not have a greater risk of hospitalization if there is continuity in the provision of comprehensive mental health care (Herz *et al.*, 1977; Creed *et al.*, 1989). The ability for the patient to maintain normal social role performance despite the presence of symptoms can be protective and stabilizing for the patient and for the family (Cooper, 1961). The effective management of acute episodes and of subacute and chronic conditions usually involves the provision of a calm, supportive interpersonal environment, psychological treatment strategies for coping with distressing symptoms and judicious psychopharmacological interventions. There is no evidence to suggest that this management is more effective when administered in a hospital than it is within suitable locations in the community. On the contrary, community locations have been shown to be at least equally effective (Mosher and Keith, 1980). Mental health services provided in the home can enhance the effectiveness of interventions (Stein and Test, 1980; Test and Stein, 1980; Fenton *et al.*, 1982; Hoult *et al.*, 1983). Benefits learned in the hospital, such as coping and interpersonal skills, are not readily transferable to the natural habitat, while benefits gained from home-based care are more likely to be long-lasting and useful to all family members.

26.3.2.2 Supplying information

Reducing the confusion, guilt and sense of helplessness starts with the most basic intervention of all: informing families about illness-related issues. Managing schizophrenia is a cooperative effort between the patient, the natural caregivers and the health-care staff. It is the responsibility of the health-carer to try to build such a relationship which is often enhanced by relevant information. Educating families is best done by combining meetings where family-specific issues are brought up in the context of handouts and other suggested readings on the illness and treatment. A basic understanding of the genetic and biological pathology places schizophrenia in a medical context and depersonalizes the etiology. Defining and discussing the impairments brought on by schizophrenia is tied in with an identification of the patient's own early warning signs. This aspect of education helps in understanding impairments as useful beacons of an impending episode. Education on the medications, their mechanisms of action and their side effects provide a better sense of control, and facilitates compliance and long-term treatment planning. Such information may be supplemented with compliance training, consisting of strategies designed specifically to prompt and maintain medication adherence over a long period. The family's involvement with the illness is framed in the stress-vulnerability model, and family burden is also discussed. The notion that stresses can be managed efficiently through effective problem-solving leads into the psychosocial interventions.

26.3.2.3 Psychosocial interventions

Psychosocial intervention strategies have developed over the last three decades that address impairments and disabilities more effectively than ever before.

Case management and crisis intervention. Early efforts to provide psychosocial treatment for schizophrenia employed a problem-oriented case management approach. A case worker was assigned to help in resolving each stress as it emerged. The worker attempted to gain the assistance of various community agencies, and employed a mixture of directive advice and psychodynamic strategies with the patient to try to resolve stresses. Such programmes, even when supplemented with social and inter-personal skills training and optimal drug management, have been shown to achieve an improvement in impairments that is no better than that achieved with drug therapy alone. The combined rate of occurrence of florid exacerbations in the first year of follow-up was 38% with controlled drug therapy compared to 36% where drugs were combined with patient-oriented case management and/or social skills training (Wallace and Liberman, 1985; Hogarty *et al.*, 1986; Tarrier *et al.*, 1989). Taking into account other aspects of outcome, some of these approaches have also aimed at preventing disabilities and handicaps. Social skills training has provided some improved social functioning (Bellack *et al.*, 1984; Wallace and Liberman, 1985). The social skills approach has assumed that disability can be improved with social learning principles following an educational-rehabilitative focus, aimed at interpersonal problem-solving in specific relevant situations. Deficits in social skills can carry the patient along a vicious circle whereby daily stresses that cannot be adequately negotiated push patients closer to their stress threshold and put them at greater risk for relapse. The skills training focuses on daily stressful issues by approximating real-life situations in repeated rehearsals. Within these re-creations of situations, therapists model new behaviours, coach and give feedback to patients to mould behaviours toward more effective ways of dealing with stressful events.

Other means of improving the efficiency of stress management have included family members in learning case management skills. With the inclusion of families, both social and clinical benefits have been evident (Strachan, 1986). Family intervention approaches that have been evaluated are based on a variety of behavioural techniques.

Family management. Various attempts to integrate the family into the treatment of schizophrenia were based on changing hypotheses about the relation of family interactions to outcome. These have been reviewed elsewhere (Falloon, 1985). More recently family theorists have come to a better understanding of the role that family strengths and family stresses play in the prognosis of schizophrenia. Family-based stress-management approaches differ dramatically from traditional family therapy in many respects. Taking the stress-vulnerability model as a starting point to educate the family about schizophrenia and treatment, therapists assist patients and family members in coping more efficiently with a wide range of stressors, impairments, disabilities and handicaps associated with the illness, and with family carers' burden and stresses. Some programmes that combine education about the illness with basic case management and support to assist the family in reducing stress (Leff *et al.*, 1982; Hogarty *et al.*, 1986), have yielded remarkable results in the short term. Low rates of florid episodes are reported in the first year after this treatment (Chapter 24), and represent a three-fold greater reduction than that achieved by optimal drug therapy alone. These results of family case management are tempered by the fact that benefits have not been long-lived (Tarrier *et al.*, 1989), unless the approach was designed to indefinitely promote efficient stress management.

Falloon and associates have developed a family intervention strategy that employs Behavioural Family Therapy (BFT) as the major component of family stress management (Falloon *et al.*, 1984). In BFT, the family is seen as the problem-solving unit for stressful events. This approach translates elements of behaviour therapy into a comprehensive intervention scheme based on the stress-vulnerability model. Where psychoeducational approaches focus on a narrow range of ambient family stresses, the emphasis of BFT has been to enhance family problem-solving skills to manage a wide range of stresses including ambient stresses associated with work, recreation, social activities, household responsibilities and life events. Wherever possible, the potential for dealing with stresses by modulating responses and behaviours in day-to-day situations is favoured over avoidance of stressful situations. Stress can be reduced with more effective coping mechanisms. A behavioural family therapy manual has been developed, and therapist BFT skills have been operationalized in a scale used for feedback and for outcome research (Laporta *et al.*, 1989). Therapy is implemented by explaining the rationale for therapy to the family, in the context of the stress-vulnerability model. The therapist's role is more akin to that of a teacher and a consultant, whose aim is to empower family members to manage their ongoing difficulties and problems based on a clear evaluable model. With this role in mind, the therapist assesses each person as to goals, strengths, weaknesses and capacity for self-reinforcement. The family's communication skills are also assessed on a regular basis and therapy is planned according to progress. This assessment procedure is aimed at capitalizing on the inherent strengths of the family (Falloon *et al.*, 1986). When the assessment is completed, an initial series of sessions focusing on information, as described earlier, gives the family the opportunity to better understand the affected member, and to gain a sense of control over the illness. Therapy is then designed to promote effective family coping skills (Falloon *et al.*, in press). The central skill of problem-solving is carefully fostered in the course of BFT, and is structured for application to a wide variety of situations. Efficient family problem-solving is shaped in a stepwise manner through basic communication skills training. Communication skills are taught with the aid of prompts, handouts and in-session rehearsals. The framework of therapy and the nature of the skills are

summarized in Table 26.3. The framework for each session is equally straightforward: assessment and review of the family's goals and of the family's strengths in applying learned skills begin each session. Information regarding new skills and relevant aspects of illness follows. New skills are modelled and then practised in rehearsals until they are acquired by each family member.

Table 26.3 Framework for behavioural family therapy

1. Assessing individual/family needs, strengths, weaknesses.

2. Educating about illness and treatment-related issues.

3. Communication training:
   - Expressing positive feelings and remarks
   - Making specific requests
   - Expressing negative feelings
   - Actively listening

4. Problem-solving training:
   - Problem identification
   - Brainstorming potential solutions
   - Evaluating pros and cons of potential solutions
   - Choosing a fitting alternative
   - Planning implementation
   - Review of success

5. Out-of-session work: generalization of skills

An important aspect of BFT is the concern with generalization of acquired skills. Principles of generalization (Stokes and Baer, 1977) are applied throughout:

(1) BFT is done in the home to approximate the daily family experience as much as possible.

(2) Careful assessment is used systematically to identify therapy issues that are most relevant to the family.

(3) Behavioural rehearsals, the central means for practising new interactional skills in sessions, are used to foster effective communication even between family members who tend to interact less easily.

(4) All family members have the responsibility to convene in a weekly meeting to give each other feedback on improvements and positive behaviours and also to identify potentially problematic issues.

(5) They are also given specific instructions about practising skills outside of session time to integrate them into their everyday life.

(6) During sessions, the therapist always attempts to hand as much responsibility as possible over to family members (e.g. giving each other feedback and directing aspects of sessions).

BFT was compared experimentally with an exhaustive outpatient management programme in a group of families where one member had schizophrenia. A two-year outcome study, carefully evaluating a broad range of outcome measures, was completed by Falloon *et al.* (1984). This study concluded that BFT, in combination with optimal drug management was more effective than comprehensive individual management combined with drug management for this group of patients. The benefits persisted over the two years of treatment and follow-up (Falloon *et al.*, 1985). The patients in the group undergoing BFT had a significant reduction in the intensity of their impairments, disabilities and handicaps, and family measures indicated significant benefits for family members. A replication of these findings with a similar treatment was recently published by Tarrier *et al.* (1989). Further controlled studies are in progress in seven centres in the USA, and in Australia and Germany.

26.3.2.4 Pharmacological strategies

Acute impairments in schizophrenia may require pharmacological intervention (Chapter 19). Neuroleptics can induce at least a partial remission of florid symptoms in 75% of patients. The major disadvantage of treatment with these agents is the risk of side effects. Reducing the long-term problem of tardive dyskinesia (TD) in particular has become a priority in drug treatment planning. It is generally thought that symptoms should be controlled with the lowest possible neuroleptic dose (Davis, 1975; Chouinard *et al.*, 1979). Two strategies for reducing the dose of neuroleptic medications have been used with success. One approach, the use of *intermittent neuroleptic treatment*, involves initiating treatment as early as possible after early warning signs are identified, and maintaining treatment only until the symptoms stabilize. This minimizes the patient's exposure to the drug. Stopping neuroleptic treatment may be contraindicated in some patients known to decompensate quickly. However, there is preliminary evidence that rehospitalization may not be significantly increased when drugs are discontinued in stable schizophrenic outpatients (Herz *et al.*, 1982). Drug discontinuation regimens will clearly be more effective if the patient is compliant with treatment plans and where cooperative family members can be alert to early symptom exacerbation. Another related treatment strategy has been the *targeting of medications*: low-dose maintenance is combined with intermittent treatment targeted to periods where patients show early signs of florid symptoms (Carpenter and Heinrichs, 1983; Herz, 1986; Marder *et al.*, 1987). Accurate early detection of an incipient episode could minimize the risk of relapse while reducing the potential complications of neuroleptic treatment (Davis *et al.*, 1980; Schooler and Severe, 1984). While almost half the patients whose acute episodes remit with neuroleptic treatment suffer recurrences within a year (Schooler and Severe, 1984), continued low-dose maintenance treatment halves this recurrence rate (Davis *et al.*, 1980).

The effects of neuroleptics seem to be most evident on impairments such as hallucinations and delusions. The development of new preparations that would have more specific effects on the schizophrenic symptoms and cause fewer side effects has been slow. The advantages of the diphenylbutylpiperidines (pimozide and

451

fluspirilene) seem to be marginal (Kane and Mayerhoff, 1989). There is some hope that clozapine may have a place in the treatment of patients with tardive dyskinesia (Marder and Van Putten, 1988), but the risk of blood dyscrasias restricts its use on a regular basis.

The ancillary impairments of schizophrenia also may necessitate specific drug treatment strategies. Depression should be present for a four-week period before a decision is taken to treat it with antidepressant medications. There is some data to indicate that antidepressants may be of significant help in post-psychotic depressions, but the lack of systematic evaluation of side effects has been a major shortcoming of these studies (Siris *et al.*, 1987, 1989). Before initiating any treatment for depression, a trial of anticholinergic medications, or, when possible, a lowering of the dose of neuroleptics should be attempted to help rule out neuroleptic-induced akinesia and negative symptoms. Anticholinergic, sedative and other additive side effects of neuroleptics and antidepressants must be carefully weighed against the advantages in each individual case, and careful monitoring of the efficacy of the treatment should be followed. The negative syndrome has only recently been the subject of systematic research efforts. Pharmacological advances in the treatment of schizophrenia had been targeted most intensely on relieving positive symptoms. The effect of neuroleptics may contribute to the negative syndrome (Wing, 1978a), though more recent work shows that they may help improve these impairments (Goldberg, 1985). Here again it is advisable to find the minimal effective dose of medication.

26.4 THE BUCKINGHAM PROJECT: A COMMUNITY-BASED PREVENTIVE MENTAL HEALTH SERVICE

In 1984, a community-based service was set up as a pilot project using preventive principles. Its aim is to provide effective preventive care for people suffering from mental illness in a cost-efficient manner. The Buckingham Mental Health Service (BMHS) provides care for adults aged 16–65 in a rapidly expanding rural community of approximately 35 000 in the North Aylesbury Vale, Buckinghamshire, England. The service is designed to support the existing frameworks of family and primary health systems while providing specialized help within the community. To minimize contact with hospitals, full-time home-based intensive nursing can be provided in cases where symptoms warrant it. The costs are considerably lower than those arising from hospital-based care. Certain iatrogenic complications associated with hospitalization such as higher drug dosages, more drug-induced side-effects, understimulation and family and social-role disruptions, are significantly reduced. Health care is provided primarily by general practitioners who are in a position to detect mental disorders at an early stage.

The incidence and prevalence of florid episodes of schizophrenia appear to be substantially lower than expected rates in the Buckingham population. Indeed, preliminary data indicate a tenfold reduction in new cases of this disorder over a four-year period. This has been accompanied by a similar reduction in the rate of major recurrences in established cases. The latter finding is consistent with the results obtained from controlled studies of family-based clinical management (Falloon, 1985). However, the suggestion that early intensive intervention during the prodromal phase of a first episode of schizophrenia may forestall the course of the disorder requires careful consideration under rigorous controlled conditions.

Involving the psychiatric services at an early stage in the evolution of a mental disorder detected by a primary care physician requires good cooperation with the community's medical practices. The ability to respond to community needs is adjusted through regular meetings with the GPs within their practices and in occasional meetings between all the BMHS staff and the area's GPs and nurses. Special sessions are scheduled to educate these agencies in the recognition of early signs of mental illness through videotape presentations, handouts and ongoing discussions. When a GP sees a patient presenting with such symptoms, a mental health nurse may be consulted for a full assessment at all times. Mental health personnel trained in specialized assessment and intervention are fully integrated into the primary care teams, sharing premises and taking clinical responsibility for consulting and tending to all persons suffering from mental disorders.

The assessment of possible pathology, impairment, disability and handicap is done using operationalized tools. For the assessment of impairments in schizophrenia, the Present State Examination (Wing *et al.*, 1974), Brief Psychiatric Rating Scale (Overall and Gorham, 1962), and Early Signs of Schizophrenia Questionnaire (Herz and Melville, 1980) are used, along with the Clinical Global Assessment Scale. A mini-mental state exam (Folstein and McHugh, 1975) may also be indicated. If depressive feelings are present, they are quantified with the Hamilton Depression Scale (Bech *et al.*, 1975) and Beck Depression Inventory (Beck and Beamesderfer, 1974). The mental health personnel are trained in the use of these scales to a high standard of reliability, similar to that employed in research studies. Disability and handicap are assessed by several means. The Charing Cross Health Index (Rosser and Kind, 1978), and the Family Burden Scale (Falloon, 1985) are used. Also, a needs-based behavioural analysis of significant disabilities, handicaps, stress factors and vulnerabilities is completed for each case. The caregivers' standpoint in understanding the situation is considered with equal emphasis; the impact of the illness on their personal goals, and their capacity to assist in the treatment are key issues in devising an effective intervention plan.

Interventions are planned to make the best use of family and individual strengths. A detailed plan is worked out after full assessment and team discussions which aims to prevent long-term morbidity and enhance the quality of life of each of the family members. Such a plan always integrates a psychosocial intervention and specific drug therapy when indicated. The assessment and interventions are almost always home-based. The outcomes of such goal-oriented interventions, though tailored to the specific needs of the person or family seeking help, can be measured and progress is carefully followed.

Information about the illness and its treatment is an essential part of all intervention plans. A family's attitude toward treatment is likely to be much more positive if there is an understanding of the illness. Also, the rationale for most intervention strategies proceeds logically from illness-related information. Initially therapists use prepared handouts and discussions to cover important aspects of the disorder; as a rule specific information on emergent aspects of the illness is needed throughout therapy. Psychosocial interventions integrate case-management approaches with family-centred management. Behavioural psychotherapy offers a range of cost-effective intervention strategies that can be applied to the treatment of schizophrenia as well as that of other stress-related disorders. Treatment may include, at different stages of the illness, daily activity schedules, drug therapy and compliance training, anxiety and depression management, or specific social skills training. Behavioural family therapy, focusing on stress-management and problem-solving training is usually an integral part of therapy. Most interventions integrate the whole family, and where patients live alone or in non-family households, involved key persons in their social networks are integrated into the programme.

Long-term management planning is required for schizophrenia as it is for many disorders with a persistent or recurrent course. After an intensive initial treatment phase, contact is maintained at a lesser frequency; this seems to facilitate professional assistance in resolving ongoing emergent stresses that could otherwise lead to a relapse. As previously discussed, a framework of early intervention and prevention implies a heightened sensitivity to early signs of stress and recurrence of impairments. Prompt intervention at this stage does not appear to result in overtreatment, but rather to shorter periods of distress. Long-term management includes low-dose drug therapy in many cases, ongoing education about the nature of the illness, and training in stress-management skills. These include communication skills and problem-solving skills. Assertive outreach is done where persons fail to attend treatment sessions or reviews, and therapists are available in the evenings and weekends to meet special patient and carer needs. The ongoing intervention plan for each case is given a detailed three-monthly review by the multidisciplinary team comprising the service. Interventions are evaluated against changes in clinical status and the attainment of individual goals; a plan may be changed if it has not been efficient in attaining these objectives.

The mental health carers must respond to the needs of the patients and their caretakers, to the needs of the community's health professionals, and to the mandate of the Buckingham Project to offer cost-effective goal-oriented treatment. They are not immune to becoming overburdened themselves. The project has built-in strategies to help them feel both stimulated and supported. Ongoing education, exchanges, supervision and feedback for all the mental health carers occurs in regular discussions and weekly teaching sessions. Didactic sessions alternate with more informal group discussions and case presentations. Weekly training of therapists through workshops ensures the maintenance of a high standard of care.

The stress-vulnerability model easily admits the integration of psychosocial and pharmacological management, as discussed earlier. Drugs are targeted to help manage certain impairments and disabilities while minimizing the patients' exposure to them. Problems of compliance are often less important when patients and families understand the rationale for drug treatment; knowledge about possible side effects prior to their appearance makes these untoward symptoms less frightening.

26.5 CONCLUSION

The recent developments in the management of schizophrenia are best understood as having followed in the wake of the stress-vulnerability model and of the application of preventive principles to this disorder. These concepts have led to a complementarity of psychosocial and biological interventions in schizophrenia, and have completely revolutionized our view of the families and carers of patients as resourceful units in the community. Psychosocial interventions that enhance mental health through stress-management and problem-solving have been effective, in combination with drug therapy, in improving the social, interpersonal and symptomatic prognosis of affected patients. Better knowledge of the effects and side effects of anti-psychotic drugs has led to their more judicious use. Also, refinements in the assessment of early warning signs, and a better understanding of psychological strengths and weaknesses, have promoted a use of preventive concepts in working toward more efficient interventions.

These approaches have been conducted under research conditions with good results. Their practicability and usefulness on a longer term basis have been put to the test in the community-based pilot Buckingham Project. There are important concepts and research findings that point to the usefulness of preventive principles in the management of patients with schizophrenia and their carers. With an adequate structuring of such services, it is possible to reduce the need for hospital-based care, improving the prognosis of patients and families while lowering the total costs of mental health care.

REFERENCES

Andreasen, N.C. and Olsen, S. (1982) Negative vs. positive schizophrenia: Definition and validation. *Arch. Gen. Psychiatry*, **39**, 709–94.

Bech, P., Gram, L.F., Dein, E. *et al.* (1975) Quantitative rating of depressive states. *Acta Psychiatr. Scand.*, **51**, 161–70.

Beck, A.T. and Beamesderfer, A. (1974) Assessment of depression: The depression inventory: Psychological measurements in psychopharmacology. In *Modern Problems in Pharmacopsychiatry*. P. Pichot (ed), S. Karger, Basel, pp. 151–69.

Bellak, A.S., Turner, S.M., Hersen, M. and Luber, R.F. (1984) An examination of the efficacy of social skills training for chronic schizophrenic patients. *Hosp. Community Psychiatry*, **35**, 1023–8.

Black, D., Yates, W.R. and Andreasen, N.C. (1988) Schizophrenia, schizophreniform disease and delusional (paranoid) disorders. In *Textbook of Psychiatry*. J.A. Talbott, R.E. Hales and S.C. Yudofsky (eds), The American Psychiatric Press, Washington, 357–402.

Bleuler, M. (1978) *The Schizophrenic Disorders: Long-term Patient and Family Studies*. Yale University Press, New Haven.

Brown, G.E. and Birley, J.L. (1968) Crisis and life change and the onset of schizophrenia. *J. Health Soc. Behav.*, **9**, 203–14.

Brown, G.W., Bone, M., Dalison, B. and Wing, J.K. (1966) *Schizophrenia and social care.* Maudsley Monograph #17, Oxford University Press, London.

Carpenter, W.T. and Heinrichs, D.W. (1983) Early intervention, time limited targeted pharmacotherapy of schizophrenia. *Schizophr. Bull.*, **9**, 533–42.

Carpenter, W.R., Heinrichs, D.W. and Alphs, L.D. (1985) Treatment of negative symptoms. *Schizophr. Bull.*, **11**, 440–52.

Chouinard, G. and Jones, B.D. (1980) Neuroleptic-induced supersensitivity psychosis: Clinical and pharmacologic characteristics. *Am. J. Psychiatry*, **137**, 16–21.

Chouinard, G., Annable, L., Ross-Chouinard, A. and Nestoros, J. (1979) Factors related to tardive dyskinesia. *Am. J. Psychiatry*, **136**, 79–83.

Cowen, E.L. (1983) Primary prevention in mental health: Past, present and future. In *Preventive Psychology, Theory, Research and Practice*. R.D. Feldner, L.A. Jason, J.N. Moritsugu and S.S. Farber (eds), Pergamon Press, New York, pp. 11–25.

Cooper, B. (1961) Social class and prognosis in schizophrenia. *Br. J. Prev. Soc. Med.* **15**, 17–41.

Creed, F., Black, D. and Anthony, P. (1989) Day hospital and community treatment for acute psychiatric illness. *Br. J. Psychiatry*, **154**, 300–10.

Creer, C. and Wing, J.K. (1974) *Schizophrenia at Home.* National Schizophrenia Fellowship, London.

Davis, J.M. (1975) Overview: Maintenance therapy in psychiatry: I. Schizophrenia. *Am. J. Psychiatry*, **132**, 1237–45.

Davis, J.M., Schaffer, C.B., Killian, G.A. *et al.* (1980) Important issues in the drug treatment of schizophrenia. *Schizophr. Bull.*, **6**, 70–8.

Day, R. (1981), Life events and schizophrenia: The triggering hypothesis. *Acta Psychiatr. Scand.*, **64**, 97–122.

Day, R., Nielsen, J.A., Korten, A. *et al.* (1987) Stressful life events preceding the acute onset of schizophrenia: A cross national study from the WHO. *Culture Med. Psychiatry*, **11**, 123–205.

Doane, J.A., Falloon, I.R.H., Goldstein, M.J. and Mintz, J. (1985) Parental affective style and the treatment of schizophrenia. *Arch. Gen. Psychiatry*, **42**, 34–42.

Fadden, G., Bebbington, P. and Kuipers, L. (1987) Caring and its burdens: A study of the spouses of depressed patients. *Br. J. Psychiatry*, **151**, 660–7.

Falloon, I.R.H., Boyd, J.L. and McGill, C.W. (1984) *Family Care of Schizophrenia.* Guilford Press, New York.

Falloon, I.R.H., Boyd, J.L., McGill, C.W. *et al.* (1985) Family management in the prevention of morbidity in schizophrenia: clinical arcane of a two-year longitudinal study. *Arch. Gen. Psychiatry*, **42**, 887–96.

Falloon, I.R.H. (ed), (1985) *Family management of schizophrenia: A study of the clinical, social, family and economic benefits.* Johns Hopkins University Press, Baltimore.

Falloon, I.R.H., Laporta, M. *et al.* (in press), *Managing Stress in Families*. Routledge, London.

Falloon, I.R.H., Pederson, J. and Al Khayyal, M. (1986) Enhancement of family giving support versus treatment of family pathology. *J. Family Ther.*, **8**, 339–50.

Fenton, W.S. and McGlashan, T.H. (1989) Risk of schizophrenia in character disordered patients. *Am. J. Psychiatry*, **146**, 1280–4.

Fenton, F.R., Tessier, L., Struening, E.L. *et al.* (1982) *Home and hospital psychiatric treatment*. Croom Helm, London.

Flach, F. (ed) (1988) *The Schizophrenias*. Directions in Psychiatry Monograph Series 4, W.W. Norton & Company, New York.

Folstein, M.F. and McHugh, P.R. (1975) 'Mini-mental state': A method of grading the cognitive state of patients for the clinician. *J. Psychiatr. Res*, **12**, 189.

Goldberg, S.C. (1985) Negative and deficit symptoms in schizophrenia do respond to neuroleptics. *Schizophr. Bull.*, **11**, 453–6.

Goldstein, J.M. and Caton, C.L.M. (1983) The effects of the community environment on chronic psychiatric patients. *Psychobiol. Med.*, **13**, 193–9.

Group for the Advancement of Psychiatry Committee on the Family (1989) The Challenge of Relational Diagnoses: Applying the psychosocial model in DSM-N. *Am. J. Psychiatry*, **146**, 1492–4.

Hahlweg, K. and Markman, H.J. (1988) Effectiveness of behavioral marital therapy: Empirical status of behavioral techniques in preventing and alleviating marital distress. *J. Consult. Clin. Psychol.*, **56**, 440–7.

Hatfield, A.B. (1983) What families want of family therapists. In *Family Therapy in Schizophrenia*, W.R. McFarlane (ed), Guilford, New York, pp. 41–68.

Heinrichs, D.W. and Carpenter, W.T. (1985) Prospective study of prodromal symptoms in schizophrenic relapse. *Am. J. Psychiatry*, **142**, 371–3.

Herz, M.I. (1986) Toward an integrated approach to the treatment of schizophrenia. *Psychother. Psychosom.*, **46**, 45–57.

Herz, M.I., Endicott, J. and Spitzer, R.L. (1977) Brief hospitalization: A two-year follow up. *Am. J. Psychiatry*, **132**, 502–7.

Herz, M.I. and Melville, C. (1980) Relapse in schizophrenia. *Am. J. Psychiatry*, **137**, 801–5.

Herz, M.I., Szymansky, H.V. and Simon, J. (1982) Intermittent medication for stable schizophrenic outpatients: An alternative to maintenance medication. *Am. J. Psychiatry*, **139**, 918–22.

Hogarty, G.E., Anderson, C.M. and Reiss, D.J. (1987) Family psychoeducation, social skills training, and medication in schizophrenia: The long and short of it. *Psychopharmacol. Bull.*, **23**, 12–13.

Hogarty, G.E., Anderson, C.M., Reiss, D.J. *et al.* (1986) Family psychoeducation, social skills training and maintenance chemotherapy in the aftercare treatment of schizophrenia. *Arch. Gen. Psychiatry*, **43**, 633–42.

Hoult, J., Reynolds, I., Charbonneau-Powis, M. *et al.* (1983) Psychiatric hospital versus community treatment: The results of a randomized trial. *A. N.Z. J. Psychiatry*, **17**, 160–7.

Kane, J.M. and Mayerhoff, D. (1989) Do negative symptoms respond to pharmacological treatment? *Br. J. Psychiatry*, **155** (Suppl. 7), 115–18.

Kane, J.A., Rifkin, A. and Woerner, M. (1986) Dose response relationships in maintenance drug treatment for schizophrenia. *Psychopharmacol. Bull.*, **6**, 205–35.

Kreisman, D.E. and Joy, V.D. (1974) Family response to the mental illness of a relative: A review of the literature. *Schizophr. Bull.*, **10**, 34–57.

Leff, J. and Vaughn, C. (1985) *Expressed emotion in Families*. Guilford Press, New York.

Leff, J., Kuipers, L., Berkowitz, R. *et al.* (1982) A controlled study of social interventions in the families of schizophrenic patients. *Br. J. Psychiatry*, **141**, 121–34.

Leff, J. and Vaughn, C. (1985) *Expressed emotion in Families*. Guilford Press, New York.

Liberman, R.P. (1988) Coping with chronic mental disorders: A framework for hope. In *Psychiatric Rehabilitation of Chronic Mental Patients*. R.P. Liberman (ed), American Psychiatric Press, Washington, DC, pp. 1–28.

Marder, S.R. and Van Putten, T. (1988) Who should receive clozapine? *Arch. Gen. Psychiatry*, **45**, 865–7.

Marder, S.R., Van Putten, T., Mintz, J. *et al.* (1987) Low and conventional dose maintenance therapy with fluphenazine decanoate. *Arch. Gen. Psychiatry*, **44**, 518–21.

Miklowitz, D.J., Goldstein, M.J., Doane, J.A. *et al.* (1989) Is expressed emotion an index of transactional process? I. Parents' affective style. *Family Process*, **28**, 153–67.

Mosher, L.R. and Keith, S.J. (1980) Psychosocial treatment: Individual, group, family and community support approaches. *Schizophr. Bull.*, **6**, 10–41.

Newton, J. (1988) *Preventing Mental Illness.* Routledge and Kegan Paul, London.

Nuechterlein, K.H. (1987) Vulnerability models: State of the art. In *Searches for the Cause of Schizophrenia.* H. Hafner, W. Gattaz and W. Jangerik (eds), Springer-Verlag, Berlin, pp. 297–316.

Nuechterlein, K.H. and Dawson, M.E. (1984) A heuristic vulnerability-stress model of schizophrenia. *Schizophr. Bull.*, **10**, 300–12.

Overall, J.E. and Gorham, D.R. (1962) The brief psychiatric rating scale. *Psychol. Rep.*, **10**, 799–812.

Price, R.H. and Smith, S.S. (1985) *A guide to evaluating prevention programs in mental health.* US Department of Health and Human Services Publication, National Institute of Mental Health, Rockville.

Raeburn, J.M. and Seymour, F.W. (1977) Planning and evaluating community health and related projects: A systems approach. *A. N.Z. Med. J.*, **86**, 188–90.

Rappaport, J. (1981) In praise of paradox: A social policy of empowerment over prevention *Am. J. Community Psychol.*, **9**, 1–27.

Rosser, R. and Kind, P. (1978) A scale of valuations of states of illness. *Int. J. Epidemiol*, **7**, 347–58.

Schooler, N.R. and Severe, J.B. (1984) Efficacy of drug treatment for chronic schizophrenic patients. In *The Chronically Mentally Ill: Research and Services.* M. Mirabi (ed), Spectrum, New York, pp. 125–42.

Shanahan, W., Laporta, M. and Fallon, I.R.H. (1989) *Prevention of psychiatric morbidity in the community.* Presented at the Stoke Mandeville Hospital Postgraduate Medical Centre Annual Research Review.

Shepherd, M., Watt, D., Fallon, I. and Smeeton, N. (1989) The natural history of schizophrenia:

A five year follow-up of outcome and prediction in a representative sample of schizophrenics. *Psychol. Med. Monogr.* **Suppl. 15**, 1–46.

Siris, S.G., Adan, F., Cohen, M. *et al.* (1987) Targeted treatment of depressive like symptoms in schizophrenia. *Psychopharmacol. Bull.*, **23**, 85–9.

Siris, S.C., Adan, F., Strachan, A. *et al.* (1989) Comparison of 6 with 9 week trials of adjunctive imipramine in postpsychotic depression. *Compr. Psychiatry*, **30**(6), 483–8.

Stein, L.I. and Test, M.A. (1980) An alternative to mental hospital treatment: I. Conceptual model, treatment program and clinical evaluation. *Arch. Gen. Psychiatry*, **37**, 392–9.

Stokes, T.F. and Baer, D.M. (1977) An implicit technology of generalization. *J. Appl. Behav. Anal.*, **10**, 349–67.

Talbott, J.A. (ed) (1978) *The chronic mental patient: Problems, solutions and recommendations for a public policy.* American Psychiatric Association, Washington, DC.

Tarrier, N., Barrowclough, C., Vaughn, C. *et al.* (1989) Community management of schizophrenia; A two-year follow-up of a behavioural intervention with families. *Br. J. Psychiatry*, **154**, 625–8.

Test, M.A. and Stein, L.I. (1980) Alternative to mental hospital treatment. III. Social cost. *Arch. Gen. Psychiatry*, **37**, 409–12.

Van Putten, T., Mutalipassi, L.R., and Malkin, M.D. (1974) Phenothiazine-induced decompensation. *Arch. Gen. Psychiatry*, **30**, 102–5.

Ventura, J., Nuechterlein, K.H., Lukoff, D. and Hardesty, J.P. (1989) A prospective study of stressful life events and schizophrenic relapse. *J. Abnorm. Psychol.*, **98**, 407–11.

Wallace, C.J. and Liberman, R.P. (1985) Social skills training for patients with schizophrenia, a controlled clinical trial. *Psychiatry Res.*, **15**, 239–47.

Wing, J.K. (1978a) *Reasoning about Madness.* Oxford University Press, London.

Wing, J.K. (1978b) Social influence on the course of schizophrenia. In *The Nature of Schizophrenia.* L.C. Wynne, L. Cromwell Rue, S. Matthysse, M.L. Toohey, B.J. Spring and J. Sugarman (eds) Wiley, New York, pp. 599–616.

457

Wing, J.K., Cooper, J.E. and Sartorius, N. (1974) *The Measurement and Classification of Psychiatric Symptoms: An Instruction Manual for the PSE and CATEGO Programme.* Cambridge University Press, London.

Zubin, J. and Spring, B. (1977) Vulnerability: A new view of schizophrenia. *J. Abnorm. Psychol.,* **86**, 103–26.

Index